Mohl/Zarb/Carlsson/Rugh

A Textbook of Occlusion

A Textbook of Occlusion

Edited by:

Norman D. Mohl, D.D.S., M.A., Ph.D.
School of Dental Medicine
State University of New York at Buffalo

George A. Zarb, B.Ch.D., M.S., M.S., D.D.S., F.R.C.D.(C)
Faculty of Dentistry
University of Toronto

Gunnar E. Carlsson, L.D.S., Odont.Dr.
Faculty of Odontology
University of Göteborg

John D. Rugh, Ph.D.
Dental School
The University of Texas
Health Science Center at San Antonio

quintessence books

Quintessence Publishing Co., Inc. 1988
Chicago, London, Berlin, São Paulo, Tokyo, and Hong Kong

Library of Congress Cataloging-in-Publication Data

A Textbook of occlusion.

Bibliography: p.
Includes index.
1. Malocclusion. 2. Occlusion (Dentistry) I. Mohl, Norman D. [DNLM: 1. Dental Occlusion. 2. Malocclusion—diagnosis. 3. Malocclusion—therapy. 4. Stomatognathic System. 5. Temporomandibular Joint Diseases—diagnosis. 6. Temporomandibular Joint Diseases—therapy. WU 440 T355]
RK523.T44 1988 617.6'43 87-29238
ISBN 0-86715-167-6

3rd Printing, 1991

Lithography: Industrie- und Presseklischee, Berlin
Composition: Midwest Technical Publications, St. Louis, MO
Printing and binding: Edwards Brothers Inc., Ann Arbor, MI
Printed in U. S. A.

Contents

Chapter 1	**Introduction to Occlusion**	**15**
	Occlusion defined	15
	The masticatory system	17
	Introduction to terminology	19
	PART I Anatomy and Physiology of the Masticatory System	25
Chapter 2	**Evolution and Comparative Anatomy of Vertebrate Masticatory Systems**	**27**
	The lower vertebrates	27
	The mammals	31
	The primates and humans	35
Chapter 3	**Development of the Occlusion**	**43**
	The primary dentition: From the 1st to the 5th year	43
	The mixed dentition: From the 6th to the 12th year	43
	Development of intermaxillary relations	47
	The permanent dentition: Variation is the rule	48
	Growth of the jaws	52
	Interrelations of form and function during development of the face and dentition	55
Chapter 4	**The Dentition**	**57**
	Occlusocranial relationships	58
	The dental arches	58
	The neutral zone	61
	Occlusal surfaces and contacts	62
	Occlusal relationships	62
	Occlusal morphology	65
	Guidance and determinants of occlusion	66
	Self-protective features of the dentition	67
	Esthetics	69

Chapter 5	**The Periodontium**	**71**
	Structure of the periodontium	71
	Functions of the periodontal ligament	77
	Sensory innervation of the periodontal ligament	78
	Role of periodontal sensory receptors in occlusion	79
	Response to physiological occlusal forces	79
Chapter 6	**The Temporomandibular Joint**	**81**
	Development of the temporomandibular joint	81
	Gross structure and function	83
	Histologic structure and function	90
	Blood and nerve supply	95
	Adaptation	95
	Osteoarthrosis	96
Chapter 7	**The Musculature**	**97**
	Muscles in general	97
	Muscles involved in mandibular function	103
	Neurosensory receptors in muscle	106
	Electromyography and muscle activity	108
Chapter 8	**The Neuromuscular System**	**115**
	Simple reflexes	116
	Jaw reflexes	118
	Facial reflexes	120
	Tongue reflexes	120
	Vagal reflexes (larynx, pharynx, palate)	121
	Regulation of reflex activity	121
	Synergies	124
	Rhythmic mastication	125
	Postural rest position of the mandible	128
Chapter 9	**Mandibular Movements**	**129**
	Border movements	129
	Functional movements	134
	Clinical significance of tooth and joint morphology	135
	Articulators and study casts	137
	Mounting casts on articulators	140
Chapter 10	**Mastication**	**143**
	Mandibular movement	143
	Condylar movement	145
	Masticatory forces	147
	Masticatory efficiency	148
	Development and learning of mastication	149
	Neurological control of mastication	150
	Muscle activity associated with mastication	151

Chapter 11	**Deglutition, Respiration, and Speech**	**153**
	Deglutition	153
	Respiration	155
	Speech	156
Chapter 12	**Concepts of Occlusion**	**161**
	Early concepts	163
	Concepts applied to the natural dentition	166
	The demise of balanced occlusion	168
	Influence of physical anthropology	170
	Current concepts	171
	PART II Occlusal and Dysfunctional Problems of the Masticatory System	177
Chapter 13	**Diagnostic Rationale: An Overview**	**179**
	Theoretically ideal occlusion	180
	Physiologic occlusion	181
	Nonphysiologic occlusion	182
	Therapeutic occlusion	184
Chapter 14	**Examination and Differential Diagnosis of Occlusal Problems**	**185**
	Examination of the occlusion	185
	History and clinical examination of the masticatory system	198
Chapter 15	**The Dentition: Occlusal Variations and Problems**	**209**
	Loss of tooth substance	209
	Tooth loss	212
	Morphological malocclusion	217
	Functional malocclusion	218
	Morphological malocclusion predisposing to functional malocclusion	223
	Diseases and trauma affecting the dentition	224
	Effects of prior dental treatment	225
Chapter 16	**The Periodontium: Responses to Occlusal Forces**	**227**
	Occlusal trauma	227
	Clinical diagnosis of occlusal trauma	229
	Occlusal trauma in the presence of periodontitis	230
	Therapeutic considerations	230
Chapter 17	**The Temporomandibular Joint: Problems Related to Occlusal Function**	**235**
	Degenerative joint disease	235
	Rheumatoid arthritis	239
	Traumatic joint disease	242
	Internal derangement	244
	Congenital anomalies	247
	Postnatal growth disturbances	247

Chapter 18	**Occlusal Parafunction**	**249**
	Nocturnal bruxism	249
	Diurnal parafunction	256
	PART III Management of Occlusal and Dysfunctional Problems	263
Chapter 19	**Therapeutic Concepts: An Overview**	**265**
	Objectives of treatment	266
	Structural occlusal problems	266
	Temporomandibular disorders	268
	Treatment sequence	270
Chapter 20	**Interocclusal Appliance Therapy**	**271**
	Theories of interocclusal appliance therapy	271
	Splint designs	274
	Overall clinical effectiveness of interocclusal appliances	275
	Symptom-specific effectiveness	277
	The stabilization splint	280
Chapter 21	**Occlusal Adjustment Therapy**	**285**
	Theories of occlusal adjustment	285
	Traumatic tooth contact recognition	287
	Indications and objectives for occlusal adjustment of the natural dentition	292
	Occlusal adjustment procedures	293
	Sequence of occlusal adjustment procedures	300
Chapter 22	**Prosthodontic, Operative, and Orthodontic Therapy**	**305**
	Prosthodontic therapy	305
	Operative therapy	321
	Orthodontic therapy	324
Chapter 23	**Behavioral Therapy**	**329**
	Foundations for successful therapy	329
	Modification of specific behaviors	331
	Procedures for general relaxation therapy	336
	Patient selection for behavioral programs	337
Chapter 24	**Physical Therapy**	**339**
	The role of physical therapy in temporomandibular disorders	339
	Exercise therapy	340
	Anesthetic adjuncts to exercise therapy	344
	Physical agents for analgesia	346
	Heat	348
	Manipulation	349
	Acupuncture	349

Chapter 25 **Pharmacological Therapy** **351**
Bases for pharmacological management 351
Pharmacological agents 352
Other pharmacological agents 355
Drug abuse and detoxification 356
Placebos 356

Chapter 26 **Surgical Therapy** **359**
Timing of orthognathic surgery in growing and nongrowing patients 361
Orthognathic surgical procedures 367
Skeletal disharmonies and temporomandibular disorders 373
Temporomandibular joint problems 373

Chapter 27 **Occlusion and Temporomandibular Disorders: A Prologue** **377**
Temporomandibular disorders 380

References 385

Index 405

Contributors

Kenneth Abramovitch, D.D.S., M.S.
Assistant Professor
Division of Oral Diagnosis/Radiology, Faculty of Dentistry, Dalhousie University, Halifax, Nova Scotia

G. Robert Bradley, D.D.S.
Resident in Advanced Education
General Dentistry Program, Department of General Practice, The University of Texas Health Science Center at San Antonio

Gunnar E. Carlsson, L.D.S., Odont. Dr.
Professor and Chairman
Department of Prosthetic Dentistry, Formerly Professor and Chairman, Department of Stomatognathic Physiology, Faculty of Odontology, University of Göteborg

Glenn T. Clark, D.D.S., M.S.
Professor
Section of Gnathology and Occlusion, School of Dentistry, Center for the Health Sciences, University of California at Los Angeles

Robert M. Davidson, D.D.S., M.S.
Research Assistant Professor
Department of Oral Biology, School of Dental Medicine, State University of New York at Buffalo

Douglas A. DePorter, D.D.S., Ph.D.
Professor
Department of Periodontics, Faculty of Dentistry, University of Toronto

M. Franklin Dolwick, D.M.D., Ph.D.
Professor and Chairman
Department of Oral and Maxillofacial Surgery, College of Dentistry, University of Florida

Aaron H. Fenton, D.D.S., M.S., F.R.C.D.(C)
Associate Professor
Department of Prosthodontics, Faculty of Dentistry, University of Toronto

L. F. Greenwood, B.D.S., D.D.S., Ph.D.
Associate Professor
Department of Prosthodontics, Faculty of Dentistry, University of Toronto

John M. Gregg, D.D.S., M.S., Ph.D.
Private Practice
Blacksburg, Virginia

Torgny Haraldson, L.D.S., Odont. Dr.
Associate Professor
Department of Stomatognathic Physiology, Faculty of Odontology, University of Göteborg

Bengt Ingervall, L.D.S., Odont. Dr.
Professor and Chairman
Department of Orthodontics, School of Dentistry, University of Bern, Bern, Switzerland

Rodney W. Johnson, D.D.S
Private Practice
Kingsville, Texas

Sigvard Kopp, L.D.S., Odont. Dr.
Professor and Chairman
Department of Stomatognathic Physiology, Faculty of Odontology, School of Dentistry, University of Lund, Malmö, Sweden

Robert P. Langlais, D.D.S., M.S.
Professor
Department of Dental Diagnostic Science, The University of Texas Health Science Center at San Antonio

Willard D. McCall, Jr., Ph.D.
Professor
Department of Oral Medicine, School of Dental Medicine, State University of New York at Buffalo

Hugh F. MacKay, D.D.S., M.Sc.
Associate Professor
Department of Prosthodontics, Faculty of Dentistry, University of Toronto

William A. Miller, B.D.S., M.S.
Professor
Department of Stomatology and Interdisciplinary Sciences, School of Dental Medicine, State University of New York at Buffalo

Norman D. Mohl, D.D.S., M.A., Ph.D.
Professor
Department of Oral Medicine, School of Dental Medicine, State University of New York at Buffalo

Richard Ohrbach, D.D.S.
Postdoctoral Fellow
Department of Oral Medicine, School of Dental Medicine, State University of New York at Buffalo

Richard R. Riggs, D.D.S.
Private Practice
Dallas, Texas

John D. Rugh, Ph.D.
Professor
Department of Oral and Maxillofacial Surgery, The University of Texas Health Science Center at San Antonio

Brian R. Smith, D.D.S.
Resident in Oral and Maxillofacial Surgery
Baylor College of Dentistry, Dallas, Texas

Joseph E. Van Sickels, D.D.S.
Associate Professor
Department of Oral and Maxillofacial Surgery, The University of Texas Health Science Center at San Antonio

George A. Zarb, B.Ch.D., M.S., M.S., D.D.S., F.R.C.D.(C)
Professor and Chairman
Department of Prosthodontics, Faculty of Dentistry, University of Toronto

Preface

The subject of Occlusion, perhaps because of its central role in the practice of dentistry, has had an interesting and controversial history. Numerous theories, concepts, techniques, and inventions have been adopted over the years in an effort to relate form and function, explain cause and effect, develop diagnostic criteria, and promulgate treatment philosophies, standards, and methods. Many of these ideas have survived and continue to be applied today. To a very large extent they came about because of insights resulting from clinical observations and experience. This should not necessarily be denigrated—empiricism has led to much progress in the diagnosis and treatment of a broad range of diseases and disorders. Historically, the clinician could not always wait for objective evidence before responding to the immediate needs of a patient with tangible disease or injury. And indeed, many early empirically based treatments appeared to be successful.

One reason a successful clinical outcome is so satisfying is that it reinforces one's preconceived hypothesis or insight. Unfortunately, clinical success, however noteworthy, *is not scientific proof of cause and effect.* The bleeding of patients by physicians for hundreds of years seemed effective because most people survived their illness or injury anyway. More immediately, an occlusal splint that eases a patient's discomfort does not prove that the etiology of that discomfort was occlusal.

We recognize and respect that empiricism and subjectivity are, and will remain, important parts of patient care. Questions involving orofacial esthetics, how best to develop rapport with a chronic facial pain patient, and when and how to deal with the unique features of a specific dentition do not easily lend themselves to objective scientific scrutiny. Subjectivity and individual perceptions are thus inevitable.

Nevertheless, it is our contention that the subject of Occlusion does have a biological basis, and that application of the scientific method can, and should be, applied to its study. We are now in an era of science and technology and the subject of Occlusion has felt the impact. Jaw tracking devices, portable electromyographic units, and high-resolution imaging machines are only a few of the developments that have enhanced our study of Occlusion. More important is the relatively new application of scientific methods to issues that have heretofore been regarded as sacrosanct. The use of normative data to describe structural and functional variability, of control groups in treatment efficacy studies, and of double-blind research protocol in clinical investigations are examples of how objective inquiry can be applied to empirically derived theories about Occlusion. We contend that the scientific method has and will continue to alter many of our traditional perceptions, and that all ideas, whatever their lineage, should be questioned and redefined based on objectively derived and replicable data. Failure to do so will invariably lead to the demise of any substantive interest in this important area of dentistry.

It is within this context that *A Textbook of Occlusion* has been written. In a very real sense, this book represents a departure from the way many of the issues of Occlusion have been perceived. Our primary objective is to present tangible, useful, and clinically relevant information to be used by the dental student, dental educator, and dental practitioner. There are, however, some important secondary objectives. These are to build and sustain a rational biological basis for the study of Occlusion, to enhance the objectivity of clinical observations and their interpretations, and to emphasize the need for increased scientific inquiry into the many old and new questions that exist.

We have not produced this textbook in order to promulgate, advance, or defend any particular concept or idea. We claim no special insight. We go on record as stating that we will embrace any concept that has been derived from objective data and that is capable of being replicated. Thus, we readily concede that a number of the ideas discussed in this textbook will be superseded in the years ahead. As long as the process takes place within the framework of nondoctrinaire, unbiased, and unemotional inquiry, it is to be welcomed, not repelled.

In reading this textbook, one may notice the dearth of unequivocal statements to support its positions. This is by design—and we recognize that it may make readers somewhat uncomfortable. Because so many dental therapeutic procedures require constant attention to detail, absolute standards are often sought. Absolutes provide comfort and security, but they cannot, at this time, be applied to the diagnosis and treatment of occlusally related problems. We have come to understand the enormous range of structural variability among human masticatory systems, that what individuals do with their occlusions may be more important than structural relationships, and that this system, like all musculoskeletal systems, often adapts to changing structural and functional demands. We are not implying that therapy, once initiated, should not adhere to strict technical standards. However, arriving at the decision of when to treat, and toward what end, deserves a less rigid outlook at the present time.

The reader will also note that, although traditional and important structural characteristics, relationships, and therapies are presented, a number of nonstructural relationships and treatment modalities are included as well. This reflects our interpretation of the current scientific literature that structural or positional occlusal factors do not precipitate parafunctional activity such as bruxism, but that such activity has the potential to produce a range of sequelae that includes pain, impaired function, and structural changes of the occlusion or other components of the masticatory system. This evidence seems compelling enough to have led us to include discussions of some nonstructural therapies that are aimed at the control of parafunctional activity or to the relief of its undesirable consequences. It is our view that, if positive evidence continues to be forthcoming, these nonstructural therapies will gradually be added to the dentist's armamentarium for the management of occlusal and related orofacial problems.

In preparing this textbook, the editors and contributors received invaluable help from many people. These include secretaries, typists, medical illustrators, photographers, reviewers, and consulting colleagues. They are too numerous to mention individually. Nonetheless, we wish to sincerely thank each of them for diligently using their skills on our behalf.

Chapter 1

Introduction to Occlusion

Norman D. Mohl

Occlusion defined

The literal definition of the term *occlusion* is "the act of closure or state of being closed," and, relative to dentistry, "the relation of the maxillary and mandibular teeth when in functional contact during activity of the mandible" (Dorland's, 1985). These definitions, although accurate, are much too narrow and do not truly define the field. A more comprehensive definition:

> The relationship between all the components of the masticatory system in normal function, dysfunction, and parafunction, including the morphological and functional features of contacting surfaces of opposing teeth and restorations, occlusal trauma and dysfunction, neuromuscular physiology, the temporomandibular joint and muscle function, swallowing and mastication, psychophysiological status, and the diagnosis, prevention, and treatment of functional disorders of the masticatory system (Jablonski, 1982)

Thus, the subject of Occlusion encompasses all factors that serve to bring about, affect, influence, or result from mandibular position, function, parafunction, and dysfunction. It implies much more than the occlusal contact relationships of the dentition and includes reference to a dynamic biomechanical musculoskeletal system: the masticatory system. Therefore, one can only understand Occlusion with a comprehensive view of the subject. This includes knowledge of biological evolution, development, histology, anatomy, biomechanics, physiology (particularly neuromuscular physiology), adaptation, pathology, the behavioral sciences, and clinical diagnosis and therapy. Because the term *occlusion* can have a somewhat narrow connotation, alternate terms are sometimes employed in an attempt to broaden the definition of the field (e.g., stomatognathic physiology). However, the word *occlusion* is the one most commonly employed by the dental profession, and it is an appropriate term *provided one views the subject in its broad context.*

The principal objective of the teaching of the field of Occlusion is to provide dental students and practitioners with theoretical and applied knowledge necessary for patient care. As already suggested, this involves a multidisciplinary presentation of the scientific and clinical factors underlying our understanding of mandibular function and dysfunction. This goal is consistent with the view that the primary purpose of dentistry is to maintain the functional integrity of the masticatory system.

Within this context, two important secondary objectives deserve to be mentioned. First, the subject of Occlusion serves as a natural interface between certain of the biologic and behavioral sciences and the clinical sciences. The teaching of this subject should serve to enhance this interface. Thus, this textbook leans heavily on information from these disciplines that is relevant to the overall subject.

Second, Occlusion is in the unique position to provide a common pool of information that can be used by all of the clinical disciplines of dentistry. The subject of Occlusion is, in the view of many, the medium that brings all branches of dentistry together (Ricketts, 1969). The teaching of this subject, therefore, should serve to encourage the common interest of the various disciplines.

Because each clinical area of dentistry deals with Occlusion to some extent, varied disciplines have taught and will continue to teach some aspect of this subject. This is not to be discouraged. However, because each clinical discipline brings its own needs and perspectives to the subject, parochialism, conflicting philosophies, or at least a lack of cohesion, often exist in the teaching of this subject in the dental curriculum. It is only natural, for example, that the orthodontist concerned with the development of the natural occlusion will view the field differently than a prosthodontist, who will tend to see the subject in terms of replacement of the edentulous or partially edentulous dentition.

The general practitioner has a particular need to view the subject of Occlusion in cohesive and comprehensive terms because it is in the general practice environment that all of the elements of dentistry are most tangibly integrated. Thus, the study of Occlusion in its broadest sense has a vital and direct relationship to the general practice of dentistry. The purpose of this textbook is to serve as an essential support vehicle to the integrated, cohesive, and comprehensive teaching of this subject to students of dentistry, and to provide useful information to practicing dentists as well.

This book is organized for use in a series of courses in Occlusion. Part I is intended as required reading to accompany a preclinical first-year or introductory course in Occlusion. This section deals with the normal anatomy and physiology of the masticatory system.

Part II is designed to serve in the same capacity for a second-level course in the dental curriculum. It entails a discussion of the definition and diagnoses of occlusal and dysfunctional problems of the masticatory system.

Part III follows in this natural sequence of teaching dentistry, dealing with therapy for occlusal and dysfunctional problems. It would, therefore, be used as required reading in the clinical years of the curriculum.

A series of courses in Occlusion should enhance, not necessarily replace, current courses or textbooks in any of the existing biological or behavioral sciences, or those used in the teaching of the important clinical disciplines. It is expected that the student will have a solid foundation in the anatomical sciences, particularly dental anatomy, head and neck anatomy, histology, and embryology, prior to taking an introductory course in Occlusion.

This approach to the teaching of Occlusion is consistent with a report by the American Dental Association's Council on Dental Education (1976), which recommended that dental schools establish coordinated teaching programs in Occlusion. Many dental schools now have such programs, spanning several years of the dental curriculum. Of 51 U.S. dental schools reporting from 1980 to 1981, 29 (56.9%) had separate departments, autonomous divisions, or departmental sections devoted to this subject (Esposito, Farman, and Veal, 1983). This textbook should provide major educational support for such programs and assist in the development of new programs.

The American Association of Dental Schools (1983) has developed "Curricular Guidelines in Occlusion." They follow in part:

> The study of occlusion involves the entire stomatognathic system. The understanding of the interrelationships between the teeth, periodontal tissues, bones, joints, muscles, and nervous system during the full range of mandibular movement as well as the normal functional movements is essential. The acceptable contact relationships of the teeth during these movements and the instrumentation and techniques required to reproduce these relationships during restorative procedures should be presented.
>
> Once the healthy functioning stomatognathic system and the acceptable contact relationships of the teeth are understood, the knowledge, techniques, and procedures for the diagnosis and treatment of the potentially pathologic and pathologic conditions can be

presented. This includes: *(1)* etiologic factors leading to the pathologic state, *(2)* the neuromuscular physiology leading to the pathologic state, *(3)* effects of parafunction or pathofunction to the teeth, periodontal tissues, muscles, and joints, *(4)* diagnostic aids, *(5)* diagnosis of the potentially pathologic and pathologic conditions, *(6)* methods of treatment, *(7)* the integration of these methods into a comprehensive treatment plan, *(8)* clinical experience in diagnosis and treatment of occlusion-related problems. Some content material can be covered in courses other than occlusion but should be considered part of the total occlusion curriculum.

The occlusion curriculum should be presented throughout the four years of undergraduate training. Occlusion directly correlates the basic science disciplines and the preclinical and clinical disciplines. The initial phase of the occlusion curriculum should be initiated as early as possible after anatomy and histology of the stomatognathic system have been presented. Neuroanatomy and physiology could be presented prior to or in conjunction with appropriate aspects of this portion of the occlusion curriculum. Instrumentation and techniques in replacement or reproduction of occlusal relationship should be presented prior to restorative preclinical courses. The portion of the occlusion curriculum that involves the diagnosis and treatment of the pathologic and dysfunctional occlusions can be presented after or in conjunction with other preclinical courses and prior to clinical experience. The clinical portion should be integrated into the clinical experience of disciplines for comprehensive patient treatment.

Because the subject of Occlusion is so broadly defined, its educational goals and recommended curriculum are so diffuse, and its application to dental practice is so closely integrated with all clinical disciplines, a textbook on this subject risks encompassing almost all of dentistry. This is clearly untenable and would not serve this book's purposes. Therefore, it deals only with those topics and concepts that are most directly related to occlusal and mandibular form and function, and to diagnostic and therapeutic modalities that are important to *all* dentists but do not fall under the aegis of one clinical specialty. Thus, this textbook does not repeat in detail concepts or treatment procedures that are unique to existing clinical disciplines of dentistry and that are readily available in other discipline-based textbooks. However, subjects that are not within the purview of existing dental disciplines are dealt with in some detail. Topics such as the functional anatomy of the temporomandibular joint, occlusal form and function, occlusal adjustment of the natural dentition, interocclusal appliance therapy, and behavioral aspects of mandibular function are examples of topics presented in more detail.

It is not the purpose of this textbook to present just one point of view or to be an advocate for any particular occlusal concept or treatment modality. The only "school of thought" that is promulgated is one that has some basis in objective scientific inquiry or is at least within the mainstream of current thought within dentistry. In this regard, certain decisions have had to be made regarding some aspects of therapy, such as occlusal adjustment. Such decisions have been made with the realization that our current knowledge may be incomplete and that other empirical techniques may provide equally beneficial results. In this regard, the reader, particularly the dental student, is encouraged to question the basic foundation of each premise presented in this textbook. This admonition was very well stated by Calder (1979), who wrote, "As individuals, scientists can be as pigheaded about their ideas as anyone else, but science itself perishes as soon as 'authority' takes charge. A continual influx of young people ready to contradict their teachers keeps it alive."

The masticatory system

The masticatory system can be regarded as a functional unit within the context of other overlapping functional entities comprising the head and neck and, indeed, the entire body. Its principal components include the dentition; the periodontal supporting structures; the maxilla and mandible; the temporomandibular joints; the mandibular musculature; the muscles of the lips, cheeks, and tongue; the soft tissues that invest these structures; and the innervation and vasculature supplying all of them. In addition to mastication, the primary functions associated with the masticatory system include respiration, deglutition, and speech. The system may also engage in occlusal parafunction, which includes such activities as clenching or grinding of the teeth (bruxism), fingernail biting, thumb-sucking, and pipe smoking, to name a few. And the role of the masticatory system in the perceived esthetics of the individual cannot be disregarded because this factor is often a very important element in patient care.

Morphological variability

It is assumed that the dentition has ceased to be a selection factor in the process of human biological evolution. As long as the vital functions of respiration and digestion are subserved, the specific anatomical characteristics of the oral structures no longer have the impact on survival they once had in anthropoids and prehominids, and still have in extant primitive human societies. This factor has permitted an expanding gene pool to occur which, in turn, has been expressed in the enormous variability seen among human beings. One need only think of the gross differences in tooth morphology, arch configuration, and relative jaw size between patients to appreciate the extent of this variability. Thus, *no one anatomical or functional description can apply to every human masticatory system*. Variability can only be contended with by the development of clinical judgment and skills and recognition of the uniqueness of each patient. Rigid clinical dogma to be applied to all patients is not warranted, *particularly when specific scientifically derived cause-and-effect relationships have not yet been determined*.

Structural and functional adaptation

The evidence is quite clear that the masticatory system has available to it a wide range of adaptive modalities involving virtually all components of the system. These adaptations can be functional and/or structural and may respond to transient and/or permanent demands. Because this system, like any biological system, can undergo change, it should not be viewed as a rigid, unyielding, immutable entity. Such views are often accompanied by a rigid, dogmatic approach to therapy that may not be warranted under individual circumstances. This does not imply that therapy, once instituted, should not be performed with care and precision in keeping with accepted therapeutic principles. The question, rather, is whether a fixed, predefined concept should be applied dogmatically to all patients and in all situations.

The masticatory system must also be viewed within the context of the overall physical and emotional health of the patient. The ability to adapt is intimately involved with the patient's general well-being. Functional or parafunctional forces in one person may produce a tissue response, a sign, or a symptom that is different from that produced in another individual. This again reinforces the observation that the masticatory system cannot be considered an isolated autonomous functional entity.

Although the epidemiology of disorders under the broad subject heading of Occlusion is beyond the scope of this book, it should be noted that structural occlusal problems, occlusal parafunction, mandibular dysfunction, and temporomandibular disorders are very common in all cultures and among all age groups. One need only consider the large number of young people who seem to require orthodontic intervention, the vast number of adults who have mutilated, partially lost, or completely lost dentitions, and the many people who have signs and symptoms of pain or compromised function involving the masticatory system, to appreciate the extent of the problem.

A review of epidemiological studies by McLain and Proffitt (1985) led them to conclude that "the majority of children, adolescents, and adults, particularly in the United States and Western Europe, have irregular teeth and/or occlusal relationships that differ from the ideal." Although one may question the criteria used in defining malocclusion in such studies and also note that current evidence for a direct association between malocclusion and oral health problems remains tenuous, it is still evident that many people seek and obtain treatment for correction of malocclusion. Much of this treatment, particularly orthodontics, may be initiated for esthetic considerations alone (Isaacson, 1985). This is not surprising because "there is clear evidence that dental and facial esthetics play a significant role in self-esteem and self-image" (McLain and Proffitt, 1985).

The high incidence of partial or total loss of the natural dentition is fairly well documented, especially in Western countries. When these data are added to those of individuals who have mutilated dentitions due to caries, attrition, trauma, aging, or other causes, the incidence of occlusally related dental problems is dramatically increased. With regard to the prevalence of temporomandibular pain or dysfunction, a review of the best available data by Solberg (1983) led him to observe that "epidemiological studies have demonstrated a moderate level of awareness of symptoms of TM disorders among otherwise healthy persons of both sexes and varying ages."

Although complete estimates for all types of occlusal and mandibular function problems are not available, it is clear that, collectively, these conditions comprise a significant proportion of dental or dentally related problems and account for a large number of patients who seek oral health care. From this we can assume that the personal, social, and financial cost to the public in seeking to treat these conditions is enormous, and that, therefore, the conditions are a significant public health problem. We must learn as much as possible about these problems for improved diagnoses and more cost-effective and better treatments.

Introduction to terminology

Consistent terminology is important to our ability to communicate. The terms used in this textbook have been selected because they are the most commonly employed, are descriptive and, we hope, unambiguous, and are consistent with the current state of our knowledge.

The terminology and concepts presented here serve as an introduction to the field and as a frame of reference for the initial study of Occlusion. Numerous additional terms will be introduced in subsequent chapters.

Mandibular position

Centric occlusion. The position of the mandible when the relationship of opposing occlusal surfaces provides for maximum planned contact and/or intercuspation. Because this is a tooth-determined position, sufficient teeth must be present for the mandible to be placed in this position *(intercuspal position [ICP], acquired occlusion, habitual occlusion, convenience occlusion).*

Centric relation. 1. "The most retruded relation of the mandible to the maxillae when the condyles are in the most posterior unstrained position in the glenoid fossae from which lateral movement can be made, at any given degree of jaw separation" *(ligamentous position, terminal hinge position)* (Academy of Denture Prosthetics, 1977). 2. The relationship of the mandible to the maxillae when the mandibular condyles are in their most superior position, with the central bearing area of the articular disks in contact with the articular surface of the condyles and with the articular eminences. In this position, the condyles may or may not be in their most retruded position, depending on the degree of restraint provided by the temporomandibular ligaments.

Note: Although the above two definitions are somewhat different, both agree that centric relation is determined by the structural features of the temporomandibular joint, and not by the dentition. In most individuals, the position of the mandible in centric relation, by either definition, is slightly behind its position in centric occlusion. The concept embodied in the second definition is the one that will be used in this textbook in place of the first, more "traditional," definition. See chapter 6 for a more detailed discussion.

Retruded contact position (RCP). The position of the mandible determined when the mandible is in centric relation, and in which closure is made to initial occlusal contact.

Intercuspal position (ICP). See *centric occlusion*.

Muscular contact position (MCP). The position of the mandible when it has been raised by voluntary muscular effort to initial occlusal contact with the head erect. In an asymptomatic individual the muscular contact position will ordinarily be consistent with the intercuspal position. One may demonstrate this consistency by noting the ability to accurately and repeatedly tap the teeth directly into the intercuspal position when the head is erect.

Occlusal vertical dimension. The vertical dimension of the face as determined by a midline vertical measurement of the face between two arbitrary points above and below the mouth when the mandible is in centric occlusion. By convention, when the term *vertical dimension* is used alone it is usually taken to mean occlusal vertical dimension *(vertical dimension of occlusion)*.

Postural rest position. The "resting" position of the mandible when an individual is sitting or standing in an upright position, as determined by the muscles and other tissues that attach to the mandible *(rest position, "physiologic" rest position, postural position, clinical rest position)*. It should be noted that postural rest position is not a position of minimal muscle activity but requires a small amount of elevator muscle contraction to maintain the mandible in this position. Electromyographic (EMG) rest position implies minimal muscle activity. The mandible is usually several millimeters more "open" in this position than in postural rest position.

Rest vertical dimension. The vertical dimension of the face when the mandible is in postural rest position.

Interocclusal distance. The distance, commonly 2 to 4 mm, between the occluding surfaces of the maxillary and mandibular teeth when the mandible is in postural rest position; the difference between occlusal vertical dimension and rest vertical dimension *(freeway space, interocclusal gap or space)*. Thus, assuming a relatively fixed postural rest position, any increase in occlusal vertical dimension would diminish the amount of interocclusal distance, and vice versa.

Mandibular movement

Disclusion. Nonocclusion or the loss of occlusal contact between opposing teeth during tooth-guided movements or positionings of the mandible. For example, if the mandible is moved forward from centric occlusion so that the opposing incisors are in occlusion and the posterior teeth are no longer in contact, the posterior teeth are said to be in disclusion. The term is not applied when the mandible is opened and all teeth are out of occlusal contact.

Hinge movement. The movement in space characterized by two divergent points moving around a central axis of rotation.

Hinge axis. An imaginary line between the mandibular condyles around which the mandible can rotate without translatory movement *(transverse hinge axis)*.

Translatory movement. The movement in space characterized by linear motion with no axis of rotation. Such movement may follow a straight path *(rectilinear translation)* or a curved path *(curvilinear translation)*.

Protrusion. Movement of the mandible forward or in an anterior direction with an anterior translation of both condyles. Thus, when the mandible is moved forward from centric occlusion, with or without occlusal contact, it is said to be in protrusion.

Retrusion. Retraction or posterior movement of the mandible from any given point.

Lateral excursion. Sideward movement of the mandible from a median occlusal position and characterized by a forward, inward, and downward translation of the contralateral condyle. Thus, when the mandible is moved into a left lateral excursion, the left condyle rotates and the right condyle translates in a forward, inward, and downward direction on its articular eminence.

Working side. The lateral segment of the dentition toward which the mandible moves during lateral excursion *(functioning, ipsilateral, laterotrusive).* Thus, if the mandible moves into left lateral excursion, the left side of the dentition is termed the *working side.*

Nonworking side. The side opposite the working side during lateral excursion *(nonfunctioning, contralateral, balancing, mediotrusive).* Thus, if the mandible is moved into a left lateral excursion, the right side of the dentition is the nonworking side.

Bennett movement. The bodily lateral movement or lateral shift of the mandible toward the working side that occurs during lateral excursion *(Bennett shift, side shift of the mandible).* Thus, as the mandible is moved into left lateral excursion, in addition to rotation of the condyle on the (left) working side and translation of the (right) nonworking side condyle, the mandible (and therefore both condyles) will shift bodily to the left by a small amount in most individuals.

Condylar guidance. The influence on mandibular movements by the direction of condylar movement during translation of the condyles as determined by the anatomical features of the temporomandibular joint. For example, during protrusion, the degree of downward movement of the condyles that occurs during their forward translation will depend on the height and amount of convexity of the articular eminences. Thus, very steep eminences will cause (guide) the condyles to move downward to a greater degree than if the eminences were less steep.

Condylar inclination. That part of the condylar guidance formed by the inclination of the condyle path as it translates forward and downward on the articular eminence. The example given above represents condylar inclination.

Condylar angulation. That part of the condylar guidance formed by the angulation of the nonworking side condyle path as it translates forward and inward during lateral excursion (Bennett angle). More specifically, it is the angle at which the nonworking side condyle moves medially during lateral excursion. Because the amount of Bennett movement is directly related to the amount of condylar angulation, it is often referred to as the Bennett angle. This can easily be seen on any semiadjustable articulator.

Anterior guidance. The influence on mandibular movements by the relative overlap of the anterior teeth as determined by the lingual surfaces of the maxillary anterior teeth and the incisal edges or labial surfaces of the mandibular anterior teeth. For example, a dentition characterized by maxillary anterior teeth that have a severe vertical overlap (overbite) over the mandibular anterior teeth when the mandible is in centric occlusion will cause (guide) the anterior part of the mandible to move downward at a steep angle during protrusion, lateral excursion or lateroprotrusive movements. Likewise, little vertical overlap of the maxillary anterior teeth over the mandibular will not necessitate such a downward movement of the mandible; hence, a reduced anterior guidance.

Incisal guidance. That part of the anterior guidance that occurs during protrusive movements of the mandible and is influenced by the relative overlap, position, and anatomy of the maxillary and mandibular incisors.

Canine guidance. That part of the anterior guidance that occurs during lateral excursion of the mandible and is influenced by the relative overlap, position, and anatomy of the maxillary and mandibular canines on the working side.

Dentition

Supporting cusps. Those cusps that are in primary occlusal contact in centric occlusion and help support occlusal vertical dimension, usually the lingual cusps of maxillary teeth and buccal cusps of mandibular teeth *(centric holding cusps).*

Guiding cusps. Those cusps that do not primarily support occlusal vertical dimension in centric occlusion but have the potential for occlusal "guiding" contact during lateral excursion of the mandible, usually the buccal cusps of maxillary teeth and lingual cusps of mandibular teeth *(nonsupporting cusps).*

Plane of occlusion. An imaginary surface that is related anatomically to the cranium and that theoretically touches the incisal edges of the incisors and the tips of the occluding surfaces of the posterior teeth. It is not a plane in the true sense of the word, but represents the mean of the curvature of the surface.

Compensating curve. The curvature of the alignment of the occlusal surfaces of the teeth that is present to compensate for the curved movement patterns of the mandible *(Monson curve).* When viewed laterally it is referred to as the *curve of Spee,* and when viewed in the frontal plane, as the *curve of Wilson.* These curves are not the same in different areas of the occlusion, and no common center, radius, or circumference exists in the natural dentition.

Overbite. The extension of the maxillary teeth over the mandibular teeth in a vertical direction when the opposing posterior teeth are in contact in centric occlusion *(vertical overlap).*

Overjet. The projection of the maxillary anterior and/or posterior teeth beyond their protagonists in a horizontal direction when the mandible is in centric occlusion *(horizontal overlap).* The anterior guidance will be greatly influenced by the relative amount of overbite and overjet. For example, much overbite and little overjet of the maxillary incisors relative to the mandibular incisors will result in a great deal of incisal guidance, and vice versa.

Occlusal stability. Absence of the tendency for teeth to migrate within a dentition other than slow physiologic compensatory movements usually resulting from normal tooth wear.

Reference planes

Frankfort plane. A horizontal plane passing through the lowest point in the margin of the left orbit *(orbitale)* and the highest point on the margin of the left and right external auditory meatus *(porion).*

Axis-orbital plane. A horizontal plane passing through the transverse hinge axis and the orbitale point.

Occlusal concepts

Mutually protected occlusion. An occlusion that provides for maximum occlusal contact on certain teeth or groups of teeth whereas other teeth have light contact or are in disclusion during centric occlusion or excursive movements of the mandible. In centric occlusion, the posterior teeth provide maximum occlusal loading and, in a sense, protect the anterior teeth; during protrusion, the incisors occlude and the other teeth do not; in lateral excursion, the working side teeth occlude while the nonworking side teeth are in disclusion. This concept is most often seen and applied to the adult natural dentition (see chapter 12 for detailed discussion).

Canine protected occlusion. A modification of the mutually protected occlusion in which the canine teeth on the working side serve to disclude all other teeth during lateral excursion of the mandible.

Group function occlusion. A modification of the mutually protected occlusion in which the canines and one or more adjacent pairs of posterior teeth on the working side are in simultaneous occlusal contact during lateral excursion of the mandible.

Balanced occlusion. An occlusion in which balanced and equal contacts are maintained throughout the entire arch during all excursions of the mandible. In the pure form, a balanced occlusion implies simultaneous occlusal contact on both working and nonworking sides during lateral excursion *(cross-arch balance),* occlusal contact between opposing buccal cusps and opposing lingual cusps on the working side during lateral excursion *(cross-tooth balance),* and simultaneous occlusal contact of anterior and posterior teeth during protrusion *(protrusive balance).* This concept, or modifications thereof, are usually reserved for complete denture prosthodontics (see chapter 12 for detailed discussion).

Theoretically ideal occlusion. A preconceived theoretical concept of occlusal structural and functional relationships that includes idealized principles and characteristics that an occlusion should have. It does not represent the norm in a statistical sense and only occasionally represents the occlusal characteristics of any given individual. The concept is used as a series of idealized parameters against which variations may be compared (see chapter 13 for detailed discussion).

Physiologic occlusion. This concept refers to an occlusion, usually adult, that deviates in one or more ways from the theoretically ideal, yet is well adapted to that particular environment, is esthetically satisfactory to the patient, and has no pathological manifestations or dysfunctional problems. It represents a state of harmony and does not require therapeutic intervention.

Nonphysiologic occlusion. This concept involves the presence of signs or symptoms of pathology, dysfunction, or inadequate adaptation of one or more components of the masticatory system that can be attributed to faulty structural relationships or to mandibular functional activity; thus, therapy may be indicated.

Malocclusion. Any occlusion in which the structural characteristics are beyond those established for a theoretically ideal occlusion. Although the prefix *mal* means bad or ill, the term malocclusion does not necessarily imply that such an occlusion is nonphysiologic or that therapy is indicated. Thus, the presence of a malocclusion does not mean that therapy is necessarily required, particularly in adults, because such an occlusion may be physiologic.

Therapeutic occlusion. An occlusion that has been modified by appropriate therapeutic modalities in order to change a nonphysiologic occlusion to one that, at the least, falls within the parameters of a physiologic occlusion, if not the theoretically ideal. Such an occlusion may contain structural modifications not necessarily found in nature, in order to optimize the health and adaptative potential of the masticatory system.

Summary

This chapter has presented a comprehensive definition of the subject of Occlusion as well as a rationale for its inclusion in the dental curriculum. The essential functions and components of the masticatory system have been reviewed while emphasizing its morphological and functional adaptability and its morphological variability. An initial list of terms and concepts has been presented as an introduction to this subject and as a frame of reference for the study of Occlusion.

PART I
Anatomy and Physiology of the Masticatory System

This section introduces the student of Occlusion to the normal anatomy and function of the masticatory musculoskeletal system, as well as to its essential components. The information included in this section is vital to an understanding of the diagnosis and management of occlusal and dysfunctional problems that are presented in subsequent sections of this textbook. Gaining thorough knowledge of normal anatomy and physiology cannot be overemphasized if one is to comprehend the clinical issues and concepts that comprise the subject of Occlusion. Fundamental knowledge based on objective scientific inquiry is essential to understanding the clinical aspects of this subject, particularly in a field that is undergoing rapid change in its clinical information, its concepts, and its rationales and modes of patient management. Accordingly, Part I contains these chapters:

Evolution and Comparative Anatomy of Vertebrate Masticatory Systems
Development of the Occlusion
The Dentition
The Periodontium
The Temporomandibular Joint
The Musculature
The Neuromuscular System
Mandibular Movements
Mastication
Deglutition, Respiration, and Speech
Concepts of Occlusion

Chapter 2

Evolution and Comparative Anatomy of Vertebrate Masticatory Systems

William A. Miller

When studying the human masticatory system in health or disease it is essential to recognize its evolutionary history, how it got the way it is, and what biological forces and factors are involved in its function. To view the human body in any of its functions as distinct from other mammals is to court misunderstanding of the real nature of that functional system. Thus, some understanding of the evolution and comparative anatomy of the masticatory system can often yield important insights into normal and potentially abnormal function in humans.

The lower vertebrates

The earliest known vertebrates, alive almost 500 million years ago, were *jawless* fish *(Agnatha)* that were probably bottom or filter feeders. Morphologically they were quite similar to contemporary lampreys. Coexisting with the later jawless fish were other primitive fish that had distinct, although not well-developed, jaws—the *placoderms.* They had fewer gill slits and arches anteriorly, and the original third branchial arch became modified to form primitive upper and lower jaws and jaw joint. These fish, now extinct, had oral tooth structures as well as body armor (Romer, 1966).

The two major extant fish groups—the cartilaginous and bony fish—probably arose from a common stock, but the dentitions of these two groups are different. In the cartilaginous group (sharks and rays, etc.) the teeth are homodont, haplodont, and polyphyodont, and are attached to the jaws by an expanded basal plate embedded in a fibrous band that lies over the jaw cartilages. The teeth develop in well-defined tooth families with the oldest member being functional and the others in a graded sequence of development on the lingual or palatal side below (Fig. 2-1). Tooth shedding and replacement are not random but are precisely sequenced events in the alternate tooth families. Many of the sharks are predatory, and their teeth form a battery of sharp narrow blades ideal for slicing and tearing flesh even from living prey—hence the severe wounds inflicted during the rare shark attack on humans (Hillsbery, 1982). The jaw joint is composed of a fibrous/fibrocartilaginous union between the articular "bone," which is cartilage, and the posterior end of the skull so that opening and closing is essentially hingelike.

Bony fish have more teeth than cartilaginous fish. As well as being on the edge of the jaws proper, these teeth are found in the roof of the mouth (vomer and palatine bones), on the primitive rodlike tongue region, and down into the pharynx, where a quite sophisticated pharyngeal dental mill is found in some species (Greenwood, 1964; Liem, 1986). The teeth are arranged in many families with distinct groups related to each tooth-bearing bone. The teeth are frequently replaced in alternate tooth-family sequences—the functioning teeth of tooth families 1,3,5,7, etc., as one sequence; 2,4,6,8, etc., as the other sequence. Separate bones have their own distinct patterns. Thus, even the adjacent premaxilla and maxilla may be different (Miller

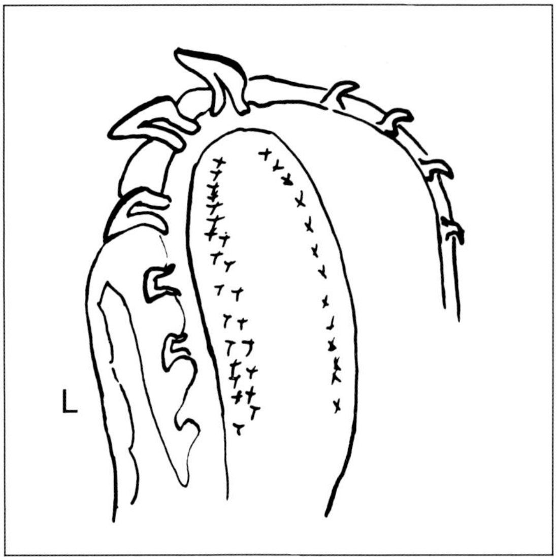

Fig. 2-1 Drawing from serial sections of developing dogfish teeth. Note that teeth start to develop on the lingual side *(L)* of the cartilaginous jaw, migrate toward the periphery, and are finally shed. Toothlike structures are also seen on the outer side of the jaw. Original magnification ×25.

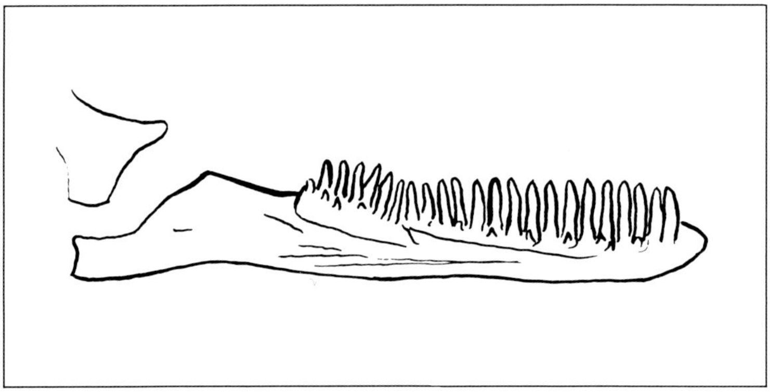

Fig. 2-2 Tracing of radiograph of *Necturus maculosus* (mudpuppy) lower jaw. Functioning teeth each have one distinct successor at the base of the tooth. Note the jaw articulation at the posterior end of the jaw.

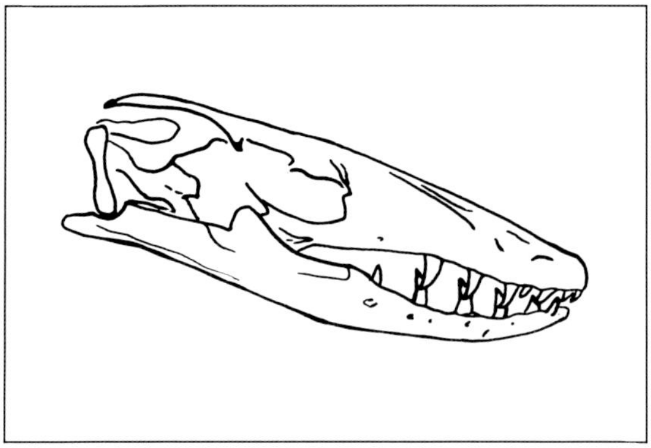

Fig. 2-3a Skull of *Varanus,* a monitor lizard. Note the reduced number of sharp, pointed teeth.

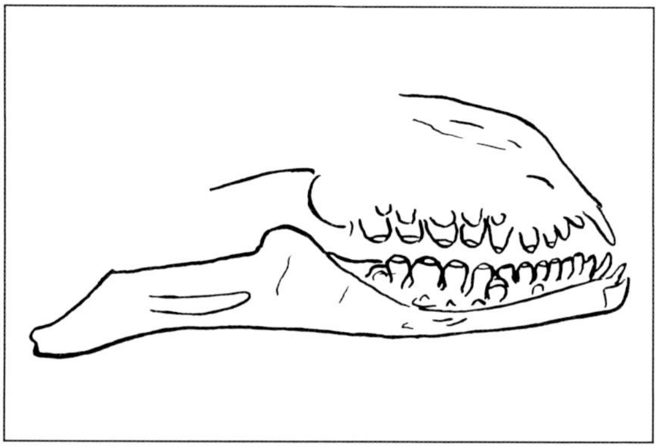

Fig. 2-3b Skull of the herbivorous blue tongue lizard. Note the rounded tooth surfaces in functioning and succeeding teeth.

and Radnor, 1973). Teeth are generally attached via a bony ankylosis to the jaws, although some bony fish have a modification of this, whereby some teeth fold back to allow prey to pass into the mouth, then flip back up to prevent its escape (Widdowson, 1946; Peyer, 1968). The jaw joint is between the articular bone of the lower jaw and the quadrate at the posterior end of the skull. It is a true diarthrodial synovial joint with hyaline cartilage covering the articulating bone surfaces.

It was from another group of primitive bony fish, which includes the lung fish, that the vertebrates emerged onto land in Devonian times. The crossopterygian fish, having retained a primitive lung, also had a strongly developed vertebral column, fins with an internal bony support, and large internal nares—and were able to make the first vertebrate invasion of the land to exploit its food resources. They had large fanglike teeth that were replaced alternately. The related, extant coelacanth *(Latimeria chalumnae)* has been shown to have true ectodermal enamel (Miller, 1969; Smith, 1978), a characteristic of the later vertebrates. Terrestial amphibians subsequently evolved marked strengthening of jaws and associated musculature and attachment of upper jaw to the skull, while the vertebral column, girdles, and limbs evolved to produce an effective, if clumsy, mode of terrestial locomotion.

Modern amphibians are highly specialized and modified. Some frogs and toads, for example, have few if any teeth (Lawson, 1966), whereas salamanders have many teeth with alternate tooth replacement (Miller and Rowe, 1973). In amphibians the jaws function as simple hinges with a strong snapping action aided by a strong hyoid system depressing the floor of the mouth (Bramble and Wake, 1985). The articulation is by the articular bone of the lower jaw to the quadrate region of the skull. The bones of the lower jaw are fewer than in fish, and the dentary bears most of the teeth (Fig. 2-2).

Reptiles, in turn, evolved from a group of primitive, ancestral amphibians. The teeth and bones of the skull in stem reptiles were well developed and quite similar in arrangement to their amphibian forebears. Later reptiles evolved modifications that resulted in a generally stronger skull and, therefore, a more efficient prey-grasping apparatus.

The reptiles eventually filled most ecological niches, including the air, and dominated both terrestial and aquatic environments. Some of their descendants are the edentulous, warm-blooded, and feathered modern birds. Both meat-eating and herbivorous forms occurred, and a whole order was both fishlike and fish eating *(Ichthyosauria)*. Thus, adaptations of the dentition related to diet occurred frequently in the Reptilia (see Romer, 1966, and Peyer, 1968, for many examples).

The modern reptiles may be predatory, for example, crocodilians and monitor lizards (*Varanus;* Fig. 2-3a), or they may be mollusc or fruit eaters, for example, the blue tongue lizard of Australia (Fig. 2-3b). The dentition and jaws are modified accordingly. Sharp teeth and strong jaws are characteristic of crocodilians with clearly defined replacement systems (Edmund, 1962; Miller and Radnor, 1970).

Although the dentition and some muscle attachments vary in the reptiles, the joint between lower jaw and skull is still between the articular bone—the only bone of the lower jaw that is cartilaginous and derived from Meckel's cartilage—and the quadrate bone of the skull: the articular-quadrate joint. The reptilian ear, posterior to the joint, consists of one bone, the stapes derived from the hyoid arch.

The jaw mechanics of reptiles are not particularly efficient. The muscles of closure are all attached well behind the dentition so that forces on the joint and at the region of muscle contraction are greater than at the working region in the dentition. As a consequence, the joint is relatively massive. Jaw opening is brought about by muscles attached to the posterior of the skull and the retroangular process at the back of the lower jaw. There is no mastication as such, and digestion does not begin until food reaches the stomach as a relatively large mass.

Many features distinguish mammals from reptiles, but those of the head, jaws, and teeth were as critical as any in ensuring the evolutionary advantage of the mammals.

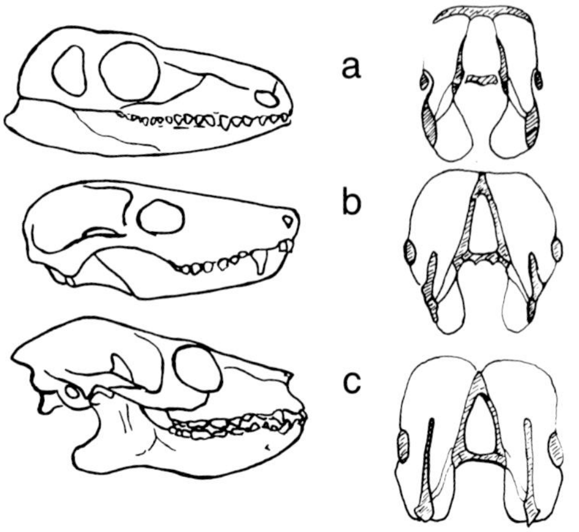

Fig. 2-4 Schematic drawings of lateral view and transverse sections of skulls: reptile *(a)*, mammal-like reptile *(b)*, and primitive mammal *(c)*. Note changes in muscle form with increasing complexity of jaw and dentition. (Redrawn from several sources.)

With prolonged intrauterine growth and subsequent suckling in mammals, the period of growth when a young animal has to fend for itself is greatly reduced. Hence the need for continual changes and enlargement of a functioning dentition is lessened, and fewer generations of teeth are required. Instead of being polyphyodont, mammals are mostly diphyodont.

Primitive mammals arose prior to the dominant giant reptiles of the Jurassic and Cretaceous periods, from the previously dominant mammal-like reptiles. These in turn had evolved from stem reptiles, several groups of which had approached the mammalian condition.

It has been suggested that it is the evolution of the mammalian jaws and jaw joint along with the changes in ear structure that are key to mammalian success (see Crompton and Parker, 1978, for review). These changes resulted in a dentition that could masticate food into small and more readily digestible pieces before swallowing. These appear to have been strong selection factors for nocturnal animals, which had to feed frequently and efficiently to maintain the high metabolic rate and constant body temperature needed to withstand the cooler nighttime when reptilian competitors were less active.

Fossil evidence shows that there was a gradual increase in size of the tooth-bearing bone of the lower jaw—the dentary—and reduction in the posterior bones, including the articular bone, which became incorporated into the mammalian middle ear as part of the incudomallear joint (Fig. 2-4).

The dentary—a membrane bone—gradually extended posteriorly until it came into contact with the squamosal portion of the temporal bone—also a membrane bone—where a new jaw joint, the temporomandibular joint (TMJ), eventually was established (Fig. 2-4). Recall that other synovial joints are cartilage-derived. Thus, both components of this joint are membrane-derived and distinct from the cartilaginous origin of primary joints. In humans early intrauterine jaw movements probably occur through the incudomallear (articular: quadrate) joint (Scott and Symons, 1977).

At the same time, there were modifications to the upper jaw to allow the development of the secondary palate; posteriorly, soft-tissue changes related to the separation of respiration and deglutition also occurred so that a young animal could breathe and suckle at the same time, and an adult breathe and masticate together. In addition, the development of true lips, a mobile tongue, and more complex salivary glands that secreted a saliva containing digestive enzymes all improved masticatory and digestive efficiency.

All muscles related to mastication became attached to the one moving bone that bore teeth, the dentary. At the same time the teeth became not only fewer in number with reduced replacements, but also individually larger and more complex. The homodont, haplodont reptilian cheek teeth gradually evolved to consist of a series of cusps, initially in the mesial and distal regions of the crown, but later forming a triangle of cusps called the *trigon* (*trigonid* in lower molars). Cusps were subsequently added posteriorly to the lower molars to form a "heel," or *talonid.*

Thus, primitive molar cuspal morphology was established; this molar is termed *tribosphenic*.

The muscles of mastication were radically changed. In reptiles there was a small pretemporalis muscle. This gradually enlarged and its attachment to the skull extended to change the direction of action to include anteroposterior as well as vertical vectors. The masseter muscle is found only in mammals. It developed to form a sling on the outside of the dentary, and so increased both the force that could be exerted and the lateral stability of the whole masticatory system (Fig. 2-4). On the medial side of the dentary, the greatly increased pterygoid muscles further contributed both to the force that could be applied and to the stability of the lower jaw. Not only were there enlarged and new muscles, the direction of action of the original muscles was changed.

Thus, there were several factors influencing the size of the dentary in particular. It should be realized that although bone (and tooth) is the tissue responsible for most fossil evidence, and so has the appearance of permanence, biologically bone is a plastic tissue, responding to the changes to which it is subjected rather than being the cause of these changes. Soft tissues such as muscle and possibly the developing pulpal/mesenchymal component of the teeth (increased tooth size) are probably what directed dentary changes. Thus, the great increase in the temporalis muscle (adductor) resulted in dramatic changes in the temporal roof of mammal-like reptiles (Fig. 2-4) as well as the later bowed formation of the mammalian zygomatic arch and the formation of the coronoid process (Barghusen and Hopson, 1979). The development of the mammalian masseter muscle, in turn, affected the form of the dentary and its angular process.

Throughout the period of giant reptile dominance, mammals survived as small rat-sized animals that were probably nocturnal. The environmental pressures were such that cunning, associated with increased brain size; a means of controlling metabolic rate, to be active during cool nights and, hence, warm blooded (homeothermic); and a keen sense of smell were all of great evolutionary advantage.

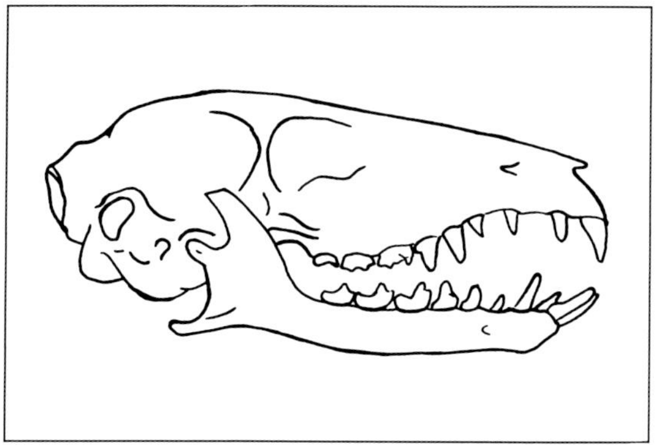

Fig. 2-5 Tracing of radiograph of the tree shrew *Tupia glis*. Note the sharp teeth with interdigitation and the talonid on the lower molars. (Courtesy of Dale Fish, Ph.D.)

The mammals have a long evolutionary history. The changes that led to mammalian characteristics occurred over a long period and through many stages; we might think of the age of mammals as the last 70 million years, when they have been the dominant vertebrates. This is in fact only the last third of mammalian evolutionary history (Lillegraven et al., 1979).

Recent studies (Fish and Mendel, 1982) have shown that the tree shrew, *Tupia glis*, which has a dentition remarkably similar to the early mammals, is able to modify its masticatory cycle depending on whether it is chewing soft food (banana), hard food (chow), or an insect (Fig. 2-5). This implies that the flexibility of the masticatory cycle allows for a variety of evolutionary pathways, and also that it is soft tissue factors that are key to evolutionary success, rather than the hard tissues, which are all that may be observed in the fossil record. This concept has already been alluded to in discussing the skull changes that occurred in the mammal-like reptiles (see Fig. 2-4).

The mammals

The principal features of mammalian dentitions include the following: *(1)* a distinct heterodonty where incisors, canine, and cheek teeth are usually clearly distinguished, and *(2)* a dentition that is usually diphyodontic, consisting of two generations of teeth—deciduous and permanent. Exceptions do occur: rodents are monophyodont, and certain mammals, such as some macropod marsupials and the manatee, have far more than the classic number of molar teeth (Sanson, 1978, 1982; Domning and Hayek, 1984). Another universal feature is that the teeth are attached by a thecodont gomphosis; this means that the teeth are held by their roots in a socket by a fibrous attachment—the periodontal ligament.

The periodontium consists of collagenous fibers, sometimes distinctly separated into bundles, running between the root cementum and the socket wall. Between the principal collagen bundles are varying small amounts of loose connective tissue and ground substance, which respond to variations in pressure (Picton and Wills, 1978). There are also many proprioceptive nerve fibers that terminate around the principal fibers of the ligament. This characteristic mammalian ligament enables tooth contact, and hence jaw position, to be monitored. The nerve endings respond to changes in the collagen fiber tension, whereas the interstitial regions act with a dampening effect on displacement. This soft tissue component is the final and, perhaps, the most important link in the development of a precise masticatory system. We have seen how the dentition, particularly molar cusp anatomy, became more elaborate, and how the jaw joint and the associated musculature changed and became more sophisticated; the mammalian periodontal ligament may be considered the final "tuning component" for the control of mammalian mastication.

In addition to these dental distinctions, mammalian masticatory systems are also distinguished from those of other vertebrates by having *(1)* a well-developed secondary palate, *(2)* separation of masticatory and respiratory pathways, *(3)* distinct lips (and cheeks) that are mobile and possibly prehensile in the acquiring of food, *(4)* a highly evolved tongue that together with the lip and cheek musculature controls the food bolus over the molar teeth during mastication, and *(5)* salivary glands that secrete a saliva that not only serves a lubricating function but also contains digestive enzymes.

The dental formula for true mammals (eutheria) is

$$i\frac{3}{3}c\frac{1}{1}pm\frac{4}{4}m\frac{3}{3}\times 2=44.$$

Very few living mammals have these characteristics for each quadrant: three incisors, one canine, four premolars with deciduous molar predecessors, and three molars without predecessors or successors. In humans the formula is

$$i\frac{2}{2}c\frac{1}{1}pm\frac{2}{2}m\frac{3}{3}\times 2=32,$$

and in the rat it is

$$i\frac{1}{1}m\frac{3}{3}\times 2=16.$$

There are three basic types of mammalian dentition: *(1)* those for eating meat (carnivores), including fish and insects (insectivores); *(2)* those for eating vegetation, either as grass, leaves, bark, fruit, nuts, etc., or combinations of these (herbivores and rodents); and *(3)* those that are able to cope with both meat and vegetation (omnivores). Each shows characteristic modifications of the teeth themselves, skull, jaw, associated musculature, and the TMJ. It should not be forgotten that the whole of the digestive tract, indeed the whole organism, is adapted in relation to diet and the obtaining of that diet. Thus, lions do not have hooves, nor do horses have claws.

Carnivores

Meat eating requires that prey be caught and killed, which, in turn, requires sharp claws and an appropriately modified dentition. The most prominent features are *(1)* in both sexes, enlarged canine teeth behind relatively small incisor teeth (as contrasted to many primates, where

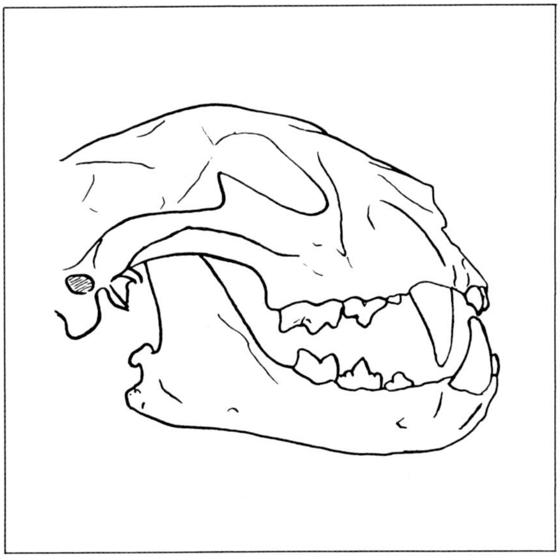

Fig. 2-6a Skull of leopard, slightly disarticulated. Note the large canine teeth and the few but elongated cheek teeth. The condyle is level with the lower molars and the skull is short.

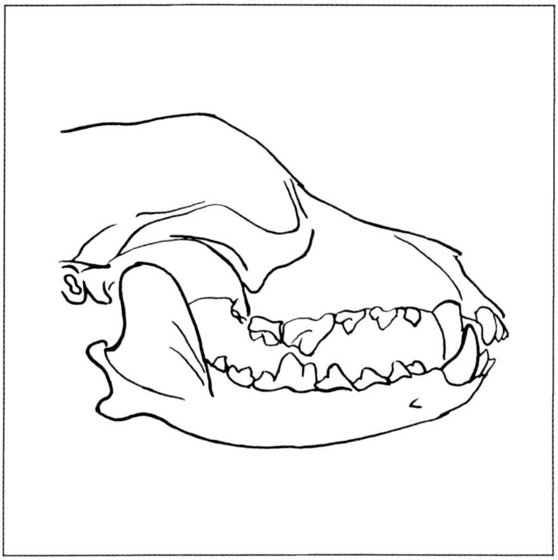

Fig. 2-6b Skull of dog. Compare with Figs. 2-6a and 2-7. The jaw is longer, there is less reduction in tooth number, and canine tooth enlargement is less pronounced.

only the male has very large canines), and *(2)* fewer cheek teeth, particularly in the cats, which have only one lower first molar or upper last premolar in each quadrant, called carnassial teeth, enlarged and flattened buccolingually to form a long sharp blade (Fig. 2-6a). The TMJ is approximately level with the occlusal plane, a feature that allows maximum gape with minimal distal displacement of the angular process, which might interfere with the airway. Because the major function of the joint is to maintain stability once the prey has been caught (because it may still be struggling), the squamosal portion is greatly strengthened. The muscles associated with jaw closure and their regions of attachment to the jaws and skull are enlarged. Enlargement of the temporalis muscle is a distinct carnivore feature (Noble, 1979). The condyle tends to be cylindrical and elongated transversely. All of these anatomical features add strength and stability to the joint. During closure there is a sliding contact between opposing carnassial teeth, which permits a shearing and slicing of meat. (Watch a cat chew a piece of raw meat.)

The dogs show less reduction in cheek tooth number than do the cats, and the modifications to the rest of the skull and TMJs are less extreme (Fig. 2-6b). There is less reduction in molar number associated with retention of an occlusal surface in the molar behind the carnassial, so that the animal is also able to crack bones, a feature that is even more accentuated in scavengers such as the hyena, where no true carnassial teeth are seen.

Modifications to the TMJ may also be quite varied in response to function; thus the North American badger has a very strongly developed glenoid fossa, which totally resists dislocation of the condyle unless fractured.

Herbivores

Two main groups of mammals have evolved to exploit a vegetable diet. One is the genuine herbivores such as the sheep, deer, horses, and rhinoceros; the other is the rodents, not discussed in this chapter.

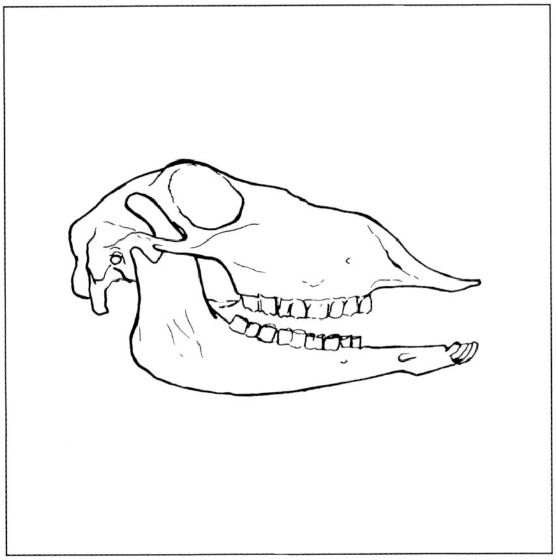

Fig. 2-7 Skull of sheep. Note the long jaws and well-developed nasal complex. The upper incisors do not develop and a fibrous gum pad replaces them. The cheek teeth are hypsodont, and the occlusal surfaces folded (selenodont). The condyle is well above the occlusal plane and the coronoid process is well developed.

The herbivores require a means of obtaining leaves (or fruit) and then a means of grinding them for digestion. It should be realized that grass eaters (grazers) also have to contend with tooth wear caused by the phytoliths of grass, which may be up to 18% dry weight. In addition to this, the hard cellulose cell walls of plants must be broken down. With vegetable diets the gut becomes lengthened and specialized in some region to allow bacterial fermentation. The multiple stomach chambers and cud chewing in ruminants is one such adaptation; the enlarged cecum and associated refection of fecal pellets found in rabbits (lagomorphs) and rats (rodents) is another. These behavioral patterns have been known to seriously affect studies of transmission of oral bacteria in experimental animals.

The anterior teeth are modified in several ways. In perissodactyls (single-toed ungulates, e.g., horses) an edge-to-edge incisal relationship has evolved with the incisal edges flattened and frequently invaginated to increase the opposing surface areas and maintain the roughness/abrasiveness of the contacting surfaces. In the artiodactyls (even-toed ungulates, e.g., sheep and goats) the upper incisors have been lost and replaced by a fibrous gum pad (Fig. 2-7). Leaves or grass are grasped by a long, almost prehensile, tongue and then cut between lower incisors and the upper gum pad.

The herbivores tend to retain most of the mammalian cheek tooth number and have modified them by various infoldings and invaginations. The premolars also have become more molarlike; all of these features increase the size and efficiency of the molar mill. Thus, in sheep and deer, characteristic selenodont cheek teeth are found, and the molars of the horse have occlusal foldings of enamel and dentin, along with coronal cementum. It should be pointed out that the ridges are at right angles to the direction of the predominantly lateral movement of the jaw. The exposed enamel, dentin, and cementum wear at different rates and so maintain tooth abrasiveness. The elongated (hypsodont) crowns allow maintenance of the abrasiveness over the animal's lifetime.

In association with these kinds of dental modifications, the mandible has a high condylar process so that the TMJ is well above the occlusal plane (Fig. 2-7). The glenoid fossa is shallow, and the joint ligaments relatively lax but strong. Muscle development is such that lateral and/or propalinal (front to back) movements are emphasized. The temporalis muscle is relatively small, whereas the masseter muscle is very large (Noble, 1979). These features serve to increase the effective force on the tooth row, although the wide gape is no longer possible.

Another feature of herbivores is the long snout. Behind the incisor teeth is a long gap (diastema) so that cheek teeth are separated from the anterior teeth. Associated with this is a well-developed nasal region and an excellent sense of smell, which is extremely important to a grazing animal in danger of predation. This in turn affects the jaw mechanics by extending the lever arm. Sheep are excellent examples of artiodactyl herbivores (Fig. 2-7).

Omnivores

The most successful omnivore are humans. The ability to eat a variety of diets gives great flexibility in choice of environment and hence adaptability to these environments. Perhaps the best known omnivore after humans is the pig (an ungulate); indeed the flesh of both is supposed to taste very similar, and this relates to their similar omnivorous diets.

The dental and skeletal features are those of *minimal* specialization. All of the teeth in the tooth row are similar in size. Incisors are not reduced, and canines are not greatly enlarged other than in the males of some species (sexual dimorphism). The cheek teeth are also of similar size, with rounded even cusps (bunodont teeth).

While humans are the exception, because of the upright stance, the jaws tend to be moderately long but without a distinct break in the tooth row as is found in herbivores. The TMJ is unspecialized and able to move in a variety of directions. The articulation is flat and the capsule lax but thickened, providing both strength and a wide range of movement. Wild pigs are able to grub for and eat roots (their canines are adapted for digging) and nuts, but they also eat carrion (dead animals), having no trouble with flesh or bones.

The primates and humans

The primates have been treated separately because they are a very old order and yet contain the most highly evolved mammal—humans—as well as living examples of many of the earlier grades of primate evolution.

The most primitive primate, the tree shrew, has been classified at times as an insectivore. The dentition is primitive in that the tribosphenic molar is retained. It has been shown, as discussed previously, that the masticatory system can function very efficiently with a wide variety of food types (see Fig. 2-5) (Fish and Mendel, 1982). The forelimb terminates in a grasping, primitive hand used not only for locomotion but also for acquiring food (Romer, 1966). They have claws and not nails. Tree shrews are crepuscular (twilight) to nocturnal and usually arboreal. This has resulted in large eyes that face forward instead of sideways, as in most mammals. Even in this "earliest" of primates the brain size is greater in proportion to body size than in other orders of mammals. This has always been a primate characteristic; relying on wile and cunning rather than on potentially restricting anatomical adaptations has been perhaps the main reason for primate success (Le Gros Clark, 1965).

The prosimian primates, such as the lemurs, lorises, and tarsiers, were widely distributed over the tropical regions on the earth during the Eocene, 60 million years before present (mybp), but are now very restricted. Their dental characteristics show a reduction in length of tooth row and snout region. They have grasping hands with nails, frequently make use of a crouching upright posture, and rely on sight rather than smell, their large eyes being on the front of the face. These are all primate characteristics. Consequent to this and associated with arboreal life is the development of stereoscopic vision. The diet is mixed and includes insects, small reptiles, fruits of many types, and leaves. Generally, the dentition is unspecialized and the TMJ permits both lateral and protrusive movements. The temporalis, masseter, and pterygoid muscles are not particularly emphasized.

Monkeys may be divided into two groups, both originally arboreal. New World monkeys, or platyrrhines (ceboidea) and Old World monkeys, or catarrhines (cercopithecidae).

New World monkeys have flat noses, as their scientific name suggests. The dental formula is

$$i\frac{2}{2}\,c\frac{1}{1}\,pm\frac{3}{3}\,m\frac{3}{3}\,.$$

The three premolars are of similar size and shape. These animals are highly adapted for arboreal life, and, along with grasping hands and feet, the tip of the tail may also be prehensile. When examining the skull of a *Platyrrhina* one is struck with its roundness, which implies a relatively large brain, and by the fact that the external auditory meatus is very short so that the ear ossicles are clearly visible within the middle ear. Fruit- and leaf-eating forms are found with appropriate modifications, particularly in the cusps of the molars. The gut is also appropriately modified to digest tough leaves.

The Old World monkeys have faces that are more pointed than their New World relations. A sharper nose points downward, again referred to in their name, *Catarrhina.* Along with primitive apes, they probably arose during the Oligocene (40 to 35 mybp). They too were primarily arboreal but with different adaptations, the most noticeable being gluteal callosities, which were perhaps related to sitting in branches. The thumb and big toe are both opposable. The premolars are reduced to two, as in humans, while the incisors remain two flat, spadelike teeth. The canines show varying degrees of sexual dimorphism, which is thought to be partly related to the degree of social organization within a troop; the difference is most marked in species with well-defined social structures and dominant males. Contemporary monkeys and apes all show some social organization, which implies cooperative action in defense and in procuring food (Jolly, 1985). Extinct forms are presumed to have been social to varying degrees.

The early monkeys and their descendants have molars with four cusps in a square pattern. The cusps are modified in leaf eaters and are sharper, as opposed to fruit eaters, where the cusps are more rounded.

It is believed that the seasonality of fruit, along with its typical coloring, resulted in the development of color vision in monkeys and apes in order to more efficiently collect fruits. Fruit eating has also recently been associated with higher metabolic rates and increased brain size (Martin, 1981). Fruit eating also had effects on the dentition and skull in that the incisors became larger and more vertically placed in the jaws. This in turn made the forces of occlusion more vertical. The stresses on the skull changed, resulting in the development of the postorbital septum, a distinctive higher primate characteristic (Cachel, 1979). Perhaps associated with periods of food gathering interspersed with food eating and care of young was the development of large cheek pouches in contemporary Old World monkeys and possibly in their ancestors. The anterior lower premolar is elongated anteriorly so that the upper canine occludes with a resulting shearing force between it and the lower canine; this is referred to as a *sectorial premolar.*

Early apes were distinguished dentally from the contemporary early monkeys by differently shaped lower molars, which had five cusps, the fissures between forming a *Y-5* pattern. This is also called the *Dryopithecus* pattern, from the earliest fossil in which the shape was observed. Their tooth rows were parallel and their palates flat. It has been suggested that the monkey four-cusped molar is the more recent adaptation (Simons, 1981), related to increased reliance on an arboreal way of life and its associated diet.

Modern apes are able to live in trees; they get around by using their long forearms to swing or move from branch to branch, a process called brachiation. The small species (gibbons and siamangs) are awkward on the ground, but the larger ones (gorillas, chimpanzees, and orangutans) move rapidly by knuckle walking. They are social animals with long periods needed for raising their young. The diets are varied; both fruit and leaves, as well as other small mammals, are taken. Chimpanzees have been observed to hunt collectively for small herbivores and even for young monkeys; cannibalism has also been observed (Goodall, 1977). The dentition is relatively unspecialized, although a sectorial lower premolar is seen (Fig. 2-8). The canines are enlarged in both sexes, but with distinct sexual dimorphism. The mandibular molar tooth rows are parallel to one another, whereas the maxillary molar row converges posteriorly and the palate is flat. The glenoid fossa is shallow.

There was one early group of apes *(Ramapithecus),* thought to be ground dwelling, which was different. The dental arch was parabolic and the palate slightly arched (Simons, 1968, 1981). The teeth were of relatively even size in that the canine, in particular, was not much larger than the first premolar. Structurally their teeth were different in that the enamel was very thick, particularly in the molars (Gantt, 1977). All of these features are recognized as distinctly human and distinguished from the other apes and the monkeys.

The importance of these ramapithecine hominids is currently open to a great deal of discussion and controversy. Is this convergent evolution? Is the enamel thickness merely related to a diet of dense hard structures like nuts, as suggested by Molnar and Gantt (1977), while its wear patterns suggest a different kind of diet (Teaford and Walker, 1984)? The problem is that later ramapithecines are contemporary with animals thought to be in the hominid line, and the fossil evidence is incomplete for this period—large time gaps occur at very critical periods, particularly between 12 mybp and 4 mybp. Recent, as yet incompletely reported, data indicate close similarities between some ramapithecines and early australopithecines (Simons, 1981).

If this chapter had been written 10 to 15 years earlier the next segment would not have been included, and our interpretation of early human evolution would have been quite different. Indeed, it is constantly changing as new evidence and interpretations occur (Delson, 1985, 1986; Walker et al., 1986).

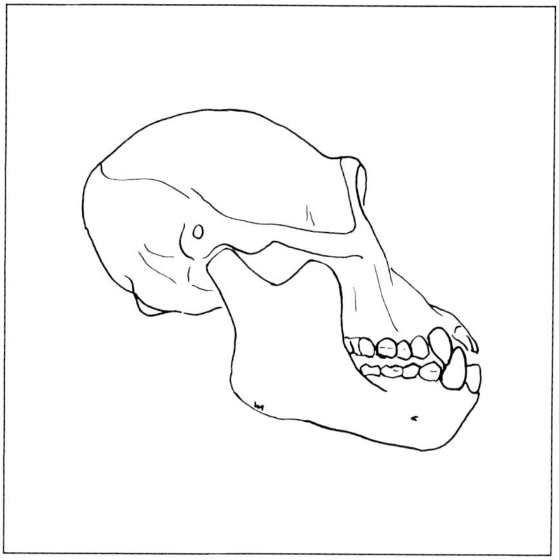

Fig. 2-8 Skull of chimpanzee.

Bipedal hominids

The discovery of several specimens of a small fossil hominid (primate) in the Hadar region of Ethiopia in the 1970s has dramatically changed our concepts of the timing and the order of changes in human evolution. That the hominid that made the footprints at Laetoli and the hominid discovered at the Hadar (Johanson and White, 1979) walked bipedally and upright, there is no dispute (Lovejoy, 1979, 1981; Charteris et al., 1982). Footprint type, stride analysis, and shape of pelvis (particularly increases in width) indicate an upright bipedalism although this is now realized to be intermediate between the apes and humans (Stern and Susman, 1983). Prior to this conclusive evidence it was generally assumed that hominids other than true *Homo sapiens* had been stooping individuals with various shuffling gaits, and that brain enlargement was the initial change in hominid evolution. "Lucy," a 40% complete hominid who lived about 3.7 mybp, walked upright but had a small brain (Johanson and Edey, 1981).

The jaws and teeth of the earliest hominid so far discovered, *Australopithecus afarensis* (Johanson et al., 1978), are in some ways similar to both extinct and extant apes (Fig. 2-9). The palate was flat and the tooth rows parallel with the upper row convergent posteriorly. There was a small diastema between upper lateral incisor and canine, but the canine was relatively small, although its wear facets were quite similar to those of extant apes. Features of the facial skeleton were similar to apes but less pronounced in *A. afarensis* (White et al., 1981; Kimbel et al., 1984). However, the canine was much reduced and has been compared to features seen in some of the ramapithecines (Simons, 1981). Mandibular bone and tooth-row features are also considered to be quite similar (White et al., 1981), in particular the first premolar, which was not sectorial, but frequently unicuspid. The glenoid fossa has been well preserved and found to be

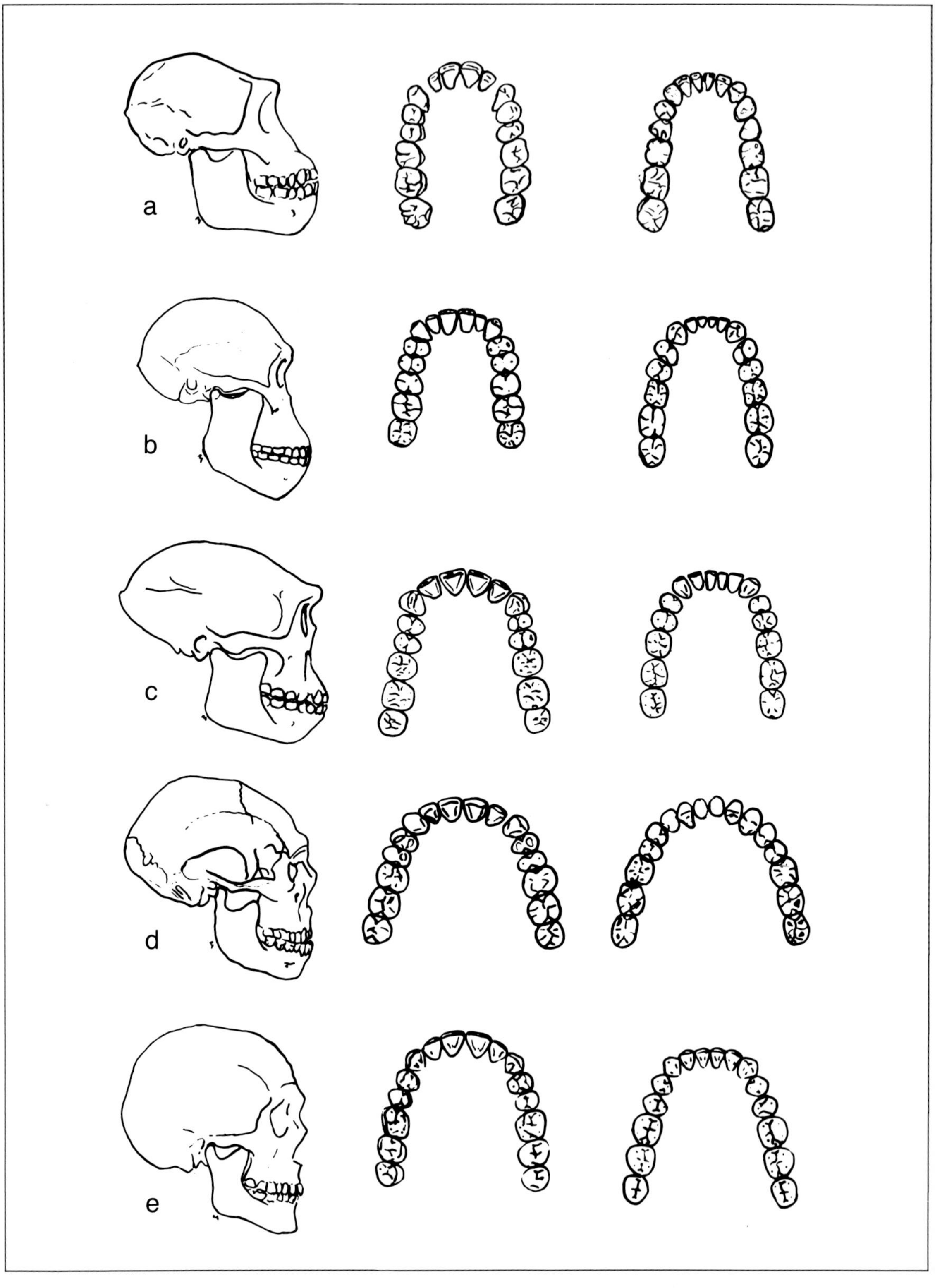
a
b
c
d
e

relatively shallow and similar to the ape condition. Another feature that has caused considerable controversy is the very distinct sexual dimorphism in *A. afarensis,* which has led some authorities to suggest there were two distinct species. However, comparison both with extant hominids such as the chimpanzee, or extinct hominids such as *Homo erectus,* show this dimorphism to be within the normal range for both species.

Scientists' classification of the australopithecines has been greatly revised of late. It is now believed that from *A. afarensis* two clades (groups) arose. One, parallel to the main hominid line—*Australopithecus africanus,* first discovered in 1925—in turn led to a very robust form, *Australopithecus robustus*. The other led to the first true member of the genus *Homo: Homo habilis* (Fig. 2-9) (Johanson and White, 1979).

There was a gradual relative reduction in the incisal segment from *A. afarensis* to *A. africanus* to *A. robustus* to *Australopithecus boisei*, with increased molarization of premolars (McHenry, 1984). In *A. robustus* the small incisors formed an almost flat row across the front of the palate, while the premolars and molars were massive—an adaptation to an abrasive vegetable diet quite similar to that which occurred in the giant panda (DuBrul, 1979). Tooth wear was more evenly distributed, more severe, and flatter than in *Homo* species. The zygomatic arch became more pronounced, changing the overall shape of the face. The canine fossa decreased in size, and the shortening of the palate along with increased stresses due to molarization of premolars was associated with bony thickening on each side of the nasal aperture (Rak, 1985). As in the gorilla, the increased attachment of the temporalis muscle resulted in sagittal crests, particularly in the bigger individuals—presumably the males. At the same time the mandibular body became deeper and the ramus higher, thus changing the relationship of tooth row to TMJ; the bone was generally thicker and more robust. However, the TMJ had a deep mandibular fossa and steep articular eminence, as in later *Homo* species (White et al., 1981). Thus the *A. robustus* line of hominid evolution eventually came to an end because of overspecialization and inability to compete with the other line of hominid evolution, the genus *Homo*.

The *A. afarensis* to *Homo habilis* transition, although as yet not well documented by the fossil record, shows a gradual evening-out of the whole dentition with diminution of its relative size (McHenry, 1984), loss of the incisor-canine diastema, a more parabolic dental arch, lessening of subnasal prognathism (Rak, 1985), and lessening of the zygomatic arch. The canines were still slightly larger than in modern humans, but the mandibular first premolars had a distinct second cusp on the distolingual side. The mandible was also less robust and its anterior surface more upright, although no true chin was seen.

The *Homo* line is distinguished by *encephalization*—increase in cranium size—seen initially in *H. habilis,* but much increased in the subsequent species, *H. erectus* and *H. sapiens* (Fig. 2-9). Frontal bones showed marked glabellar prominence in *H. erectus,* and the parietal bones became somewhat bossed. Occipital expansion occurred, and the associated bones became more rounded. Thus, the relative proportion of cranium to jaws has changed in humans due to both an increase in cranium size and decrease in jaw size.

Fig. 2-9 *(left) Left column:* skulls; *center column:* upper dentition; *right column:* lower dentition. *Australopithecus afarensis (a); A. africanus (b); H. erectus (c); H. sapiens neandertalensis (d); H. sapiens sapiens (e).* (These were redrawn and modified from various sources and are not to the same scale.) Note the following changes: *(1)* the proportion of jaw to skull; *(2)* the shape of the skull, particularly the cranium; and *(3)* the shape of the dental arches and tooth proportions from parallel in *A. afarensis,* with the distinct precanine diastema, through the increasing width and parabolic forms of the *Homo* series. In *H. sapiens neandertalensis* there is distinct prognathism of both lower jaw and upper jaw and space behind third molars.

H. habilis ("handy man") fossils are associated with primitive stone tools, although the likelihood of other nonpreserved tools should not be overlooked. No such artifacts have so far been found with any of the australopithecines.

It is not the purpose of this review to discuss combining or separating the species of the genus *Homo*. Certain very distinct types can be observed at different geological times. How gradual the change was and whether differences warrant species distinction are not our concern here. However, one should be aware that ideas on human evolution have been in a state of ferment for the last 20 or more years and will continue to be for quite some time (Delson, 1985).

The next distinct subhuman/human type was *H. erectus,* appearing about 400,000 years ago. Remains were found initially in Java by Dubois, and later in China, Europe, and Africa. Cranial capacity is much enlarged over *H. habilis,* approaching 1,000 ml, and the skull is noticeably longer (Fig. 2-9). The whole body size had also increased. Glabellar prominence was greatly accentuated. Although the cause of this is disputed, it is most likely related to stresses in the anterior part of the skull associated with heavy mastication.

The dentition was quite similar to that of modern humans but was larger in proportion to body size. However, as distinct from modern humans, the third molar was larger than the second, which was larger than the first; and the canine was proportionally bigger. Hence, there was distinct prognathism, but without a chin.

The outstanding features associated with *H. erectus* are the use of stone tools, the use of fire, and the cooperative hunting of large animals. Culture had started to develop, and one of its features was primitive cooking associated with greater ease of mastication. Having a good dentition was no longer completely necessary for survival, and the freeing of the human dentition from evolutionary pressure was accentuated, a process that Kraus et al. (1969) suggest may have started with the acquiring of upright posture and bipedalism. However, the more recent findings that these were very early events in human evolution make this theory less likely.

Tool use was refined over many thousands of years and there was also the gradual transition—several intermediate skull types were found—to a more modern cranial capacity (Trinkaus and Howells, 1979).

The Neanderthals *(Homo sapiens neandertalensis)* ranged over Europe, Asia, and down into Africa, and were highly successful for about 100,000 years. During the last great ice age, particularly in Europe, Neanderthals were active and successful in a very harsh environment. During this period, however, the European group is thought to have become isolated from the main genetic pool of evolving *H. sapiens* and to have evolved into a heavy-boned, heavy-browed group of individuals termed "classic" Neanderthals (Trinkaus and Howells, 1979).

Although the dentition was essentially similar to that in modern humans, the prognathism of the jaws was so marked that a lateral view of the skull shows a distinct gap between the distal surface of the third molar and anterior surface of the ascending ramus of the mandible (Fig. 2-9). No chance of impacted third molars here! Some Neanderthal molars show elongated crowns, termed the hypsodont or taurodont molars. This feature was found in Krapina Neanderthals and sometimes is seen in modern humans (Miller, 1968). In the Middle East the increase in robustness of skull structure did not occur. In fact, forensic reconstruction techniques have shown that these individuals looked remarkedly like modern humans (Rensberger, 1981).

H. sapiens ("thinking man") apparently appeared quite rapidly in Europe around 33,000 years ago and somewhat earlier in the Middle and Near East (Trinkaus and Howells, 1979) while the Neanderthals disappeared. The exact nature of this change is still under study. Thus, modern humans have a relatively short history, but roots that reach far back in time. It has been suggested that the more gracile *H. sapiens* form derived from the adoption of a less tough diet, possibly associated with early cooking. Recent data, however, do not support this (Schoeninger, 1982).

The modern spectrum of human races, grouping around the three major types, Mongoloids,

Negroids, and Caucasoids, but with many intermediates, appears to be a recent phenomenon with antecedents that reach far back into time. As the successful *H. sapiens* spread into a wide variety of habitats, minor adaptive body changes occurred that were related to temperature and light extremes. However, all modern humans are classified as *H. sapiens*.

Summary

The purpose of this chapter has been to demonstrate the biological spectrum of the masticatory system. Throughout evolution it can be seen that function and form have gone hand in hand, be it in the bottom-feeding ray or the fruit-eating monkey, slightly yet significantly different from its leaf-eating neighbor.

The forces that shaped our masticatory system have been at work for millions of years, and although evolutionary selection no longer directly effects the dentition per se, the imprint of this history is still very evident.

Chapter 3

Development of the Occlusion

Bengt Ingervall

The primary dentition: From the 1st to the 5th year

The first primary (deciduous) teeth to erupt are generally the mandibular central incisors, at about 8 months of age. These teeth are followed by the rest of the maxillary and mandibular incisors, and at 16 months of age by the primary first molars (Fig. 3-1). The establishment of occlusion of the first molars is an important event in occlusal development because occlusal height and intercuspation become established for the first time. The primary dentition is usually complete around $2^1/_2$ years of age with the eruption of the maxillary second molars.

The dental arches of the primary dentition are more rounded than those of the permanent dentition, as described in chapter 4 (Fig. 3-2). The incisors are more upright than in the permanent dentition, the average overjet and overbite being around 3.0 mm and 2.5 mm, respectively.

The anteroposterior intermaxillary relation of the primary posterior teeth has, in most children, a so-called mesial step between the distal surfaces of the second molars (Fig. 3-3a). This means that the mandibular posterior teeth, as in the neutral* permanent dentition, are more anteriorly situated than the maxillary teeth. A large minority of children, however, have a flush terminal plane, i.e., the distal surfaces of the deciduous second molars are in the same frontal plane (Fig. 3-3b). A smaller percentage of children have a distal step (Carlsen and Meredith, 1960). A distal step implies a relatively more posterior position of the mandibular than of the maxillary teeth (Fig. 3-3c).

During the first years of life there is considerable growth of the jaws and alveolar processes. This growth provides space for the developing primary dentition and results, in most children, in a small surplus of space (i.e., small spaces between the primary teeth). The largest spaces are often found mesial to the maxillary primary canines and distal to the mandibular canines; they are called *primate spaces* (Fig. 3-4) (Baume, 1950). After the eruption of all primary teeth, no great changes of the dentition are seen clinically, except for a progressive wear of the teeth. The attrition on primary teeth is often marked (Fig. 3-5).

The mixed dentition: From the 6th to the 12th year

Around the age of 6 years the permanent first molars erupt and primary mandibular central incisors are exfoliated (Fig. 3-6). The primary incisors are replaced by their succedaneous permanent teeth at 6 to 8 years of age. Variations in the order of eruption in the early mixed dentition from that given in Fig. 3-6 frequently occur between the mandibular first molar and central

*The term *neutral occlusion*, or *Class I occlusion*, indicates a normal mesiodistal or anteroposterior relation of the mandibular arch to the maxillary arch.

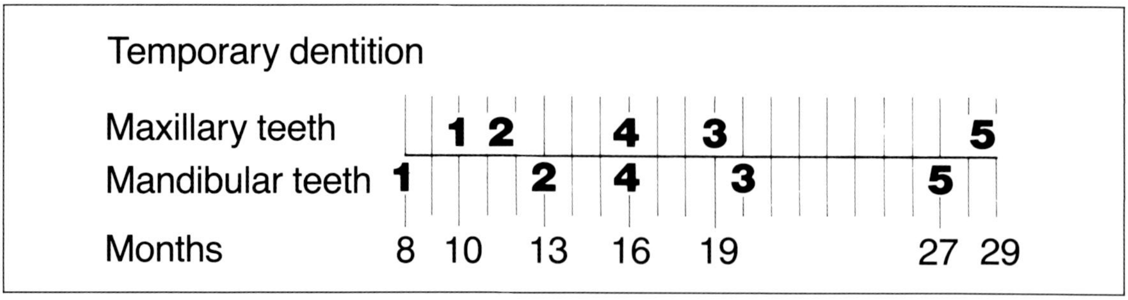

Fig. 3-1 Mean time and order of eruption of the primary teeth. Mean eruption time (from 8 to 29 months) of each maxillary and mandibular tooth in sequence of eruption. Note: central incisor *(1)*; lateral incisor *(2)*; canine *(3)*; first molar *(4)*; second molar *(5)*.

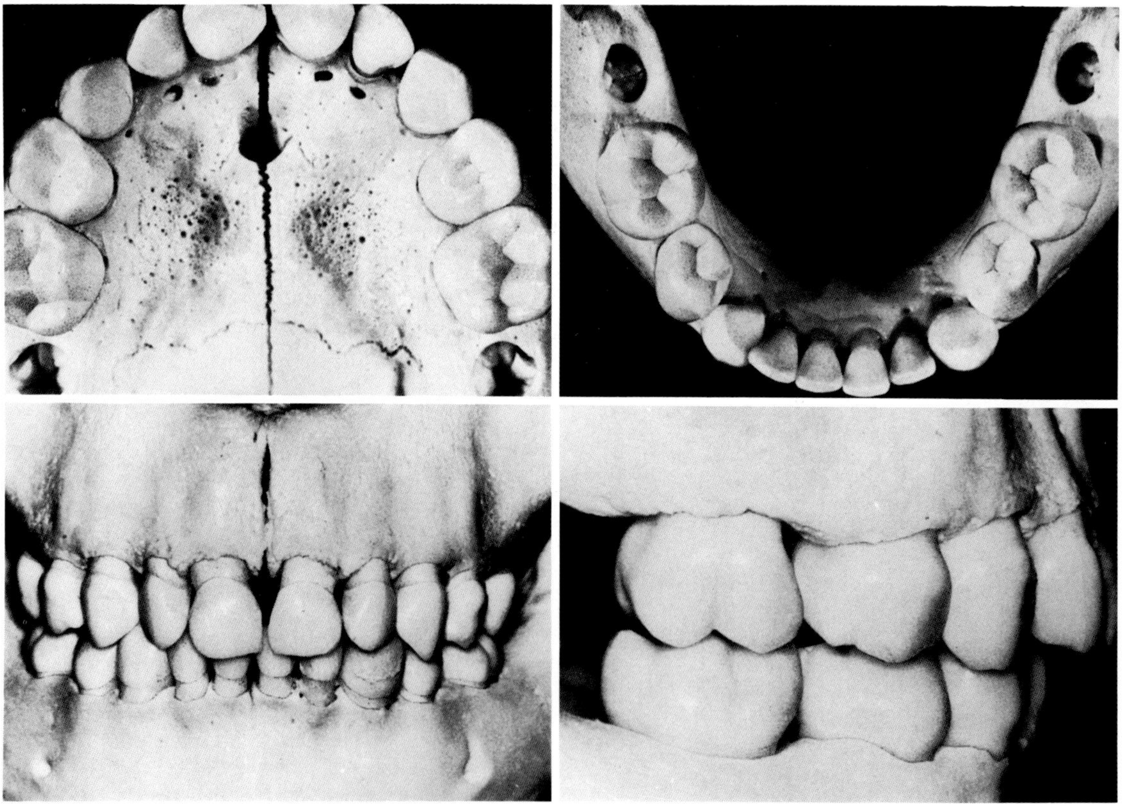

Fig. 3-2 Dental arches and occlusion of the primary dentition. *(top left)* Maxillary arch. *(top right)* Mandibular arch. *(bottom left)* Facial view. *(bottom right)* Lateral view.

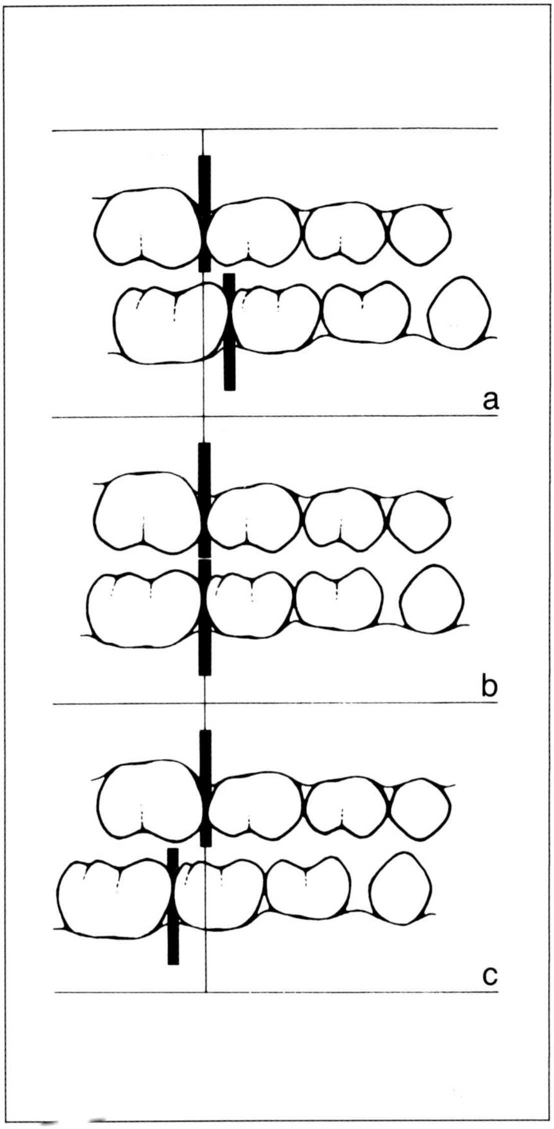

Fig. 3-3 Relation between maxillary and mandibular posterior teeth. Mesial step *(a)*; flush terminal plane *(b)*; distal step *(c)*.

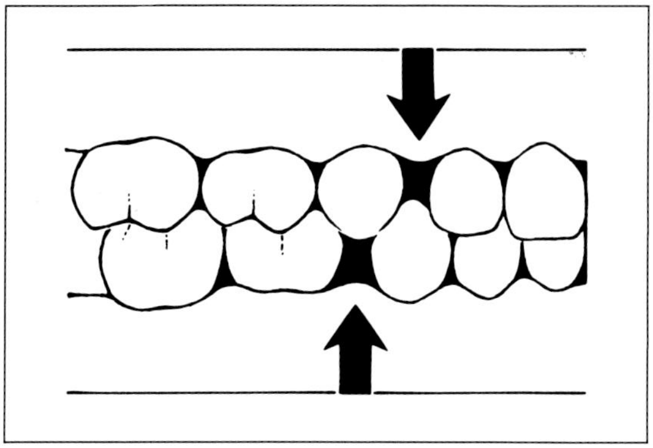

Fig. 3-4 Primate spaces of the primary dentition in the maxillary arch anterior to the canines, and in the mandibular arch posterior to the canines.

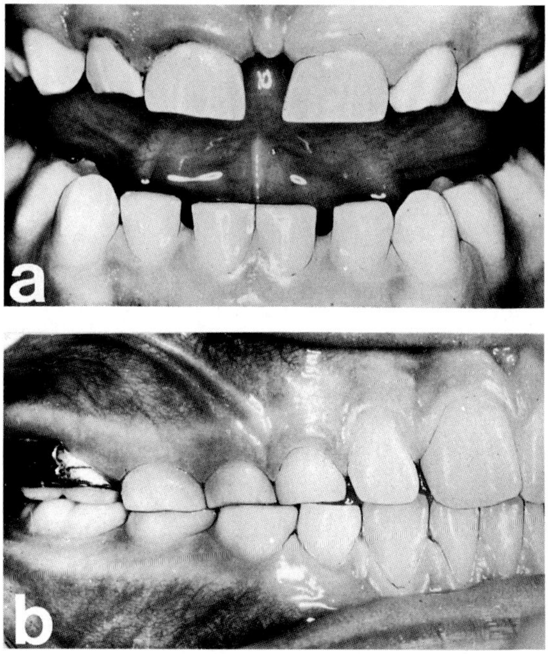

Fig. 3-5 Attrition of primary anterior teeth *(a)* and posterior teeth *(b)*.

incisor. In many children the mandibular central incisor is the first permanent tooth to erupt.

After the eruption of the first permanent molars and the incisors there is a "quiet" period in the mixed dentition from 8 to 10 years of age, when exfoliation of the primary canines and molars starts. After eruption of the permanent second molars at 12 years of age there is again a long pause until the third molars finally erupt around the age of 20.

Common variations in the order of eruption of the permanent teeth in the late mixed dentition period are between the mandibular second premolar and second molar, the premolar, in many

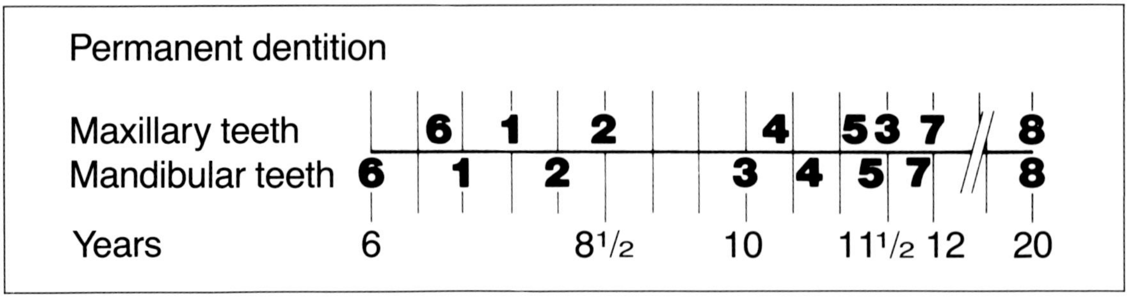

Fig. 3-6 Mean time and order of eruption of the permanent teeth. Note: central incisor *(1)*; lateral incisor *(2)*; canine *(3)*; first premolar *(4)*; second premolar *(5)*; first molar *(6)*; second molar *(7)*; third molar *(8)*.

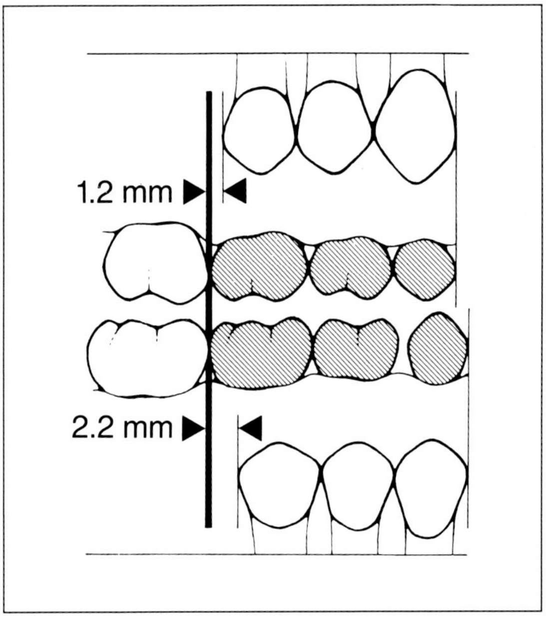

Fig. 3-7 Leeway space in maxillary and mandibular dental arches upon exfoliation of the primary molars.

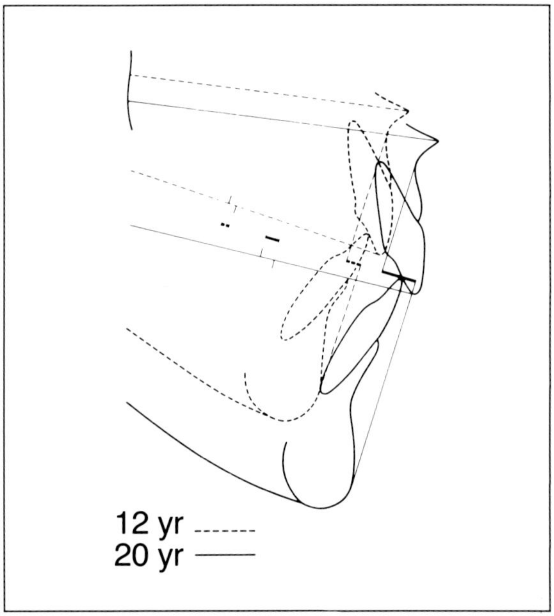

Fig. 3-8 Change in sagittal jaw relation and in molar relation from 12 to 20 years of age. (Courtesy of H.U. Paulsen, D.D.S.)

cases, erupting after the molar. Common variations in the maxilla are between the second premolar (tooth 5), the second molar (tooth 7), and the canine (tooth 3). In many children the order of eruption is 3, 5, 7 or 5, 7, 3, in addition to the 5, 3, 7 sequence given in Fig. 3-6.

In contrast to the primary teeth, there is for the permanent teeth a sex difference in the time of eruption; the permanent teeth erupt on the average 4 months later in boys than in girls.

The permanent incisors and canines are wider than the corresponding primary teeth. Space for these permanent teeth is provided by *(1)* the small surplus of space found in most primary dentitions, *(2)* greater labial inclination of the maxillary permanent than of the primary incisors, and *(3)* a small increase in dental arch width during eruption of the permanent anterior teeth (Moorrees and Reed, 1965). The primary molars, on the other hand, are smaller than the succedaneous premolars. Exfoliation of the primary posterior teeth, therefore, provides surplus space of importance for the establishment of normal intercuspation (see following).

Development of intermaxillary relations

As they erupt, the permanent first molars follow the distal surfaces of the primary second molars. If there is a mesial step between these teeth, the permanent molars can, more or less, erupt into a neutral intermaxillary relation. If, on the other hand, the intermaxillary relation between the distal surfaces of the primary molars produces a flush terminal plane, the permanent first molars will erupt into a cusp-to-cusp position (see Fig. 3-3b). A neutral relation between the permanent molars, that is, with the mandibular molar one cusp width more mesial than the maxillary, can be established by the following mechanisms:

1. *Closure of the mandibular primate space.* When the permanent first molars erupt, they exert a forwardly directed pressure on the primary molars. This pressure will elicit mesial migration of the primary mandibular molars because these teeth have a possibility of migrating into the primate space located distally to the canine.

2. *Utilization of the "leeway" space upon exfoliation of the primary molars.* The difference in the sum of the mesiodistal widths of the two primary molars and the two premolars is at least 1 mm greater in the mandible than in the maxilla (Fig. 3-7). Upon exfoliation of the primary molars the mandibular permanent molars can migrate mesially somewhat more than the maxillary molars.

3. *Relatively more growth of the mandible than of the maxilla.* The mandible is, at birth, less developed than the maxilla. During postnatal growth the mandible must catch up with the maxilla. The mandible grows more and finishes its growth later than the maxilla (Bjork and Palling, 1955). The greater mandibular growth will carry mandibular teeth more anteriorly than the maxillary teeth, resulting in a slight shift of their relationship (Paulsen, 1971) (Fig. 3-8).

The possibility that the primary second molars have a relation with a distal step is unfavorable for development of a neutral occlusion. A distal step between the primary molars means that the permanent molars will erupt into postnormal* occlusion (see Fig. 3-3). When such a relation is once established, the chances for spontaneous improvement to neutral occlusion are small (Frohlich, 1961). The cuspal occlusal locking in most cases effectively hinders a change from the postnormal relationship to a neutral occlusion.

About 75% of children whose permanent first molars erupt into a cusp-to-cusp relation undergo a favorable transition into neutral occlusion, while the rest of the cases develop into postnormal occlusion (Carlsen and Meredith, 1960). Reasons for postnormal development may be different directions of growth of the jaws (influence mechanism 3, mentioned above) or local factors, such as the order of exfoliation of the maxillary and mandibular primary second molars (influence mechanism 2).

Thus, the occlusal relationships of the permanent first molars are important in determining the intermaxillary relations of the other permanent molars. Another important tooth that decides the occlusal relations of later erupting teeth is the first premolar.

Teeth often erupt into an end-to-end or cusp-to-cusp relation, with their further eruption guided into proper intercuspation by the inclined planes of the cusps. It is the obligation of the child's dentist to supervise the development of the occlusion. In the case of an end-to-end eruption of the teeth, slight selective grinding of cuspal planes can guide the teeth in the proper direction. Negligence in the undertaking of such procedures may result in an improper mesiodis-

*The term *postnormal,* or *distal occlusion* or *Class II occlusion,* indicates that the mandibular dental arch is posterior to the maxillary arch—the mandibular first molar is distal to its normal position relative to the maxillary first molar.

tal or buccolingual relation of several pair of opposing teeth.

The generally greater postnatal growth of the mandible than of the maxilla also implies a decrease of the overjet during the growth period. This decrease is marked during the first 6 months of life. Despite a transient increase in overjet during the primary to mixed dentition period, there is a steady reduction in overjet from childhood through adolescence (Leighton, 1977). In the longitudinal sample of Bjork (1953), for example, the average overjet in boys decreased from 4.1 mm at 12 years of age to 3.4 mm at 20 years. There was also a corresponding decrease in overbite from 2.6 to 2.1 mm.

As in adults, the retruded contact position of the mandible can be precisely recorded in children from the age of 5 years (Ingervall, 1968). The average distance between the retruded contact and intercuspal positions in children is about 1 mm, with a range of variation from 0 to 2 mm—values completely in accordance with those in adults. This holds true also for children with their primary dentitions (Ingervall, 1968).

During lateral gliding movements most children with a mixed dentition have multiple tooth contacts on the working side and simultaneous contact on the nonworking side, as is often found in young adults (Ingervall, 1972a). There is, however, a difference between children and adults in the type of working side contact. Before the permanent maxillary canines are in full occlusion, contact on the working side is found most frequently between the permanent first molars; later on, however, it is between the canines (Ingervall, 1972a). The contact on the nonworking side is usually found on the most posteriorly erupted tooth, that is, it changes in location from the permanent first molar to the third molar as the dentition develops.

The permanent dentition: Variation is the rule

The descriptions of overjet and overbite given above, as well as that of the dentition in the following chapter, refer to the so-called normal or ideal occlusion. *The dentition of most individuals differs, however, in one or more respects from this theoretically ideal occlusion.*

Deviations from the ideal (or normal) occlusion—malocclusions or anomalies*—may be grouped into three main categories: *(1)* dentitional, *(2)* occlusal, and *(3)* space anomalies (Bjork et al., 1964). *Dentitional anomalies* refer to the individual teeth, and include aberrations in the formation, eruption, and alignment of the teeth. *Occlusal anomalies* refer to the sagittal, vertical, and transverse intermaxillary relation, and *space anomalies* to spacing or crowding in the dental arches. The total frequency of anomalies is high in most ethnic groups but the proportion of the three different categories may vary (Bjork and Helm, 1969). In Danes with a mixed or young permanent dentition, over 75% had at least one type of anomaly: 30% to 40% were dentitional (more in boys than in girls), about 50% were occlusal, and about 50% were spatial (Helm, 1968, 1970).

Recorded incidence of malocclusion depends on the criteria used for recording. To illustrate what deviations can be considered outside the accepted range of variation, we'll examine the criteria for recording occlusal anomalies in the Danish studies above. Occlusal anomalies in the sagittal plane were: extreme maxillary overjet (6 mm or more), mandibular overjet (0 mm or a negative value), and distal or mesial molar occlusion (a deviation of one half a cusp width or more) (Figs. 3-9 and 3-10). Vertical occlusal anomalies were: anterior deep bite (overbite of 5 mm or more), posterior open bite (an absence of contact between posterior teeth), and anterior open bite (overbite of 0 mm or a negative value) (Fig. 3-11). Occlusal anomalies in the transverse plane were lingual crossbite, when the buccal cusp of a maxillary posterior tooth occluded lingually to the buccal cusp of the opposing mandibular tooth, and buccal crossbite, when the lingual cusp of a maxillary posterior tooth

*The term *anomaly* means a marked deviation from the normal standard.

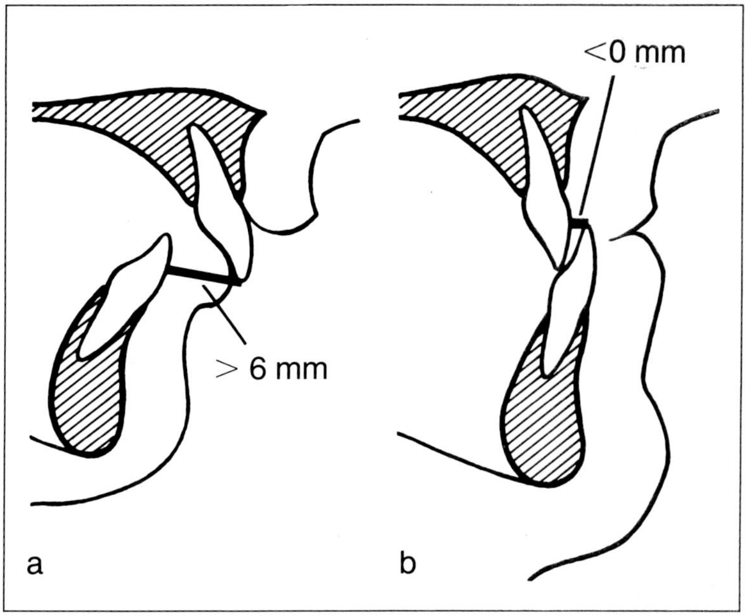

Fig. 3-9 Criteria for recording of extreme maxillary overjet *(a)* and mandibular overjet *(b)*.

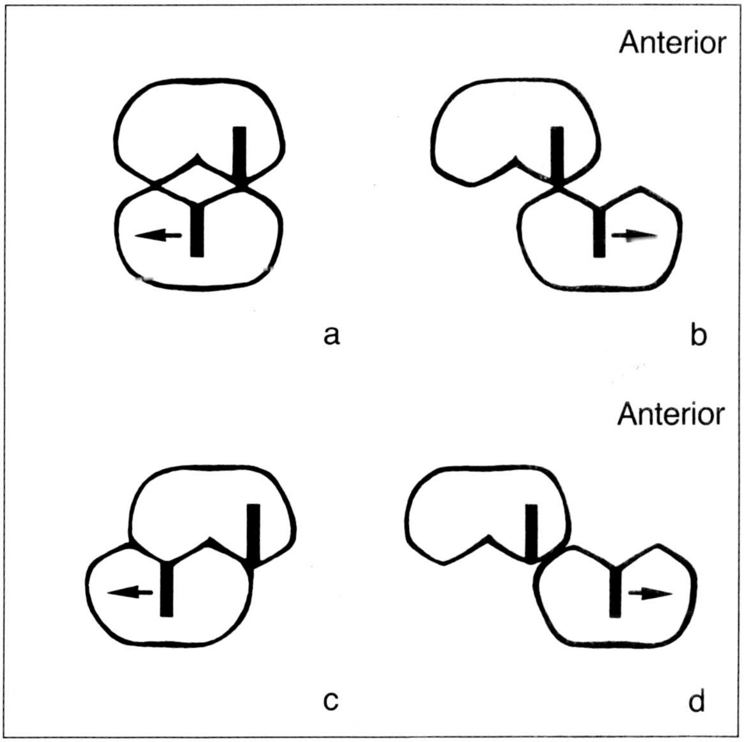

Fig. 3-10 One-half cusp width distal *(a)* and mesial *(b)* molar occlusion, and full cusp width distal *(c)* and mesial *(d)* molar occlusion.

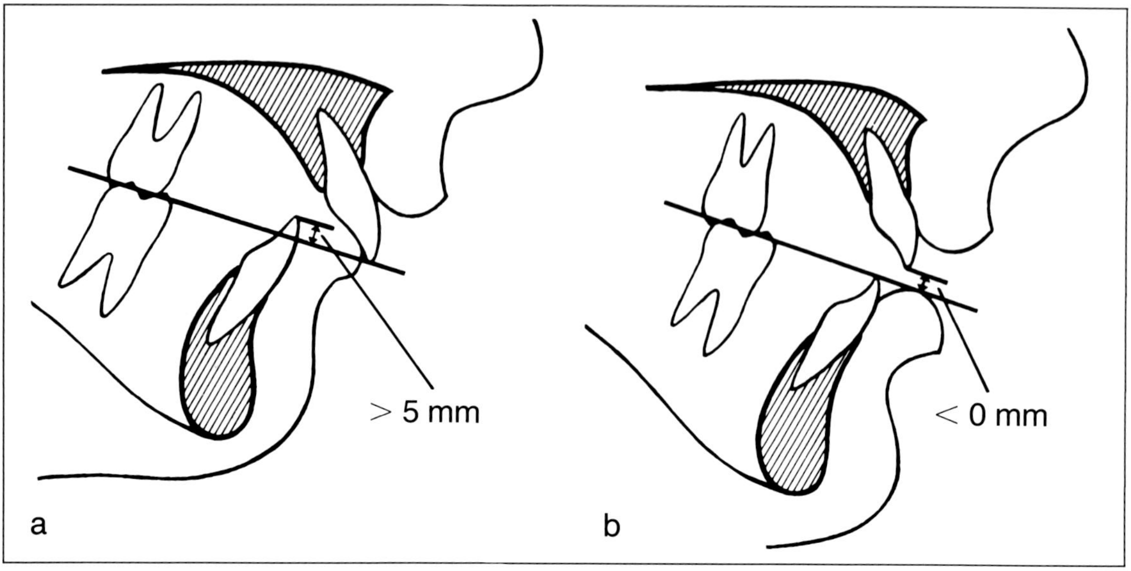

Fig. 3-11 Criteria for recording of anterior deep bite *(a)* and anterior open bite *(b)*.

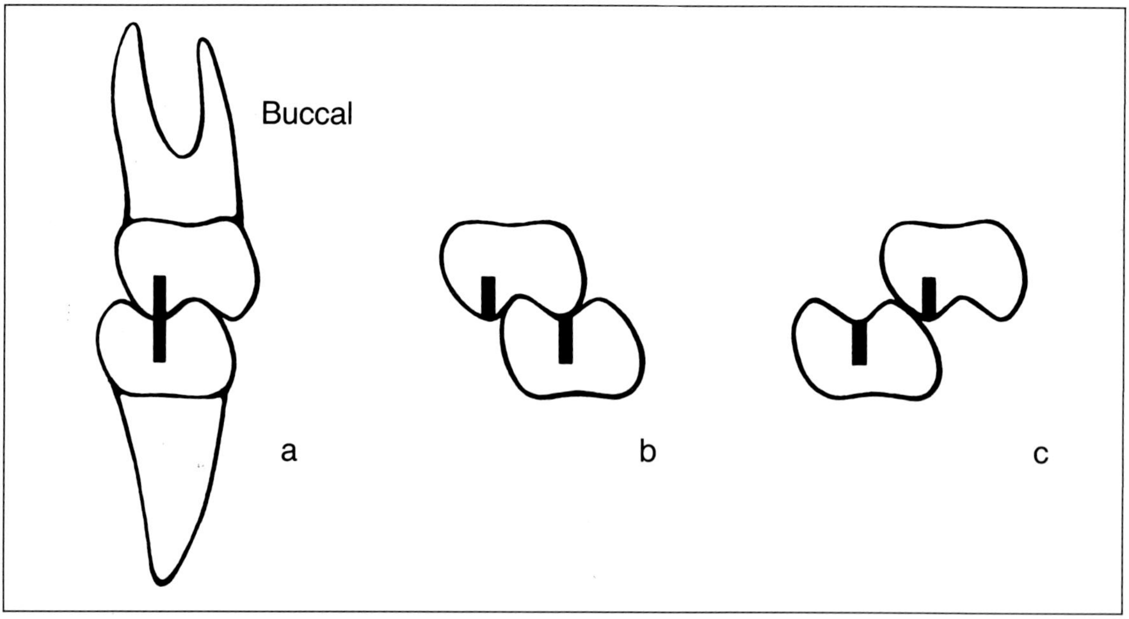

Fig. 3-12 Normal transverse relation of posterior teeth *(a)*. Lingual *(b)* and buccal *(c)* crossbite of posterior teeth.

Table 3-1 Prevalence of occlusal anomalies in 565 Danish boys and 675 Danish girls aged 9 to 18 years (Helm, 1968, 1970) and in 301 Swedish men aged 18 to 21 years (Ingervall, 1974)

Anomaly	Boys	Girls	Men
	percent		
Sagittal			
Extreme maxillary overjet	16.0	13.0	11.0
Mandibular overjet	1.0	0.3	2.0
Distal molar occlusion (unilaterally or bilaterally)	23.0	26.0	34.0
Distal molar occlusion (bilaterally)	10.0	12.0	13.0
Mesial molar occlusion (unilaterally or bilaterally)	4.0	5.0	12.0
Mesial molar occlusion (bilaterally)	1.0	2.0	6.0
Vertical			
Anterior open bite	2.0	2.0	4.0
Posterior open bite	0.4	0.0	—
Anterior deep bite	23.0	15.0	10.0
Transverse			
Crossbite	9.0	14.0	19.0
Scissors (deep-shearing) bite	7.0	8.0	8.0

occluded buccally to the buccal cusp of the opposing mandibular (Fig. 3-12).

The prevalence of each type of occlusal anomaly in orthodontically untreated Danish children and adolescents (Helm, 1968, 1970) and in Swedish young adults (Ingervall, 1974), recorded with the same methods, are given in Table 3-1. The two sets of data are probably representative of the Scandinavian population for the ages represented. The differences in malocclusion frequency between the two groups may be due to real differences or to unavoidable minor differences between observers in the application of the recording method. A source of real difference between the two groups is, without doubt, age. For example, a decrease in the prevalence of extreme maxillary overjet and an increase in mandibular overjet is to be expected with age due to greater mandibular growth.

A study of Table 3-1 should convince the reader that a great variation in occlusal conditions is to be expected within a population, even one with intact dentitions.

The cause of the high prevalence of anomalies is, above all, genetic factors governing such

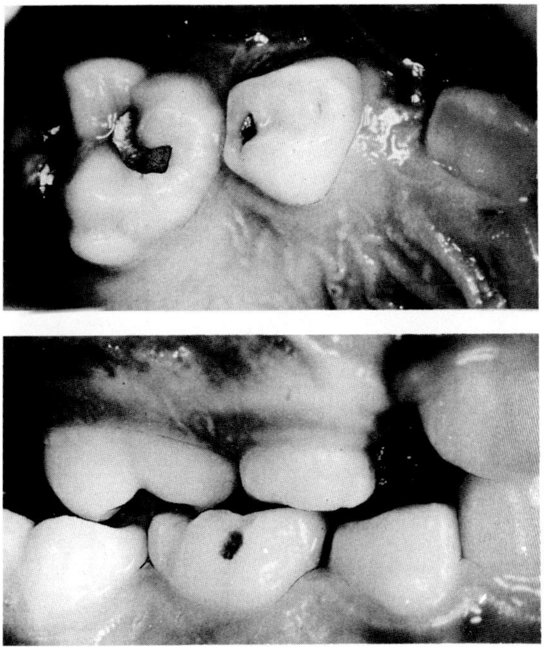

Fig. 3-13 Effect of premature loss of primary maxillary second molar. The permanent first molar has migrated, tipped mesially, and rotated. *(top)* Occlusal view. *(bottom)* Facial view.

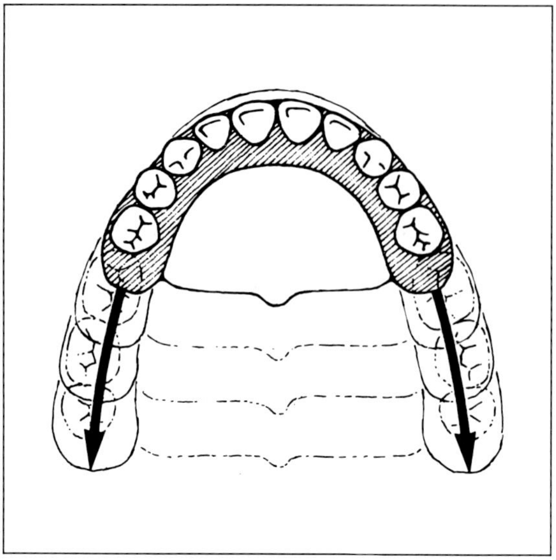

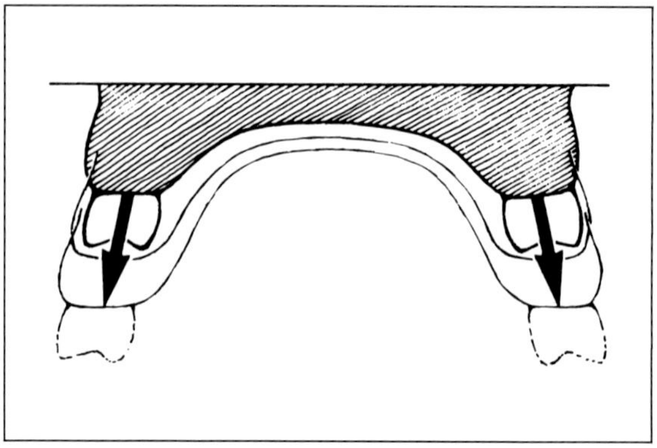

Fig. 3-14 *(left)* Lengthening of the maxilla by apposition of bone to the maxillary tuberosities.

Fig. 3-15 *(above)* Growth in height of the maxillary alveolar processes.

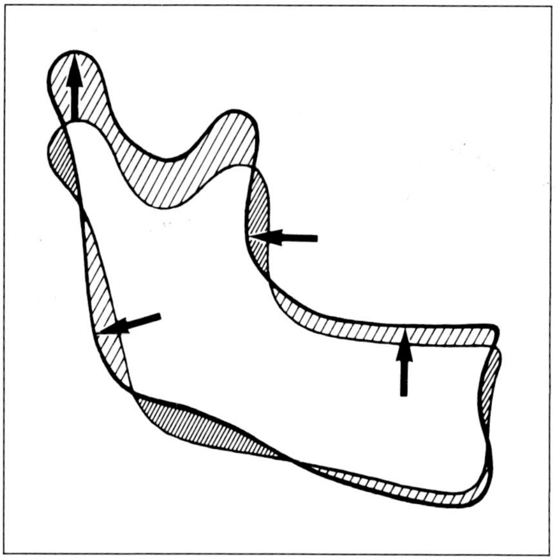

Fig. 3-16 Growth of the mandible. Note bone apposition at the posterior borders and bone resorption at the anterior borders of the rami.

things as the size of the teeth and jaws and the growth of the face. A disadvantageous combination of genetic input from the two parents can easily be thought of as responsible for malocclusion in their child. Environmental influences during the development of the dentition are, however, of great importance as well.

Numerous environmental factors can give rise to malocclusion, for example, the premature loss of primary molars due to dental caries. Worst in this respect is the premature loss of the primary second molar, which can lead to mesial migration, rotation, and tipping of the permanent first molar (Fig. 3-13). The teeth anterior to the extraction gap may migrate distally because of the loss of continuity in the dental arch. The forces of eruption and of occlusion will cause the adjacent teeth to migrate into the gap. The result will be loss of space for the succedaneous teeth as well as changed intermaxillary relations.

Growth of the jaws

The general direction of growth of the face in relation to the skull and the cranial base is inferiorly and anteriorly (see Fig. 3-17). The dentition is transported inferiorly and anteriorly, concomi-

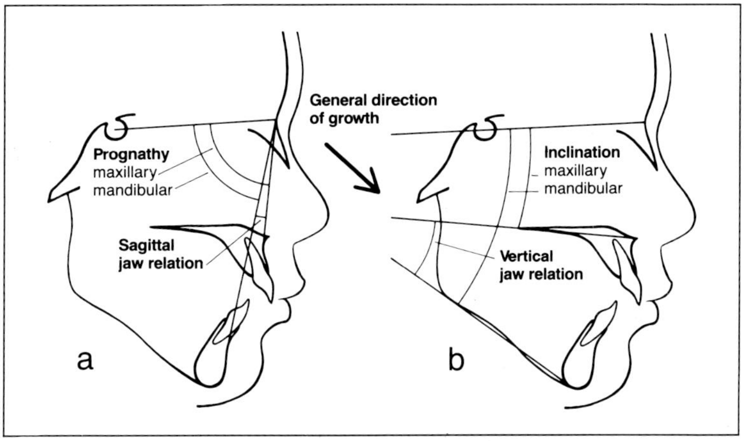

Fig. 3-17 Measurement of prognathism *(a)* and inclination *(b)* of the face in cephalometric profile radiographs.

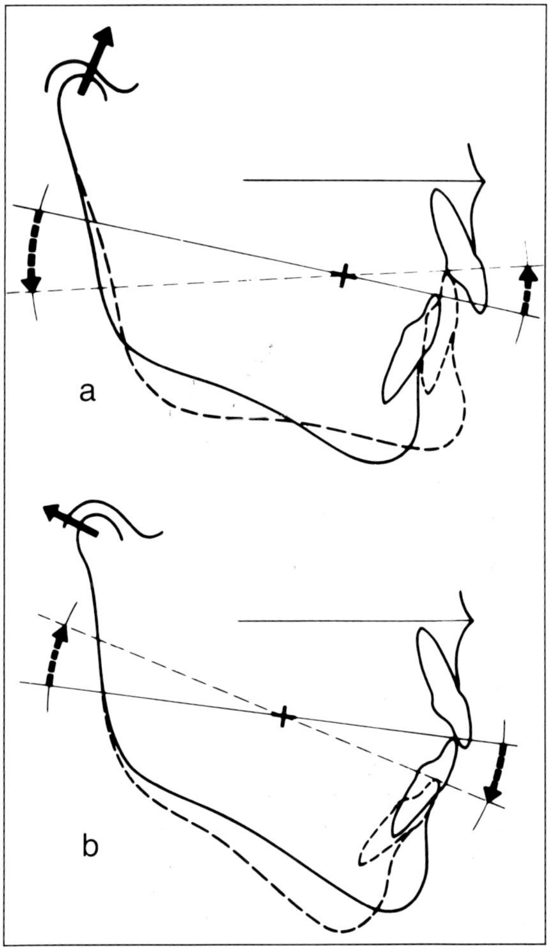

Fig. 3-18 Anterior *(a)* and posterior *(b)* rotation of the mandible during growth, with development of anterior deep bite and anterior open bite. (Courtesy of A. Bjork, D.Odont.)

tantly with an enlargement of the jaws and alveolar processes that creates space for the developing dentition.

Growth in maxillary length takes place almost exclusively as apposition of bone to the maxillary tuberosity, thereby lengthening the alveolar processes (Fig. 3-14). Because the alveolar processes diverge posteriorly, the bony apposition at tuberosities will also contribute to widening of the tooth-bearing portion of the maxilla. Another source of increase in width is growth in the midpalatal suture of the maxilla. Widening can also occur as the result of slight lateral direction of the vertical growth apposition at the maxillary alveolar process as the teeth are erupting (Fig. 3-15).

The surface apposition of bone on the alveolar processes and at the maxillary tuberosities is accompanied by growth in the sutures between the maxilla and adjacent bones of the nasal septum. Remodeling changes of the zygomatic process and orbital and nasal floors also occur at this time.

Growth of the mandible takes place mainly in the condyle and as surface apposition at the posterior border of the ramus and the alveolar processes (Fig. 3-16). The growth in the condyle and at the ramus lengthens the mandible and is accompanied by resorption of bone at the ante-

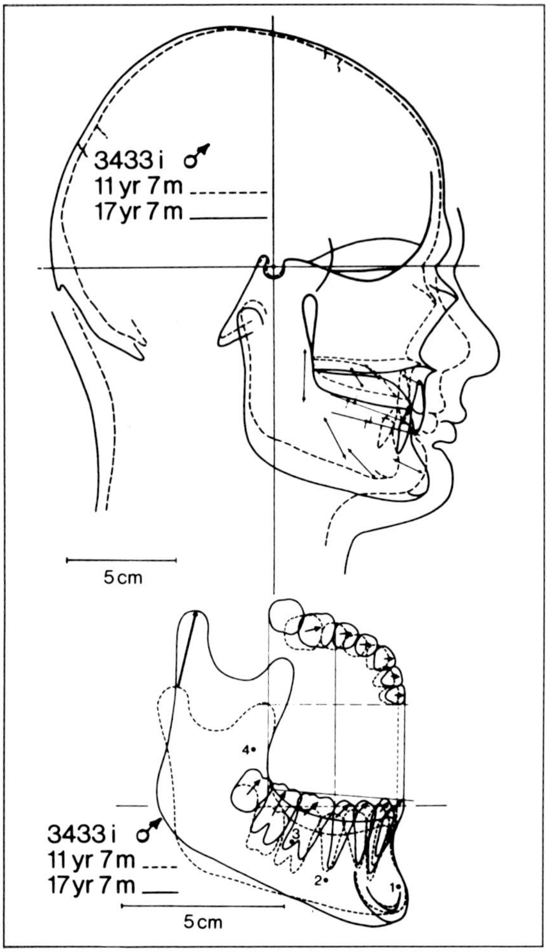

Fig. 3-19 Development of anterior deep bite in case of anterior rotation of the mandible during growth. (Courtesy of A. Bjork, D.Odont.)

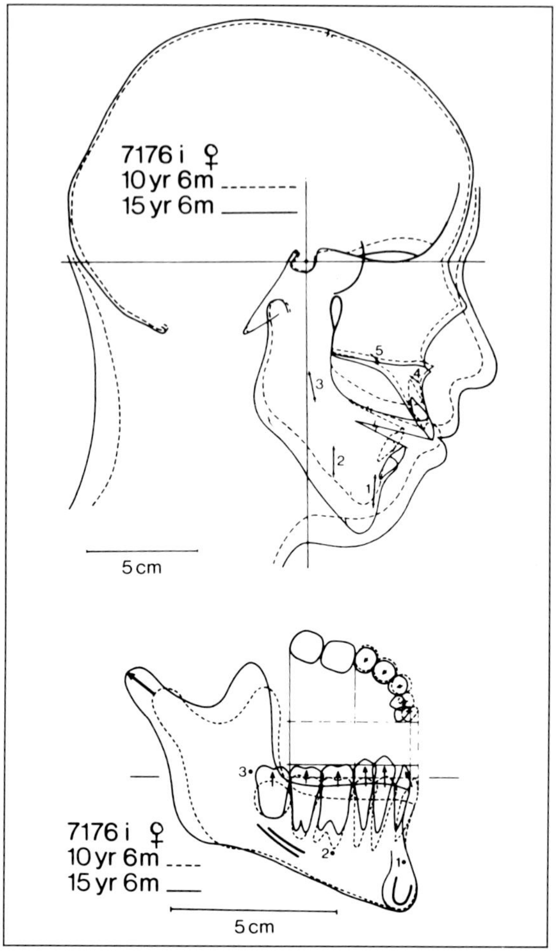

Fig. 3-20 Development of anterior open bite in case of posterior rotation of the mandible during growth. (Courtesy of A. Bjork, D.Odont.)

rior ramal border, which lengthens the alveolar processes. This lengthening provides space for the developing dentition.

Cephalometric radiology and the use of intrabony metallic implants as fixed landmarks (Bjork, 1955) have made possible longitudinal studies of the formative development of the face. The form of the face is largely dependent on the anteroposterior position of the jaws in relation to the cranial base (prognathism of the face), and the vertical relation between the jaws and the cranial base (inclination of the face) (Fig. 3-17).

The most important factor in the formative development of the face is the direction of growth of the mandibular condyle. If this direction is superior and slightly anterior, the mandible will rotate anteriorly; this may be accompanied by development of an anterior deep bite (Fig. 3-18a). If the condyle grows posteriorly, the mandible rotates posteriorly and an anterior open bite can develop (Fig. 3-18b). The appearance of the face in cases with extreme anterior and posterior rotation of the mandible is shown in Figs. 3-19 and 3-20.

Interrelations of form and function during development of the face and dentition

Hereditary factors are probably most important for determining the direction of growth of the face. It is yet uncertain to what extent normal function influences the amount and direction of jaw growth. It is possible that strong masticatory muscles contribute to the development of the face—a relationship has been demonstrated among facial form, bite force, and the electromyographically recorded activity of masticatory muscles during biting and chewing (Ringqvist, 1973; Ingervall and Thilander, 1974; Ingervall, 1976). Individuals with greater bite force and high muscle activity have a face shape described as rectangular (Ingervall and Thilander, 1974), similar to that shown in Fig. 3-19. Individuals with less bite force have a triangular face shape, similar to that shown in Fig. 3-20.

It is not known whether the muscle force is the primary factor deciding the facial form or whether the shape of the face secondarily gives rise to strong or weak muscle force. Observations of variations in facial form in groups of individuals with strong and weak muscles suggest that the muscles have a primary influence (Ingervall and Helkimo, 1978).

There is also a relationship between facial form and the height of the articular eminence of the temporomandibular joint—and, thereby, the inclination of the condylar path (Ingervall, 1972b). The condylar inclination is steeper with the rectangular type of face and shallower in the triangular facial type. The contrasting facial types in two young men with steep and shallow condylar inclinations, respectively, are shown in Fig. 3-21.

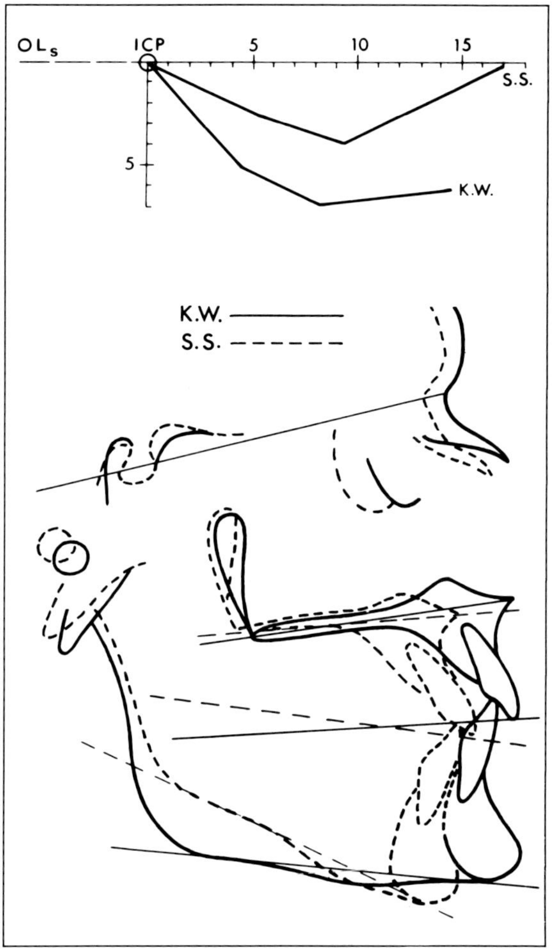

Fig. 3-21 Facial form of two young men with steep and shallow condylar inclinations, respectively.

Although the influence of normal function on human jaw growth is in many respects unknown, the outcome of some forms of deviating function is well documented. Perhaps the most common type of oral parafunction in childhood is finger- or dummy (pacifier)-sucking. Prolonged finger-sucking that continues until school age will change the forms of the jaw and the dental arches, producing increased overjet, anterior open bite, crossbite, and distal occlusion in many children (Fig. 3-22).

Another deviant function known to influence the development of the dentition is mouth-breathing. Habitual mouth-breathing is usually due to an obstructed airway in the nose or nasopharynx. In order to get a free airway through the mouth, the person has to extend the head and lower the mandible and the position of the tongue. This changes the normal balance of the muscles surrounding the dentition, resulting, in

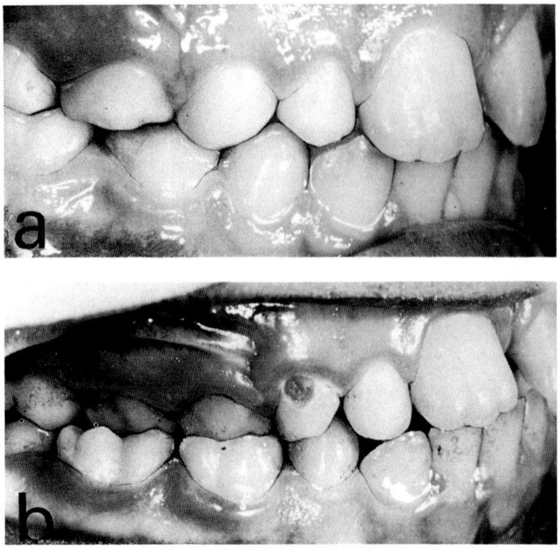

Fig. 3-22 Effect of finger-sucking as demonstrated in a pair of monozygotic twins. Normal occlusion in twin without finger-sucking *(a)*. Occlusion in finger-sucking twin; note distal relation of molars and crossbite *(b)*.

many cases, in crossbite of posterior teeth and in less labial inclination of the incisors (Linder-Aronson, 1970).

Summary

This chapter has reviewed the developmental stages through which the dentition and jaws pass in order to achieve the adult occlusion. It has been emphasized that a great amount of variability exists at all stages of development. The degree of variability and many of the intrinsic and environmental factors that influence the developmental outcome have been discussed. A few of those noted were differential growth pattern of the jaws, finger-sucking, and premature tooth loss. Numerous examples of the types of structural variations that may be found in the developing and, therefore, the completed dentition have been given. The reader should now have an understanding of the typical sequence of occlusal development so as to be able to assess the relative degree of variation that is so often exhibited in individual patients.

Chapter 4

The Dentition

Gunnar E. Carlsson, Torgny Haraldson, and Norman D. Mohl

"Normal" and "ideal" are terms often used in the description of the adult natural dentition. Normal generally implies ordinary, average, or the absence of disease, whereas ideal means conforming to a predetermined standard of perfect, harmonious tooth relationships. Both of these terms usually refer only to static, rather than to functional, conditions. Moreover, they are difficult to use because the terms are easily subject to individual interpretations (Krogh-Poulsen, 1973; Ramfjord and Ash, 1983).

It must be recognized that the size and shape of dental arches and alignment of teeth vary considerably between persons with healthy dentitions. It has even been maintained that malocclusions could be regarded as normal because they are more commonly found in the population than "normal" occlusions, are rarely predisposed to dental disease, and, in most cases, are not associated with masticatory dysfunction (Berkovitz et al., 1978). In the case of the so-called ideal occlusion, perfect conformity to a set of rigid predefined idealized standards is only occasionally seen in a patient population, even assuming that the specific characteristics of such an occlusion could be agreed upon. Because of this, authors such as Berkovitz et al. (1978) prefer the concept that

> If there is an ideal occlusion, at present it can only be defined in broad functional terms. We believe that the characteristics of an ideal occlusion are those
>
> 1. Where the teeth are aligned such that the masticatory loads are within physiological range and act through the long axes of as many teeth in the arch as possible.
> 2. Where lateral jaw movements occur without undue mechanical interference.
> 3. Where, in the rest position of the jaw, the gap between teeth, the freeway space, is adequate for the individual concerned.
> 4. Where the tooth alignment is aesthetically pleasing to their possessor.

As stated by Goldman and Cohen (1968), "There is little evidence to tell us of the precise and exact manner in which teeth should be aligned in *Homo Sapiens*." Thus, current knowledge does not yet give a firm basis for ideal relationships between form and function of the dentition; more and more, the emphasis is placed on functional aspects of occlusion rather than on the specific anatomical tooth relationships (see chapters 9 and 12). Therefore, any description of the adult natural dentition must be viewed within the context of expected variability and with the understanding that, *in the final analysis, optimal function and absence of disease is the principal characteristic of a good occlusion.*

It is within this framework that the foregoing characteristics of the dentition are described. In any description of the adult natural dentition, some standards must be employed as a basis for communication, hence "ideal" or "normal" characteristics are referred to. However, such characteristics are utilized only as a basis for assessing the degree of variation from the standard. It must be emphasized that the range of anatomical variation among humans is exceedingly great and, most importantly, that such variations are not necessarily unhealthy, abnormal, or pathological. *By itself, anatomical variation does not imply that treatment is indicated.* The issues of diagnostic and therapeutic criteria will be discussed in more detail in chapter 13 and in subsequent chapters. In this chapter, some anatomical characteristics of the natural dentition will be described. These will include

1. Occlusocranial relationships
2. The dental arches
3. The neutral zone
4. Occlusal surfaces and contacts
5. Occlusal relationships
6. Occlusal morphology
7. Guidance and determinants of occlusion
8. Self-protective features of the dentition
9. Esthetics

Occlusocranial relationships

It is impossible to describe an ideal relationship of the dentition and the occlusion to other cranial structures. However, certain averages can be noted as a means to introduce some of the landmarks used by dentists to assess patterns of craniofacial growth and development, and to compare degrees of variability among individuals. In the patient these assessments are done by standardized lateral radiographs of the head (cephalometric radiographs). Tracings of such radiographs permit analysis of static positional relationships of the structures depicted (Fig. 4-1). The details of such an analysis are more properly discussed in orthodontics courses and textbooks. However, a few of the most commonly used relationships are included here because they are relevant to the overall subject of Occlusion. The averages given were reported by Downs in 1948.

Plane of occlusion. Often defined as an imaginary surface that is related anatomically to the cranium and that theoretically touches the incisal edges of the incisors and the tips of the occluding surfaces of the posterior teeth. Due to the compensating curve, it is not a plane in the true sense of the word, but represents the mean of the curvature of the surface. It is frequently used to help to anatomically relate the dentition to other craniofacial structures. On an articulator, the plane of occlusion is often related to the *axis-orbital plane* (orbitale point to transverse hinge axis of condyle). In orthodontics, it is usually related to the *Frankfort plane* (orbitale to porion). The relationship of the occlusal plane to either of these reference planes will depend upon the skeletal configuration of the face; a short square face has nearly parallel planes, and a long, narrow face has a large angle between them. On the average, the cant of the occlusal plane is +9.3° in relation to the Frankfort horizontal plane, with a range of +1.5° to +14° (Downs, 1948). Thus, the plane of occlusion is ordinarily not parallel to the true horizontal plane when the head is erect.

Mandibular plane. Plane formed by the tangent to the lower border of the mandible. The mandibular plane angle averages +21.9° (17° to 28°) to the Frankfort plane (Downs, 1948). This relationship is commonly used as a diagnostic aid in orthodontics because it helps in evaluating the relative heights of the anterior and posterior parts of the facial skeleton.

Facial plane. Plane that contains the *nasion* (point where nasal and frontal bones meet) and the *pogonion* (most anterior midline point on the mandible). The average facial plane angle is 87.7° (82° to 95°) to the Frankfort plane (Downs, 1948). This angle is used to measure recession or prominence of the chin. The facial plane may also be used as a reference against which to compare the anteroposterior positions of the incisor teeth and alveolar processes.

The dental arches

A complete adult natural dentition consists of 32 teeth, equally divided between the two dental arches. Because the third molars are missing for various reasons in many individuals, a complete

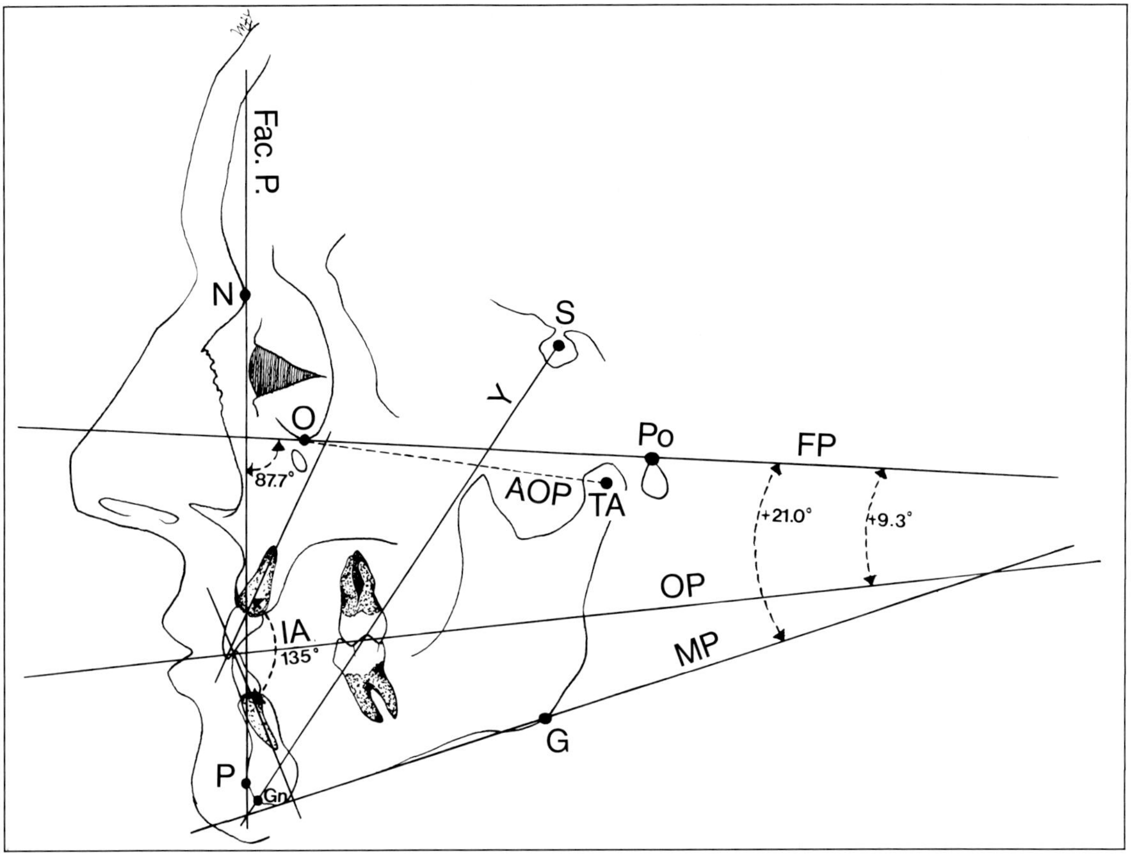

Fig. 4-1 A tracing adapted from an average cephalometric radiograph with some common craniofacial landmarks, planes, and relationships noted. The Frankfort plane *(FP)* is determined by the orbitale *(O)* and the porion *(Po)* at the superior margins of the external auditory meatuses. Using this plane as a reference, it may be noted that the occlusal plane *(OP)* averages +9.3°, the mandibular plane *(MP)* averages +21.0°, and the facial plane *(Fac. P.)* running from nasion *(N)* to pogonion *(P)* averages 87.7°, according to Downs (1948). The "Y" axis runs from the center of the sella turcica *(S)*, through the buccal groove of the maxillary first molar, to gnathion *(Gn)*. The angle of the mandible is represented by gonion *(G)*. The long axes of the central incisors are shown with an average interincisal angle *(IA)* of 135°. In an articulator, the occlusal plane *(OP)* is often related to the axis-orbital plane *(AOP)*, running from orbitale *(O)* to the terminal hinge axis *(TA)*. The *AOP* is close to, but not identical to, the Frankfort plane.

dentition is often defined in clinical studies as comprising 28 teeth.

Even if the size and shape of the arches vary between individuals, the maxillary arch generally takes the form of a half ellipse, whereas the mandibular arch resembles a parabola (Figs. 4-2a and b) (Krogh-Poulsen, 1958). Ideally, the teeth of each arch are symmetrically distributed around the median (mid-sagittal) plane. In this way the dentition can be divided into four quadrants with eight teeth in each: two incisors, one canine, two premolars, and three molars. This division is the basis for most of the tooth designation systems (Figs. 4-3a and b).

On the basis of form and function, the dental arches may be divided into different segments (see Figs. 4-2a and b). The anterior segment is a curve extending from canine to canine across the

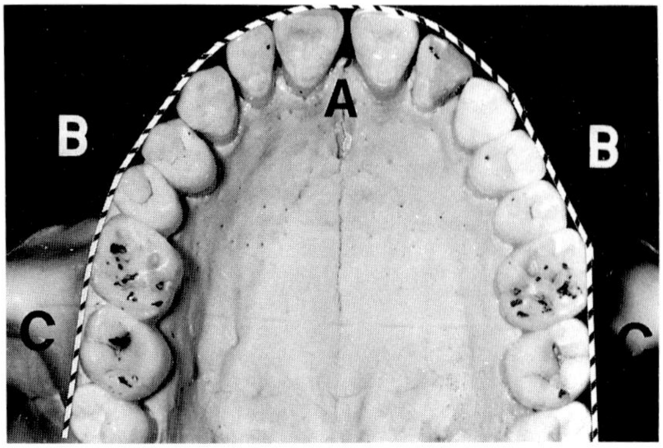

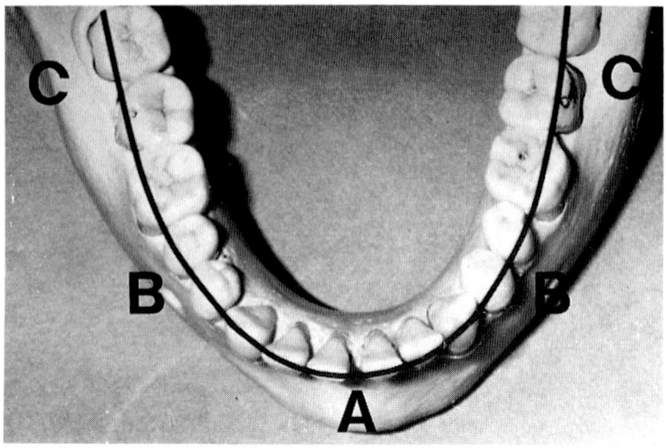

Figs. 4-2a and b Occlusal view of the dental arches (from a skull) with the anterior *(A)*, middle *(B)*, and posterior *(C)* segments marked.

Maxillary

18	*17*	*16*	*15*	*14*	*13*	*12*	*11*
8.5	9.0	10.0	7.0	7.0	7.5	6.5	8.5

48	*47*	*46*	*45*	*44*	*43*	*42*	*41*
10.0	10.5	11.0	7.0	7.0	7.0	5.5	5.6

Mandibular

Fig. 4-3a The right quadrants of the dentition. The relative relationship between the maxillary and mandibular permanent teeth in intercuspal position. The teeth are designated according to the FDI two-digit system (in italics). The average mesiodistal diameter (in millimeters) is given below the tooth number.

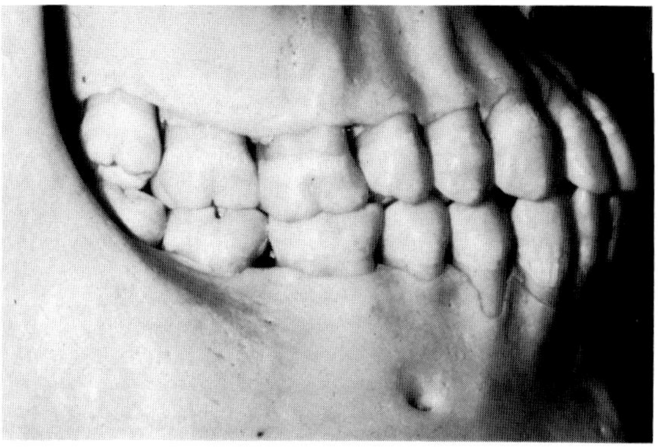

Fig. 4-3b The corresponding natural teeth of a skull.

midline. The medial, or premolar, segment is a straight line from the distal aspect of the canine to the mesial aspect of the first molar. A straight line from the medial aspect of the first premolar posteriorly describes the posterior, or molar, segments.

The teeth are aligned in the dental arches with varying degrees of inclination, both mesiodistally and buccolingually (Dempster et al., 1963). When viewed laterally, a line from the tip of the canine touching the tips of the buccal cusps of the posterior teeth will usually describe a relatively smooth curve, the *curve of Spee* (Fig. 4-4). In the transverse (frontal) plane, the alignments of the long axes of the posterior teeth cause the occlusal surfaces of the mandibular molars to be directed somewhat lingually, whereas those of the maxillary molars are directed somewhat buccally. For each pair of left and right posterior teeth, a transverse occlusal curve, the *curve of Wilson*, can be described (Figs. 4-5a and b). This curve is more exaggerated in the third molar area than in the first molar area. As described in chapter 12, it was once suggested that the curves

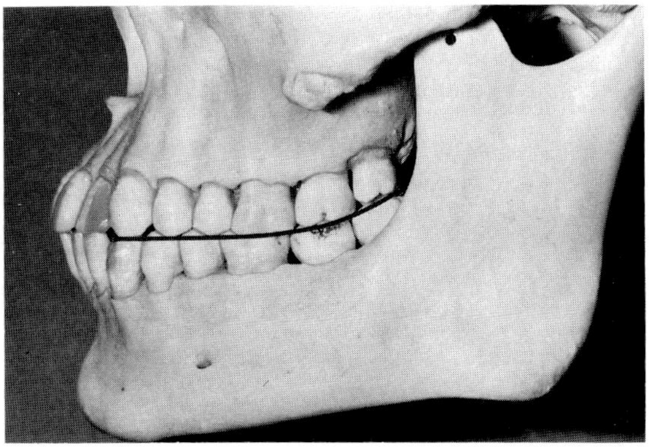

Fig. 4-4 The curve of Spee: a line from the tip of the canine touching the tips of the buccal cusps of the posterior teeth (drawn on jaws of a skull).

Figs. 4-5a and b Occlusal curves of Wilson.

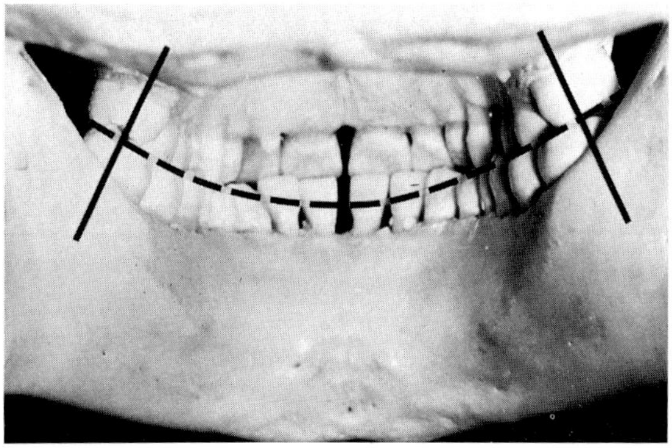

Fig. 4-5a A curve drawn on the third molars (of a skull).

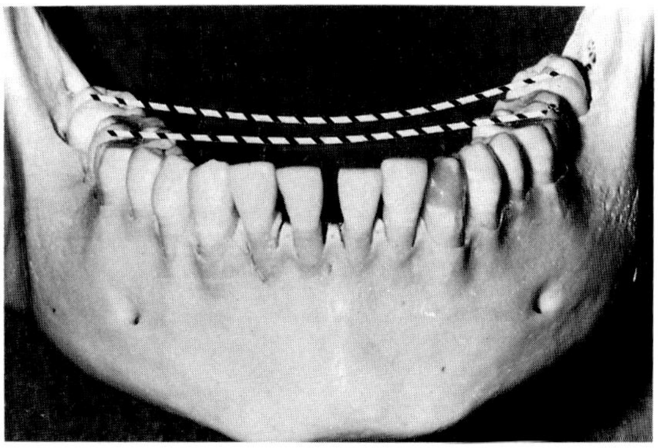

Fig. 4-5b Curves on the first and third molars of the mandible. Note the difference in the curves.

of Spee and Wilson are related three-dimensionally so that all the cusp tips and incisal ridges of all the teeth are aligned on the curved surface of a sphere *(sphere of Monson)*. However, attempts to demonstrate such spherical curves in the natural dentition have failed (Kraus et al., 1969).

The neutral zone

The dental arches are situated in a space bounded by the lips and cheeks externally and the tongue internally (Figs. 4-6a to c). In this space, called the *neutral zone* or *neutral space,* there is an equilibrium of muscular forces if the lip-cheek-tongue system is in balance. Equal forces acting on the teeth from lingual and facial sides helps the teeth to attain a position of relative stability. An imbalance of the system can unfavorably influence the position of teeth in the dental arches.

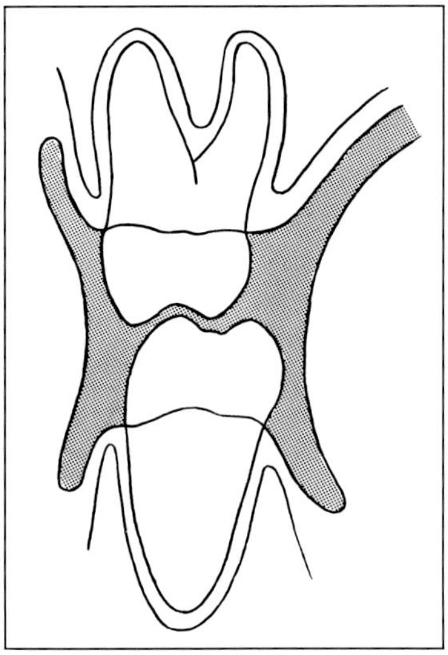

Fig. 4-6a The neutral zone (stippled area) in the molar region.

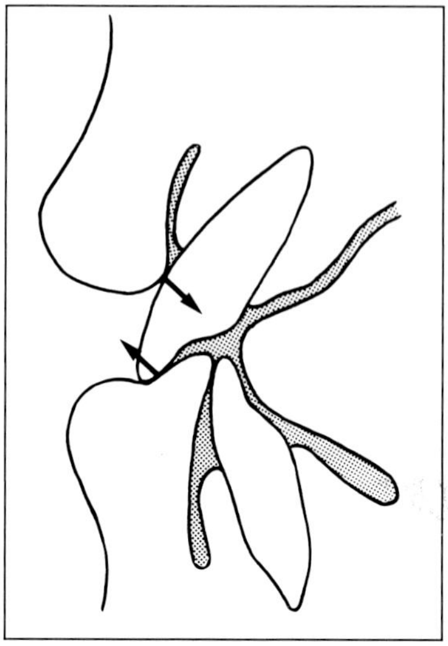

Fig. 4-6b Disturbance of the equilibrium of the neutral zone in the incisor region by the lower lip.

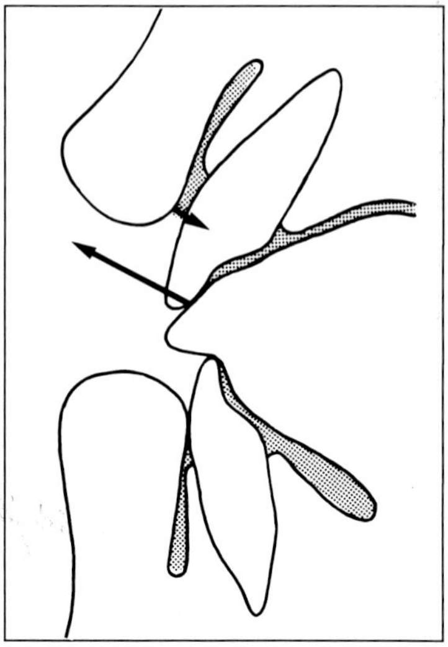

Fig. 4-6c Disturbance by the tongue.

Occlusal surfaces and contacts

In their unworn state the anatomical structures on the occlusal surfaces of the teeth—cusps, ridges, grooves, fossae—are rounded. In occlusal function they meet opposing tooth surfaces at many points, or small contact areas. As attrition occurs during function, these rounded occluding structures become broader and somewhat flattened area-to-area occluding surfaces (see chapter 15). A common pattern of attrition is the more rapid wear of maxillary lingual and mandibular buccal cusps relative to the other cusps.

The mesiodistal distances between buccal cusps are progressively shorter from the canines distally to the third molars. The height of the cusps also gradually decreases from the canines posteriorly. These characteristics are largely related to different movement trajectories of the anterior and posterior portions of the mandible. The greater anterior cusp height, for example, corresponds to the more vertical path of the anterior teeth during jaw closing as compared to the path of the molars. These anatomical arrangements are also related to efficiency and force distribution during masticatory function. The smaller surfaces of the sharp incisal edges and canine cusps give a relatively higher cutting pressure per unit area than the larger but shorter and blunter molar cusps, despite the fact that maximum bite force in the incisor area is much lower than that in the molar area.

Occlusal relationships

Several mandibular positions with occlusal contacts will be described in subsequent chapters. The following refers to the maximal intercuspation of the teeth, usually called the *intercuspal position* or *centric occlusion,* and often described as the terminal position of physiologic jaw closure.

In a classical arrangement, all teeth in the ideal dentition, except the mandibular central incisor and the maxillary third molar, have contacts with two teeth in the opposing arch (see Fig. 4-3). Because the maxillary arch is slightly larger than the mandibular arch, each tooth will oc-

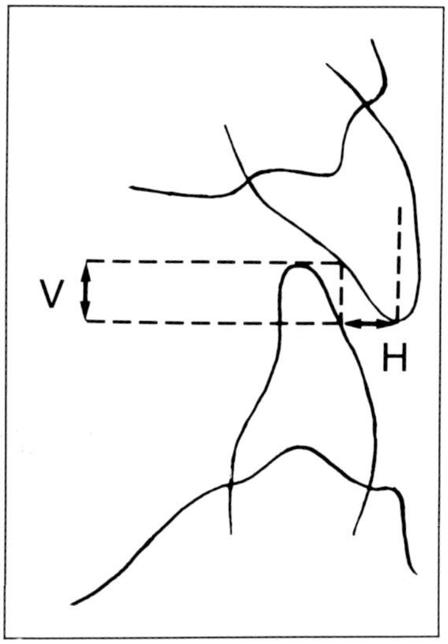

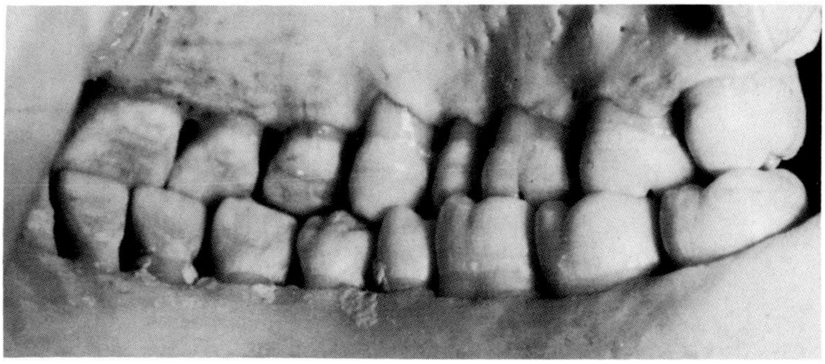

Figs. 4-7a and b Overbite and overjet.

Fig. 4-7a *(left)* The labiolingual incisor relationships in intercuspal position (ICP) vertically *(V)* and horizontally *(H)*.

Fig. 4-7b *(above)* The horizontal and vertical relationship between the teeth on the right side in the lingual view.

clude against its corresponding mandibular tooth and the tooth distal to it. For example, the maxillary first premolar will contact both the first and second mandibular premolars. The differences of arch sizes and tooth alignments result in an overlap of the mandibular arch by the maxillary arch such that the most inferior parts of the maxillary teeth extend a little beyond their mandibular antagonists.

In the incisor region, this relationship is of special interest. The maxillary incisors overlap the mandibular antagonists both horizontally and vertically (Figs. 4-7a and b). The horizontal overlap is termed *overjet* and the vertical overlap is called *overbite*. Frequent measurements in natural dentitions for both overjet and overbite are 1 to 3 mm. The influence on mandibular movements, such as protrusion, by the lingual surfaces of the maxillary incisors and the incisal edges of the mandibular incisors is termed the *incisal guidance*. Figure 4-7a shows that an increase in the overbite of the incisors will require the anterior portion of the mandible to move farther down during protrusion due to increased incisal guidance. An increased incisal overjet will have the opposite effect; that is, incisal guidance will be reduced. This same concept may be applied to the overbite-overjet relationship of the canines *(canine guidance)* and the posterior teeth *(posterior guidance)* during lateral excursion of the mandible.

In centric occlusion, the cusps of the mandibular teeth interdigitate maximally with their maxillary antagonists. The classical anatomical relationship is that, in this position, the lingual (palatal) cusps of the maxillary teeth and the buccal cusps of the mandibular teeth have maximal and simultaneous contact on both sides of the arch. Since these cuspal contacts provide the major support of occlusal vertical dimension, they are referred to as *supporting cusps* or *centric-holding cusps*. Normally, the supporting cusps of all posterior teeth occlude with marginal ridges, except for the distobuccal cusps of mandibular molars and the mesiolingual cusps of maxillary molars, which occlude with the central fossae of their respective antagonists (Figs. 4-8a and b). Except for the mandibular canine, all of the mandibular anterior teeth occlude against maxillary inclined surfaces that are

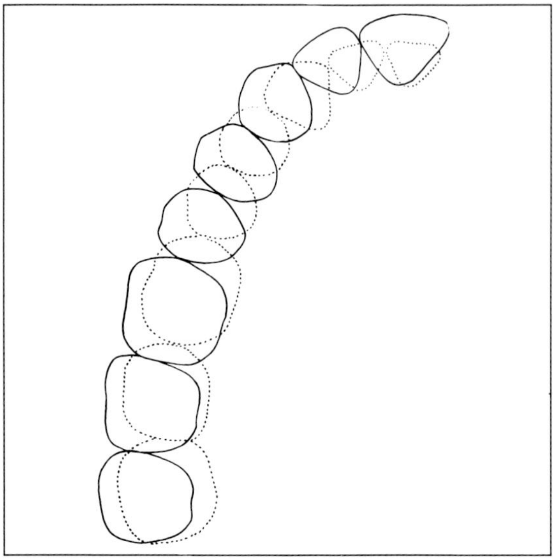

Fig. 4-8a The relationship between the maxillary and mandibular permanent teeth in ICP. Superimposition of the occlusal surfaces of the maxillary arch *(full lines)* on the mandibular arch *(broken lines)*.

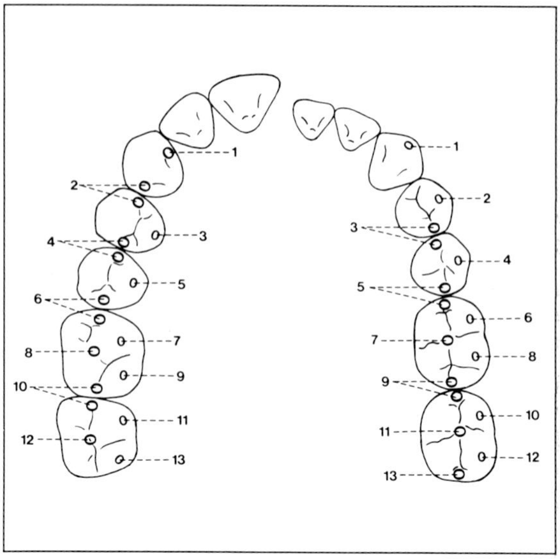

Fig. 4-8b Location of centric stops in an "ideal occlusion" (maxillary arch to the left, mandibular arch to the right). The cusp, fossa, and ridge relationships between the antagonistic teeth are indicated by like numbers.

Figs. 4-9a and b Occlusal contacts in a natural dentition (of a skull) with evidently stable occlusion (see Fig. 4-3b).

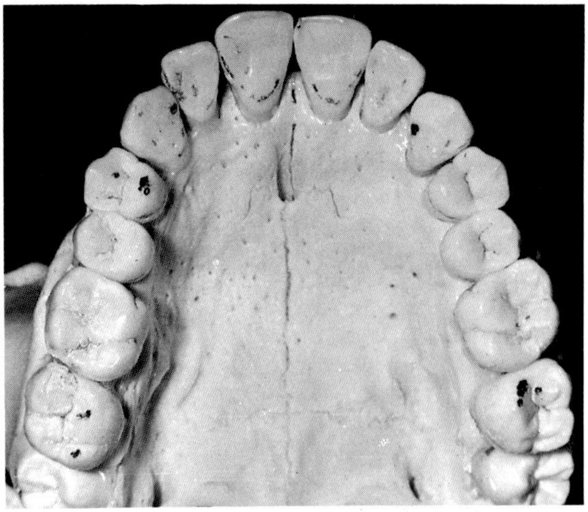

Fig. 4-9a Marking with a thin occlusal folium (0.008 mm thick) gives only few contacts.

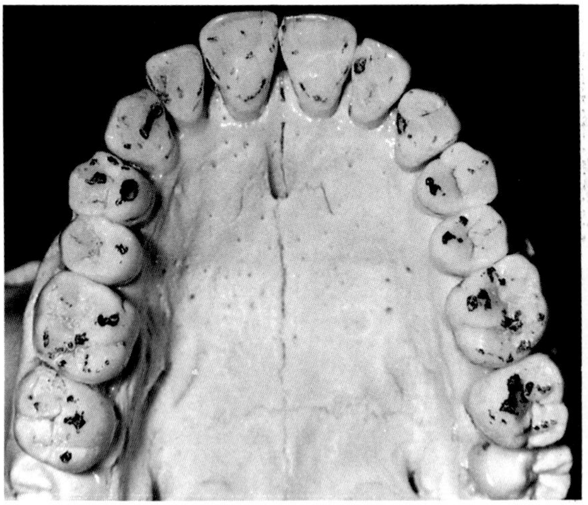

Fig. 4-9b Marking with a thicker articulating paper (0.1 mm) indicates a broader distribution of contacts in the same case.

not organized in a way that optimally supports occlusal vertical dimension and the occlusal forces generated in centric occlusion. Thus, in centric occlusion, the anterior teeth normally have very light occlusal contacts.

The buccal cusps of the maxillary teeth and the lingual cusps of the mandibular teeth do not support occlusal vertical dimension while in centric occlusion—hence the term *nonsupporting cusps*. They have the potential of occluding when one side becomes the working side during lateral excursion; because they may influence or "guide" such movement, they are sometimes referred to as the *guiding cusps*.

These classical contact relationships help to maintain occlusal stability in centric occlusion. The loss of supporting cusps can cause occlusal instability, since teeth may extrude, rotate, or otherwise migrate into new positions in the arch. It should be observed, however, that occlusal stability may be maintained even without these morphologically ideal cusp relations. This is based on the observation that the occlusal contacts in centric occlusion in the natural dentition usually are much fewer than anticipated for a theoretically ideal occlusion (Woda et al., 1979). The anterior teeth in a natural dentition, for example, are often slightly out of occlusal contact in centric occlusion; minor malocclusions with deviations from ideal tooth relationships may well have enough occlusal contacts to achieve intercuspal stabilization. It must also be remembered that the number of occlusal contacts in centric occlusion depends on biting force—more contacts are recorded when the individual is biting hard than when lightly bringing the jaws together (Riise and Ericsson, 1983). The occlusal marking material used for recording of occlusal contacts also influences the results of such recordings (Figs. 4-9a and b).

Occlusal morphology

The marginal ridges and inner inclines of the cusps of a posterior tooth form the *occlusal table* (Figs. 4-10a to c). This area between the cusp tips and cusp ridges of the buccal and lingual cusps forms only 50% to 60% of the overall buccolingual dimension of the crown of the tooth (Kraus et al., 1969). The occlusal table is centered over the root of the tooth so as to be in the best functional position to withstand occlusal forces. The supporting cusps articulate within the opposing occlusal table as they determine the occlusal vertical dimension in the intercuspal position. Because the supporting cusps bear most of the vertical occlusal load in this position, they are located nearer to the center of the tooth than are the nonsupporting, or guiding, cusps. This is particularly evident in the mesiolingual cusps of the maxillary molars and the buccal cusps of the mandibular posterior teeth compared with the nonsupporting cusps of those teeth. A variable 1-mm zone on the outer inclines of the supporting cusps also helps to support the intercuspal position; it is frequently referred to as the *functional outer aspect* (Kraus et al., 1969). This narrow zone is just lingual to maxillary supporting cusps and just buccal to mandibular supporting cusps.

The opposing areas that may be contacted by the supporting cusps during lateral excursion are called *guiding inclines*. On the working side, these inclines are typically located on the lingual aspects of the maxillary buccal cusps and the buccal aspect of the mandibular lingual cusps and have the potential for contact only during excursive movements. These cusps are usually sharper than the more rounded supporting cusps. Their potential contact patterns in eccentric movements are described further in chapter 9.

Although there is little specific relationship between the morphologies of the temporomandibular joint and the occlusion, certain general features are common to both. For example, the parabolic curve of the human dental arches is compatible with the posterior "bowing out" of the mandible. Lines connecting the buccal and lingual cusps of the posterior teeth will not be perpendicular to the mid-sagittal plane. They will, however, tend to be parallel to the long axes of the condyle, articular eminence, and fossa of the joint (Fig. 4-11).

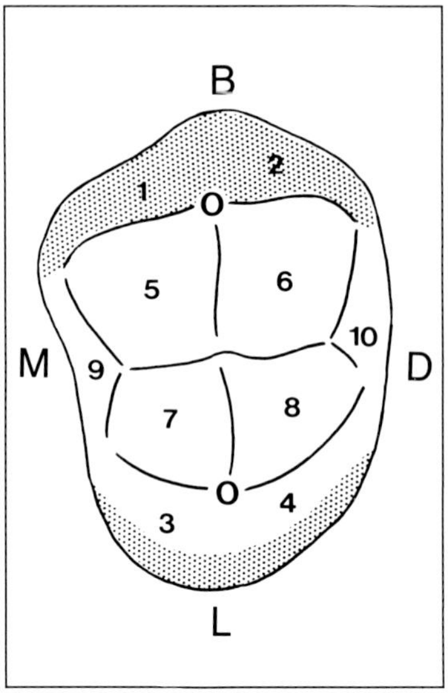

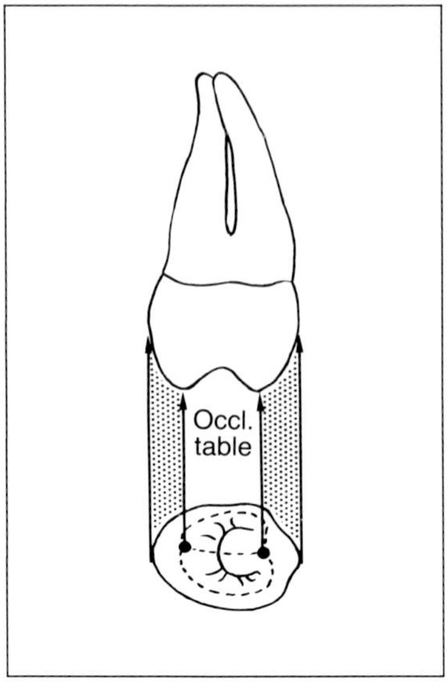

Fig. 4-10a *(left)* Landmarks of the occlusal surface of a maxillary premolar: mesial *(1)* and distal *(2)* outer aspects of the buccal *(B)* cusp; mesial *(3)* and distal *(4)* outer aspects of the lingual *(L)* cusp; mesial *(5)* and distal *(6)* inner aspects of the buccal cusp; mesial *(7)* and distal *(8)* inner aspects of the lingual cusp; mesial *(9)* and distal *(10)* marginal ridges. Areas 5 to 10 form the occlusal table.

Fig. 4-10b *(right)* Occlusal table.

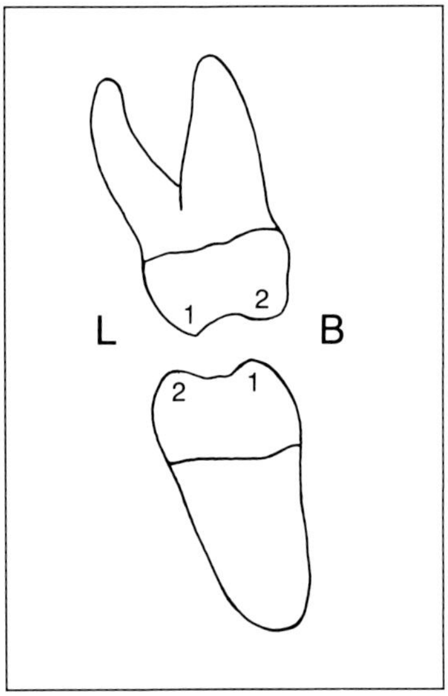

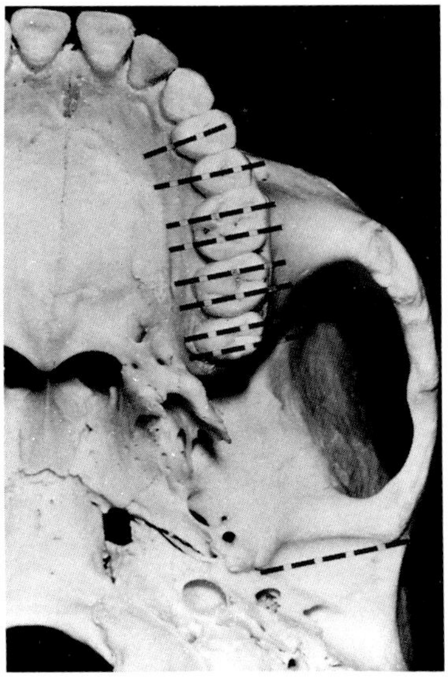

Fig. 4-10c *(left)* Supporting *(1)* and guiding *(2)* cusps of posterior teeth. Lingual *(L)*; buccal *(B)*.

Fig. 4-11 *(right)* A form-function relationship between occlusion and TMJ is indicated by the nearly parallel direction of lines connecting the buccal and lingual cusps of premolars and molars, and the mediolateral direction of the articular fossa and eminence.

Guidance and determinants of occlusion

In classic textbooks on Occlusion the concept of a *balanced occlusion*—simultaneous bilateral posterior and anterior tooth contacts during all positions and movements—has been emphasized. Although this is of value in complete denture construction to help stabilize denture bases during function, it is seldom found and should not be established in the natural dentition, where the teeth are individually anchored to the jaws. A more complete explanation of the historical development of this and other concepts of occlusion can be found in chapter 12.

For creation of a balanced occlusion for a set of complete dentures in an articulator, five factors *(Hanau's quint)* have been described that presumably must be specifically related and integrated to achieve balance *(Thielmann's formula)*. These five factors, called *determinants of occlusion,* are *(1)* condylar guidance, *(2)* incisal guidance, *(3)* plane of occlusion, *(4)* compensating curve, and *(5)* cusp height. A detailed explanation of how the integration of these factors is related to balanced occlusion of complete dentures is best left to the study of that discipline. It deserves to be stated, however, that the exact integration of these "determinants of occlusion" does not apply to a natural dentition where balance is not a naturally occurring condition or a therapeutic imperative. Thus, it has little relevance here.

The fact that the determinants of occlusion are not collectivized in a precise manner in the natural dentition does not imply that each one individually does not have an influence on posterior cusp height and occlusal morphology over time. Each has some influence on the attritional pattern of the dentition, and in that sense may be considered an occlusal determinant. Although the rate of attrition will be decided by such factors as the abrasiveness of the diet, the type and frequency of bruxism, and the occlusal forces utilized, the patterns of attrition will depend on existing occlusal morphology and relationships, and on the patterns of mandibular position and movement. Although these patterns will be controlled by the neuromuscular system, they will be influenced by the structural relationships of the various components of the dentition and the rest of the masticatory system.

For example, posterior cusp height will be influenced over time by the degree of anterior guidance, both incisal and canine. A person with a steep anterior guidance (much overbite and little overjet of the anterior teeth) will have a tendency to more easily disclude the posterior teeth during eccentric movements; thus the cusps will tend to remain high as attrition occurs. On the other hand, persons with little or no anterior guidance (much overjet and/or little overbite) will, given time, tend to flatten the cusps of the posterior teeth during eccentric movements because they do not disclude as readily during functional activity. Again, no specific fixed relationships have been found that integrate all of these factors in simple mechanical models. Mandibular function with its neuromuscular controls and resultant influences on the attritional patterns of the dentition is much too complex a phenomenon to permit such a narrow interpretation of the influence of the determinants of occlusion.

Self-protective features of the dentition

It is generally assumed that teeth with proper form and alignment will help to protect their supporting structures during normal function (Kraus et al., 1969). However, the complicated functional mechanisms in the masticatory system and the limited research on form-function relationships make our knowledge in this field incomplete. Therefore, only a few items will be discussed here.

Protection to the gingival tissues. Normal masticatory function is often said to be necessary for adequate stimulation of the gingival tissues. With a unilateral chewing habit, the unused side has been observed to accumulate more plaque and calculus than the functioning side (Kraus et al., 1969). However, according to current knowledge in periodontology, proper oral hygiene will help to maintain good gingival health, and the influence of masticatory function is, therefore, relatively small compared with that of effective plaque control.

Crown form and gingival response. The facial, lingual, and interproximal contours of the teeth usually exhibit a gentle convexity. The height of the faciolingual coronal contours of all teeth except the lingual surfaces of the mandibular posterior teeth are usually in the gingival one third of their crowns. Because of the lingual inclinations of the mandibular posterior teeth, particularly the molars, the heights of contour are generally in the middle one third on the lingual sides of these teeth. Interproximal crown form usually creates contact areas between adjacent teeth that are located more facially than lingually, and more occlusally than gingivally. Thus, lingual embrasures usually are larger than facial embrasures, and gingival embrasures are bigger than occlusal embrasures.

The marginal ridges of adjacent teeth should ordinarily be at the same heights in order to reduce the likelihood of food impaction between the teeth. Such contour relationships are presumed to provide an optimal response from the gingiva, and are thus recreated when crown structure is restored. In an effort to enhance this crown form–gingival response relationship, some dentists have adopted the "protective deflective contour therapy," whereby "exaggerated contours are incorporated into artificial crowns to prevent sulcular food impaction" (Jameson and Malone, 1982). According to Jameson and Malone (1982), there is little scientific evidence to support the concept of a "protective bulge," which is rarely seen in nature and may, in fact, facilitate areas of plaque formation. Although overcontouring is probably more detrimental to gingival health than undercontouring, the latter has been associated with hyperplastic gingival tissue (Kraus et al., 1969). Interproximally, overcontouring is also usually more harmful than undercontouring, although sufficient contour should exist to create properly formed and located contact areas and embrasure spaces. It is perhaps a safe assumption that the best contour is that found in the naturally occurring dental environment; this environment should usually be replicated when the crowns of teeth are restored.

Again, adequate plaque removal procedures and toothbrush massage will easily resolve the possible negative influences of *minor* variations in buccolingual crown contour. Perhaps more important than the crown contour is the placement of the gingival margin of the artificial crown. The least favorable results are produced by subgingival restorations near the bottom of the gingival sulcus, whereas supragingival placement does not interfere with the periodontal conditions (Silness, 1980).

Protection to the periodontium. It has generally been maintained that occlusal forces are best withstood when transmitted in an axial direction to a tooth, and that horizontal forces are not tolerated as well as vertical forces. A healthy periodontium, however, seems to adapt to any direction of functional occlusal forces, including the extreme type of jiggling studied in animal model systems (Polson and Heijl, 1980). There is now little question that occlusal forces, whatever the direction, will not cause periodontal pocket formation or a reduction in the level of connective tissue attachment. However, the magnitude and direction of such forces will adaptively influence the width of the periodontal ligament space and the qualitative histomorphologic organization of the periodontal ligament, factors that help to determine the degree of mobility of a tooth. It is generally conceded that vertical axial forces will cause less displacement of teeth than horizontally directed forces. Thus, the location and direction of occlusal contacts, not to mention the magnitude of the force, can influence a tooth's mobility. In the absence of inflammatory periodontal disease, such tooth mobility should be regarded as an adaptation to these environmental forces.

There remains some controversy over whether nonprogressive tooth mobility in the absence of periodontitis requires therapeutic intervention to reduce occlusal loading and, hence, the tooth's mobility. These issues are further addressed in chapters 5, 13, and 16.

Protection to oral soft tissues (lip, cheek, tongue). The buccal overlap of the maxillary teeth seems to be important to keep the lip and cheek away from the occlusal surfaces in function. In a similar way, the tongue is presumed to be protected by the lingual overlap. Problems with tongue- and cheek-biting can be encountered in construction of both fixed and removable prostheses when such an overlap is not incorporated. They are often transient or can be solved by changing the degree of overlap. In the natural dentition, deviations from the normal overlap relationship as seen in many malocclusions seldom produce such problems because of functional adaptation.

Esthetics

There can be little question that the dentition plays a vital role in one's facial appearance. Whether the form, position, and relationships of the dentition enhance or detract from this appearance is a matter of degree and, most importantly, of the subjective assessment of the individual. The latter is very often linked to the cultural and social environment of that person. Thus, no categorical statements can be made regarding esthetics and specific dental characteristics. Some of the general factors that have the greatest impact on esthetics can be mentioned, however. These include individual tooth crown form, color and translucency, relationship of adjacent teeth to one another, degree of anterior overbite and overjet, arch form, and dental-lip relationships. Such characteristics are viewed subjectively within the context of age, sex, and overall facial morphology and features, etc. Attempts have been made to categorize dental characteristics and their impact on esthetics, particularly in the area of complete denture prosthodontics, where it is of obvious concern. Such categorizations are not easily accomplished, however, because of the essentially individualistic perceptions of esthetic qualities. However, one thing is clear: esthetic considerations are an important ingredient of the occlusion. They will influence diagnosis, treatment planning, and the patient's perception of the success of treatment.

Summary

An idealized description of the form and structural relationships of the dentition is highly theoretical. Less than ideal morphological characteristics do not by themselves imply that function is less than optimal. In the final analysis, morphological variability and adaptative ability make it imperative that judgments of health and nonhealth be based on functional considerations.

Chapter 5

The Periodontium

Douglas A. DePorter and George A. Zarb

The periodontium comprises four specialized connective tissues: gingiva, cementum, periodontal ligament, and alveolar process. These tissues not only provide the attachment apparatus for the teeth, but also contain numerous fibers of the trigeminal nerve (cranial nerve V) that contribute to the neurosensory control of occlusal function. In this chapter we will discuss the role of the periodontium in occlusion. First, a brief review of the structure of the periodontium will be presented. The greatest attention will be directed to the periodontal ligament, because it appears to provide the major periodontal input to the control of occlusal function.

Structure of the periodontium

Gingiva

Clinically, gingiva is described as consisting of two zones, the *marginal gingiva* or *free gingiva* and the *attached gingiva* (Fig. 5-1). The marginal gingiva is the retractable cuff of gingival tissue that surrounds the neck of the tooth and, in health, forms the wall of the gingival sulcus. It adheres to the tooth surface at the base of the sulcus via the sulcular epithelium. The attached gingiva, on the other hand, comprises the bulk of the gingival tissue and provides the major protection for the underlying tissues of the periodontium. The collagen fibers of healthy attached gingiva are firmly inserted into bone and cementum as Sharpey's fibers.

Histologically, the lamina propria of the gingiva can be seen to consist primarily of collagen fibers that are organized into four major groups (Ten Cate, 1980). The fibers of the largest group, the *dentogingival group,* run from the lamina propria of both marginal and attached gingiva to the cervical cementum. The *alveologingival group* of fibers runs from the bone of the alveolar process to the lamina propria of the marginal and attached gingiva. The *circular group* of fibers runs circumferentially about the tooth within the free gingiva. The *dentoperiosteal group* of fibers extends from the cervical cementum over the crest of the alveolar process and in an apical direction so as ultimately to insert into the outer cortical plate of the alveolar process. A subgroup (not shown in Fig. 5-1) of this last group of fibers runs interdentally from the cervical cementum of one tooth to that of the adjacent tooth. These fibers are called *transseptal fibers* because they traverse the lamina propria of the interdental gingival septum.

At the level of the alveolar crest, the collagen fibers of the periodontal ligament merge with those of the lamina propria of the gingiva. For this reason, it has been suggested that the gingiva and periodontal ligament are two anatomical parts of the same functional system (Melcher and Eastoe, 1969). The functions shared by these tissues would include providing a dynamic attachment apparatus connecting the tooth to the bone of the alveolar process, absorbing the

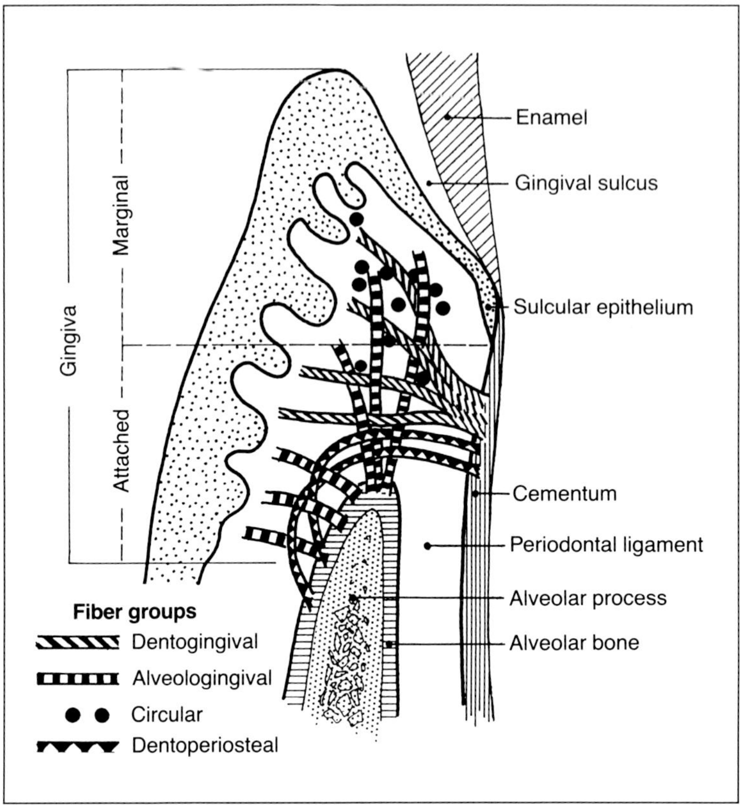

Fig. 5-1 Organization and interrelationships of gingival collagen fibers.

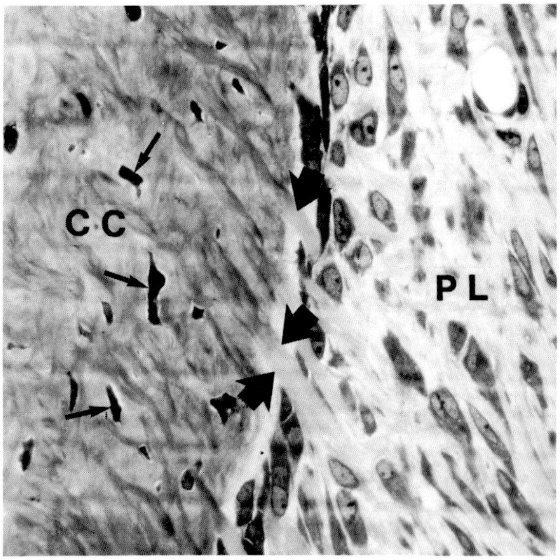

Fig. 5-2 Histological section of rat periodontium showing cellular cementum *(CC)* and Sharpey's fibers *(large arrows)*, cementocytes *(small arrows)*, and periodontal ligament *(PL)*. Original magnification ×900.

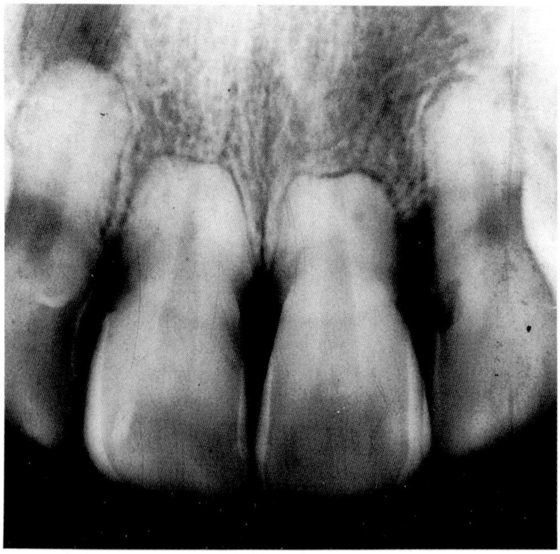

Fig. 5-3 Radiographic view of extensive external root resorption following the application of excessive orthodontics forces to the affected teeth. (Courtesy of F. Kellman, D.D.S.)

forces generated by occlusal contact, and providing neurosensory input for the control of normal occlusal function.

Cementum

Cementum is a mineralized connective tissue, the organic component of which comprises collagen and a number of noncollagenous components, including glycosaminoglycans and glycoproteins (Melcher and Eastoe, 1969). The collagen fibers of cementum include both intrinsic collagen fibers originally produced by cementoblasts, and extrinsic collagen fibers originally produced by fibroblasts of the developing periodontal ligament. These extrinsic fibers are also called Sharpey's fibers, and are the continuation of the principal fibers of the periodontal ligament (Fig. 5-2). They form the attachment of the ligament to the root surface.

There are two types of cementum: cellular and acellular. A thin layer of acellular cementum usually covers up to one half of the cervical root dentin (see Fig. 5-6). Cellular cementum contains cementocytes within lacunae (Fig. 5-2), and is deposited on the majority of the root surface, including forming a covering on the layer of acellular cementum, especially toward the root apex. Acellular cementum consists primarily of mineralized extrinsic or Sharpey's fibers, while cellular cementum has both extrinsic and intrinsic fibers. The intrinsic fibers and superficial portions of the extrinsic (Sharpey's) fibers of cellular cementum become mineralized, while the central cores of the extrinsic fibers do not.

Cementogenesis continues at intervals throughout life, especially in the more apical regions of the root. Unlike bone, however, cementum is an avascular tissue and does not seem to undergo extensive remodeling. As new layers of cementum are laid down, the older cementocytes in the deeper aspects of the cellular cementum lose their nutritional support and become nonvital. Also unlike bone, cementum is usually resistant to resorption. While the forces of normal occlusion do not normally lead to cementum resorption, the application of heavy forces, for example, orthodontic, can cause extensive resorption of cementum and dentin. It seems likely that the periodontal ligament provides some inhibitory effect that under normal conditions prevents root resorption. However, any alteration of the normal homeostasis of the periodontal ligament, as might occur in some types of orthodontic therapy, may lead to an interruption in this inhibitory effect and result in varying degrees of root resorption (Fig. 5-3). The resorptive cells apparently arise from precursor cells in the periodontal ligament.

Alveolar process

The bone that surrounds and supports the teeth comprises the alveolar process. It is dependent on the presence of natural teeth for its existence, as it is gradually resorbed once the teeth have been extracted. The anatomy of the bone of the alveolar process is variable. In the posterior areas the alveolar process consists, both buccally and lingually, of outer and inner cortical bony plates with varying amounts of cancellous bone between them. In anterior regions, there may be little or no cancellous bone between the two cortical plates. The inner cortical plate has been variously referred to as alveolar bone, bundle bone, or the cribriform plate, and is thought to represent the lamina dura seen in radiographs of teeth (Fig. 5-4). This is a layer of cortical bone that forms the wall of the tooth socket, and into which the principal fibers of the periodontal ligament are inserted (Fig. 5-5). It is perforated by many small canals through which blood vessels, nerves, and lymphatic vessels gain access to the periodontal ligament (Fig. 5-6). Unlike cementum, alveolar bone is constantly being remodeled in response to normal occlusal forces enabling adaptive tooth movements to occur (Fig. 5-7). In keeping with the terminology used elsewhere in this book, we will often refer to this remodeling activity and that of the periodontal ligament as *adaptive responses*.

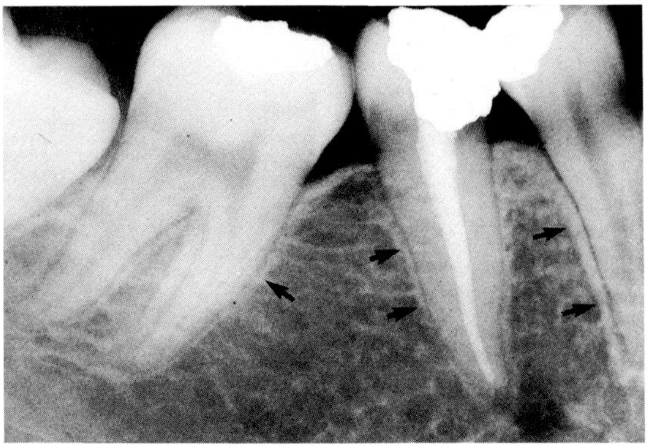

Fig. 5-4 Radiograph of normal lamina dura of varying thickness *(arrows)*. (Courtesy of B. Friedland, D.D.S.)

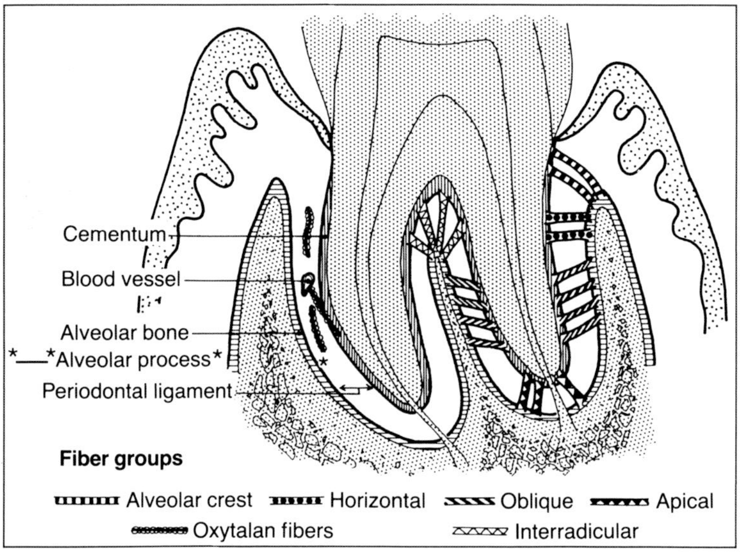

Fig. 5-5 The principal fiber groups of the periodontium—their orientation and relationship to each other and to oxytalan fibers.

Periodontal ligament

The band of soft connective tissue that connects the tooth root to the alveolar bone is the periodontal ligament. In humans it ranges in width from 0.15 to 0.38 mm, but appears to narrow with age (Melcher, 1980). It is termed a ligament because it consists of dense, regular bundles of collagen fibers. However, unlike a typical ligament, it is highly cellular, highly vascular, well innervated, and metabolically very active.

The periodontal ligament consists largely of cells and extracellular substances. The latter comprises collagen and a number of noncollagenous components, including oxytalan fibers, glycosaminoglycans, and glycoproteins.

The collagen fibers (also termed the principal fibers) of the periodontal ligament are organized into a number of groups recognizable in the light microscope (see Fig. 5-5). These groups of fibers are the alveolar crest group; the horizontal group; the oblique group, which constitutes the bulk of the ligament fibers; the apical group; and, in the case of multirooted teeth, the interradicular group. The fiber bundles of these groups run from cementum to alveolar bone, and are

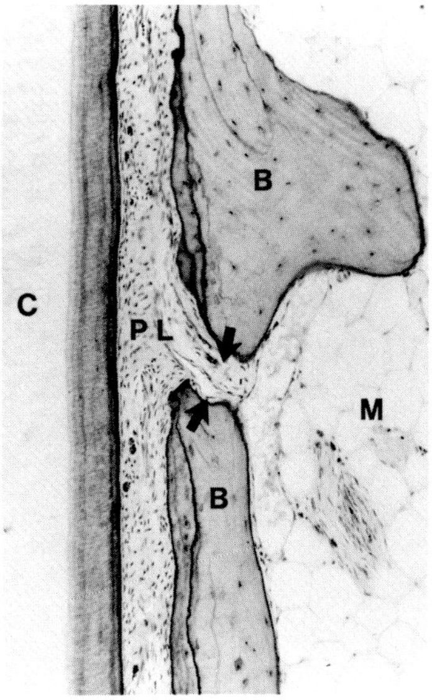

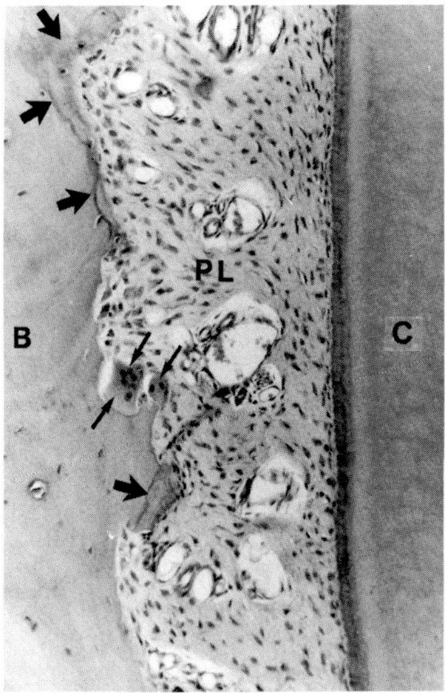

Fig. 5-6 *(left)* Histological section of human periodontium showing: acellular cementum *(C)*; alveolar bone *(B)* and its perforation by small canals *(arrows)* through which blood vessels, nerves, and lymphatics gain access to the periodontal ligament *(PL)*; and bone marrow *(M)*. Original magnification ×200.

Fig. 5-7 *(right)* Histological longitudinal section of human periodontium showing: remodeling of the alveolar bone *(B)* of the socket wall; osteoclast *(small arrows)*; and reversal line *(large arrows)*. Note the irregular nature of the bone margin. Note also the high vascularity of the periodontal ligament *(PL)*. Cementum *(C)*. Original magnification ×280.

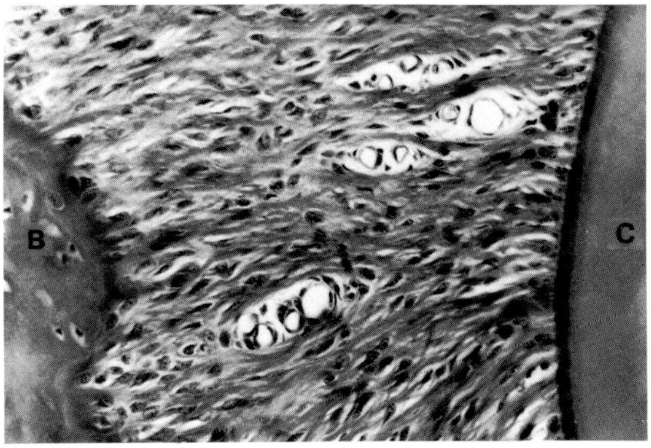

Fig. 5-8 Longitudinal section of human periodontium near the crest of the alveolar process. Note the orientation of collagen fibers (horizontal and oblique) with respect to cementum *(C)* and bone *(B)*, and their insertion into these tissues as Sharpey's fibers. Original magnification ×600.

inserted into these two hard connective tissues as Sharpey's fibers (i.e., the "extrinsic" fibers of cementum and bone) (Fig. 5-8).

In addition to collagen fibers, the periodontal ligament also contains significant amounts of oxytalan fibers, which seem to be unique to this tissue and are thought to consist of immature elastin. Unlike the principal fibers of the ligament, oxytalan fibers are not organized into regular bundles that run from tooth to bone. Instead, they tend to run as single fibers or small groups of fibers that may be attached at one end to blood vessels and at the other end to cementum or bone. It is speculated that they play some role in controlling vessel size in the ligament by maintaining tension on the vessel wall.

The noncollagenous component of the extracellular compartment of periodontal ligament, often termed the *ground substance,* fills all the interstices between cells, fibers, vessels, nerves, and other identifiable components of the ligament. It provides a milieu suitable for cell migration and diffusion of nutrients and end products of metabolism between blood vessels and cells. Biochemical investigations have shown that the noncollagenous component of periodontal liga-

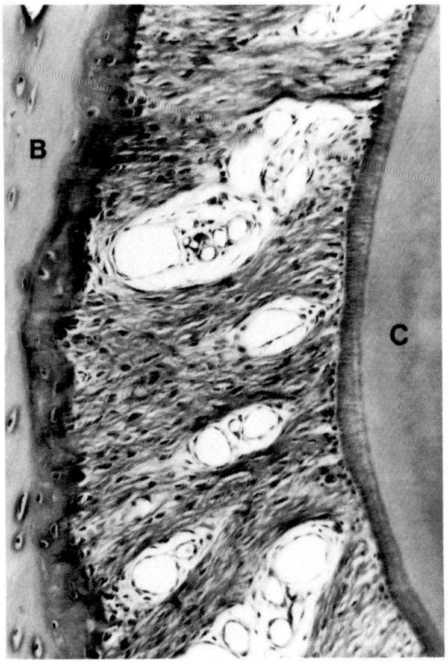

Fig. 5-9 Horizontal section of monkey periodontium to demonstrate the extensive vascularity of the periodontal ligament. The main vessels run vertically within the ligament and are seen here in cross section. Bone *(B)*; cementum *(C)*. Original magnification ×125.

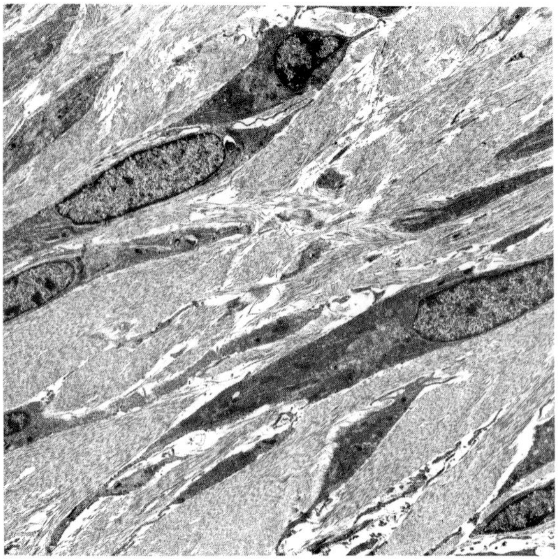

Fig. 5-10 Low-power electron micrograph of rat periodontal ligament showing the orientation of fibroblasts with respect to the fibrils of the major fiber bundles. The cells have numerous cellular processes that interdigitate with each other. Original magnification ×35,500.

ment consists of glycosaminoglycans, glycoproteins, and glycolipids. Little is known about the structure and organization of these noncollagenous moieties, especially in relation to the other components of the ligament, because it is technically difficult to preserve them in the electron microscope. However, it is known that many of these macromolecules are highly hydrated in vivo; this feature is thought to contribute to the ability of the ligament to absorb the stress of occlusal function.

Little is known about the blood supply of the human periodontal ligament. However, it is known from latex perfusion experiments that the arterial blood supply of the monkey periodontal ligament arises from branches of vessels in the gingiva and alveolar process (Kindlova, 1965). Branches of gingival vessels enter the ligament at its coronal aspect. Branches of intraalveolar vessels, which themselves arise from the superior alveolar and inferior alveolar arteries, enter the ligament in the horizontal plane by passing through foramina in the cribriform plate (see Fig. 5-6). Once within the ligament the main arterioles run vertically, often in close proximity to the alveolar bone (Fig. 5-9). However, they give off branches that subsequently form an extensive capillary network that appears to be more prominent on the alveolar-bone half of the ligament and to be particularly well developed in the apical and cervical regions of the ligament. The arterioles also form numerous anastamoses with the venous system, and the latter drains vertically towards the apex of the root.

The cells of the periodontal ligament are many and varied. They include osteoblasts and osteoclasts lining the alveolar-bone aspect of the ligament, cementoblasts lining active sites on the cementum side of the ligament, clusters of epithelial cells (the epithelial cell *rests of Malassez*), macrophages, fibroblasts, and undifferentiated mesenchymal cells. The undifferentiated mesenchymal cells are pluripotent, primarily located in perivascular locations, and thought to provide precursor cells for renewal of all of the connective tissue cells in the ligament (Gould et al., 1977, 1980).

Despite the fact that the periodontal ligament contains dense, highly organized bundles of collagen fibers, it is by no means an inactive tissue. Indeed, at least in experimental animals, the periodontal ligament has been shown to have an extremely high level of collagen turnover and remodeling, characteristics that allow considerable adaptive change during function.

The cell responsible for the turnover and remodeling of the collagen fibers of the periodontal ligament is the fibroblast. The fibroblast seems to be responsible for both the synthesis and the degradation of ligament collagen. Fibroblasts of the ligament tend to be oriented parallel to the fiber bundles and to have numerous interdigitating cell processes (Fig. 5-10). Collagen is synthesized and secreted by the fibroblast as procollagen molecules—these subsequently become altered by extracellular enzymes (procollagen peptidases) to form collagen molecules, which aggregate with one another to form collagen fibers. While some controversy does exist on how the fibroblast degrades collagen, numerous authors have suggested that this degradation occurs close to, or within, the fibroblast by means of fibroblast-synthesized enzymes such as collagenase and some lysosomal enzymes.

For many years, it was widely held that adaptation of the periodontal ligament occurred primarily in its central portions. The term *intermediate plexus* was introduced to denote this hypothetical area of active remodeling. The cementum- and bone-related regions of the ligament were considered to be relatively inactive. More recent work, however, suggests that adaptive change is relatively uniform throughout the ligament. The alveolar bone itself also undergoes constant remodeling or adaption under conditions of normal function (see Fig. 5-7).

To summarize, the periodontal ligament comprises a layer of soft connective tissue that connects the tooth root to its bony socket. It contains a perivascular source of undifferentiated mesenchymal cells, and it is metabolically very active. Interestingly, the periodontal ligament seems to have control mechanisms to prevent is obliteration by osteogenesis or cementogenesis. For this reason, ankylosis of normally functioning teeth is rare. If, however, ligament is lost from the root surface—for example, following traumatic tooth avulsion and replantation—the root commonly undergoes ankylosis and extensive root resorption unless vital ligament tissue can be retained on the root at the time of replantation.

It must be emphasized that the ligament does not function independently of the other tissues of the periodontium. These four specialized tissues form a functional unit in which responses to diverse stimuli in individual tissues will frequently overlap.

Functions of the periodontal ligament

The periodontal ligament seems to play three major functional roles in occlusion: absorption of occlusal forces, permitting adaptive tooth movements, and providing neurosensory input.

The periodontal ligament has long been known to function in the absorption of forces generated by normal occlusion. Because of the arrangement of the principal fibers of the ligament, it was originally thought that they were well suited to resist axial and horizontal forces by fiber tension. It was suggested that the fibers might follow a wavy course at rest but become stretched when occlusal forces were applied. However, this concept is not supported by experimental evidence (Ten Cate, 1980).

Physiological experiments suggest that the ligament functions as a viscoelastic cushion with at least two components. First, the blood vessels of the ligament act as a hydraulic damper system, giving the ligament elasticity. Whereas at rest the blood vessels maintain a positive hydraulic pressure within the ligament space, when a force is applied to a tooth a partial collapse of the blood vessels occurs, resulting in localized areas of ligament compression and permitting tooth movement away from the direction of force.

Second, the ground substance of the ligament binds large amounts of water from the tissue fluid, giving the ligament a viscous quality. With the application of occlusal force, the ground substance and its bound water are easily displaced to nonloaded regions of the ligament and even through the many foramina in the alveolar bone. The net effect of the blood vessel alterations and extracellular fluid displacement is dissipation of the applied forces. As stated above, deformation of the alveolar bone may also contribute to this cushioning effect. When the forces are removed, the tooth rebounds to its preloaded position as the blood and then the ground substance and tissue fluids redistribute themselves.

The second major function of the periodontal ligament is to permit adaptive tooth movements. As indicated, the ligament is a very active tissue with a high rate of turnover and remodeling. This property permits tooth movements (e.g., eruptive and mesial drifting) required to compensate for occlusal and interproximal wear on the crowns. Unfortunately, it also allows for the tipping, drifting, and supraeruptive movements that often accompany the loss of adjacent or opposing teeth.

The periodontal ligament also acts as a neurosensory organ to modulate masticatory forces and to prevent overloading of the periodontal apparatus. It can also play a role in a child's learning to masticate.

Sensory innervation of the periodontal ligament

The periodontal ligament is innervated primarily via the inferior alveolar (mandibular teeth) and superior alveolar (maxillary teeth) branches of the trigeminal nerve. Nerve fibers enter the periodontal ligament in two ways. Bundles of nerve fibers enter the periodontal ligament space in the region of the root apex and branch out in a coronal direction. These fibers are joined by others that enter the ligament in the horizontal plane by passing through foramina in the alveolar bone (see Fig. 5-6). These latter fibers also send branches in an apical or coronal direction. At the crest of the alveolar process all these fibers join with others of periosteal origin to innervate the gingiva.

Many of the nonspecialized, or free, nerve endings are thought to be pain receptors, whereas others are associated with blood vessels and may represent autonomic nerve fibers with a vasomotor function. It has also been suggested that some free endings may be mechanoreceptors, specialized to respond to the non-noxious sensations of touch and pressure.

The specialized nerve endings are thought to be mechanoreceptors. They exhibit their maximum activity when a stimulus is applied in one direction (Anderson, 1969). Physiological experiments have indicated that there are both rapidly and slowly adapting mechanoreceptors. Rapidly adapting mechanoreceptors fire only a few nerve impulses when a stimulus is applied, while slowly adapting mechanoreceptors fire throughout the stimulus application.

The function of the periodontal ligament mechanoreceptors is to mediate tactile sensibility of the teeth and related sensory functions, such as oral stereognosis, which is the ability to recognize the size, shape, thickness, hardness, and texture of objects placed in the mouth. Pulpal receptors do not seem to play a major role in this function since the tactile thresholds of vital and endodontically treated teeth are similar (Linden, 1975). However, sensory receptors in the gingiva, oral mucosae, tongue, and temporomandibular joint (TMJ) contribute to this function (Dubner et al., 1978). For example, TMJ infiltration with local anesthetic will increase the threshold for discriminating the sizes of objects placed between the teeth.

In addition to their role in tactile sensibility, periodontal ligament mechanoreceptors also help to modulate a variety of reflex motor functions involved in occlusion, swallowing patterns and habits, speech, and protective reflexes of the orofacial region (Dubner et al., 1978). The role of these receptors in controlling occlusal function are discussed in the next section.

Role of periodontal sensory receptors in occlusion

It appears that the control of functional jaw movement in occlusion involves interrelated sensory input from receptors in the muscles of mastication, tendons, TMJ, and the periodontium (Kawamura, 1967). Periodontal receptors are most likely involved in limiting biting force by inhibiting muscle activity in the mandibular elevators (masseter, temporalis, medial pterygoid, and, perhaps, the superior head of the lateral pterygoid muscles) once initial tooth contact occurs. Periodontal receptors are also involved in the sudden cessation of chewing that occurs when the teeth strike a hard object in a food bolus such as a piece of bone or grit, a nociceptive reflex. Some experimental evidence suggests that periodontal receptors can initiate a jaw opening reflex (Hannam and Matthews, 1969). This seems to be an important mechanism when the teeth contact a hard, foreign object during chewing, and involves pain receptors as well as mechanoreceptors.

Periodontal receptors also seem to be involved in initiating the so-called silent period in the jaw-closing muscles after tooth contact. The silent period is a brief (5 to 60 ms) disappearance of electromyographic activity in the contracted elevator muscles that occurs at the point of tooth contact in both humans and experimental animals (Ahlgren, 1969). It may be preceded by a brief excitatory period in the same muscles, which probably involves a monosynaptic reflex and is thought to be initiated by periodontal mechanoreceptors (Goldberg, 1971; Sessle and Schmitt, 1972). The silent period immediately precedes the onset of the jaw-opening reflex (Yemm, 1972a), and may represent a period of neurologic rest It is important to note that other, nonperiodontal receptors may also induce both a monosynaptic reflex and the silent period (Dubner et al., 1978). This fact may help to explain why the silent period remains relatively normal in the absence of a true periodontium in edentulous patients whose mouths have been restored using osseointegrated dental implants (Haraldson and Ingervall, 1979). The silent period is discussed further in chapters 7 and 8.

In addition to inhibiting the jaw-closing reflex and initiating the monosynaptic reflex and silent period, periodontal mechanoreceptors may also help to limit the maximal clenching force that can be developed between antagonistic teeth (Van Steenberghe and deVries, 1978a and b). Receptors in other locations, such as the TMJ, may also be important to this limiting. In experimental trials with humans, the maximal clenching force increases progressively with repeated successive clenchings. This would suggest that, as the tooth is intruded into its socket and the viscoelastic periodontium is deformed, the periodontal mechanoreceptors become progressively less sensitive, permitting larger clenching forces to develop. This adaptive mechanism may have clinical significance in parafunctional activities such as bruxism, when it may permit forces that are potentially destructive for periodontium and tooth structure to develop.

Periodontal receptors can also modify the path of mandibular closure, although the exact mechanism is not completely understood. If, for example, a premature tooth contact develops in a patient's occlusion, periodontal receptors associated with the affected tooth may mediate an alteration in the closing pattern in order to avoid the prematurity.

Response to physiological occlusal forces

As indicated above, both vertical and horizontal forces of occlusion are absorbed largely by the displacement of blood and fluids to nonloaded regions of the ligament and through foramina in the alveolar bone. Clearly, some accompanying distortion of the alveolar bone must also occur, depending upon the intensity and duration of the applied forces. Force removal results in alveolar bone recoiling to its preloaded position and fluid returning to the ligament space.

Histologically, the character of the tissues of

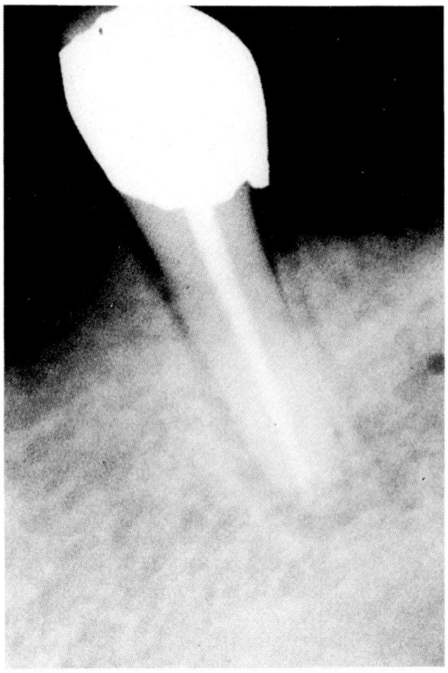

Fig. 5-11 Radiograph of a premolar in hyperfunction. Widening of the periodontal ligament space mesially can be seen.

the periodontium reflects the amount of force currently being applied to the teeth. Noticeable changes occur in these tissues with a significant increase or decrease in occlusal forces. If occlusal forces are increased above normal but within physiologic limits (hyperfunction), for example following the placement of an inadequately carved amalgam restoration, there can be as much as a 50% increase in ligament width, and an accompanying increase in ligament collagen density. The bony trabeculae supporting the alveolar bone also increase in number and thickness, which can be manifested as sclerotic changes in and around the lamina dura. Some of these changes can be observed in radiographs (Fig. 5-11). Conversely, a reduction in occlusal forces (hypofunction), as occurs following the reduction or removal of opposing teeth, results in opposite changes: significant thinning of the periodontal ligament, reduction in ligament collagen density, and decrease in number and thickness of supporting bony trabeculae.

Summary

The specialized tissue components of the periodontium, together with its innervations, underscore the versatile role of this attachment mechanism. Among the important functions are absorbing occlusal forces, permitting adaptive tooth involvement, and providing neurosensory input to the central nervous system. Because of the influence of the periodontal receptors on masticatory muscle activity, and hence on occlusal function, special emphasis has been given to the neurosensory role of the periodontium.

Chapter 6

The Temporomandibular Joint

Norman D. Mohl

The temporomandibular joint (TMJ) is the freely movable (diarthrodial) articulation between the condyle of the mandible and squamous portion of the temporal bone. It is a true synovial joint, and it has much in common with the other synovial joints of the body. However, it does possess certain unique developmental, anatomical, and functional characteristics that distinguish it from most other joints of this type. For example, it is the only joint system with a rigid end point of closure—specifically, the calcified occlusal surfaces of the teeth. The nature of the occlusion may, therefore, influence the joint's function. Also, since the left and right condyles are part of the same movable mandible, the TMJ of one side cannot function without movement of the contralateral joint. The term *craniomandibular joint,* or *articulation,* is sometimes used to emphasize this bilateralness (DuBrul, 1980).

The TMJ is a complex articulation. An articular disk completely divides the joint space into separate superior and inferior compartments. Functionally, it may be classified as a hinge joint with a sliding socket. A hinge (ginglymus) movement predominates in the inferior compartment between the condyle and disk, while a sliding (arthrodial, gliding, translatory) movement predominates in the superior compartment between the disk and the articular eminence of the temporal bone. Typically, it is the only joint that can be dislocated without extrinsic forces acting upon it (Gardner et al., 1963).

Unlike most synovial joints, the articular surfaces of the TMJ are not composed of hyaline cartilage. These surfaces, as well as the central portion of the articular disk, consist of a nerve-free, nonvascular dense fibrous connective tissue (Moffett, 1962; Hylander, 1979b; Öberg and Carlsson, 1979; DuBrul, 1980). Areas with a few cartilage cells surrounded by a scanty cartilage matrix may often be found in the dense fibrous connective tissue, particularly in older joints. Such articular areas are termed *fibrocartilage.* The unique histologic features of the TMJ are to a large extent related to its distinctive embryology, which, in turn, is directly related to the specific evolutionary processes that led to the appearance of the TMJ in mammals (see chapter 2).

Development of the temporomandibular joint

Temporomandibular joint components

As if to reflect its late appearance in evolution, the TMJ develops very late in embryonic life (Symons, 1952; Macalister, 1955; Moffett, 1957, 1962, 1966; Furstman, 1963; Yuodelis, 1966). In a 7-week-old human embryo, the elbow, hip, knee, and shoulder joints are already well along in development while the TMJ is barely making its initial appearance (Moffett, 1966). At this stage, Meckel's cartilage is present as a cartilaginous bar from the region of the future chin to the area of the future middle ear. It serves as a temporary reinforcement of the first

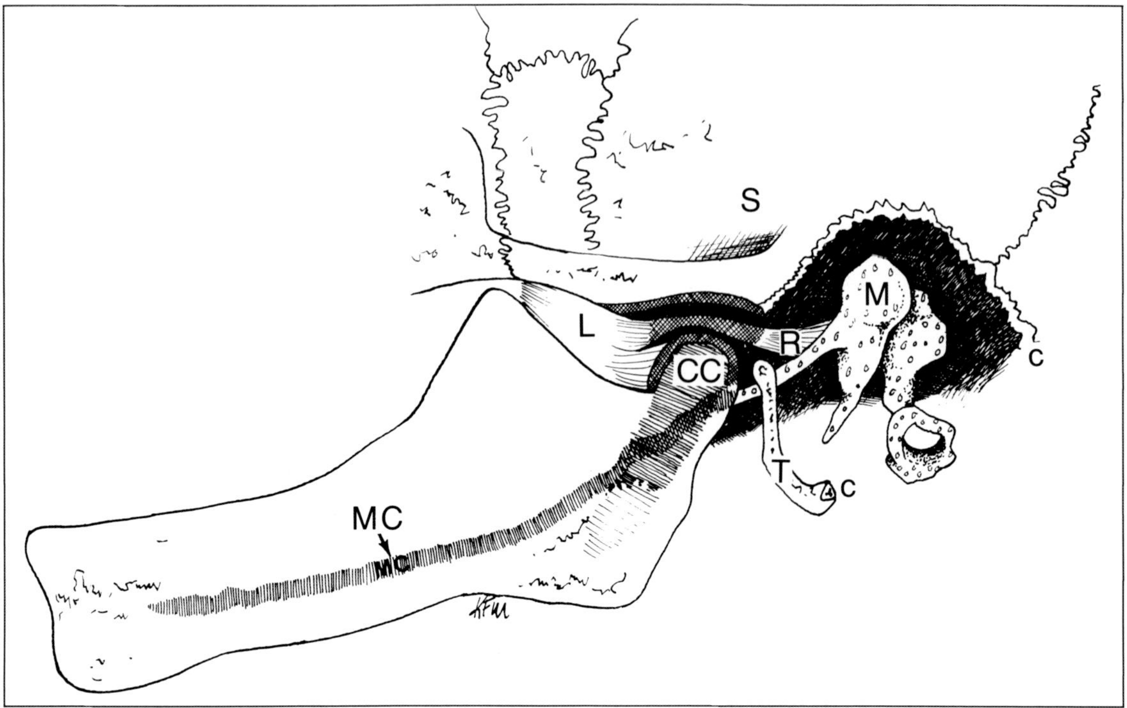

Fig. 6-1 Composite schematic drawing of major structures involved in the development of the TMJ, with cut areas *(c)* to reveal the ossicles in the middle ear cavity. Note Meckel's cartilage *(MC)* located medial to the developing mandible and continuous with the malleus *(M)*; the developing tympanic *(T)* and squamous *(S)* parts of the temporal bone; and part of the tendon of the lateral pterygoid muscle *(L)* continuous with the articular disk, the retrodiscal ligament *(R)*, and the malleus. Cross-hatched areas represent the dense fibrous connective tissue comprising the disk and the articular layers over the condyle and articular eminence. The condylar cartilage *(CC)* is located under the condylar articular tissue and shows a zone of erosion inferiorly where the cartilage is being replaced by bone.

branchial arch. Its posterior end serves as a temporary hinge articulation between the developing mandible and the cranium. This temporary joint is homologous with the premammalian articular-quadrate jaw joint.

After the principal structures of the TMJ are formed (12 weeks), most of Meckel's cartilage disappears. Its posterior portion, however, becomes, from anterior to posterior, the sphenomandibular ligament, the anterior ligament of the malleus, and the malleus. Thus, the temporary jaw joint loses its association with the mandible and becomes incorporated into the mammalian middle ear as the incudomalleolar joint (Fig. 6-1).

The bony components of typical hyaline cartilage synovial joints have a primary cartilage model and develop by endochondral ossification. However, the mandible (dentary bone) and squamous and tympanic parts of the temporal bone are membrane bones without primary cartilage precursors. Although the developing condyle contains cartilage, it is considered to be secondary cartilage because it originates within the local mesenchymal condylar blastema and not as part of the original, or primary, cartilage basicranium or branchial arches. And unlike primary cartilage, it does not function as a principal determinant of the amount and direction of growth. Rather, it functions more passively as a response to growth conditions determined elsewhere. Thus, as the mandible is carried inferiorly and anteriorly within the developing craniofacial complex, the condyle, with its secondary "growth" cartilage, grows adaptively superiorly and posteriorly in order to maintain an optimal relationship to the developing temporal squama.

Also unlike the components of typical hyaline cartilage synovial joints, which develop from a single continuous blastema, the mandibular and temporal components develop separately and then approach each other—not unlike the dentary meeting the squamosum during its evolution. This situation does not produce the counterpressure on the intervening mesenchyme that is believed to be responsible for the progressive chondrification of articular structures in hyaline cartilage synovial joints (Whillis, 1940). Thus, the intervening mesenchyme develops into dense fibrous articular tissue as the mandibular condyle grows superiorly toward the temporal bone.

In its early stage of development, the tendon of the lateral pterygoid muscle runs through the future joint area and inserts on the posterior portion of Meckel's cartilage that will become the malleus. As the condyle and temporal squama develop and move toward one another, the developing lateral pterygoid tendon becomes entrapped within the joint and contributes to the formation of the articular disk (Harpman and Woollard, 1938). As a result, the articular disk is also composed of dense fibrous connective tissue, as is the articular tissue over the temporal squama and that over the mandibular condyle.

As development continues, the condylar cartilage becomes replaced by bone until, at birth, a thin layer of cartilage remains over the bony condyle and under the dense fibrous connective tissue articular layer. During prenatal development and postnatal growth of the condyle, no secondary center of ossification appears in this cartilage. Thus, there is no typical bony epiphysis or cartilaginous epiphyseal plate in the developing condyle as one would expect to find in growing long bones. Consequently, clinical radiographs of the TMJ cannot be used to assess whether growth potential is still present in the condyle. Based on postmortem histologic evidence, it is believed that the last remnant of the original condylar cartilage disappears sometime after 16 to 17 years of age (Wright and Moffett, 1974).

Temporomandibular joint–otological relationships

It has been claimed that, because of the common development of the TMJ and certain middle ear structures, a permanent physical connection is maintained between these areas in the adult—that problems of the joint may be manifested in the ear. It has been claimed that the disk-to-malleus relationship is retained in adults and that movement of the articular disk will cause the malleus, incus, stapes, and tympanic membrane to move (Pinto, 1962). However, more recent evidence reveals that such movement cannot occur (Coleman, 1970; Marshall, 1975; Komori et al., 1986). One relationship of interest is the innervation of the tensor tympani muscle by the mandibular division of the trigeminal nerve—there is some evidence that clenching of the teeth will be accompanied by contraction of this muscle (Djupesland, 1967). The tensor tympani muscle, which attaches to the malleus, is a rudimentary muscle of mastication, having been involved in movement of the premammalian jaw joint. However, despite these anatomical relationships, any use of this information to attempt to explain subjective clinical otologic symptoms is entirely speculative. Only otolgia (ear pain) referred from masticatory structures, including the TMJ, can be explained on the basis of common sensory innervation of the two areas.

Gross structure and function

Condyle

The condyle is generally convex in the frontal plane and strongly convex in the parasagittal

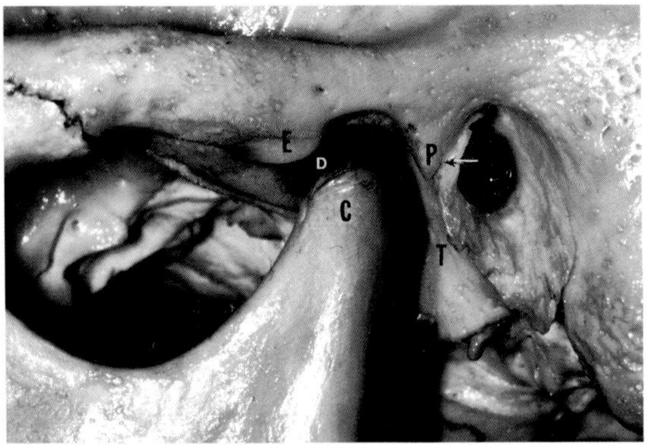

Fig. 6-2 Lateral view of skull showing condyle *(C)*, articular eminence *(E)*, articular disk *(D)*, postglenoid process *(P)*, tympanic plate *(T)*, and squamotympanic fissure *(arrow)*. The mandible has been placed in centric occlusion. Note the position of the condyle and disk relative to the articular eminence and glenoid fossa.

plane. Its adult anteroposterior dimension averages 0.8 to 1.0 cm; mediolaterally it is about twice this dimension. It is not symmetrical. The medial pole of this semicylindrical body projects well beyond the medial surface of the ramus, while the lateral pole extends only slightly laterally. A shallow concavity, the pterygoid fovea, is located on the anteromedial aspect of the mandibular neck. It is here that the inferior head and most fibers of the superior head of the lateral pterygoid muscle insert on the mandible (DuBrul, 1980; Mahan et al., 1983; Meyenberg et al., 1986). When the mandible is in the maximum intercuspal position (centric occlusion), the articular surface of the condyle faces the posterior slope of the articular eminence rather than the deepest portion of the mandibular (glenoid) fossa. That the condyle does not articulate within the depth of the fossa is often misunderstood when one examines a dry skull with wire springs attaching the mandible to the cranium. A more accurate relationship of condyle to temporal bone may be seen after removal of these wires by, assuming there are occludable posterior teeth, holding the mandible in the position of maximum intercuspation (Fig. 6-2).

There is a large degree of variation among human condyles, both in shape and in the angle at which the condyle is related to the ramus of the mandible (Yale et al., 1966). In any individual, the left condyle may not have the same form as the right condyle. The long axis between the medial and lateral poles of each condyle are generally perpendicular to the plane of the ramus and, because the rami diverge posteriorly in the human mandible, the axes of both sides are not parallel. They form an obtuse angle of around 145° to 160° when projected medially and posteriorly (Hylander, 1979b; DuBrul, 1980) (Figs. 6-3a and b).

Thus, conventional radiographs of the TMJ must be taken with an oblique projection in order to attempt to obtain an undistorted anteroposterior view of condylar form and position. The most commonly employed conventional technique is called lateral transcranial radiography, and involves a projection whereby the central beam is directed toward the film-side condyle from about 5 cm *above* and 2.5 cm *behind* the opposite external acoustic meatus (Blaschke and White, 1979). It should be noted, however, that this radiographic technique only depicts the superior surface of the most lateral aspect of the bony condyle (Weinberg, 1973; Omnell, 1980). This technique is not a reliable method to assess the relative amount of "joint space" between the condyle and fossa (Fig. 6-4).

Articular disk

The articular disk is a firm but flexible structure that will accommodate to the incongruities that exist between the shape of the articular surface of

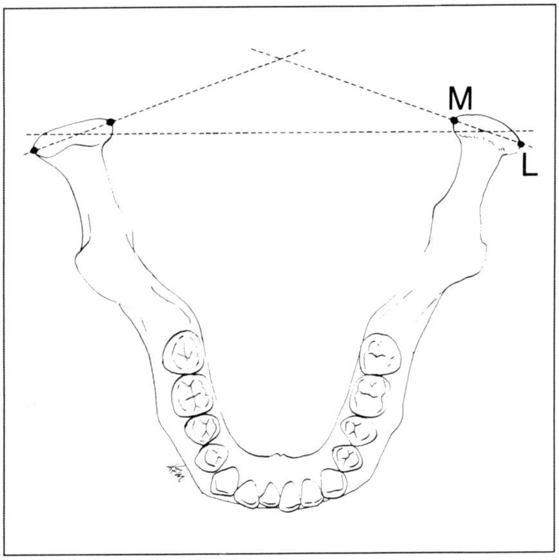

Fig. 6-3a *(left)* Note that lines projected through the lateral *(L)* and medial *(M)* poles of the condyle meet medially and posteriorly at an obtuse angle of 145° to 160°. The lateral pole lies anterior to, and the medial pole posterior to, the intercondylar transverse axis.

Fig. 6-3b *(below)* On mandibular opening, the lateral pole moves inferiorly and posteriorly relative to this axis *(rod)*, whereas the medial pole moves superiorly and anteriorly. The opposite occurs during mandibular closure.

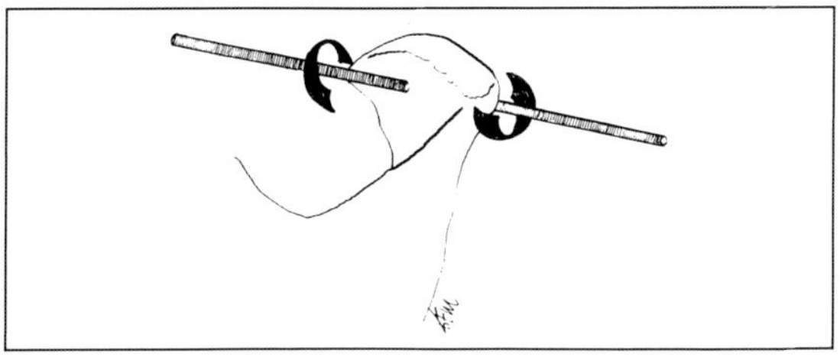

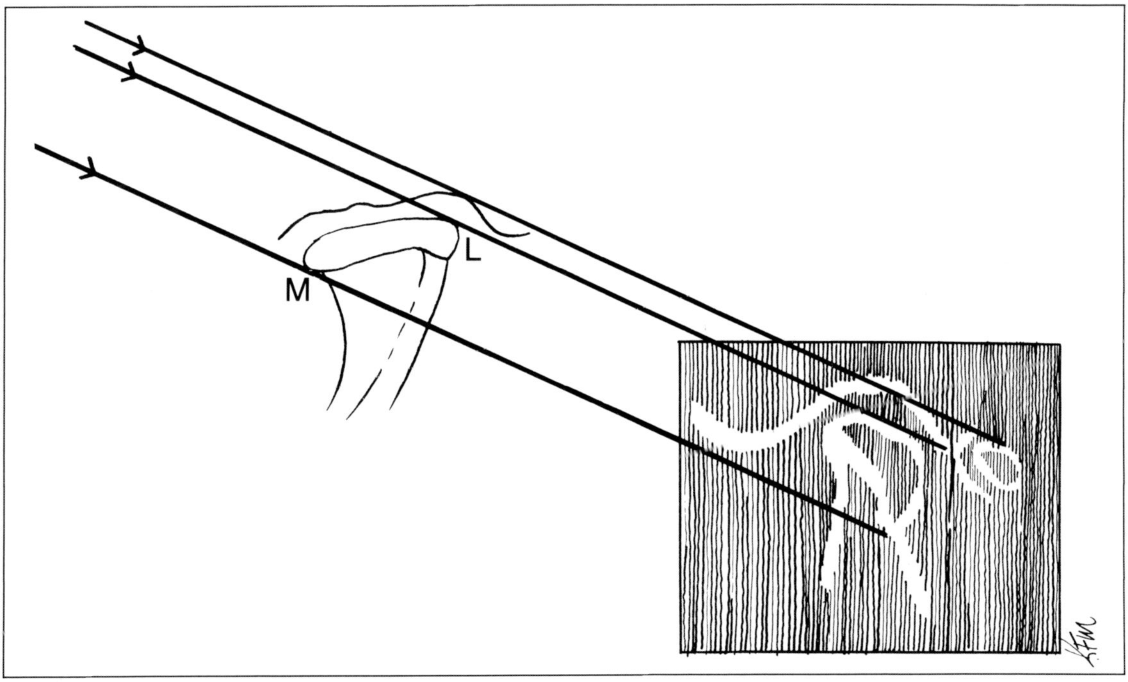

Fig. 6-4 Schematic drawing illustrating angulation of transcranial radiograph beam (on left) passing through the TMJ and being projected onto a simulated radiographic film (on right). Note the location of the area above the lateral pole *(L)* and the relative location of the medial pole *(M)* on the radiograph. Slight changes in the radiographic angulations can change the relative size of the "joint space" on the radiograph. (Adapted from Weinberg, 1973, and Omnell, 1980.)

the condyle and that of the articular eminence. It will change its shape and position relative to these structures during condylar movement. While the disk merges with the joint capsule around its periphery, it is firmly and independently attached to the condyle at its medial and lateral poles. A layer (lamina) of collagen fibers from the inferior-posterior area of the disk to the posterior surface of the condyle provides another definitive attachment. The disk is not directly attached to the temporal bone. Thus, it will move with the condyle as the latter translates in relation to the articular eminence. Posteriorly, the disk is contiguous with the loosely organized structure called the retrodiscal pad. Although most of the superior head of the lateral pterygoid muscle attaches directly to the condyle, there is some secondary attachment to the fused capsule and disk anteromedially.

The central area of the disk, sometimes referred to as the intermediate zone, is thinner than its periphery (Rees, 1954). It is through this area that the condyle normally exerts pressure against the articular eminence. The thickest part of the disk is the posterior border or band that typically envelops the most superior portion of the condyle when the mandible is in the intercuspal position.

Articular eminence

The articular eminence runs obliquely from the posterior root of the zygomatic arch to the medial aspect of the joint. It is strongly convex anteroposteriorly, and slightly concave mediolaterally. The posterior slope of the eminence is much steeper than the gradual slope anterior to the crest of the eminence; the latter is referred to as the *preglenoid plane*. During closing, muscular activity will pull the condyle/disk superiorly and posteriorly along this slippery incline toward centric relation. During voluntary wide opening of the mouth, the condyle will move to the height of the crest of the eminence and, in most healthy individuals, will go well anterior to the crest (Ricketts, 1950; Sheppard and Sheppard, 1965; Wooten, 1966). Thus, in the absence of symptoms, such movement should not be regarded as pathological or dysfunctional.

Because of the convexity of the articular eminence, the condyles must move inferiorly in a curvilinear path as they translate anteriorly during protrusion of the mandible. For the same reason, the nonworking side condyle moves anteriorly, medially, and inferiorly during lateral excursion of the mandible. This helps to disclude the posterior teeth during protrusion and the nonworking side teeth during lateral excursion—the so-called *Christensen phenomenon*. This inferior and anterior inclination can be recorded, and is referred to as the *condylar inclination*.

It is obvious that the condylar inclination of an individual will depend on the height and convexity of the articular eminence. But there is no positive evidence to indicate that the form of the eminence is directly related to specific occlusal relationships (Angel, 1948; Ricketts, 1950; Moffett, 1962). Because the articular eminence is not very evident at birth, and, in many children, is not fully developed during the first decade of life, the condylar inclination may be relatively shallow while the primary and early mixed dentitions are present. Thus, disclusion of the primary molars and permanent first molars may be less likely to occur during mandibular protrusive and lateral movements. Along with bruxism and minimal anterior guidance, this may explain why the occlusion of the primary molars may become flattened prior to exfoliation, and, as is observed in many 7-year-old children, the permanent first molar may be worn flat within 1 year after it has erupted (Ricketts, 1966).

Mandibular fossa

The mandibular fossa is the concave area bounded medially by a narrow bony wall, anteriorly by the posterior slope of the articular eminence, and posteriorly by the postglenoid process, or tubercle. The postglenoid process is an inferior extension of the temporal squama directly posterior to the most lateral part of the fossa and anterior to the opening into the external acoustic meatus. The tympanic plate lies posteriorly to this process and the rest of the mandibular fossa lies medially. It meets the squamosum at the squamotympanic fissure, which runs mediolaterally behind the depth of the fossa. In its medial portion, a small fingerlike projection of the petrous portion of the temporal bone may be seen in the fissure. Thus, the medial part of the squamotympanic fissure becomes further divided into a petrosquamosal fissure anterior to and a petrotympanic fissure posterior to this small projection.

The chorda tympani nerve and the anterior tympanic artery and vein pass through the petrotympanic fissure. This fissure is well posterior to the boundaries of the mandibular fossa and attachment of the posterior joint capsule; the chorda tympani nerve and accompanying blood vessels are *not* within the anatomical or functional confines of the TMJ and are well protected from any impingement by the condyle. As in the case of the condyle and articular eminence, much morphologic variation exists with regard to the mandibular fossa (Ricketts, 1950). The roof of the fossa is thin, frequently translucent to light, and not built to withstand loading from the condyle (Hylander, 1979b). The postglenoid process is also nonarticulating in humans (DuBrul, 1980). The joint capsule attaches to its entire anterior surface, and a portion of the retrodiscal pad is interposed between it and the condyle. Thus, the condyle does not normally make contact with the postglenoid process even during complete retrusion of the mandible (DuBrul, 1980).

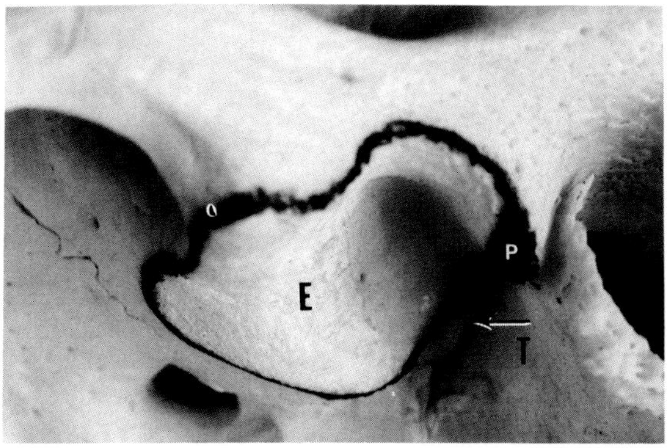

Fig. 6-5 The attachment of the articular capsule drawn on the temporal bone. Note that it encompasses the entire articular eminence *(E)*. Posteriorly it attaches to the tip and anterior surface of the postglenoid process *(P)*, and to the anterior lip of the squamotympanic and petrosquamosal fissures. It does not have a primary attachment to the tympanic plate *(T)*. The petrotympanic fissure *(arrow)* with its exiting chorda tympanic nerve is outside the anatomical and functional limits of the TMJ.

Articular capsule

As in any synovial joint, the capsule defines the anatomical and functional boundaries of the TMJ. The rather thin, relatively loose fibrous articular capsule surrounds the articular surface of the condyle and blends with the periosteum of the mandibular neck. It attaches separately just below the attachments of the articular disk, at the medial and lateral poles of the condyle. On the temporal bone, the articular capsule completely surrounds the eminence, and is well anterior to its crest. Laterally, it adheres to a small bony elevation, the articular tubercle, on the outside of the root of the zygomatic process, and runs along the lateral edge of the eminence, mandibular fossa, and postglenoid process. Posteriorly, it attaches to the tip and anterior surface of the postglenoid process and extends medially along the raised anterior lip of the squamotympanic and petrosquamosal fissures. Its medial attachment runs along the sphenosquamosal suture. Anteromedially it is not a discrete structure, since it is in this area that some fibers of the superior head of the lateral pterygoid muscle attach to the fused capsule and disk.

From this description it can be seen that the area enclosed by the joint capsule belongs entirely to the squamous portion of the temporal bone, and that the tympanic portion lies completely posterior to the joint (Fig. 6-5). Thus, Moffett (1962) has noted that the tympanic part of the temporal bone "can be dissected away without destroying the integrity of the joint and without opening the joint capsule."

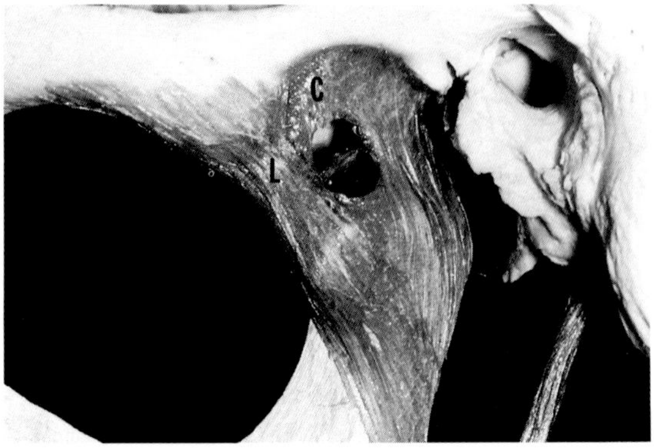

Fig. 6-6 Lateral view of TMJ showing joint capsule *(C)* and superficial oblique fibers of the TM ligament *(L)*. A hole has been cut through the capsule and ligament.

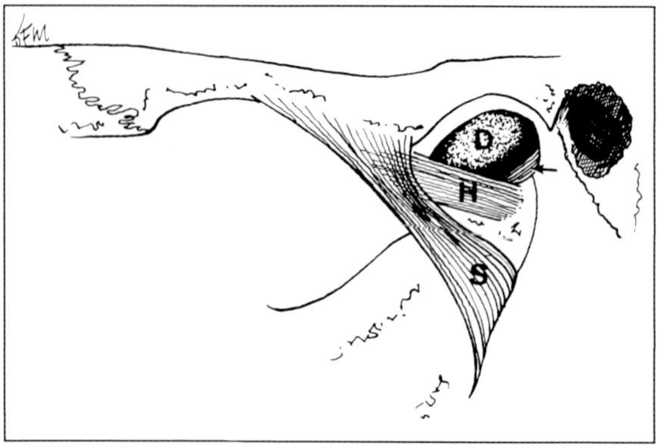

Fig. 6-7 Schematic drawing of lateral view of TMJ illustrating superficial oblique fibers of the TM ligament *(S)*, and its deeper horizontal band *(H)* attaching to the lateral pole *(arrow)*, and to the posterolateral part of the articular disk *(D)*. (Adapted from DuBrul, 1980.)

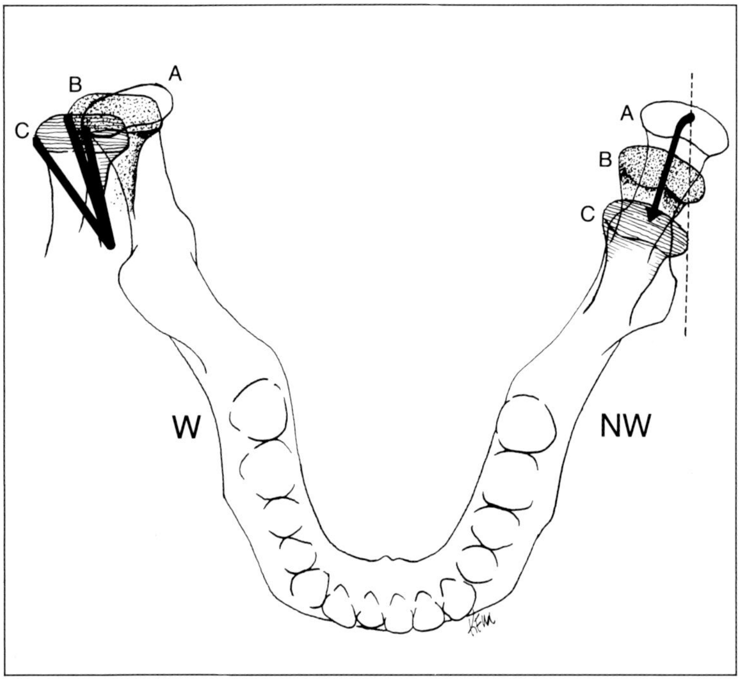

Fig. 6-8 Schematic drawing illustrating effect of the horizontal fibers of the TM ligament on the working side *(W)* condyle during lateral excursion. As the nonworking side *(NW)* is pulled anteriorly and inward by its lateral pterygoid muscle from positions *A* to *B* to *C*, the working side condyle attempts to rotate around a vertical axis. However, the attachment of the TM ligament to the lateral pole of the condyle "checks" the posterior movement of this pole as the condyle moves from position *A* to *B*. Continued lateral excursion occurs as the working side condyle, and thus the entire mandible, moves laterally to position C under the passive restraining influence of the TM ligament (the Bennett movement). The medial contour of the nonworking side TMJ permits the side shift to occur. (Adapted from DuBrul, 1980.)

Temporomandibular ligament

The articular capsule is reinforced laterally by the TM (lateral) ligament. A comparable reinforcement is not present on the medial side of each joint. According to DuBrul (1980), the TM ligament is composed of a superficial fan-shaped layer of obliquely oriented collagen fibers and a deeper, narrow band of such fibers that runs in a more horizontal direction. The superficial portion attaches broadly to the outer surface of the root of the zygomatic arch and converges to attach to the condyle inferior to and posterior to its lateral pole. The deeper band joins the articular tubercle to the lateral condylar pole and posterolateral portion of the articular disk (DuBrul, 1980) (Figs. 6-6 and 6-7). It deserves to be noted that a preliminary report by Savalle (1984) suggests that this ligament may not exist as a discrete structure in some TMJs.

The principal biomechanical function of the TM ligament, acting singly or with its contralateral mate, is to "check" or limit movements of the condyle-disk complex. One such function is to limit retrusion of the condyle against retrocondylar structures. With relaxation of the lateral pterygoid muscle it is possible to retrude the mandible to a position which, in most people, is slightly posterior to the intercuspal position. This most retruded position has been referred to as the *ligamentous position* of the mandible because it is thought to be determined by the left and right TM ligaments (Brill et al., 1959). Because further retrusion is not permitted beyond this position, it is regarded as a border position of the mandible. As such, it is reproducible, recordable, and not much influenced by transient postural factors (Posselt, 1952). When the mandible is placed in this position by posteriorly directed *external* forces, the condyles and disks may not always be seated superiorly and anteriorly against the posterior slope of their articular eminences. Therein lies much difficulty in attempting to define the term *centric relation*.

Centric relation of the mandible is a position often used in therapy. This position implies that both condyles and their normally positioned disks are located superiorly in the fossae while still maintaining contact with the posterior slopes of the articular eminences. Centric relation can thus be defined as "the most superior position of the mandibular condyles with the central bearing area of the disk in contact with the articular surface of the condyle and the articular eminence" (Gilboe, 1983). The horizontal fibers of the TM ligaments may or may not be "taut" in this position. If they are, centric relation will also be a ligamentous retruded border position. If not, slight further retrusion behind centric relation will be possible when the mandible is pushed posteriorly. *Thus, centric relation may or may not be the same as the ligamentous position.*

Mandibular movement

The mandible can be guided to open and close for a short distance with a retruded hinge movement, the tranverse axis of the hinge running approximately through both condyles (DuBrul, 1980). If one were to depress the mandible in a hinge movement in this manner, opening would only proceed until an average distance of around 19 mm existed between the posterior teeth (Posselt, 1952). Continued opening on this hinge would cause the mandible to infringe upon the vital submandibular and retromandibular structures of the neck. This is of particular importance in humans because of our erect posture and vertically placed vertebral column. Such a continued hinge movement is prevented by the TM ligaments, an adaptation that appears to be unique in humans (Burch and Lundeen, 1971). Thus, the human mandible, even when guided, cannot open all the way purely with a hinge movement. Forward translation of the condyles must occur in order to depress the mandible to its full extent (Posselt, 1952) (see chapter 9).

When the mandible is moved along a border pathway into lateral excursion, the condyle on the working side twists slightly on its disk as it attempts to rotate around a vertical axis located slightly posterior to the condyle. However, because of the insertion of the TM ligament at the lateral pole of the condyle, this pole is limited in its attempt to rotate posteriorly (Fig. 6-8). As explained by DuBrul (1980), in order for lateral excursion to continue, the working side condyle, and thus the entire mandible, must move laterally under the passive restraining influence of the TM ligament on the working side. This side shift, or *Bennett movement,* although influenced by the working side TM ligament and permitted by the medial contour of the nonworking side joint, is actually produced by activity of the lateral pterygoid muscle of the nonworking side (DuBrul and Menekratis, 1981).

The Bennett movement may be defined as the side shift of the mandible toward the working side during lateral excursion. During lateral excursion, the nonworking side condyle moves anteriorly, inferiorly, and medially. The medial movement can be recorded and is seen to form an angle with a parasagittal plane. This is referred to as the *condylar angulation,* or *Bennett angle.* A large angle will be related to a large Bennett shift during lateral excursion; a small angle will be associated with little or no side shift.

The TM ligament also serves to prevent the condyle from being displaced away from the articular eminence, a situation that is only possible under certain extreme circumstances (Hylander, 1979b). Thus, this ligament is the final restraining influence on condyle/disk movement in a variety of mandibular border positions.

Two accessory ligaments are associated with the TMJ. One is the sphenomandibular ligament, which attaches on and around the lingula of the mandibular ramus inferiorly and to the spine of the sphenoid and the squamotympanic and petrotympanic fissure areas superiorly. The stylomandibular ligament, a portion of the deep cervical fascia, attaches around the angle of the mandible and medial pterygoid fascia and runs superiorly and posteriorly to the styloid process. These ligaments appear to have little or no significant biomechanical influence on mandibular movements or position (DuBrul, 1980). Another accessory ligament, the medial retrodiscal ligament, attaches the most medial portion of the disk to the most medial area of the squamotympanic fissure. It is composed of fibroelastic tissue and is a remnant of the diskomalleolar band, which connected the lateral ptyergoid tendon to the malleus in fetal life (Harpman and Woollard, 1938; Rees, 1954).

Histologic structure and function

Articular tissue

As already noted, the articular tissues of the TMJ are composed of dense fibrous connective tissue and/or fibrocartilage—not hyaline cartilage (Figs. 6-9 and 6-10). The reason for this is based on unique developmental characteristics and certain functional advantages. Hyaline cartilage is uniquely constructed to withstand compressive and torsional loading; it is less able to withstand shearing forces (Moss, 1966). Dense fibrous connective tissue, on the other hand, can tolerate shearing forces much better than compressive forces. Under normal circumstances, with a full complement of teeth and no excessive muscular activity, shearing forces probably predominate over compression forces in the human TMJ. Thus, under optimal conditions, dense fibrous connective tissue is the appropriate functional tissue for the TMJ.

Biomechanics

The fact that the articular tissues of the TMJ are composed of dense fibrous connective tissue instead of hyaline cartilage once led observers to claim that it is not a "weight-bearing" joint and that no compressive loading occurs, even under ideal conditions (Robinson, 1946). However, research has shown that such claims are not correct. As in all diarthrodial joints, the musculature pulls across the joint (DuBrul and Menekratis, 1981). Even the oblique or horizontal alignment of the middle and posterior fibers of the temporalis muscles produce forces that are mostly superior, since its fibers bend around the root of the zygomatic process before inserting on and around the coronoid process. As Sicher and DuBrul (1975) have stated, "Only their direction below this pulley is significant" (Fig. 6-11).

Furthermore, there is ample evidence to indicate that the human mandible functions within the constraints of a Class III lever system and that forces produced by muscle contraction result in

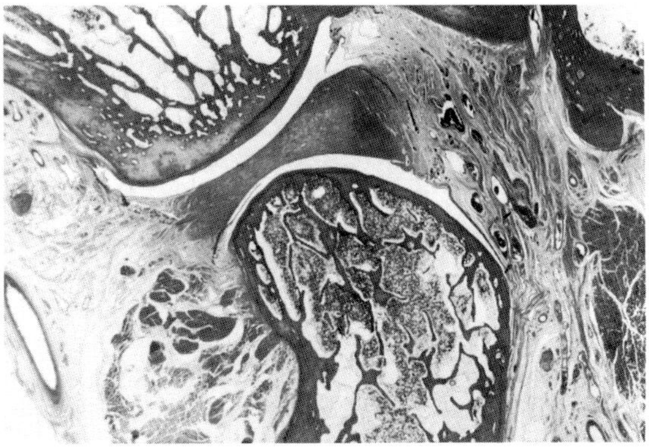

Fig. 6-9 Parasagittal section of TMJ from a 67-year-old male with a complete natural dentition. Note the condyle and articular eminence with the biconcave articular disk interposed. The retrodiscal pad, with its loose connective tissue and large blood-filled spaces, is seen to attach to the posterior part of the disk anteriorly, to the posterior aspect of the condyle inferiorly, to the joint capsule posteriorly, and to a part of the surface of the mandibular fossa superiorly. Forces within the joint produced by muscular activity are located between the condyle, disk, and eminence, which are best suited to withstand and adapt to such forces.

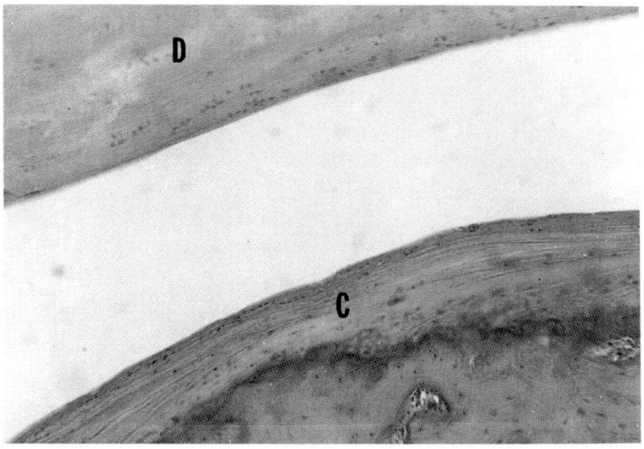

Fig. 6-10 Unlike most synovial joints, the TMJ is composed of dense fibrous connective tissue and not hyaline cartilage. This avascular, noninnervated connective tissue covers the articular eminence and the condyle *(C)*, and comprises the central load-bearing area of the articular disk *(D)*.

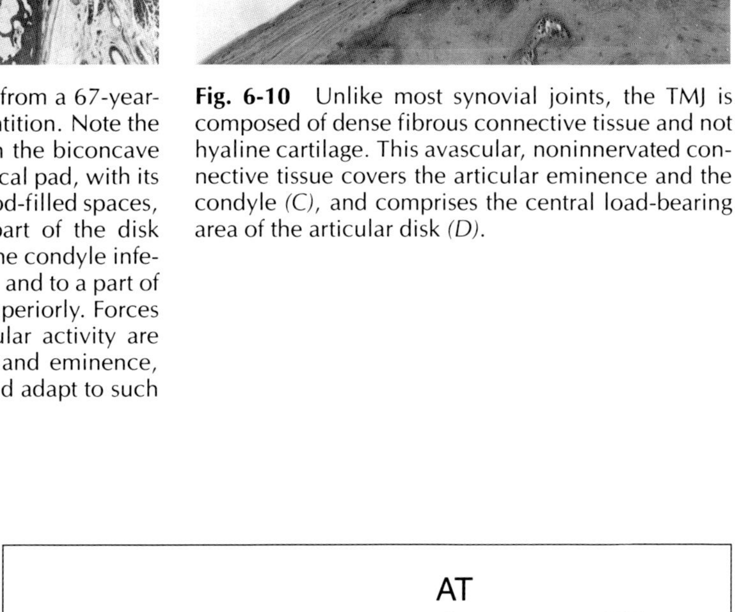

Fig. 6-11 Relative position of the vectors produced on the mandible by the muscles of mastication: lateral pterygoid *(LP)*; anterior border of masseter *(M)*; anterior border of medial pterygoid *(MP)*; anterior fibers of temporalis *(AT)*; and posterior fibers of temporalis *(PT)* with its effective pull in a posterior and superior direction. Note that all muscle pull (force) is between the dentition (resistance) and the condyle (fulcrum), creating a Class III lever system. In this biomechanical system, muscular force is always shared between the dentition and the joint. The amount of sharing, however, depends upon relative distances from the force. Thus, more force can be applied to the first molars relative to the condyles and central incisors. Likewise, less force can be applied to the central incisors relative to the condyles and first molars.

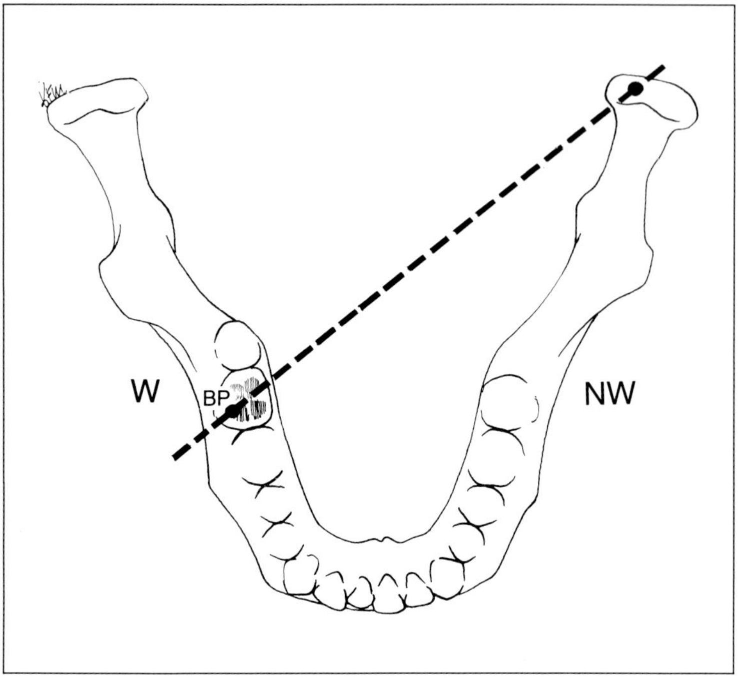

Fig. 6-12 In lateral excursion, the mandible may be regarded as a loaded bent beam with the axis of the beam *(interrupted line)* running between the bitepoint *(BP)* on the working side *(W)* to the condyle on the nonworking side *(NW)*. Thus, the nonworking side condyle is loaded in lateral excursion. The working side condyle will also be loaded if the total vectors of muscle contraction are *posterior to* the axis of the beam, which they are, under most circumstances. Should such vectors be applied anterior to the axis, as when the bitepoint is moved distally to the third, and possibly second, molar, the working side condyle will be "distracted" away from its articular eminence. (Adapted from Walker, 1978.)

loads both on the dentition and within the joint (Barbenel, 1969; DuBrul, 1980; Hylander, 1975, 1979b) (Fig. 6-11). Indirect analyses and direct measurements of these loading phenomena have been accomplished in primates and humans (Hekneby, 1974; Roydhouse, 1955; Hylander, 1978, 1979a; Smith, 1978; Brehnan et al., 1981; Smith et al., 1986; Ito et al., 1986). In addition, studies involving three-dimensional photoelastic stress analysis to visualize the intensity and direction of stresses within the condyle have demonstrated that stresses do occur under occlusal loads and that the stress trajectories are consistent with known trabecular patterns within the condyle (Standlee et al., 1977, 1981).

Clinical examples also illustrate that the mandibular musculature pulls the condyles up firmly against the temporal component of the joint. That the last molars will be the only teeth in occlusal contact following bilateral condylar fractures, or as condyles erode from pathologic conditions, may be explained as "experiments of nature" that only help prove the point. This phenomenon has also been demonstrated experimentally after bilateral condylectomy in rhesus monkeys (Poswillo, 1972). In a Class III lever system, any situation that would increase the resistance arm (tooth-to-TMJ distance) relative to the effort arm (muscle-to-TMJ distance) will lead to increased load at the fulcrum (TMJ). Thus, persistent occlusal forces only on incisors, such as after loss of posterior teeth, would cause the condyle to exert an increased load against the articular eminence than would be the case when biting on the molars. Similarly, the replacement of these missing posterior teeth by prosthetic appliances may reduce the magnitude of such loading. However, complete distraction of the condyle away from the articular eminence does not seem possible *once intrinsic muscular forces are applied.*

In addition, it is believed the mandible functions as a loaded beam during asymmetric occlusal positions, the axis of the beam running obliquely between the occlusal bitepoints on the working side and nonworking side condyles (Fig. 6-12). Thus, both of these areas are definitely loaded to some extent during closing muscle activity (Walker, 1978). The working side condyle would also be loaded in this model if the muscle activity vectors are *posterior* to this axis—a situation determined by the location of the bitepoint.

Theoretically, if the bitepoint is far enough back on the working side, the muscle action vectors would be exerted anterior to the axis of the loaded beam, and unloading of the working side condyle could occur. Studies in monkeys have found that the working side condyle may become unloaded during biting on the working side third molars. This condyle remains loaded, however, when occlusal forces are generated on the premolars or first and second molars (Hylander, 1979a). It has also been reported that, in humans, biting on a supracontact in the third molar area can produce an unloading and distraction of the working side condyle (Koerber, 1971; Ito et al., 1986).

Thus, while there is little question that shearing forces are a predominant feature of the TMJ, there is also sufficient evidence to indicate that the human mandible functions within the parameters of a lever system and that *the condyles are loaded to varying degrees depending on the occlusal contact position and the amount and direction of mandibular musculature contraction*. The important question is not whether the TMJ is loaded, but to what degree, that is, the frequency, duration, magnitude, direction, and location of biomechanical loading within the joint. The health of the joint will, to a large extent, depend on these forces and on the adaptive responses of the articular tissues to them.

An examination of the histologic structure of the TMJ reveals the general location of loading forces, whether shear, compression, or torsion (see Fig. 6-9). The relatively thick layer of avascular, noninnervated dense fibrous connective tissue in the central part of the articular disk, on the anterior and superior surfaces of the condyle, and on the posterior slope and crest of the articular eminence, is strong evidence that load is generated from the condyle through the central portion of the disk to the articular eminence. With increasing function, these areas of articular tissue may demonstrate the presence of chondrocytes, lacunae, and the pericellular proteoglycan characteristics of cartilage matrix.

It is generally believed that proteoglycans are responsible for the ability of articular surfaces to resist temporary compressive forces (Kempson et al., 1976). This resistance or compressive stiffness probably occurs because of the spatial arrangement of the proteoglycan-collagen network, and because of the ability of proteoglycans to imbibe and retain extracellular water by osmotic forces, thus having a "cushion" effect. The proteoglycan components apparently responsible for this are long carbohydrate chains called glycosaminoglycans (GAG). The presence and amount of GAG relative to its collagen matrix in articular tissues is a measure of the resilience of the tissue and of the location and degree of compressive loading in a joint (Matthews, 1952).

Histochemical studies have produced data concerning the topographic distribution of sulfated GAGs in human TMJs (Kopp, 1976, 1978). These substances are found to be present mostly in the articular tissues on the anterior part of the condyle, in the central portion of the articular disk, and on the articular eminence, particularly its lateral portions. Such findings are entirely consistent with our understanding of the locations of loading in the TMJ. As Kopp (1978) states, "This distribution also supports the view that the mandibular condyle articulates predominantly in the lateral part of the joint leaving the medial part of the temporal eminence relatively unloaded." The explanation for this is that the lateral pole of the condyle lies anterior to a transverse condylar rotational axis while the medial pole lies posterior to this axis. As the condyle rotates during depression of the mandible, the lateral pole, which lies in front of the axis, moves inferiorly and posteriorly as the medial pole moves superiorly and anteriorly.

The condyle and its attached disk remain in close apposition to the articular eminence during opening, albeit a shift of contact occurs from the lateral aspect to the medial aspect. During closing, the reverse occurs (see Fig. 6-3). Thus, the lateral aspect of the condyle is "closer" to the articular eminence in a closed mandibular position—a position in which the most strenuous muscular forces are expressed during mastication and bruxism. This is probably one important explanation of why GAGs and regressive remodeling predominate on the lateral aspect of the articular eminence, why the disk is thinnest laterally, and why a failure of adaptation to loading, namely degenerative joint disease (osteoarthrosis), is first seen in the lateral aspects of most TMJs (Moffett et al., 1964; Öberg et al., 1971; Hansson et al., 1977; Hansson and Öberg, 1977). It appears that shear, compressive, and torsional forces of a more persistent character would be generated on more localized areas of articular tissue in the lateral aspect of the TMJ.

It is a characteristic of articular tissues that, if a load is applied slowly or kept constant, deformation of the tissue will continue to increase in time as the fluid is squeezed out (Frankel and Nordin, 1980). Such stress concentration is curtailed in normal functional conditions in the human TMJ because of its anatomical configuration. Even slight opening and closing movement of the mandible shifts the loaded areas mediolaterally as well as anteroposteriorly between condyle, disk, and articular eminence. It seems clear that the health of the articular tissue in the TMJ is highly dependent upon *unsustained* loading, that is, on the rate and duration of which forces are applied and removed.

Other articular structures

The discussion of histologic structure so far has concentrated on the anterior portions of the joint, where the functional forces are generated. By contrast, other areas of the joint reveal much different histologic and, by implication, functional characteristics. The periphery of the articular disk, including its thickened anterior and posterior portions, is also composed of dense fibrous connective tissue. However, these areas are innervated and vascularized (Thilander, 1964; Boyer et al., 1964). The bone in the depth of the mandibular fossa is covered by a thin layer of vascularized connective tissue similar to normal periosteum. This fact, and that the bone which separates the depth of the mandibular fossa from the middle cranial fossa is very thin lamellar bone with no osteons, is strong evidence that the condyle does not exert forces directly into the depth of the fossa.

Attached to the posterior end of the disk and filling the rest of the fossa posterior to the condyle is a thick pad of specialized loose connective tissue called the *retrodiscal pad* (see Fig. 6-9). This pad attaches to the posterior joint capsule (Choukas and Sicher, 1960; Hylander, 1979b; DuBrul, 1980). The retrodiscal pad is highly innervated and contains many large blood-filled endothelium-lined spaces. It gives the disk the ability to move anteriorly with considerable freedom, and is well suited to fill the space in the fossa vacated by the condyle as it moves anteriorly (Rees, 1954; DuBrul, 1980). Even a cursory histologic examination of the retrodiscal pad will reveal that it is not designed to withstand loading of any type. Thus, it does not play a significant role in limiting posterior movement of the condyles (Parsons and Boucher, 1966).

A synovial membrane composed of a thin layer of vascularized connective tissue lines the inner surfaces of the joint capsule, the superior and inferior surfaces of the retrodiscal pad, and all surfaces not under shearing or compressive load (Hylander, 1979b). Thus, a synovial lining does *not* cover the condyle, articular eminence, or superior and inferior surfaces of the articular disk. The synovial membrane may form folds over the retrodiscal pad when the condyle and disk are retruded; this area will unfold when the disk moves anteriorly. Small projections called synovial villi may also extend into the superior and inferior joint compartments anteriorly or at other locations (see Fig. 6-9).

The function of the synovial membrane is to produce the synovial fluid within each compartment. This fluid is composed of tissue fluid with a higher concentration of hyaluronic acid, and a few cells (Moffett, 1962). Neither joint compartment contains much synovial fluid, but the small amount present functions very effectively. Its lubricating characteristics are highly efficient—friction within the joint is usually reduced to negligible levels. Synovial fluid also participates in the nutrition of the avascular articular tissues within the joint.

Blood and nerve supply

Branches of the two terminal ends of the external carotid artery, namely the maxillary and superficial temporal arteries, provide the vascular supply to the TMJ. More specifically, these are the deep auricular, anterior tympanic, and middle meningeal arteries posteromedially; the deep posterior temporals and masseteric arteries anteriorly; and other unnamed articular branches posterolaterally (Moffett, 1962). These multiple branches form an extensive capsular plexus around the joint, supplying the joint capsule, synovial membrane, retrodiscal pad, and periphery—but not the center—of the articular disk (Choukas and Sicher, 1960; Boyer et al., 1964). It is obvious that an excellent system of collateral circulation exists for the TMJ.

The nerve supply that serves the posterior, lateral, and medial portions of the joint capsule is primarily from the auriculotemporal nerve (Thilander, 1961). Accessory articular branches arise from the masseteric, deep temporal, and pterygoid nerves. The innervation is to the same areas of the joint that are vascularized (Moffett, 1962). Because all of these nerves are branches of the mandibular division of the trigeminal nerve, the innervation of this joint is in accordance with Hilton's law, which in effect states that a nerve trunk which supplies a joint also supplies its overlying skin and the muscles that move it. The position of the auriculotemporal nerve medial and posterior to the neck of the mandible prevents impingement on this important structure by the condyle, even in the most extreme border positions.

Neurosensory receptors, both free nerve endings and specialized endings, are present in the joint capsule and ligaments, particularly in the lateral and posterior aspects of the joint. These receptors also participate in the perception of pain, and, of particular significance, help to monitor both position and movement of the mandible. Thus, the neurosensory receptors associated with the TMJs acting in conjunction with muscle and intraoral receptors are important to one's perception of mandibular position. Although much is yet to be learned about the precise role of these receptors in mandibular function, there is at present convincing evidence that they do play a modulating role in cyclical movement and that they make a continuous contribution to the reflex control of mandibular movement in humans (Klineberg, 1980).

Adaptation

It has long been recognized that articular tissue has a slow turnover of its cells and intercellular ingredients throughout a lifetime, and that the underlying bone remodels as an adaptation to biomechanical needs (Moffett et al., 1964). The extent to which this occurs, if at all, in the adult TMJ is still being investigated and debated. However, in human autopsy and radiographic studies, there has been consistent evidence that adaptations occur in a great many adult TMJs (Moffett et al., 1964; Blackwood, 1966a, 1966b; Mongini, 1972, 1975; Carlsson and Öberg, 1979). Although specific etiological factors are still not completely understood, it is clear that the adult human TMJ is not an immutable structure. As with other synovial joints, it is capable of adaptation to biomechanical stresses and perhaps to metabolic requirements.

Adaptation can be accomplished by alterations in the composition of the soft articular tissues and associated metaplastic change of that tissue. It can also occur by the mechanism of remodeling. This may involve internal remodeling, which includes restructuring of osteons in the compact bone underneath the articular layers as well as reorientation of the trabecular pattern of the underlying cancellous bone. External remodeling may also occur. This involves an initial proliferation of the articular tissues accompanied by changes in the external form of the subarticular bone. As already discussed, dense fibrous connective tissue, of which collagen is the principal ingredient, is not built to withstand compressive loading very well. Thus, as such stresses are introduced from normal and/or excessive mandibular function, chondrocytes are differentiated that produce the intercellular substances typical of cartilage, specifically, sulfated GAGs. Since these substances have the ability to imbibe and retain water, it helps the articular tissue to resist the loading. The amount and proportion of GAG has also been found to be relatively stable with age, which implies that mechanical loading, rather than age, is the principal variable. The frequency and location of internal remodeling in the condyle has also been reported. Such studies also support the view that this type of adaptation is more closely related to the status of the dentition than it is to age. Likewise, studies of external remodeling, principally progressive and regressive types leading to slow changes in form of the condyle and eminence, support the idea that such adaptation is influenced not simply by age but also by the condition of the dentition and related functions of the masticatory system.

It is very important to note, however, that there are limits to any adaptive response. One cannot assume that the TMJ will always adapt to all functional, dysfunctional, or therapeutic situations. Such adaptation is slow and not necessarily predictable. Therefore, one should not depend upon this phenomenon as a way for the adult joint to "self-correct" to less than optimal therapeutic maxillomandibular relationships. The alveolar processes and periodontal supporting apparatus are much more responsive to adaptive requirements than is the TMJ. Thus, in therapy it is best to have the occlusion meet the requirements of the joint, particularly when it is healthy. Expecting the joint to meet the conditions of sustained loading may lead to osteoarthrosis.

Osteoarthrosis

Osteoarthrosis (degenerative joint disease) involves a breakdown of articular tissue with associated uncontrolled remodeling of the underlying bone. It is a noninflammatory process, although secondary inflammation in the form of a synovitis may sometimes result from the degenerating products of the disease. Osteoarthorsis is a failure to adapt to primarily local uncompensated biomechanical factors. It seems to begin in areas of local abuse where the normal nutrition of the articular tissues is compromised. Glycosaminoglycans, instead of being increased, are lost. The GAG : collagen ratio becomes less able to withstand biomechanical stresses, particularly compressive loading. Loss of the surface tangential layers, fibrillation, fissuring, and exfoliation of articular tissue occurs and may be accompanied by eburnation of the underlying bone and by an active uncompensated remodeling process.

Osteoarthritic lesions are most frequently found in the lateral portion of the TMJ. This may include perforation of the articular disk, which, when present, is almost always located in the lateral part of its thinner central area. These observations are consistent with the view that this area of the joint is subjected to the greatest load. For a more thorough discussion of this subject, the reader should review chapter 17.

Summary

This chapter has included a review of the development of the TMJ—an important subject if one is to better understand the morphology and histology of this joint. The subsequent discussion has given particular emphasis to the relationships between structure and function. A thorough knowledge of these relationships is essential if one is to fully comprehend normal anatomy and physiology, adaptive processes, and dysfunction and pathology of the TMJs.

Chapter 7

The Musculature

Willard D. McCall, Jr.

Muscle provides the prime moving force for all actions in the body. The cardiac muscle pumps blood, the gastrointestinal muscles propel the food through the digestive tract, limb muscles provide locomotion, and jaw muscles produce chewing. The importance of muscle to the human organism can scarcely be exaggerated.

Clinical problems commonly treated by dentists, such as bruxism and temporomandibular (TM) disorders, involve the mandibular musculature.

This chapter is organized into four main sections covering the muscles in general, muscles involved in mandibular function, neurosensory receptors in muscles, and electromyography and muscle activity.

Muscles in general

Muscles are usually divided into three types: *(1)* cardiac, *(2)* smooth, and *(3)* striated or skeletal. The first two are important to the function of the heart and the hollow organs; striated muscle is found in the skeletal system, and so will be the only muscle type considered here.

The purpose of muscle is to provide force. This force, depending on the load, then produces movement. The only force an individual muscle can provide is a pull, a contraction, or a tension. It cannot push, expand, or lengthen actively. To anchor the muscle and move the part of the organism it serves, skeletal muscle is anchored at each end. The end that is fixed is called the *origin* and the end that is more movable is called the *insertion*.

The color of the muscle tissue is roughly correlated with its physiological use. Muscle that is more pale or "white" is usually used for rapid or phasic movements and fatigues quickly. Darker or "red" muscle is usually used for postural or tonic activities and resists fatigue. Redness arises from the myoglobin content. The masseter and temporalis muscles, for example, are pale, have a rate of contraction among the fastest in the body, and have fatigue and enzyme properties consistent with phasic muscles (Bishop, 1982).

The muscles of mastication, however, do not fit well with the classifications developed for limb muscles (Burke et al., 1973). The jaw-closing muscles (masseter, temporalis, and medial pterygoid) have few of the powerful, high-threshold, fatigue-sensitive motor units, but instead have predominantly the low-threshold, fatigue-resistant motor units (Eriksson et al., 1983). The fiber types in the lateral pterygoid are similar to the jaw-closing muscles (Eriksson et al., 1981), whereas the digastric is most similar to limb muscles in that it contains about one third Type I (low-threshold, fatigue-resistant), one third Type IIA (high-threshold, fatigue-sensitive), and one third Type IIB (high-threshold, fatigue-resistant) motor units (Eriksson et al., 1982). The fiber types would suggest that the digastric, not the closers or the lateral pterygoid, would be a more likely candidate for fatigue and consequent pain; clinical experience, however, shows the opposite.

Macroscopic physiological properties

The function of skeletal muscle is to contract and supply force that may then exert force on an external object, such as a bolus of food. The force may cause movement, such as elevating or depressing the mandible. Functionally, a muscle is composed of elements called motor units. The force exerted by the whole muscle depends on several factors: the frequency of motor unit activity, the number of motor units activated, the length of the muscle, the velocity at which the muscle shortens, and fatigue.

Length-tension

If the whole muscle is excited by a single electrical shock, there will be a brief rise and fall of force called a *twitch*. If the muscle is not allowed to shorten, then the contraction is called *isometric* (of equal length). The force of an isometric contraction depends on the external length fixed by the experimenter. If the muscle has slack in it, or a short initial length, little or no force will be generated. As the length of the muscle is increased from trial to trial, the resulting isometric force will increase to a maximum and then decrease (Fig. 7-1).

The forces at short and moderate muscle lengths are produced mostly by active contraction of the muscle in response to the stimulus, whereas at more extreme lengths the forces exerted are due to passive stretch of the muscle tissue. Thus, active rather than passive muscle responses would account for most of the forces produced on the bolus in the range of opening ordinarily used for functional activity.

At any given length, force is first increased by the recruitment of more motor units. Additional force would then be applied by an increase in the rate of contraction of the motor units (Basmajian, 1974).

The length at which the maximum force is obtained is called the *resting length* of the muscle by physiologists because in many animal limbs this length corresponds to the length observed in the postural position. The resting length as defined by the physiologist should *not* be confused with the *postural rest position* of the mandible as defined by the dentist. Postural position determined clinically by the dentist usually occurs with the incisors a few millimeters apart.

The position of the mandible where maximum force can be exerted is reported to be where the incisors are as much as 10 to 15 mm apart (Manns and Spreng, 1977; Manns et al., 1979, 1981; MacKenna and Turker, 1978). The clinical implication of such data would be that more force could be applied to a bolus with a certain optimal thickness than at centric occlusion where the jaw-closing muscles are shorter. Moreover, forces applied to a very large bolus, beyond the maximum of the length-tension relationship, would tend to be reduced.

Force-velocity

The experiment leading to the length-tension curve considered an isometric contraction and observed changes in force. Now consider an isotonic (of equal force or load) contraction and observe the changes in length and velocity. If a weight is hung on a passive muscle, the muscle will stretch. If the muscle is then stimulated, it will contract and lift the weight. The weight, in a single trial, will lift slowly at first, then more rapidly at an approximately constant velocity. Finally the velocity will decrease to zero as the muscle reaches minimum length.

This velocity in the middle of the shortening may be measured and plotted against the weight—that is, against the external force lifted by the muscle. The velocity is observed to decrease as the force is increased (Fig. 7-2). In other words, the heavier the load, the more slowly it is lifted, even when all other conditions such as initial length and stimulation intensity remain constant.

Normal jaw function, of course, does not include lifting external weights at constant velocities. The resistance of a bolus, however, will provide a force opposing jaw closing and the magnitude of that force may influence the velocity of jaw closing. During mastication, therefore, velocity will ordinarily begin to decrease prior to any occlusal contact as the bolus provides resis-

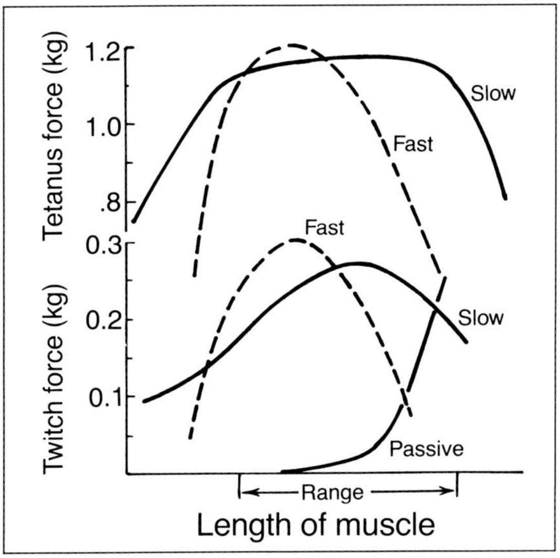

Fig. 7-1 Length-tension curve. The total force consists of passive and active parts. The passive part is determined by tissue elasticity. The active part depends on the contraction, which in turn depends on the length of the muscle. Fast and slow muscles may differ in their length-tension properties. The range over which the muscle usually operates is indicated.

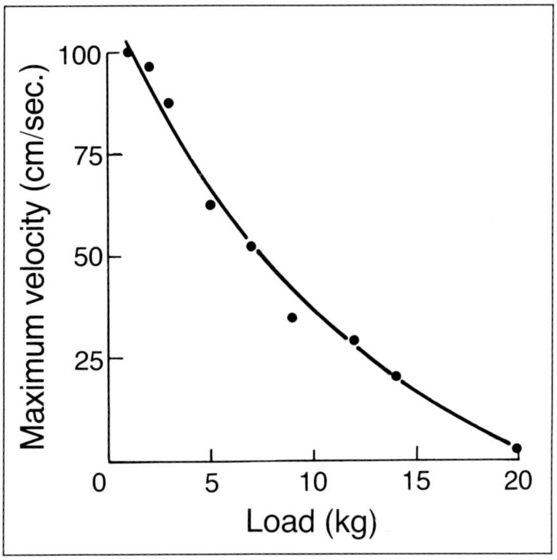

Fig. 7-2 Force-velocity curve. The greater the load placed on a muscle, the slower its maximum velocity of shortening will be.

tance to the closing movement (Hannam et al., 1977).

Twitch and tetanus

If the nerve to a muscle or the muscle itself is given a single stimulus, the force produced by the muscle rises, peaks, and descends to zero in several tens of milliseconds. This is called a *twitch*. If, on the other hand, a rapid series of stimuli are delivered to the muscle or its nerve, the force rises in staircase fashion to a plateau of force that can be maintained. This is called *tetanus*. The maximum force produced during tetanus is typically four times greater than the peak force produced during a twitch (Fig. 7-3). Tetanus as used by the physiologist to indicate contraction from a rapid series of stimuli is not to be confused with tetanus as used by the physician to indicate a tonic spasm, as in "lockjaw."

The usual mode of operation for a muscle is a shower of twitches rather than a sustained tetanus, so one would expect that the forces exerted during chewing would be far less than the maximum force possible. Experiments have confirmed this. Estimates of maximum clenching forces range from tens of kilograms to one hundred kilograms (Proffitt et al., 1983). Chewing forces, in contrast, are only a few kilograms (Anderson and Picton, 1958; Graf et al., 1974; DeBoever et al., 1978). The forces exerted during bruxism have the potential of being much greater than those exerted during mastication.

If the muscle did use tetanus, explaining a smooth contraction or a usefully smooth force would be easy. But muscles do not work that way. Muscles usually exert force by supplying a shower of twitches. Each motor unit contributes only a small amount of force (from about 10 to 200 g [Goldberg and Derfler, 1977]). If all the active motor units contracted simultaneously, our movements would be as jerky as the head of

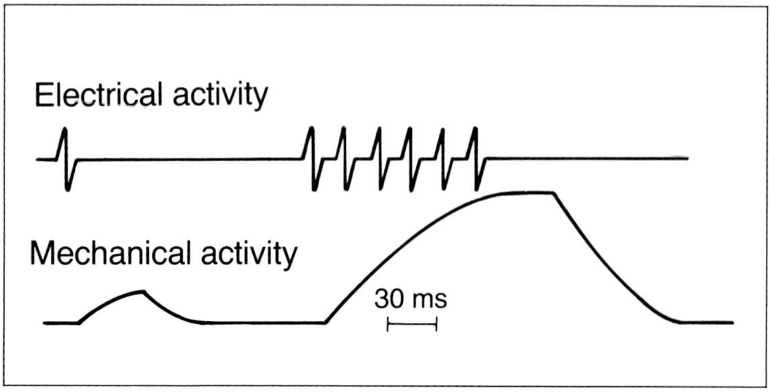

Fig. 7-3 Twitch and tetanus. A single shock leads to a twitch, shown on the left, whereas a series of shocks leads to tetanus. Notice the delay from the onset of shocks to the peak force, the greater force in tetanus than in a twitch, and the long duration of the mechanical event compared with the electrical event.

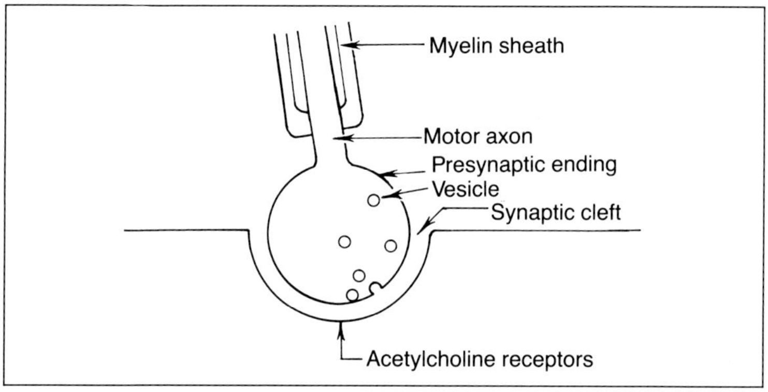

Fig. 7-4 Neuromuscular junction. An action potential causes a large number of vesicles to release their acetylcholine into the synaptic cleft, where it diffuses across to the receptors on the membrane.

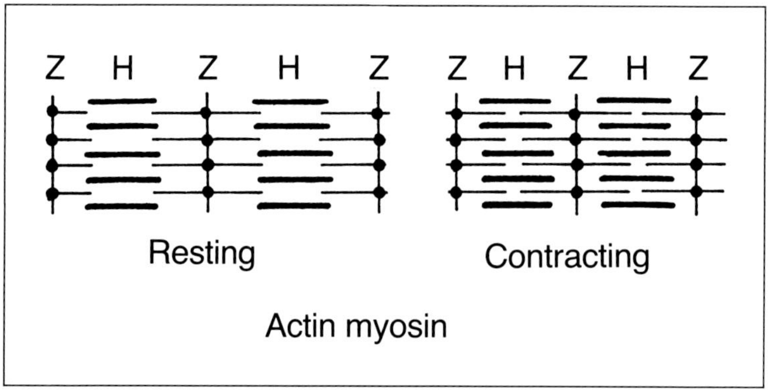

Fig. 7-5 Molecular structure of muscle. The main contractile elements of muscle are actin *(thin elements)* and myosin *(thick elements)*. Cross-linkages between these two proteins provide the force for muscle contraction. A sarcomere extends from one *Z* line to the next. The *H* band is the gap between the thin actin elements.

a walking pigeon. But the twitches occur randomly in time, so the summation of all the small twitches occurring at various times adds up to a smooth contraction and a fairly constant force.

Fatigue

Fatigue can be a difficult concept, because the notion of "tiredness" may arise in the central nervous system from feedback from peripheral receptors, in the motor system from depletion of the transmitter at the neuromuscular junction, or in the muscle itself from depletion of energy metabolites.

Scientists define concepts "operationally," that is, by the techniques used to make the measurements. Fatigue may be defined as a decrease in the tetanic force under specified rates of stimulation. All muscles will fatigue, but some will fatigue more rapidly than others.

Muscles that fatigue more rapidly usually have faster contraction times too. One can predict, based on research on limb muscles, that the faster the contraction times, the faster the onset of fatigue. Jaw muscles have contraction times among the fastest in the body (only the eye muscles are faster), so one would expect them to become fatigued quickly. If fatigue of the jaw muscles can be caused by typical jaw movements of patients, one might wonder whether these properties might lead to the pain and dysfunction experienced by some patients. Experimental bruxism studies suggest that pain and tenderness can readily be produced by the movements of jaw muscles during bruxism (Christensen, 1971).

Microscopic structure

Motor units

A motor unit is defined as a motor neuron, its axon, and all the muscle fibers (cells) supplied by that axon. In the absence of disease, an action potential in a motor neuron will propagate down the axon, down all the terminal branches of that axon, and across the neuromuscular junction, causing an action potential in the muscle fibers. Since neuron, axon, and fibers function as a single entity, they are called a motor unit.

The number of muscle fibers in an average motor unit is related to the fineness of the movement required of the muscle. For example, the muscles that move the eye have only a few muscle fibers per motor unit, whereas the muscles of the leg may have 1,000 or more. The jaw muscles fall between these, with about 700 to 900 muscle fibers per motor unit (Goodgold and Eberstein, 1978). All the muscles fibers in one motor unit are believed to be of the same fiber type, although a muscle may contain various types of motor units. The digastric muscle, as cited previously, contains equal measures of Type I, Type IIA, and Type IIB motor units.

Neuromuscular junction

The neuromuscular junction is the synapse between the motor axon and the muscle fiber (Fig. 7-4). An action potential from the motor axon causes vesicles of acetylcholine to be released from the presynaptic endings of the motor axon. The acetylcholine diffuses across the synaptic cleft to receptors located on the specialized membrane of the muscle fibers. Stimulation of these receptors by the acetylcholine increases the permeability of the muscle fibers to sodium ions, thereby depolarizing the adjacent patch of muscle cell membrane and causing an action potential to be initiated in the muscle fiber.

An essential difference between a synapse in the brain or spinal cord and the synapse at the muscle is that at the neuromuscular junction an action potential arriving from the axon always causes an action potential in the muscle (the postsynaptic cell). In the central nervous system, on the other hand, many action potentials must be summated to cause the postsynaptic cell to fire an action potential.

Molecular structure

The molecular structure of muscle consists mainly of actin, myosin, and cross-linkages between these two contractile proteins. The length-tension and force-velocity curves may be understood by reference to the actin-myosin model (Fig. 7-5).

The static length-tension properties arise from the number of cross-linkages between the two proteins. Each link is assumed to provide one small unit of force. At long lengths there is little overlap between the actin and the myosin, few cross-linkages, and little force. At progressively shorter lengths there are progressively more linkages and progressively more force. At short lengths the opposing actin structures overlap, effectively reducing the number of linkages and reducing the available force.

For the force-velocity curve, one assumes that a certain amount of time is required to make and break the cross-linkages between actin and myosin. At progressively greater velocities a progressively larger fraction of the available population of cross-linkages will be involved in making or breaking the linkages, rather than producing force.

Electrical properties

Action potentials

The membranes of nerve axons and muscle fibers are specialized to conduct action potentials. Outward-flowing current depolarizes (reduces the negative voltage across) the membrane. Increased depolarization leads to increased permeability to sodium ions, which in turn leads to increased outward-flowing current and to further depolarization. When the membrane potential reaches a voltage called the *threshold* or *critical firing level,* a self-regenerating cycle occurs and is propagated down the cell membrane as an action potential.

For a millisecond or so the sodium conductance increases, causing outward flow of sodium ions and decreased membrane potential. Then the sodium conductance decreases and the potassium conductance increases. The increased potassium conductance allows potassium ions to flow from outside to inside the membrane and to repolarize the cell, which is then ready for the next action potential cycle to occur.

The muscle action potential is identical in mechanism to the nerve action potential. The muscle cell membrane, however, is much larger and more convoluted than the nerve cell membrane, so the amount of current involved in a muscle action potential is much larger than that in a nerve action potential. This has important consequences for detecting these signals by electromyography.

Electromechanical coupling

The muscle action potential causes calcium ions to be released from the sarcoplasmic reticulum, a structure inside the membrane and parallel to the contractile proteins. The calcium ions diffuse into the contractile proteins, leading to the mechanical contraction. After the contraction the calcium ions are again acquired by the sarcoplasmic reticulum. There is a delay of some milliseconds (see Fig. 7-3) between the electrical event, the action potentials, and the mechanical event, the twitch. For example, in the masseter there is a delay of approximately 10 ms (Hannam et al., 1977) between the electromyogram observed with electrodes over the masseter muscle and the upward movement of the mandible.

Innervation

The muscles of mastication are innervated by branches of the mandibular division of the trigeminal nerve. These muscles include the masseter, temporalis, medial pterygoid, lateral pterygoid, anterior digastric, mylohyoid, tensor tympani, and tensor palatini. Certain muscles of facial expression (buccinator, posterior digastric, and platysma, for example) may also be involved; these are innervated by the facial nerve. Other cranial nerves such as the hypoglossal as well as cervical spinal are involved in oral or related functions. A more specific discussion of the nervous system will be given in chapter 8.

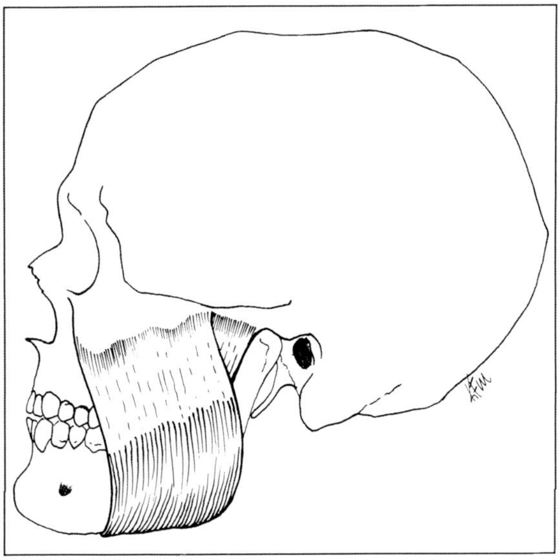

Fig. 7-6 Masseter muscle.

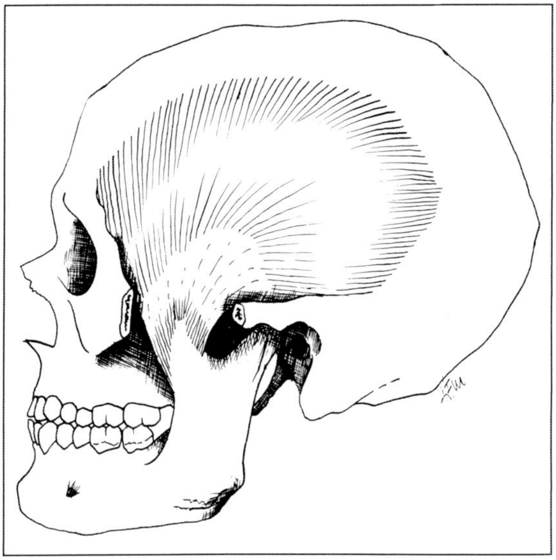

Fig. 7-7 Temporalis muscle.

Muscles involved in mandibular function

Jaw-closing muscles

The jaw-closing muscles include the masseter, the temporalis, and the medial pterygoid.

Masseter muscle

The masseter muscle has two portions, a larger superficial portion and a much smaller, deep portion (Fig. 7-6). The origin of the superficial masseter muscle is on the zygomatic process of the maxilla and the inferior border of the zygomatic arch. It has a strong and large tendinous attachment to these structures. The muscle-tendon fibers of the superficial masseter run obliquely inferiorly and posteriorly to the area of insertion on the angle of the mandible and the inferior half of the lateral side of the ramus. The fiber direction is roughly perpendicular to the plane of occlusion.

The deep portion of the masseter muscle also has its origin on the zygomatic process; it then runs vertically down to insert on the ramus of the mandible up to the base of the coronoid process.

The principal function of the masseter is to close the jaws. The deep portion of the masseter muscle, because of its different fiber orientation, also helps to retrude the mandible. The masseter muscle is a powerful elevator of the mandible and is thought to provide the bulk of the power for chewing a bolus. Innervating this muscle is the masseteric nerve.

Temporalis muscle

The fan-shaped temporalis muscle has its broad origin in the temporal fossa and the temporal fascia along the side of the head. The insertion is on the medial surface, apex, and anterior border of the coronoid process of the mandible and, via a superficial and a deep tendon, along the anterior border of the ramus of the mandible (Fig. 7-7).

The fibers of all three portions descend and converge on a tendon that passes deep into the zygomatic arch. Posteriorly this tendon bends like a pulley around the root of the zygomatic

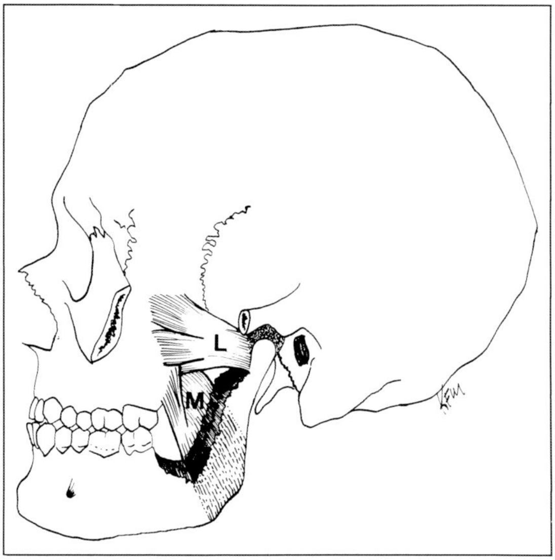

Fig. 7-8 Medial *(M)* and lateral *(L)* pterygoid muscles.

arch. This arrangement limits the angles of the force vectors that can be produced by the contracting temporalis fibers, especially its posterior fibers. (See also chapter 6; Fig. 6-11.)

The function of the temporalis muscle is to close the jaws; the posterior fibers also help retrude the mandible. Some authors believe that this muscle has an important role as a positioner of the mandible during elevation (Ramfjord and Ash, 1983). The fiber directions are somewhat different among the anterior, medial, and posterior portions of the temporalis muscle.

The temporalis muscle is innervated by the anterior and posterior deep temporal nerves.

Medial pterygoid muscle

The medial pterygoid muscle, formerly called the "internal" pterygoid, is located on the medial side of the ramus. It is similar to the superficial masseter in fiber direction, and these two muscles function synergistically to form the "mandibular sling." While an important elevator of the mandible, the medial pterygoid is not quite as powerful as the masseter. The origin of the medial pterygoid muscle is in the pterygoid fossa and on the medial surface of the lateral pterygoid plate. The triangular insertion is on the ramus and the angle of the mandible, and on the inferior and posterior aspect of the medial surface (Fig. 7-8). The innervation is from the nerve to the medial pterygoid muscle.

Jaw-opening muscles

The main jaw-opening muscles are the lateral pterygoid and anterior digastric.

Lateral pterygoid muscle

The lateral pterygoid (formerly called the "external" pterygoid) muscle arises from two heads. The smaller superior head arises from the wing of the sphenoid and from the infratemporal crest; the larger inferior head arises from the lateral surface of the lateral pterygoid plate. All the fibers pass horizontally posteriorly and laterally to insert anterior to the neck of the mandible (pterygoid fovea), with a variable number of fibers from the superior head inserting into the anteromedial margin of the articular disk (Fig. 7-8) (Meyenberg et al., 1986).

The important functions of the lateral pterygoid muscle are to open the jaws and to protrude the mandible. It is believed to be the initiator of jaw opening. On contracting unilaterally the lateral pterygoid muscle will pull the condyle and its attached disk anteriorly, lingually, and inferiorly along the posterior slope of the articular eminence, causing the mandible to move to the opposite side. It is therefore an important muscle in lateral movements of the mandible. The lateral pterygoid muscle also has an important role in determining the position of the condyle relative to the eminence, and limits the degree of condylar retrusion (Wood et al., 1986).

The two heads of the lateral pterygoid muscle act differently. The inferior head acts as a synergist with the suprahyoid group during jaw opening, whereas the superior head acts as a synergist with the elevator muscles during jaw closing or

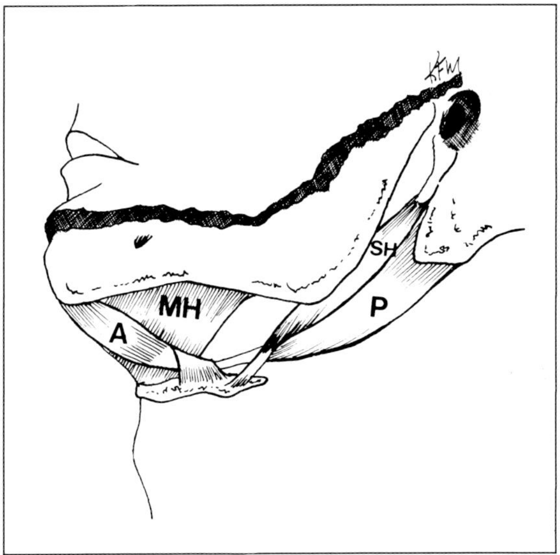

Fig. 7-9 Digastric muscle with its anterior *(A)* and posterior *(P)* bellies; mylohyoid *(MH)*; stylohyoid *(SH)*.

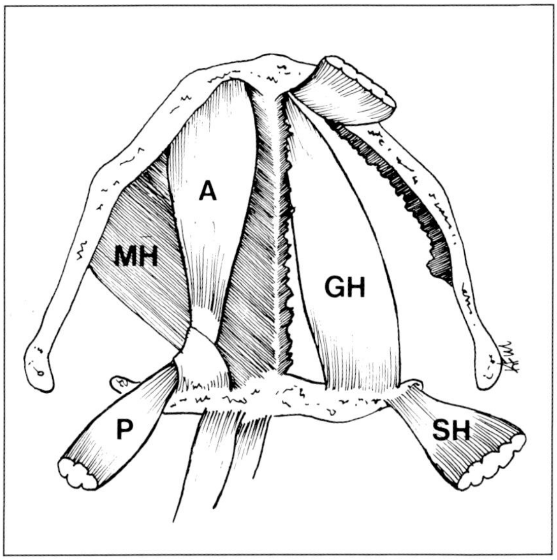

Fig. 7-10 Suprahyoid muscles viewed from below. These muscles include the anterior *(A)* and posterior *(P)* bellies of the digastric, the mylohyoid *(MH)*, the geniohyoid *(GH)*, and the stylohyoid *(SH)* muscles.

clenching (McNamara, 1973). In humans, the electrode placement cannot be verified absolutely but the reciprocal activity of the heads, consistent with McNamara's results in the monkey, has been reported in the human (Mahan et al., 1983; Wood et al., 1986; Widmer, 1987).

The lateral pterygoid muscle is innervated by the lateral pterygoid nerve.

Anterior digastric muscle

The digastric muscle (Fig. 7-9) is part of the suprahyoid group and consists of two bellies, the anterior and the posterior. The longer posterior belly arises from the mastoid notch of the temporal bone and passes inferiorly and anteriorly. The anterior belly arises from the lingual side of the inferior border of the mandible, then passes inferiorly and posteriorly. The two bellies are joined by a common tendon, which can slide through a fascial pulley attached to the hyoid bone.

The digastric muscle assists in retruding the mandible. This muscle is also active in opening the jaw, especially against resistance or during rapid opening. The anterior belly is innervated by the mylohyoid nerve from the inferior alveolar branch of the mandibular division of the trigeminal nerve. The posterior belly is innervated by a branch of the facial nerve.

Other muscle groups

Suprahyoid group

The suprahyoid muscle group (Fig 7 10) consists of the digastric, mylohyoid, geniohyoid, and stylohyoid muscles. The stylohyoid, like the posterior digastric, is innervated by the facial nerve and pulls the hyoid bone superiorly and posteriorly, as occurs during swallowing.

The mylohyoid muscle lies superior to the anterior digastric muscle and forms a muscular floor for the mouth. The origin is on the lingual surface of the mandible from the symphysis to the last molar. The posterior fibers insert on the hyoid bone. The anterior and medial fibers join at an angle with the fibers of the opposite muscle. The mylohyoid muscle is innervated by the mylohyoid nerve. Its actions are to raise the hyoid bone, the tongue, and the floor of the mouth.

The geniohyoid muscle attaches to the hyoid bone and to the inferior genial tubercle on the lingual surface of the anterior of the mandible. It is innervated by the second and third cervical nerves via branches of the hypoglossal nerve. It draws the hyoid bone and the tongue anteriorly.

The group action of the suprahyoid muscles is dual: to raise the hyoid bone and the base of the tongue during swallowing, and to help to depress the mandible during jaw opening. During elevation of the mandible they relax. The relative activity of this muscle group, along with the jaw-closing muscles, helps to determine the postural rest position of the mandible.

Infrahyoid group

The infrahyoid muscles are located below the hyoid bone and draw it inferiorly. This group includes the sternohyoid, sternothyroid, thyrohyoid, and omohyoid muscles. They are innervated by the first, second, and third cervical nerves.

Facial group

The muscles of the facial group number over 20; only the two most relevant to chewing will be considered here.

The *orbicularis oris muscle* runs transversely within the lips, some of its fibers being derived from adjacent facial muscles. The actions of the orbicularis oris muscle are to close the lips, to press the lips against the anterior teeth, and to protrude the lips. It is innervated by the buccal branches of the facial nerve.

The *buccinator muscle* is the main muscle of the cheek and forms a wide, flat, muscular, and lateral wall for the oral cavity. The origin of the buccinator muscle is on the alveolar processes of the maxilla and mandible in the region of the molars and from the pterygomandibular raphe. The fibers converge and insert anteriorly into the mucous membrane around the corner of the mouth and, via interlacing muscle fibers, into the skin of the lateral part of the lips.

The chief function of the buccinator muscle is to cause tension in the cheek, thereby moving food onto the teeth from the lateral side and preventing cheek folds from being bitten by the teeth during jaw closing. The motor nerve fibers come from buccal branches of the facial nerve.

Cervical group

Other muscle groups are indirectly involved in mandibular function. These include the trapezius, sternocleidomastoid, and anterior vertebral muscles; the lateral vertebral (scalenus) muscles; and other deep posterior cervical muscles. These muscle groups act to stabilize head posture during active contraction of the masticatory, suprahyoid, and infrahyoid muscles during mastication and swallowing.

Neurosensory receptors in muscle

Sensory information is sent to the central nervous system from receptors in muscle. These receptors include muscle spindles to signal muscle length and velocity, Golgi tendon organs to signal muscle tension, and free nerve endings to signal, among other things, pain.

Muscle spindles

Jaw-closing muscles have many muscle spindles, but jaw-opening muscles and facial muscles have few or none.

Anatomy

The muscle spindle (Fig. 7-11) is a sensory organ a few millimeters in length and about 100 μm in width, which lies parallel with the force-producing extrafusal muscle fibers. It is named for its shape: fatter in the middle and thinner at both ends (fusiform shape). Each spindle contains two types of intrafusal muscle fibers: *nuclear bag* and *nuclear chain*.

Nuclear bag intrafusal fibers have a neurosensory ending, called a primary or annulospiral ending, wrapped around their central portions. This primary ending of the muscle spindle is connected to a large-diameter *(Ia)* sensory axon. The nuclear chain intrafusal fiber has a neurosensory ending called a *secondary,* or *flower-spray* ending, which is located on either side of the central region of the fiber. The secondary ending of the muscle spindle is connected to a smaller-diameter *(II)* sensory axon. The intrafusal fibers also receive a small-diameter *(gamma)* motor (fusimotor) supply of two types: *static,* which innervates both nuclear bag and nuclear chain fibers; and *dynamic,* which innervates nuclear bag fibers only.

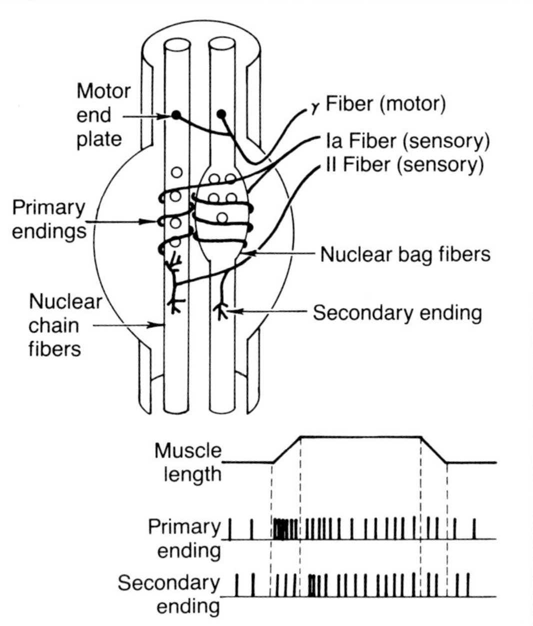

Fig. 7-11 Muscle spindle. A schematic of the anatomy is shown above; the response to changes in muscle length is shown below.

Physiology

The muscle spindle lies parallel with the muscle, so it will respond to the length of the muscle. The primary ending of the muscle spindle is sensitive to the static length of the muscle and also to change in the length of the muscle. In other words, the primary ending of the muscle spindle is sensitive to both length and velocity. The secondary ending of the muscle spindle is sensitive to length only, without significant velocity sensitivity (see Fig. 7-11).

The motor inputs to the muscle spindle, the gamma efferents, complicate the response of the sensory endings. Activity in the static gamma fibers increases the static (length) sensitivity of both the primary and secondary endings by contracting the intrafusal muscle fibers within the spindle. Activity in the dynamic gamma fibers increases the dynamic (velocity) sensitivity of the primary endings without substantially changing their static sensitivities. Gamma efferent activity therefore increases the sensitivity of the muscle to changes in length and velocity.

The sensory afferents from the muscle spindles make monosynaptic excitatory connections to jaw-closer alpha motoneurons. Thus, the extrafusal muscle fibers, the vast majority of the muscle, can be activated in three ways. First, the alpha motoneurons to the extrafusal fibers could be activated directly. Second, the gamma efferent motoneurons could be activated, leading to increased tension in the intrafusal fibers, increased response from the muscle spindle afferent endings, increased monosynaptic bombardment of the alpha motoneurons, and, finally, after this circuitous route, increased activity in the alpha motoneurons. Third, the alpha and gamma motoneurons could be "coactivated" so that the direct alpha route is used but the spindle afferents remain active during the contraction. Recent evidence is interpreted as indicating that coactivation does occur (Lund et al., 1979).

In summary, the muscle spindles *(1)* provide sensory information about the lengths and changing lengths of muscles; *(2)* receive motor control from the gamma efferents, which influences their sensitivity; and *(3)* provide important input to the motor system via the monosynaptic connections to motoneurons. Because muscle spindles are tightly connected with the motor system, they have been postulated to be the source of muscle "hyperactivity" leading to bruxism and TM disorders. These postulations should be viewed skeptically, since the evidence for such a link is minimal.

Tendon organs

Tendon organs, as the name implies, are located in the tendons of the muscles and respond to the forces generated by the muscles. The tendon organs are located in the fascicles of the tendons; an individual tendon organ will respond to contractions of some motor units and not to others. The threshold of response of the tendon organ is much lower to active contraction of a motor unit than to passive stretch of the whole muscle. Tendon organs are slowly adapting receptors like the muscle spindles and, like the secondary endings of the muscle spindles, show only minimal response to the rate of change of input.

A few tendon organs have been shown in the jaw-closing muscles of the cat (Lund et al., 1978), but their functional significance is not clear, and their existence in humans is doubtful. The inhibition of muscle activity following a tap to the chin during a jaw-clenching action in humans has been ascribed to tendon organ activation, but there are other possible causes that are supported by experimental evidence as well (Bratzlavsky, 1972).

Free nerve endings

Free nerve endings do not have specialized endings like the muscle spindles and tendon organs. The free nerve endings are located ubiquitously throughout the organism and provide receptors for nociceptive afferents. The fibers are very small and conduct very slowly compared with those from muscle spindles and tendon organs. The response of nociceptive afferents, unlike that of mechanoreceptors, does not adapt or decrease with constant input.

Electromyography and muscle activity

Electromyography (EMG) is the electrical record of the activity of a muscle. It has been, and is, a powerful tool for investigating and understanding the function of jaw muscles. Thus, an understanding of the basis, techniques, pitfalls, and applications of EMG, as well as its relevance to the study of occlusion, are important.

Basis and techniques of electromyography

Muscle action potentials generate small amounts of electrical current that not only depolarize the adjacent patch of membrane to propagate the action potentials, but also flow at considerable distances from the muscle and can be detected by electronic equipment. *Volume conduction* is the term used to describe the phenomenon of electrical signals being detected at a distance from their source through a mass of tissue.

The apparatus of EMG includes electrodes to detect the currents and potentials described above, an amplifier to make them large enough to analyze, and a display system for the operator or clinician to observe and evaluate the signals.

Electrodes

The three general types of electrodes are surface, needle, and fine wire. Surface electrodes are simply pieces of metal on the surface of the skin. These are good for observing the gross activity of the whole muscle. The disadvantages are that single motor units cannot be observed, and that more superficial muscles may confound attempts to record from deeper muscles.

Needle electrodes are usually needles with insulation covering all but the tips. The tip may then be inserted into the appropriate muscle even if the muscle is remote from the surface of the skin.

A fine wire electrode consists of two fine wires, inserted through a needle, cut, and bent. The needle is passed into the muscle and withdrawn. Hooks are made by bending the wire, and serve to retain the electrodes in the muscle. These electrodes can record the fine detail of motor unit activity often required for scientific and clinical investigation. They must be used to record the activity of deeper muscles, such as the lateral and medial pterygoids.

Amplifier

The amplifier must provide a high input impedance (that is, it must use as little as possible of the biological current produced by the muscle action potentials), provide adequate gain or amplification of the small biological signals, and have the appropriate bandwidth or frequency response. Modern electronics have made the commercially available devices adequate for the task.

Display

The display of the recorded signal may use any of several techniques. The traditional way used to be to have the EMG amplifier drive pens while paper moved past the pens. In this way, a permanent record was made for later analysis. Unfortunately, pens and other mechanical devices have a limited frequency response due to the mass and inertia of the pens—so techniques were devised to avoid this problem. One is to display the signal on an oscilloscope. A second is to record the data on a tape recorder at a high tape speed and replay the tape at a slow tape speed onto a penwriter. A third is to record the data by computer and do the data assessment on the computer.

Pitfalls and problems of electromyography

Electromyography is easy to implement and so has been very popular with dental researchers. There are, however, potential problems that one should consider. Signal contamination is one. Surface electrodes over the masseter, for example, might be recording signals from facial muscles rather than from the masseter muscle. Also, needle electrodes placed into deep muscles, such as the lateral pterygoid, should have independent confirmation of proper placement.

The vagaries of amplitude measurement are another potential problem. The amplitude of the signal recorded depends on many factors, including the number of motor units recorded, the frequency at which they fire, the distance from the motor units to the electrodes, and the spacing between the electrodes. Often these factors are difficult or impossible to control. Therefore, comparisons of EMG amplitudes should be viewed skeptically and critically when they arise from different muscles, from different subjects, or even from the same muscle on the same subject but on different days.

Electromyography should not be used to infer force, because the two are linearly related only under isometric conditions. Nor should EMG be used to infer position, since equal activity in a muscle could be obtained at any position.

Perhaps the lesson of this section is that the usefulness of EMG is increased considerably when measurements of jaw motion and bite force are obtained concurrently (Hannam et al., 1977).

Application of electromyography to occlusion

Electromyography is particularly useful in determining whether or not muscle contraction is occurring and, if it is, the temporal sequence of such activity. Thus, EMG has been used to determine the contraction sequences of the muscles of mastication during chewing.

In the field of Occlusion, EMG has been applied in at least six general areas of study: *(1)* the pattern of masticatory muscle activity during voluntary acts such as chewing and swallowing, *(2)* the pattern of activity in patients with different types of anatomical malocclusions, *(3)* postural rest position of the mandible, *(4)* TM disorders and bruxism, *(5)* jaw reflexes, and *(6)* biofeedback.

The scope of this chapter prohibits extensive details of the many ways in which EMG has been employed in dentistry; only a few examples will be given.

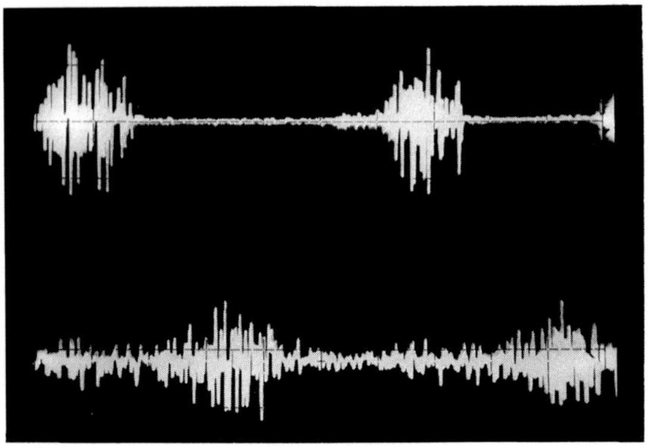

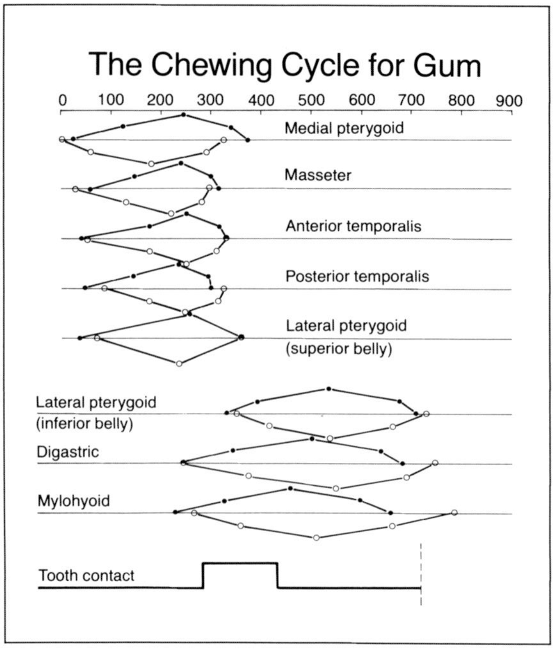

Figs. 7-12a and b Electromyography of chewing from a 10-year-old girl.

Fig. 7-12a *(above)* Electromyographic traces. Surface EMG from left masseter muscle *(top)* and suprahyoid group *(bottom)* while chewing gum. Full horizontal scale is 1 second.

Fig. 7-12b *(right)* Average timing of group. The timing of the EMG activity of the chewing, ipsilateral, or working side is shown above the line, and the activity of the nonchewing, contralateral, or nonworking side is shown below the line. As given by Møller (1966), the timing is presented as onset, 50% (on the rising side), 100%, 50% (on the falling side), and end of activity. All amplitudes are shown equal because it is difficult to compare amplitudes among muscles and among electrodes. Another omission is the relative force contributions from the different muscles; the small lateral pterygoid and digastric muscles will clearly provide less force than the large masseter, temporalis, and medial pterygoid muscles.

Chewing and swallowing

Electromyography has often been used to confirm what anatomists have concluded from gross dissection of muscles and their attachments. For example, the masseter muscle is electrically active during jaw closing. Information from EMG not available from anatomical sources includes the timing and sequence of muscle activity during functional activity such as chewing.

In the average chewing cycle for chewing gum, alternating activity in antagonistic muscles is seen (Figs. 7-12a and b). All the jaw-closing muscles are active more or less simultaneously while the jaw-opening muscles are silent, then all the opening muscles are active at once while the jaw-closing muscles are silent. Note the bilateral activity of the muscles even during unilateral chewing.

A more detailed examination of the chewing cycle reveals that activity in the medial pterygoid muscle contralateral to the chewing side begins first, followed by nearly simultaneous activity in the other closing muscles (Møller, 1966). The mean duration of the chewing cycle is about 0.7 to 0.75 seconds. Contraction of the jaw-closing muscles takes about 38% of the cycle; activity in the jaw-opening muscles begins about 0.3 sec-

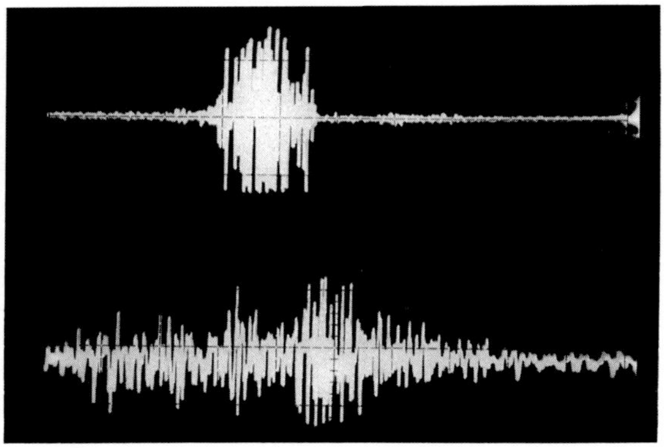

Figs. 7-13 a and b Electromyography of swallowing for same patient as in Fig. 7-12.

Fig. 7-13a Electromyographic traces. Surface EMG from left masseter *(top)* and suprahyoid group *(bottom)* while chewing gum. Full horizontal scale is 1 second.

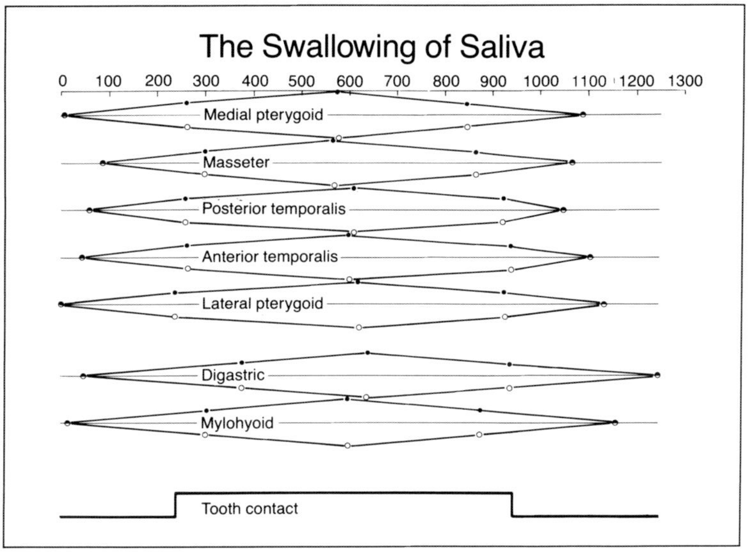

Fig. 7-13b Average timing of group. The timing of the EMG from the two sides are shown above and below the line, as in Fig. 7-12b. Swallowing is a complex process involving the masticatory muscles only at the beginning of a carefully timed reflex involving a large number of muscles.

onds after the activity in the closing muscles begins.

The peak of the EMG activity has passed prior to tooth contact in gum chewing. One might expect that the maximal activity in the closing muscles would occur during tooth contact. However, it is important to remember that the EMG activity in a muscle precedes the force production by some tens of milliseconds, and that tooth contact will occur after the teeth have penetrated the bolus.

Electromyography also reveals that the closing muscles contract during swallowing (Figs. 7-13a and b). This stabilizes the mandible so that the suprahyoid muscles can move the hyoid bone more effectively during swallowing.

In contrast to chewing, where the jaw-opening and jaw-closing muscles are active in separate parts of the chewing cycle, the activity of the opening and closing muscles during swallowing occurs at roughly the same time. Also in contrast to chewing, the duration of the activity during swallowing is much longer—over 1 second—whereas the entire chewing cycle takes only about 0.75 second divided over opening, closing, and occlusal phases.

Types of malocclusion

Although several attempts have been made to correlate muscle contraction patterns with specific types of malocclusions, such efforts have as yet failed to provide us with consistent quantifiable information. Thus, at the present time we must conclude that such patterns are not diagnostic of any particular structural occlusal relationship.

Postural rest position

The hope that EMG could be used to more precisely determine clinical or postural rest position has not been fulfilled. Studies have demonstrated that the position of the mandible when EMG activity is least involves a range of positions (Garnick and Ramfjord, 1962). Even when more precisely determined, EMG "rest" position has been found to be at a more open jaw position, about 8 or 10 mm, than clinically determined postural rest position of the mandible, about 2 to 4 mm (Rugh and Drago, 1981).

Temporomandibular disorders and bruxism

Some early studies suggested that the EMG patterns during swallowing were "unharmonious" when the subject exhibited a slide from centric relation to centric occlusion, particularly a slide that was three dimensional (Ramfjord, 1961a, 1961b). Clinical correlation also suggested that these slides served as primary occlusal triggers for bruxism and led to symptoms of pain and dysfunction. Nonworking side "interferences" were also implicated in this sequence of events. Such specific cause-and-effect relationships have not yet been replicated or quantified, and an occlusal etiology for these problems remains controversial.

Nonetheless, there is general agreement among both clinicians and investigators that masticatory muscle activity is increased in symptomatic patients as compared with normal subjects. Electromyography is the principal tool used to investigate such differences.

Jaw reflexes

Reflexes available for study by the neurologist or dentist include the monosynaptic (stretch) reflex, silent periods, the blink reflex, and the jaw-opening reflex. The compound action potential produced by the monosynaptic, or jaw jerk, reflex (Fig. 7-14a) is the simplest because it is produced by primary endings of muscle spindles, their afferents, the one synapse to the motor neuron, the motor axon, and the muscle fibers of the jaw-closing muscles. This reflex is enormously useful in neurology, but has not been shown to be useful for the study of dental maladies.

Silent periods are a transient inhibition of jaw-closing activity (Fig. 7-14b). The EMG records this as a temporary reduction or cessation of activity during an otherwise sustained contraction. If a tap to the chin is delivered during a clench, a brief inhibition of the EMG of the jaw-closing muscle may be observed. The duration of this inhibition (the silent period) has been shown in several laboratories to be longer, on the average, in a group of TM disorder patients than in a group of asymptomatic subjects or a group of successfully treated patients (Bessette et al., 1971; Widmalm, 1976; Bailey et al., 1977; Bernstein et al., 1981; Skiba and Laskin, 1981; Hussein and McCall, 1983).

There are some proven facts about silent period durations: they get shorter with successful treatment, they correlate roughly with symptom severity (McCall et al., 1978; Helkimo et al., 1979), and the variability is considerable within both individuals and groups (McCall et al., 1981). Still, much remains to be learned. For example, the neuromuscular mechanisms responsible for the prolongation of the silent period and any connection with an etiology for the dysfunction are not fully understood. Preliminary evidence, however, suggests that decreased bite force in TM disorder patients may explain their prolonged silent period durations (Donnarumma et al., 1986). Therefore, the recording of masseteric silent period duration *cannot* be used on an *individual* basis as a specific diagnostic test for TM disorder patients.

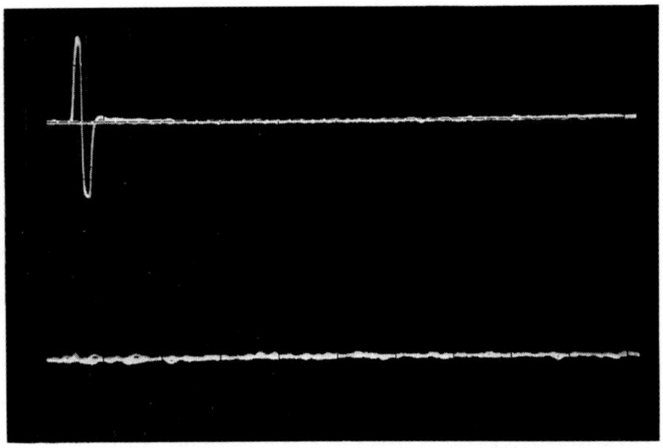

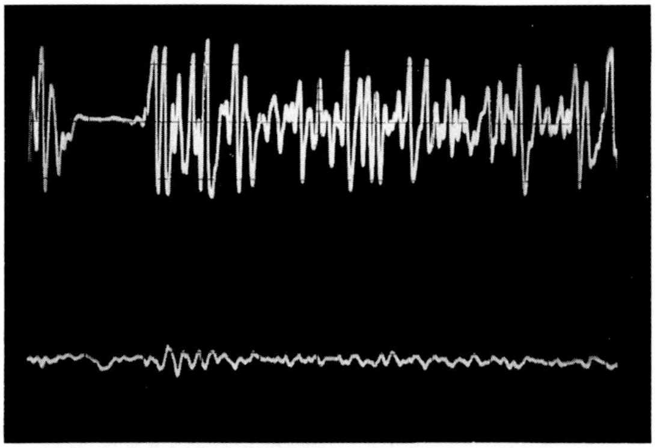

Figs. 7-14a and b Monosynaptic reflex and silent period for same patient as in Figs. 7-12 and 7-13. Surface EMG from the left masseter *(top)* and suprahyoid group *(bottom)* with subject instructed to relax (Fig. 7-14a) or to clench (Fig. 7-14b). The time scale is 200 ms full scale, and the trace was initiated by a tap to the chin.

The blink reflex is evoked by a tap or other stimulus around the eyes and observed electromyographically as activity in the orbicularis oculi muscles. This is one example of a class of reflexes that can be evoked by stimulating the trigeminal nerve and recorded from the muscles innervated by the facial nerve.

The jaw-opening reflex has been regarded as the equivalent of the withdrawal, flexion, or nociceptive reflexes of limbs. A stimulus to the orofacial area causes inhibition of jaw-closing muscles (a silent period) and excitation of jaw-opening muscles.

Biofeedback

Biofeedback may be defined as presenting to a subject a biological variable in a way in which it may be perceived consciously by the subject. For example, blood pressure may be presented as a tone that gets louder when the pressure goes up.

Biofeedback may also be used with the EMG from a jaw muscle. The EMG from a masseter muscle may be presented to a TM disorder patient, and the patient asked to relax the muscle. If the number or level being displayed decreases, the patient is praised and asked to reduce the amplitude further. The goal is to teach the patient to relax the muscle under voluntary, conscious control. A large fraction of such patients respond positively to biofeedback therapy (Carlsson et al., 1975).

Biofeedback may also be used out of the laboratory in the natural environment with miniaturized portable EMG units. Such units may be used to record masseter muscle activity during sleep to determine the amount of nocturnal bruxism of a subject. Feedback of the activity through an earphone to arouse the subject will curtail the bruxing and may help to alleviate symptoms from the bruxing. The use of EMG biofeedback in diagnosis and therapy will be discussed in greater detail in chapter 24.

Summary

It is clear that dentistry deals with maladies in addition to caries and periodontal diseases: bruxism and TM disorders are two prime examples. Muscle activity plays an essential role in these conditions. Numerous controversies have surrounded these disorders, such as the name, the etiology, the treatment, and the subdivisions of diagnosis. Well-meaning and intelligent dentists have labored in good faith for several decades without resolving all of the issues.

Much has been learned about muscle activity in the presence of these conditions, but diagnostic criteria and cause-and-effect relationships are still not clear in most instances. Only through the application of critical clinical observations and sound research based on the scientific method can these issues be resolved. There is little question that increased knowledge of the activity of the musculature will play an important role in the future practice of dentistry.

Chapter 8

The Neuromuscular System

L. F. Greenwood

How does the nervous system control the movements of the face, tongue, and jaws? We cannot yet answer this question completely, but we can put together a coherent story which is probably fairly accurate, even though it involves some conjecture.

Many of the components of the story are derived necessarily from animal studies, and the use of animals poses two problems. First, conclusions reached from animal studies cannot always be extrapolated to humans because both anatomical and physiological details differ in different species. For example, the cat is often used in studies of jaw musculature and movement. But, unlike humans, the cat has no lateral component in its jaw movements, nor does it have spindles in its small lateral pterygoid muscles. Second, for humane reasons, most neural experiments on animals are conducted under general anesthesia, which profoundly depresses the activity of the central nervous system, making interpretation of complex neural events extremely difficult.

Fortunately, chronic recording techniques in conscious animals have improved greatly, and can now monitor neural activity under almost normal conditions so that neural events may be correlated with particular behavior patterns. However, there remain many questions that cannot be addressed using these chronic techniques; so the problem of anesthesia remains with us.

Another problem in forming the full neuromuscular story in humans is the almost universal use of electrical stimulation in neurophysiological experiments. Whereas it is useful in demonstrating potential pathways and interconnections in the nervous system, it does not necessarily demonstrate what happens in a functioning organism when presented with natural stimuli.

The early days of neurophysiology were greatly influenced by Sherrington's work (1906) in which spinal reflexes were elicited in anesthetized or decerebrate cats, and "wiring diagrams" of neural influences on the motoneurons were worked out. The effects of cerebral, cerebellar, pontine, and bulbar structures were also investigated—not only their direct effects, but also their ability to modify a simple reflex response.

This work, limited though it was by crude recording devices, forms the basis of our present concepts of the nervous system. We view this system not as a complex but predictable network where a given input always elicits a given output, but as a hierarchical system where the "building blocks" of simple spinal and cranial reflexes are aggregated into more complex units of synergistic reflexes, and where central and peripheral filtering and modification of both inputs and outputs confers great flexibility on the system and allows it to respond to a given input in different ways, depending upon the prevailing circumstances (Lund and Olsson, 1983). These synergistic reflexes combine to produce automated or cyclic patterns of activity, which in turn form units of behavior in the psychological sense.

In terms of the jaws then, this chapter will begin by looking at simple reflexes such as jaw opening and jaw closing. Then it will cover how

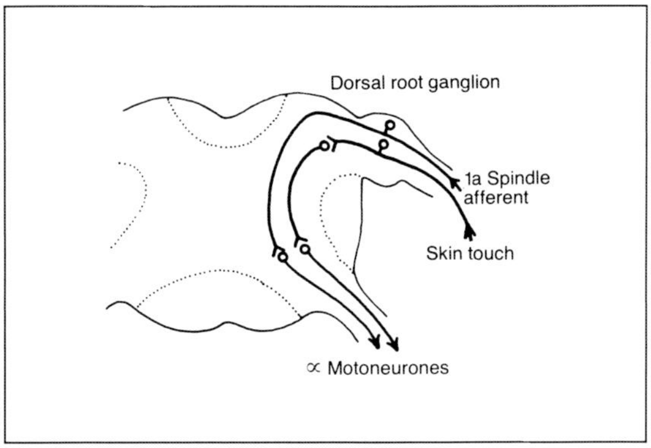

Fig. 8-1a Cross section of spinal cord. Primary afferent fiber cell bodies are contained within the dorsal root ganglion, which is outside the central nervous system (CNS). Simple reflex arcs are shown for stimulation of muscle spindles and skin mechanoreceptors.

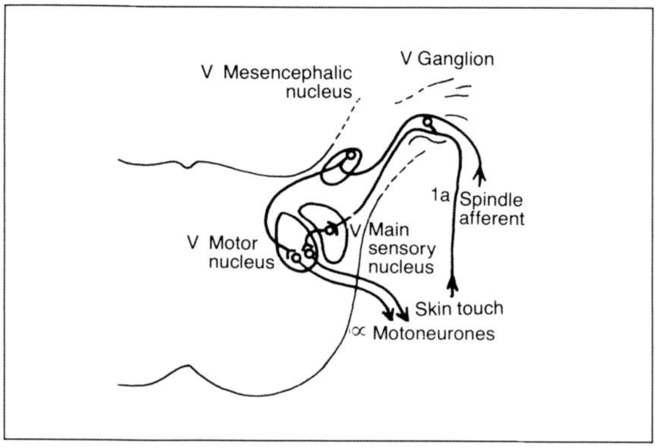

Fig. 8-1b Cross section of brain stem. Primary afferent cell bodies are contained within the trigeminal (V) ganglion (outside the CNS) and in the mesencephalic nucleus (inside the CNS). Contrast the simple reflex pathways with those in Fig. 8-1a.

these are built into more complex synergies involving more than one motor nucleus, such as gagging and spitting, which in turn are incorporated into automated sequential patterns of activity, such as mastication and swallowing. Later chapters will deal with the most complex levels of behavior, including speech.

Simple reflexes

A "simple" reflex arc consists of an afferent pathway from a receptor (e.g., in muscle, joint, skin, mucosa, or periodontium), which connects via one or more synapses to the cell body of a motoneuron in the motor nucleus of a cranial nerve. The efferent pathway is along the motoneuron fibers to the muscle fibers, where muscle contraction is initiated. There may be a direct connection, i.e., one synapse, between the afferent and efferent limbs; or one or more interneurons may be interposed, that is, two or more synapses. The reflex is called simple as long as it is confined to one motor nucleus and only a few interneurons are involved.

Simple reflexes associated with the muscles of mastication and tongue and facial muscles have essentially the same organization as simple spinal reflexes, but there are some important differences (Figs. 8-1a and b).

The cell bodies of primary afferent fibers involved in spinal reflexes are contained within the dorsal root ganglion, which is located outside the central nervous system. In the trigeminal system, the analogue is the trigeminal ganglion, which contains the majority of the trigeminal primary afferent cell bodies and is also outside the central nervous system. However, the cell bodies of trigeminal muscle spindle afferents are found in the trigeminal mesencephalic nucleus *within* the central nervous system. The cells within this nucleus have tight junctions between them, which may allow them to act in concert, either amplifying the incoming signals, or modulating them before they are transmitted onward.

In contrast to the muscles served by spinal neural segments, many oral and facial muscles have no spindles or Golgi tendon organs (see chapter 7). Muscles without muscle spindles obviously have no spindle afferents nor gamma efferents. The proprioceptive role usually played by spindles and tendon organs may be taken over by other receptors either in the muscles themselves or in the surrounding tissues, for example, the skin (Appenteng et al., 1982b) or temporomandibular joint (TMJ) (Lund and Matthews, 1981), but the neural organization is nec-

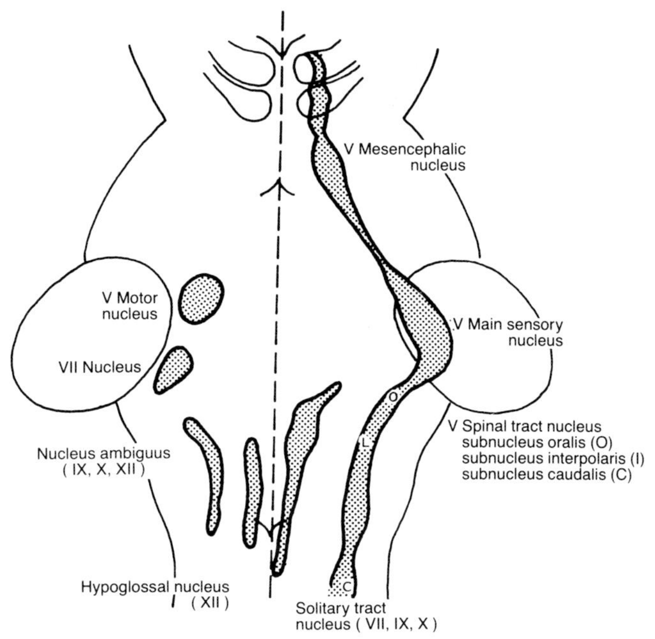

Fig. 8-2 Longitudinal section of the brain stem in the region of the pons. The sensory nuclei are shown on the right and the motor nuclei on the left for clarity, though both are present bilaterally. The roman numerals refer to the cranial nerves represented in the nuclei.

essarily different from that in the spinal cord. There is, for instance, evidence that monosynaptic reflexes may be initiated by receptors other than muscle spindles (see following).

A second organizational difference associated with the oral and facial muscles is that the alternating left side/right side pattern of activity seen in limb muscles (as in walking) is not appropriate for head and neck structures, where the two sides more often act in concert (as in jaw opening and closing). The different functional pattern does not require the reciprocal inhibition seen in the spinal cord, whereby muscle spindle afferent fibers exert opposite effects on the motoneurons of antagonistic muscles (Westerman, 1985). In fact, the lack of spindle afferents and tendon organs in many oral and facial muscles precludes such an arrangement (Lund et al., 1978).

A further basic difference between the spinal and cranial neural organization is seen in the conduction velocity of fibers with similar functions in the two areas. The classification of nerve fibers was first applied to spinal nerves and made on the basis of fiber diameter and conduction velocity. Although we refer to cranial motoneuron fibers as *alpha* and *gamma*, or to spindle afferents as *Ia*, in fact their conduction velocities appear to be slower than those of the analogous spinal fibers and are not strictly within the range of conduction velocities that their names imply. A spinal alpha motoneuron, for instance, may conduct at a rate of 50 to 100 meters per second, whereas a masseter alpha motoneuron would conduct at 25 to 50 meters per second (Greenwood and Sessle, 1976). Some of the apparent discrepancy may be explained by the difficulty of measuring the intracranial length of the fibers accurately, but the slower conduction velocities in cranial motoneurons correlate with their smaller cell body size and smaller fiber diameters.

If we now consider the arrangement of the sensory and motor nuclei of the cranial nerves within the brain stem, there are quite marked differences from the familiar H-shaped gray matter of the spinal cord cross section, with its orderly layers of sensory cells dorsally and motoneurons ventrally. The brain stem sensory and motor nuclei are not only situated very close to each other, as Fig. 8-2 shows, but they also have a rich supply of interneurons linking them. The trigeminal sensory nucleus, especially, has many interneurons not only linking it with other structures, but also running between different parts of the nucleus itself. These interconnections provide a convenient anatomical arrangement for modulation or integration of reflex activities. Thus, there are several neuroanatomical and neurophysiological differences in simple reflexes mediated via cranial and spinal nerves.

Jaw reflexes

Jaw-closing reflex

The simplest possible reflex arc in the jaws has only two neurons and therefore one synapse. This monosynaptic reflex has a very short latency of only 6 ms in humans, between the time the stimulus is applied and the time electrical activity first appears in the muscle fibers. The receptors involved are the muscle spindles in the jaw-closing muscles, which discharge in response to stretch (see chapter 7), activating the Ia afferent fibers that pass to the mesencephalic nucleus of the trigeminal nerve. The central processes of these cells synapse with alpha motoneurons in the trigeminal motor nucleus (see Fig. 8-1). Activation of the alpha motoneurons brings about muscle contraction and jaw closing. This reflex is similar to the knee-jerk reflex, and is sometimes called the jaw-jerk reflex, or masseteric or temporalis reflex, if individual muscles are being singled out. It is usually elicited experimentally by a sharp downward tap to the chin, which causes a sudden stretch of the jaw-closing muscles. This type of stimulus is rarely encountered outside the boxing ring, and the sharp phasic movement it produces is quite unlike the tonic contraction by which these muscles maintain the postural position of the jaw, which relies on simultaneous activation of both alpha and gamma efferent fibers.

Short latency (possibly monosynaptic) activation of jaw-closing muscles may also be elicited by stimulation of periodontal ligament afferent fibers (Greenwood and Sessle, 1976; Sessle, 1977), in which case the afferent cell body may be in the trigeminal mesencephalic nucleus (Larson et al., 1981), though most are in the trigeminal ganglion (Appenteng et al., 1982a) (see Fig. 8-1).

The apparently simple jaw-closing reflex has many ramifications: it can be modulated by activity in other afferent fibers and by descending influences from the cerebral cortex, cerebellum, and other central structures; and of itself sets up inhibitory effects in neighboring structures (Lund and Olsson, 1983) (Fig. 8-3).

Jaw-opening reflex

The jaw-opening reflex involves two or more synapses; its afferent arm relies on receptors in the TMJ, periodontium, oral mucosa, and facial skin, and its efferent arm consists of alpha motoneurons supplying the digastric muscle. The inferior head of the lateral pterygoid and other jaw-opening muscles may also be involved.

Jaw opening is the first craniofacial reflex to appear in the fetus (at 8½ weeks menstrual age) and was at first considered to be a nociceptive reflex analogous to the flexion-withdrawal reflex of the limbs. However, more recent studies showed that it can be elicited by quite gentle stimulation of the mechanoreceptors. The interneurons concerned lie in the descending or spinal tract nucleus of the trigeminal nerve (for receptors in the TMJ, teeth, and oral mucosa) or in the nucleus of the solitary tract (for receptors in the larynx, pharynx, and tongue).

Jaw-unloading reflex

The jaw-unloading reflex is a protective reflex in

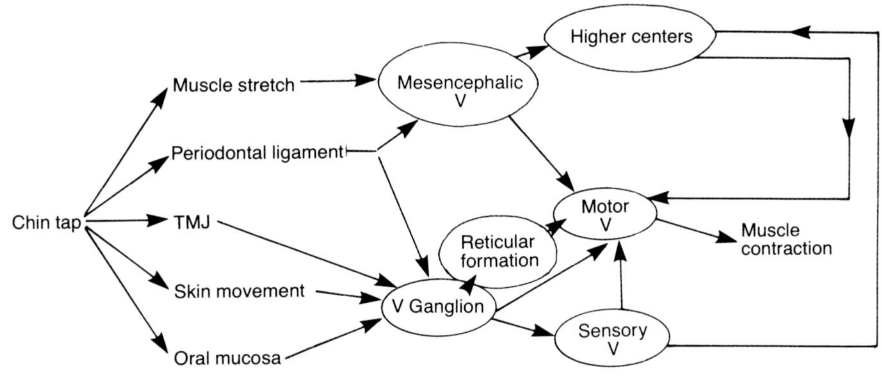

Fig. 8-3 Sequence of events in a simple jaw-closing reflex. The chin-tap stimulus activates receptors in several areas and not only results in the muscle contraction, which brings about jaw closing, but also activates higher centers that in turn influence the motoneurons via descending pathways, which are predominantly inhibitory.

that it prevents the teeth from crashing together forcibly when a hard substance held between the teeth breaks suddenly. The most common, everyday example is cracking nuts between the teeth. The shell yields suddenly but the teeth do not smash together because there is a sudden reduction of activity in jaw-closing muscles and an increase of activity in jaw-opening muscles. The receptors and interneurons involved have not yet been identified.

Horizontal jaw reflexes

The horizontal jaw reflexes are the most important clinically, because they are probably implicated in the everyday dental problems of deflective occlusal contacts and the effects of dental guidance on jaw movements. By extension, they are also likely involved in the structural changes that are thought to stem from alterations in jaw muscle function, including some malocclusions and TMJ disturbances. It is unfortunate, therefore, that very little detailed neurophysiological research has been devoted to these reflexes. The main reason for this apparent oversight is that the pterygoid muscles are small in size compared with other jaw muscles and are relatively inaccessible. Recording techniques are therefore stretched to their limits, and noninvasive techniques, such as surface electromyography (EMG), are not very useful for these types of studies. However, there are several studies that clearly demonstrate the existence of horizontal jaw reflexes without unraveling the neural mechanisms involved; most of these implicate the teeth and periodontium on the receptor side.

Stimulation of the teeth in monkeys and rabbits brings about lateral jaw movements that are correlated with activation of the lateral pterygoid muscles (Lund and Dellow, 1971; Sessle and Gurza, 1982).

In humans, EMG techniques have been used to study the asymmetrical muscle effects produced by making various changes in the patterns of tooth contact both in intercuspal position and in eccentric excursions of the mandible.

Postural activity may be increased asymmetrically by placing high restorations on molars in intercuspal position. When the interference is removed, muscle activity returns to normal (Randow et al., 1976; Funakoshi et al., 1976; Riise and Sheikholeslam, 1982). Increased muscle activity is accompanied by clinical symptoms such as pain and clicking. However, in studies where nonworking side interferences occurring naturally were removed (Ingervall and Carlsson, 1982), or where such interferences were placed experimentally (Schärer and Stallard, 1966; Graf and Zander, 1963), there was little change in muscle activity or gross clinical effects such as pain or dysfunction. Subtle changes in muscle function were revealed by more sophisticated recording techniques (Hannam et al., 1977). However, the effects of adding a working side interference were not predictable from subject to subject (Hannam et al., 1981), whereas the addition of nonworking side interferences appeared to have a significant effect on muscle activity only in eccentric clenching movements such as might be made during occlusal parafunction (Belser and Hannam, 1985).

Some early work investigated the presence or absence of silent periods in EMG activity of masticatory muscles while subjects chewed on dentitions that artificially provided canine guidance (Butler and Zander, 1968) or nonworking side interferences (Schärer and Stallard, 1966). Silent periods were seen in 40% of nonworking side contacts, 5% of working side contacts, and not at all in canine guidance contacts. The absence of silent periods was taken to show that the actions concerned were passive in nature and did not involve reflex activity. However, tooth contacts may be avoided by changes in mandibular movements that do not involve silent periods in muscle electrical activity (Storey, 1975), and so the absence of a silent period does not necessarily indicate lack of reflex participation. The larger and more acute the interference is, the greater the chance of avoidance movements—but there is no clear evidence on this point as yet.

Clark and Adler (1985) reviewed occlusal therapy and concluded that naturally occurring occlusal interferences both in maximum intercuspation and in excursive movements may, if they contact in an adverse or forceful manner, harm the periodontal tissues. The effects of iatrogenic (i.e., acutely placed) interferences depend upon their location; those interfering with maximum intercuspation can chronically alter postural muscle activity and produce dental and muscle pain, while those interfering only with excursive contacts do not usually disrupt muscle activity or the chewing cycle and are much less likely to cause clinical symptoms.

Facial reflexes

Facial reflexes are important as diagnostic tools in clinical medicine, the most common example being the use of the corneal (blink) reflex to test for depth of anesthesia. Neurological disorders such as facial palsy and trigeminal neuralgia result in characteristic changes in reflexes, and while there is as yet no clear evidence on this point, dentally important disorders of lip posture and function may be associated with facial reflex changes.

Tapping the skin of the face elicits reflex contractions in the orbicularis oculi and orbicularis oris muscles. The mechanoreceptors involved are associated with afferent trigeminal fibers whose cell bodies are in the trigeminal ganglion and relay, via interneurons in the trigeminal spinal tract, to the motoneurons in the motor nucleus of the facial nerve (nVII). It is probable that nociceptor stimulation can elicit similar reflexes since orbicularis oris contraction in particular can be initiated by stimulation of high threshold intraoral receptors.

The facial nerve contains about 20% sensory fibers, which are mainly high threshold and concerned with general visceral sensation. There are few, if any, muscle spindles in facial muscles, and their proprioceptive function is probably taken over by cutaneous receptors transmitting through the trigeminal nerve. There is therefore no monosynaptic reflex associated with facial musculature.

Tongue reflexes

The motor nerve of the tongue is the hypoglossal (nXII). The interneurons are in either the trigeminal spinal tract or the solitary tract nucleus, and the receptors concerned are found in the oral, lingual, laryngeal, and pharyngeal mucosae, periodontium, TMJ, and tongue muscle.

In humans, both the intrinsic and extrinsic tongue muscles contain many muscle spindles. The intrinsic muscles allow the tongue to change its shape, while the extrinsic muscles move it bodily up or down, from side to side, and in and out. The potentially huge number of movements possible has made it difficult to isolate the precise effect of a single stimulus on one particular muscle, and, until recently, most studies concentrated on recording gross reflex activity in the hypoglossal nerve. However, electromyographic studies of individual intrinsic muscles in monkeys and humans suggest stimuli delivered to the anterior part of the mouth bring about tongue retraction via the hypoglossus muscle, whereas stimulation of the larynx, pharynx, and TMJ mainly produce tongue protrusion via genioglossus muscle reflex activity. The retraction reflexes would help to prevent the tongue from being bitten during chewing, while the protrusive reflexes may help to preserve the airway during laryngeal or pharyngeal obstruction. A chronic obstruction with concomitant tongue protrusion may even be responsible for some anterior open-bite malocclusions (Lowe and Johnston, 1979).

Vagal reflexes (larynx, pharynx, palate)

Vagal reflexes are often neglected in dental texts. However, they are important not only because of their involvement in speech and swallowing, but because of their role in reflex protection of the airway and the alimentary tract.

Most motoneuron axons involved in these reflexes run in the vagus nerve (nX) with cell bodies in the nucleus ambiguus (see Fig. 8-2). The glossopharyngeal (nIX) and accessory (nXII) nerves also contribute. The sensory fibers derive from the glossopharyngeal and vagus nerves, with some trigeminal input. The interneurons are found principally in the solitary tract nucleus, trigeminal tract nucleus (V input), and adjacent reticular formation. If the laryngeal or pharyngeal mucosa is stimulated, there is a reflex closure of the glottis and suppression of ventilation, in addition to reflex activity in tongue, face, and jaw muscles. These protective reflexes, which would prevent aspiration of fluid or food into the lungs, are powerful and preeminent. Their existence is but one example of the wide ranging and physiologically important connections of intraoral receptors.

Regulation of reflex activity

Central regulation

In most discussions of central regulation of reflex activity, the first topic discussed is the cerebral cortex. The major emphasis is placed on the direct pathway between the cortex and motoneurons, called the *pyramidal pathway.* Most neurophysiological studies have concentrated on this system because, complex though it is, it seems straightforward by comparison with the other central motor pathway, the extrapyramidal system. The extrapyramidal system consists of phylogenetically more ancient structures such as the basal ganglia, cerebellum, reticular formation, and limbic system. A further complication is that these two central systems, pyramidal and extrapyramidal, can exert their effects on motor activity in several ways: *(1)* directly on the alpha motoneurons, *(2)* via the gamma motoneurons and the spindle afferent loop (see chapter 7), or *(3)* by gating incoming sensory information and thereby modulating the ongoing motor effect.

The early neat and tidy ideas of motor organization have become less clear-cut as a result of recent research. For example, the implications of the sensory and motor homunculi (Fig. 8-4) that discrete areas of the cerebral cortex are responsible for specific sensory or motor activities is no longer tenable because there is some overlap of function between the two areas. The "somato-

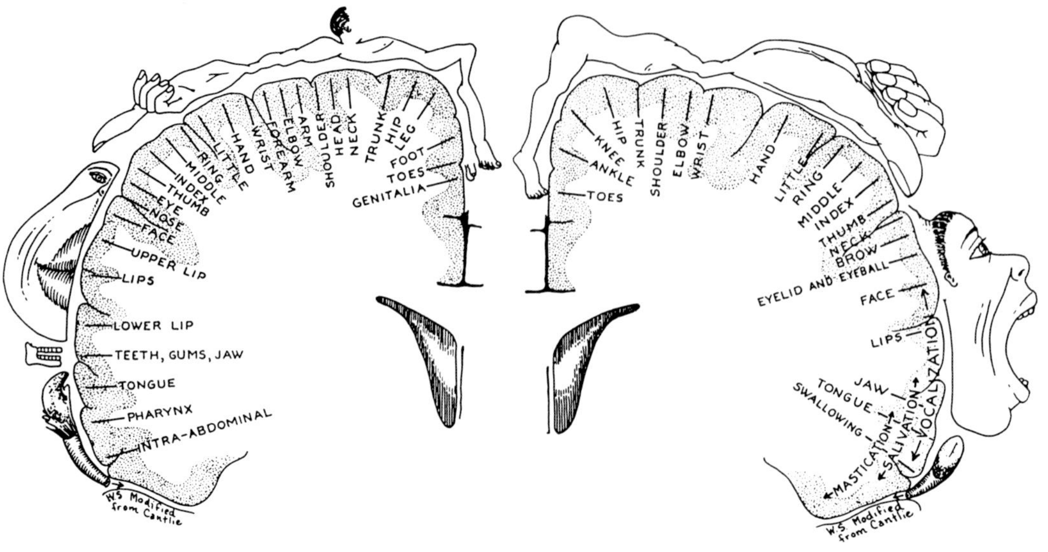

Fig. 8-4 Sensory *(left)* and motor *(right)* homunculi depict cortical areas of representation of different body parts. The oral and facial regions have large areas of representation out of all proportion to their actual size. (Modified from Everett, 1965, reprinted with permission from Lea & Febiger.)

sensory'' area, for instance, contains some neurons that are concerned with motor activities, while the ''motor'' cortex contains some sensory neurons that receive feedback from oral and facial areas and so can monitor the progress of a particular movement pattern. Studies in which cortical areas have been either stimulated, removed, or recorded from in conscious animals have shown that movements, rather than individual muscles, are represented at cortical levels and even quite complex activities such as swallowing or rhythmic alternating jaw-opening and jaw-closing can be initiated by stimulation of the appropriate cortical site. This is not to say that the cortex is the only site that can initiate these movements; even decorticate humans and animals can chew and swallow with only small apparent changes in motility.

However, our present topic is not central initiation of movement but central modulation of reflex activity. As a rough generalization, cortical activity facilitates jaw-opening reflexes and inhibits jaw-closing reflexes. Both pre- and postsynaptic influences on the trigeminal motoneurons have been demonstrated, and both alpha and gamma motoneurons are susceptible to central influences. A multitude of pathways is therefore available whereby voluntary modification of jaw reflexes can take place, but the central modulation can also be turned on by peripheral influences. For example, there is evidence in humans that feedback to cortical neurons from periodontal mechanoreceptors can induce changes in excitability of jaw muscle motoneurons (Lamarre and Lund, 1975). These long loop transcortical reflexes may be involved in the control of jaw musculature during activities such as crushing of foodstuffs, where the load is constantly changing.

The effect of cortical stimulation on jaw reflexes can also be changed by the central state of the animal. Changes in sleep state are responsible for the most profound alterations. For example, in the awake animal, cortical stimulation inhibits the masseteric jaw-closing reflex; this inhibition is reduced when the animal is asleep. Inhibition induced by peripheral stimuli is unchanged in these circumstances, showing that sleep does not produce a general reduction of conditioning effects (Chase and McGinty, 1970).

The extrapyramidal system and its effects on jaw reflexes present yet more complex interactions. Stimulation of the hypothalamus, amygdala, cerebellum, and reticular formation can modulate jaw reflexes. Again, the precise effect depends on the state of the animal. For example, in the cat, stimulation of the reticular formation in the awake animal facilitates the masseteric jaw-closing reflex, whereas the same stimulus induces inhibition of the reflex while the cat is in active (rapid eye movement) sleep (Chase et al., 1976). Another example illustrates how the response to a stimulus can be entirely changed by extrapyramidal stimulation, even to the extent of utilizing different cranial motor nuclei. In normal circumstances, touching the skin of a cat's muzzle causes the lips to close. If the hypothalamus is stimulated just before the same skin stimulus is delivered, the response changes to a jaw-opening movement coupled with a turn of the head, thus involving jaw and neck muscles, rather than facial muscles, as in the first example.

Stress and emotion also have a profound effect on jaw reflex activity. These exert their effects through subcortical centers such as the limbic system and reticular formation. Experimentally induced stress causes marked hyperactivity of the masseter muscles (Yemm, 1971a, 1971b, 1976a); even adverse comments from the dean of a dental school were enough to increase the activity of the masseter muscles in one dental student (Perry et al., 1960). The pathways by which such effects are exerted are not yet well defined, but their clinical significance is very high in conditions such as those TM disorders where there is an important psychological or psychophysiological component.

All these descending influences, whether originating in the cortex or in the extrapyramidal system, act in part by regulating incoming sensory information (see Fig. 8-3). Inhibition by cortical stimulation of transmission in the trigeminal spinal tract nucleus was first shown almost 30 years ago; investigations since then have confirmed that most descending regulatory mechanisms are inhibitory and depend on presynaptic depolarization of the primary afferent terminals, mainly on the contralateral side.

The relationships appear to be highly specific, at least in the tactile pathways, in that primary afferent fiber terminals are depolarized (i.e., inhibited) by stimulation of the same site on the cerebral cortex to which they eventually transmit their information. This arrangement allows for a negative feedback loop, which may serve to maximize discrimination of tactile stimulus edges and increase signal-to-noise ratios in the relevant pathways. But in addition to this discriminatory function, these pathways play a role in oral and facial motor control, because the tactile primary afferent fibers (among others) are involved in reflex functions. This kind of mechanism may play a part, for example, in the distraction techniques practiced by dentists when giving an intraoral injection of local anesthetic. The tactile and noxious stimulus of the needle would usually evoke a reflex withdrawal of the head, but if the dentist keeps up a soothing flow of talk while inserting the needle, the reflex withdrawal movement can be suppressed. This principle should be considered, too, in relation to altered physiological states. If the central conditions are changed—at times of great emotion or anxiety, for example—and at the same time the peripheral conditions are changed—by a painful tooth or a high restoration, for example—then the interaction of the regulatory influences could well account for altered patterns of mandibular movement.

This leads to a consideration of the modification of reflex activity by peripheral factors.

Peripheral regulation

The foregoing discussion of simple jaw reflexes illustrates how peripheral sensory stimuli can initiate motor activity in a reflex pathway. If another sensory stimulus is delivered just before the initiating stimulus, then the reflex activity evoked can be modified, that is to say, facilitated, inhibited, or even entirely suppressed. The neural mechanisms involved, which are both pre- and post-synaptic, will not be discussed here since details can be found in most neurophysiological textbooks.

Although jaw-muscle reflexes can be influenced by stimuli applied to many parts of the body, the most effective modifying or "conditioning" influences come from intraoral stimuli. These cause complex and long-lasting changes in the basic reflex pattern. *In jaw-closing muscles, the dominant effect of intraoral conditioning stimuli is inhibition.* For example, if a tooth is tapped just prior to reflex stimulation of a masseter motoneuron, the excitability of the motoneuron is briefly enhanced, then depressed, with concomitant changes in the vigor of any resulting reflex movement. If the muscle is tonically active when the conditioning stimulus is applied, the depression of activity following the brief excitation shows up in the record as a "silent period" that may last several hundred milliseconds. Similar effects can be obtained in tongue, laryngeal, and pharyngeal muscles and with a variety of conditioning stimuli of both intraoral and more remote sites such as limbs.

In jaw-opening muscles the dominant conditioning effect is facilitation. The conditioning stimuli, therefore, tend to have opposite effects on the jaw-opening and jaw-closing muscles. Similar reciprocal effects probably exist in the antagonist tongue-protruding and tongue-retruding muscles.

However, in considering the regulation of reflex activity as one conditioning stimulus followed by one initiating (or "test") stimulus, we lose sight of the real situation, which is that each motoneuron has hundreds or thousands of neurons communicating with it and that the motoneuron cell membrane sums all the inputs (some positive, some negative) from all these neurons. At a certain critical level, an action potential is produced and a motor unit in the target muscle is activated. It is not surprising then, that in order to elicit the apparently simple monosynaptic jaw-closing reflex by tapping the chin in humans, certain conditions have to be fulfilled. For example, the monosynaptic excitation is not seen unless the mouth is slightly open, and the ensuing silent period is seen only if there is tonic contraction of the masseter muscles.

The length of the silent period and the ease of elicitation of the reflex can also be manipulated by altering variables such as head position and strength and duration of the stimulus. Similar dependency on conditions is also seen in more complex jaw activities such as chewing: tactile sensitivity thresholds in humans are increased during chewing (Öwall and Møller, 1974), the phase of mastication during which a stimulus is applied may alter its effect (Forssberg et al., 1975), and stimulus effectiveness varies according to whether the side of application is the working or nonworking (Goldberg, 1972).

Synergies

We now turn to combining these building blocks of "simple" reflexes (simple insofar as they concern only one motor nucleus; their ramifications and regulation are certainly far from simple) into more complex reflex synergies, where more than one motor nucleus is involved. They include reflexes of the upper alimentary tract and upper respiratory tract, and have usefully been divided into *supportive reflexes,* which aid the intake of food, liquids, or air (as in swallowing or sniffing), and *protective reflexes,* which either prevent liquids or solids from entering the respiratory tract (as in apnea, glottic closure, or gagging) or expel foreign or noxious material from either tract (as in coughing, spitting, or vomiting) (Storey, 1975) (Fig. 8-5).

Gagging

Gagging is a useful synergy for us to consider here as representative because it often poses problems in dental treatment, especially in impression taking and design of maxillary dentures. The receptors involved are mechanoreceptors in the mucosa of the base of the tongue, palate, posterior pharyngeal wall, and pillars of the fauces. The interneurons are in the solitary tract

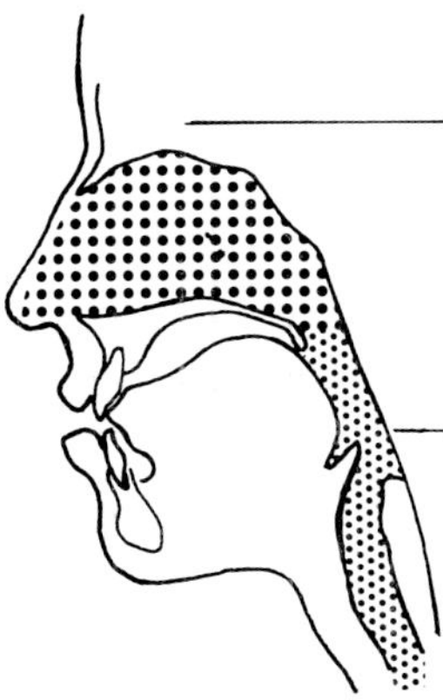

	EFFECTOR SITES	SUPPORTIVE REFLEXES	PROTECTIVE REFLEXES
UPPER AIRWAY	Nose	Sniffling	Apnea / Sneezing
	Pharynx	Airway maintenance	Sniffling
	Larynx	Airway maintenance	Apnea / Glottic closure Swallowing / Coughing
ALIMENTARY TRACT	Mouth	Suckling Mastication	Spitting
	Pharynx	Swallowing	Gagging
	Esophagus	Swallowing	Vomiting

Fig. 8-5 Supportive and protective reflexes that arise from the upper airway and alimentary tract. In the figure on the left the airway is stippled throughout; the alimentary tract is clear except in the region of the oropharynx where the airway and alimentary tract cross over. (Modified from Storey, 1976.)

nucleus and adjacent reticular formation. The motoneurons are mostly in the glossopharyngeal, vagal, facial, trigeminal, and hypoglossal motor nuclei. The motor activities of gagging and vomiting are very similar—both reverse the order of events in swallowing.

Gagging can be conditioned in the psychological sense, and the sight of a loaded impression tray may be enough to set off a susceptible patient. None of the clinical tricks used to prevent gagging is entirely effective. Since the central regulation of this synergy is quite marked, procedures that calm the patient and reduce anxiety should be generally useful, together with a variety of procedures that rely on distraction. Hypnosis and posthypnotic suggestion can be very effective on appropriate subjects.

Rhythmic mastication

At the next highest level of organization, complex synergies combine either in an automated pattern, as in swallowing, or in a rhythmically alternating pattern, as in mastication. It is apparent from the discussion of muscle activity patterns during chewing (chapter 7) that *mastication involves more than mere rhythmic alternation of opening and closing jaw movements*. The question, then, is whether these movements are programmed by a central mechanism or depend on a reciprocal interplay of simple jaw reflexes as described above.

The early view that mastication had a reflex basis has been displaced by the notion of a central pattern generator that sets up a rhythmic cycle of jaw-opening and jaw-closing movements. This basic pattern is then modified by central and reflex activity, depending upon the shape, size, and consistency of the bolus; the movements of the tongue and lips; and other variables. It is probably premature to call this central pattern generator a "chewing center," since it is not certain that it generates the horizontal jaw movements or the coordinated tongue and facial movements that are a part of chewing activity.

Stimulation and sectioning experiments locate

the pattern generator in the pontine reticular formation, but its precise location and the properties of its cells have not been established. Stimulation of the pattern generator in anesthetized animals gives rise to rhythmic opening and closing movements whose frequency is independent of the frequency of stimulation but is dependent on the level of anesthesia. It was noted above that stimulation of higher centers such as the motor cortex can also produce rhythmic opening and closing movements. However, these higher centers are not essential to the rhythmic movements, as is the pontine center. The generator can function independently of peripheral feedback, but its rate can be influenced by peripheral stimuli that can initiate mastication, such as the presence of a bolus in the mouth and the consistency of the bolus. That human beings chew soft foods faster than hard foods illustrates the effect of peripheral feedback in mastication (though, again, it must be remembered that the cyclic pattern generator is just that, and not a "chewing center").

Central regulation of cyclic jaw activity

Although there is evidence that central sites such as the cerebral cortex, basal ganglia, hypothalamus, red nucleus, cerebellum, and reticular formation can not only initiate but also modify cyclic jaw activity and feeding behavior, only the cerebral cortex has been explored in any detail in unanesthetized primates. Information from other sites is scanty and conflicting because of differences among species and levels of anesthesia. For a detailed review the reader is referred to Kubota (1976), and for brief reviews to Dubner et al. (1978) and Lund (1985).

Although studies so far have not clearly demonstrated the role of different parts of the cerebral cortex in the initiation and control of jaw movements, they have shown a remarkable number of neurons in the "motor" areas of the cerebral cortex, which receive sensory information from the oral and facial areas. These loops from the periphery to the cerebral cortex to the cyclic pattern generator to the jaw muscle motoneurons are involved not only in the control of crushing activity (covered in the section dealing with central regulation of reflex activity), but would also be concerned with the learning and maturation of jaw mobility patterns. It has been speculated, for instance, that the cyclic pattern generator for chewing in the adult develops from the pattern generator involved in suckling in the infant, the maturational changes being prompted in part by the changing peripheral feedback as the jaws and dentition develop (Dellow, 1969).

Peripheral regulation of cyclic jaw activity

Whereas peripheral influences can affect motoneuron activity directly or via loops through the cerebral cortex, they can also exert their effects at the level of the cyclic pattern generator. Animal experiments show that cyclic jaw activity initiated by stimulation of the pattern generator can be suppressed by noxious stimulation, not only of oral and facial sites, but also by stimulation of remote areas such as a limb. Low-intensity stimulation of intraoral areas facilitates the rhythmic movements.

There is also a suggestion of interactions between the "chewing" and "swallowing" centers in that strong stimulation of the superior laryngeal nerve inhibits cyclic jaw movements evoked by cortical stimulation, but facilitates cortically evoked swallowing: this arrangement has obvious protective value if swallowing, with its respiratory implications, takes precedence over chewing. However, even in the animal experiments involving centrally induced cyclic activity, it is not clear at which of the many possible levels the peripheral influences are acting.

The picture becomes still more confused when one turns to humans or the higher primates and looks at mastication itself. Changes in mastication can certainly be related to changes in peripheral input, such as alterations in food consistency (Ahlgren, 1966) or occlusal anatomy (Hannam et al., 1977), but the complexity of the neural mechanisms involved has so far precluded a precise description of how the peripheral stimuli bring about the observed changes in mastication. In addition, most studies have concentrated on the effects of intraoral and, especially, periodontal stimulation. Receptors such as those in the jaw musculature and the TMJ, which are likely to be involved in the modification of cyclic jaw activity, have so far received little attention.

Some of the apparently confusing observations in this field need a closer look. It was stated earlier that cyclic jaw activity can be initiated and maintained in the absence of all peripheral input, yet peripheral events can influence its rate. These statements are not contradictory, but merely reflect an "optional extra" in the control system—just as a car with automatic transmission may also have a couple of gears that can be operated manually.

The observation that unilateral or bilateral destruction of the trigeminal mesencephalic nucleus (which contains the cell bodies of the spindle afferents from the jaw muscles) causes little or no change in the rate of chewing, muscle EMG, or jaw movement patterns in monkeys (Goodwin and Luschei, 1975) would suggest that the muscle spindles are not involved in the control of mastication. This would back up the observation that cyclical movements continue in the absence of peripheral input. However, the changes involved may have been too subtle to be detected by such gross methods as EMG and movement recording, or other afferent systems may have compensated for the loss of the muscle spindle input. Similar arguments can be raised in the case of experiments in which various sites have been anesthetized with no apparent change in jaw muscle EMG or movements in humans (Schärer et al., 1966).

Another consideration is the ability of the brain to suppress selected incoming information; it may be that peripheral inputs that are capable of modifying cyclic jaw activity or mastication are suppressed in some circumstances, and so appear to be ineffective. An example is in the work of Öwall and Møller (1974), which showed that, during chewing in human beings, the tactile threshold of the teeth is raised by a factor of 60. More evidence comes from the work of Lund and Rossignol (1981), which was summarized and elaborated upon by Lund (1985). The jaw-opening reflex was produced in lightly anesthetized rabbits by both high- and low-intensity stimulation of intraoral and extraoral sites, while jaw movement was recorded together with EMG activity of the jaw-opening and jaw-closing muscles.

When the jaw-opening reflex was elicited by *low*-intensity electrical stimulation and the animal began to chew, the amplitude of the reflex fell. The amplitude returned when chewing ceased. The functional significance of this is that the low-threshold stimulation is of the type that would be generated during mastication by the presence of a moving bolus of food within the mouth; if a jaw-opening reflex were generated with the arrival of each stimulus, then the process of chewing would be hopelessly disrupted. The suppression of the jaw-opening reflex during chewing allows mastication to proceed.

However, the outcome was different if *high*-threshold (i.e., noxious) stimulation was used to elicit the jaw-opening reflex. In this case not only was there no reduction of the reflex amplitude when chewing started, there was even an enhancement of the reflex. Functionally, this accounts for the protective effect of reflex jaw opening when the tongue or cheek is bitten accidentally or a hard object is encountered during chewing.

A hypothetical brain-stem control system for mastication has been proposed on the basis of these and other observations (Lund, 1985) whereby useful reflexes are integrated into the total pattern while potentially disruptive ones are suppressed.

Mastication itself will be covered in chapter 10, but a brief summary of the present neurophysiological evidence is pertinent here. *The basic pattern of cyclic jaw opening and jaw closing is provided by a pattern generator in the pontine reticular formation. The generator can be activated from both central and peripheral sites, although it can act independently of either.*

The generator can be silenced by peripheral stimuli, which are potentially damaging; its rate can be altered by low-intensity peripheral stimuli, especially from the oral cavity; and its maturation is affected by peripheral feedback. Otherwise it appears to be surprisingly insensitive to peripheral low-threshold feedback, possibly as a result of the many compensatory mechanisms available or because of central suppression of incoming information.

Postural rest position of the mandible

The first question to address is whether postural rest position is actively or passively maintained. Yemm and Berry (1969) and Yemm (1976b) opt for a passive mechanism involving the elastic elements of the jaw musculature, which include the connective tissue, ligaments, and tendons. The tendency for the jaw to drop open under the influence of gravity is balanced by the elastic forces built up in the jaw-closing muscles as they are passively stretched beyond their rest positions. The evidence cited is the low level of, or perhaps lack of, EMG activity in the jaw musculature of humans at postural rest position, and the lack of change in the force needed to maintain an open jaw position immediately after an animal has been killed.

Other investigations have demonstrated EMG activity at postural rest position (e.g., Møller, 1976) and tonic activity in trigeminal motoneurons in animal experiments (Sessle and Greenwood, 1976; Sessle, 1977). Also, most people have observed that during sleep the jaw drops open. *The consensus at the moment is that mandibular postural rest position is actively determined.* The next question is, which of three possible reflex mechanisms is responsible: the monosynaptic stretch reflex, reflexes from TMJ receptors, or airway protective reflexes?

The stretch reflex has been discussed above. Its role in maintaining postural rest position would parallel the posture-maintaining role of the stretch reflex in limb muscles.

The effect of TMJ receptors on jaw postural position in the cat was investigated in 1966 by Greenfield and Wyke, who separated jaw muscles from their attachments and then recorded their EMG activity at different degrees of jaw opening; closing the jaw decreased EMG activity and opening the jaw increased it. These changes could be suppressed reversibly by infiltrating local anesthetic around the joints, which would indicate that receptors within the joint were responsible, at least to some extent, for the EMG changes.

As for the airway reflexes, clinical evidence shows that enlarged pharyngeal tonsils (adenoids) lead to mouth-breathing with a change in postural rest position, either a chronic forward posturing of the mandible or an inferior and posterior rotation of the mandible. This may be accompanied by a slight extension of the head (Mohl, 1984). The underlying mechanisms are poorly understood at this time, although it seems clear that respiratory requirements take precedence over all others.

In normal circumstances, both the stretch reflex and the TMJ reflexes are probably involved in maintaining postural rest position of the mandible, just as the analogous muscle and joint receptors are involved in maintaining limb posture. However, in situations where there is chronic embarrassment of the airway, changes in postural rest position that tend to restore airway adequacy will predominate (Storey, 1975).

Summary

A given input into the neuromuscular system may result in one of many possible outputs, depending on conditions in the rest of the system. Simple reflexes are combined and modified both centrally and peripherally to produce the complex synergistic integrated activities of the oral and facial neuromuscular system.

Chapter 9

Mandibular Movements

John D. Rugh and Rodney W. Johnson

Border movements

Mandibular movements take place within certain three-dimensional limits, as shown in Fig. 9-1. The mandible can move about 10 mm laterally, open about 50 to 60 mm, protrude approximately 9 mm, and retrude about 1 mm. It was these limits that Posselt described in 1952 and which are known as border movements of the mandible. Stated simply, border movements are the most extreme positions to which the jaw is able to move. A tracing of these borders, as in Fig. 9-1, is made by moving the mandible along its most extreme range of motions. These positions are generally considered to be relatively stable and reproducible, except under certain pathological states. Border movements have been described from the sagittal, frontal, and horizontal planes. Such movements are usually not affected by head or body posture. One should become familiar with the border movements from these three perspectives and understand the structures that are responsible for limiting jaw movement.

Sagittal plane border movements

Posselt's diagram of the sagittal plane border movements is a tracing of the maximum vertical and anterior-posterior movements of the mandibular central incisors with respect to the maxillary teeth. It is thus a map of the boundary or border movements of the mandible when viewed from one side of the head, as shown in Figs. 9-2a and b. Key structures directly affecting the border movements are also shown. The following determine border movements of the mandible in the sagittal plane: incisors, posterior occlusion, temporomandibular joints (TMJs), disk, and, not shown in Figs. 9-2a and b, the muscles and ligaments.

To better understand mandibular movements and border positions, Figs. 9-2a and b and 9-3 should be carefully studied. It is helpful to position one's jaw in the various border positions and observe structures that determine these limits. Compare these with the figures. The first and perhaps most important mandibular border position is *maximum intercuspation* or *centric occlusion*. This border position is usually defined as that point where the teeth best interdigitate, that is, where there is a maximum number of teeth contacting. The mandible is usually guided into this position during closure by occlusal inclines of the teeth (Fig. 9-2b*1*). Centric occlusion is thus the usual end point in the chewing cycle and the position at which most individuals position the mandible when swallowing. This is a tooth-determined border position, usually resulting from a long period of growth, development, and adaptation. This position may change when tooth morphology or tooth position is altered through restorative dentistry or orthodontics.

When the mandible is moved retrusively with the teeth in light contact, the anterior teeth usually separate and the incisal point moves inferiorly and posteriorly (Fig. 9-2b2). This occurs in

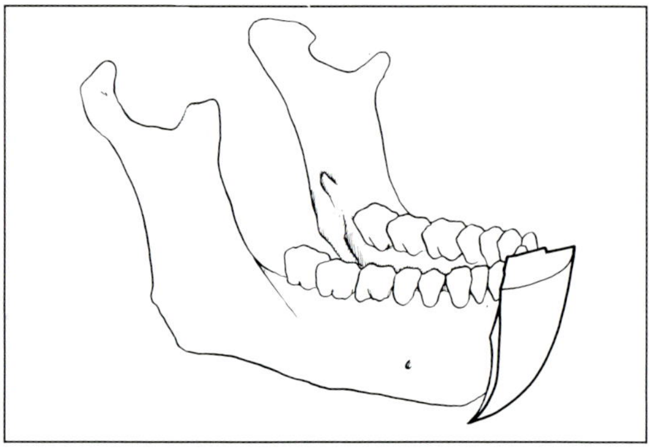

Fig. 9-1 Three-dimensional limits of mandibular movement. (Modified from Posselt, 1952.)

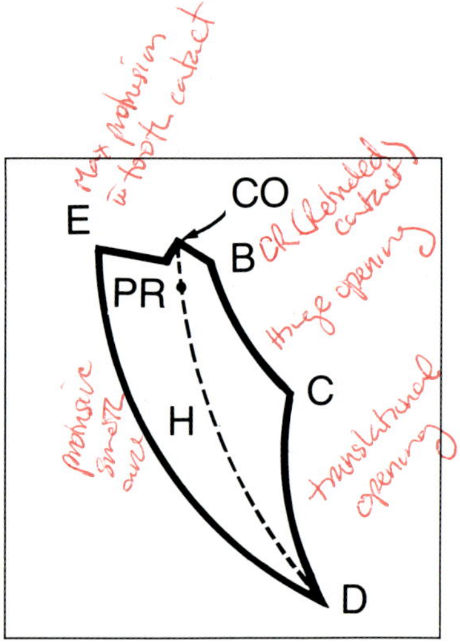

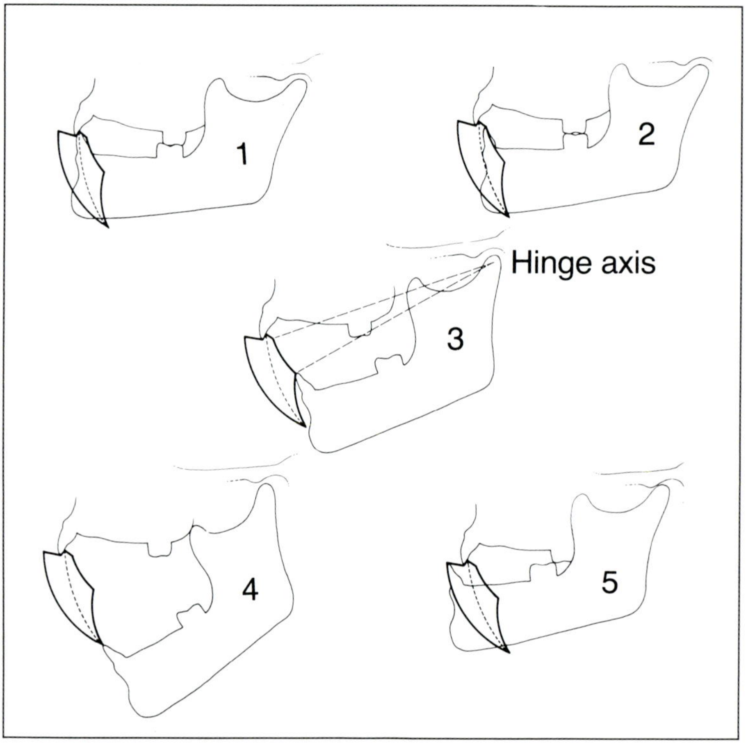

Fig. 9-2a *(above)* Mandibular border movements in the sagittal plane. Centric occlusion *(CO)* and the other most superior portions of the border movements are tooth-determined positions. Other border positions—retruded contact position *(B)*, the rotational hinge movement opening *(line B to C)*, the translation phase of opening *(line C to D)*, the protrusive smooth arc *(line D to E)* to maximum protrusion with tooth contact *(E)*—are determined by structures of the joint and associated ligaments. Review the condyle-fossa relationships at the various border positions. Note that postural rest position *(PR)* and the path of habitual closure *(H)* are not located on any of the borders.

Fig. 9-2b *(right) (1)* Note the position of the mandibular incisal point in centric occlusion. *(2)* This point moves inferiorly and posteriorly as the mandible is retruded with posterior occlusal contact. *(3)* The incisal point arcs downward and backward during retruded rotational opening. *(4)* Note the position of this point during maximum opening with condylar translation. *(5)* Maximum protrusion with tooth contact brings the incisal point to a reverse incisal overbite position.

approximately 90% of the population (Posselt, 1952). Posterior tooth contacts provide guidance, and thus dictate the angle at which this inferior and posterior movement occurs. Again, in order to better understand these various jaw positions, one will find it helpful to position the jaw in the respective positions and observe the structures that appear to be determining the jaw position.

If the mandible is retruded farther to its posterior-most, superior-most *terminal hinge position,* the limits of movement and the border position are determined by structures of the TM joint. Normally the structures that ultimately limit posterior movement are the left and right TM ligaments (see chapter 6). However, the thickened posterior edge of the articular disk may also play a role in determining this retruded border position. Some have also referred to this position as *centric relation*; however, it must be remembered that centric relation has been defined in a number of different ways (see terminology in chapter 1). The term *retruded contact position* is often used to refer to the position of the mandible when it is in centric relation and initial occlusal contact occurs. The difference between the retruded contact position and the intercuspal position is usually between 0.5 to 1.5 mm with Angle Class I occlusions. This has been referred to as the *slide in centric*.

If the condyles are held in this terminal hinge position and the mouth is opened, the superior segment of the posterior border of Posselt's diagram is recorded (Fig. 9-2b3). This portion of jaw movement is referred to as a *hinge movement,* since the jaw is rotating about a stationary hinge axis. Movement is thus primarily rotational.

As the mandible continues to open (Fig. 9-2b4), at about 19 mm between the maxillary and mandibular molars (Posselt, 1952), the condyle begins to travel or translate inferiorly and anteriorly on the articular eminence, thus the term *translation*. The fact that the human mandible cannot open all the way with a purely rotational movement is a necessary adaptation to our upright posture (see chapter 6). The posterior border of Posselt's diagram is thus a combination of terminal hinge rotation and translatory movements. The maximum average openings for healthy adults 20 years of age are 58.6 mm for men and 53.3 mm for women (Agerberg, 1974). Values are less for younger and older individuals.

The protrusive arc of jaw movement, when closing from the maximum open position, is limited by muscle and ligament, and is a smooth arc due to the condyles remaining in a translated relationship.

Finally, the most superior movements of the mandible are determined by tooth contact. When the mandible is thrust protrusively from centric occlusion and the teeth held in light contact, the mandibular incisors will typically slide anteriorly and inferiorly in contact with the lingual surfaces of the maxillary incisors. The angle at which the mandibular incisor moves is determined by the relative amount of overbite and overjet of the incisors, which determine the incisal guidance. During this movement, incisal guidance, along with its condylar inclination, will in most cases cause the mandible to open slightly, resulting in disclusion of all the posterior teeth. From an incisal edge-to-edge position, further protrusion brings the mandible into a reverse incisal overbite position (Fig. 9-2b5). The average protrusive movement is 9 mm (Agerberg, 1974).

In examining the Posselt diagram in Figs. 9-2a and b, it is important to remember that this diagram indicates the limits of mandibular movement as drawn from a point on the mandibular central incisors with respect to the maxilla. Also, it should be remembered that different phases of mandibular movement are limited by different structures. The most superior or coronal aspects are limited by tooth contact. The remaining movements are limited by joint structures and ligaments.

One final aspect of Figs. 9-2a and b is the path of habitual closure. The path of habitual closure is the tracing of the mandibular central incisors as they move from the maximum opening, through the area of clinical or postural rest position, to centric occlusion. The trajectory is a combination of hinge and translatory movement of the condyles. Since this is not a border move-

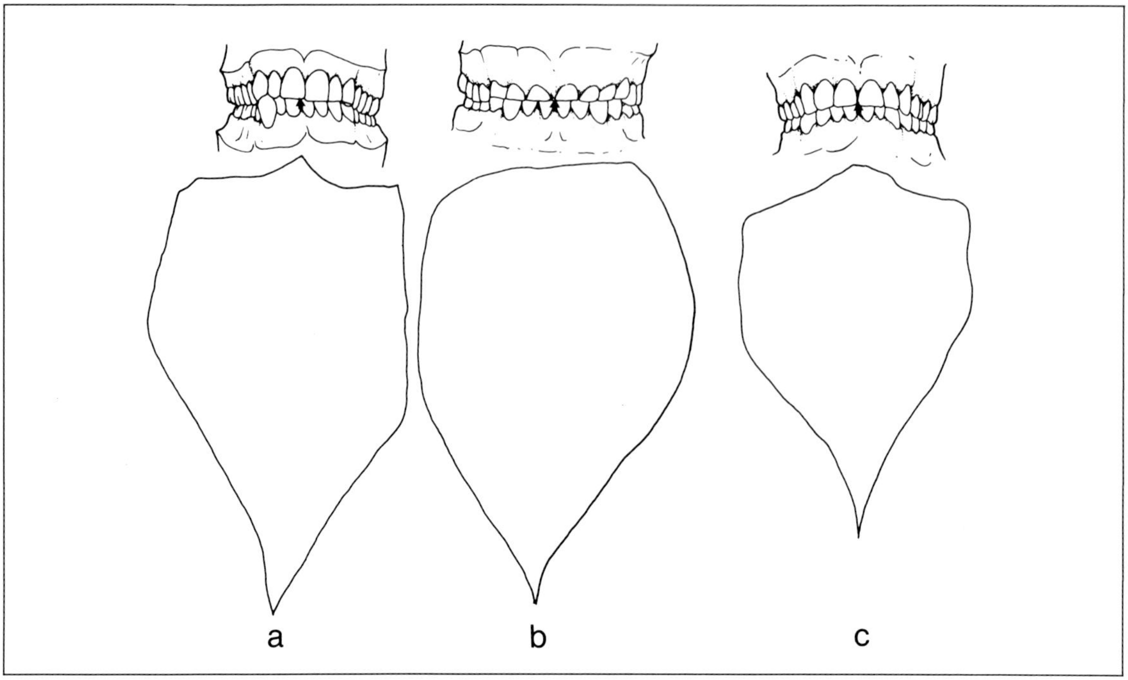

Fig. 9-3 Tracings of frontal plane mandibular border movements in three patients with different occlusal conditions. Tracing *a* is from a patient with a relatively steep occlusal guidance and a very specific intercuspal position. Tracing *b* is of a bruxer with very severe tooth wear. The tooth wear provides a relatively flat occlusion that results in a comparatively flat coronal movement tracing for this patient. Tracing *c* is a more common tracing; however, the vertical opening is somewhat restricted. (Adapted from Gibbs and Lundeen, 1982.)

ment, it is not a consistent and reproducible movement but is a function of head posture. As the head tilts forward, this arc of closure will also move anteriorly, and, as a consequence, the first tooth contacts will change before the intercuspal position is assumed (Mohl, 1984). These changes are due to gravitational influences and associated muscular responses to these gravitational effects.

Border movements in the frontal plane

Border movements of the mandible can also be viewed from the frontal plane, as shown in Fig. 9-3. As in the sagittal movements, the most coronal aspects of mandibular movement are determined by the teeth. When the mandible is moved left or right from centric occlusion with the teeth lightly touching, the inclines of the working side teeth (often the canines) guide the mandible in a lateral and inferior direction.

As shown in Fig. 9-3, the border movements vary greatly between individuals. However, they generally have the shape of a shield. The relative overlap of the occluding teeth often determines the inferior angle of movement. Notice also that the maximum lateral and vertical opening varies among individuals. The lateral movement capabilities are determined by structures of the joint, muscle, and ligaments. The border movement tracings in Fig. 9-3 show that lateral movements are less as the mandible is opened wide. Remember that the superior positions of the border movements are determined by the teeth and thus vary, depending upon the anatomy of the teeth, type of occlusion, and wear. Notice the relatively flat superior portions of the tracing of Fig. 9-3c resulting from extreme tooth wear.

Border movements in the horizontal plane

Mandibular border movements can be viewed from a horizontal plane if one imagines looking down through the head from above (Fig. 9-4). The Gothic arch tracings of Gysi (1910) recorded from this plane show lateral and anterior-posterior movements of the jaw. These tracings can be made on an intraoral plate, or extraorally using a pantographic tracing device.

The tracings usually begin with the mandible at the terminal hinge position, that is, retruded maximally (Fig. 9-4, point *a*). The incisal point moves (left) laterally and anteriorly as the right condyle translates anteriorly and inward. The right lateral border tracing is made as the incisal point moves right laterally and anteriorly while the left condyle translates anteriorly and lingually. The protrusive record is made as the mandibular jaw is thrust straight anteriorly. Thus, in the fully protruded position, both condyles have translated onto their eminences. Note that centric occlusion is usually anterior to the terminal hinge position by about 1 mm. As with the frontal and sagittal border movements, there are great individual differences in the characteristics of the Gothic arch tracings. These differences are due to individual variability in the shape and size of the condyle and fossa and to muscular and ligament characteristics (Mongini and Capurso, 1982).

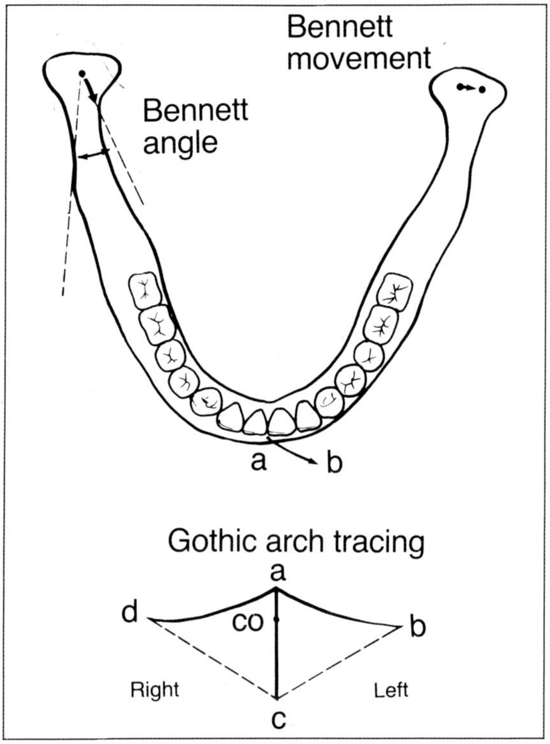

Fig. 9-4 Border movements of the mandible as viewed from the horizontal plane. Line *a–b* is recorded from the incisal point as the mandible moves left. Line *a–c* is made as the mandible is protruded. Line *a–d* represents a right lateral movement. Fully protruded position *(C)*; centric occlusion *(CO)*.

Bennett movement

The range and limitations of mandibular movement have thus far been described from the perspective of the incisal point. Mandibular movements may also be viewed from any one tooth or from either condyle. The condylar movements described so far have been translation and rotation; however, there is additional movement occurring during lateral excursions (Fig. 9-5). As the mandible moves in a right lateral excursion, there is a right lateral and anterior shift of the left condyle and a right lateral and sometimes slightly posterior shift of the right condyle. The lateral shift is known as the *Bennett movement,* which is defined as the bodily shift of the mandible toward the working side during lateral excursion. This movement takes place because of restraining influences of the temporomandibular ligament on the working side condyle and to some extent by the medial wall of the glenoid fossa on the nonworking side (see chapter 6).

The angle formed between this anterior and medial movement of the nonworking condyle and a straight protrusive movement is known as the *Bennett angle* or condylar angulation. There is a direct relationship between the degree of Bennett angle and the amount of Bennett movement. It is helpful to study the drawings of Fig. 9-5 and observe condylar movements on oneself

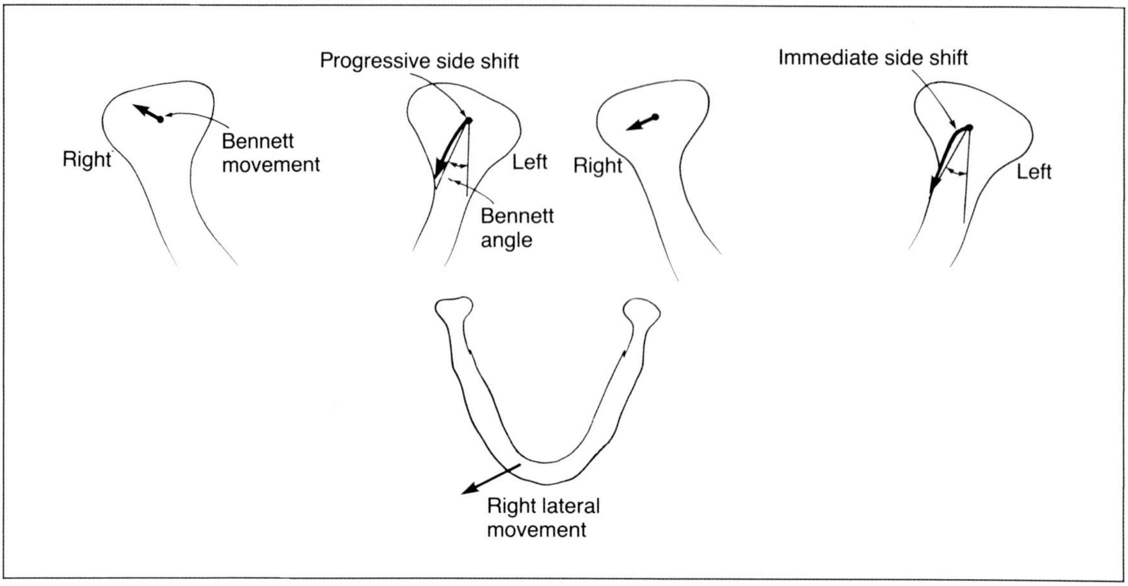

Fig. 9-5 Right lateral condylar movements in the horizontal plane showing a patient with a progressive side shift and one with an immediate side shift.

as the jaw moves laterally. The timing of the Bennett movement varies greatly between individuals. If the lateral component comes early in the movement, it is termed an "immediate" or "early" side shift. The gradual lateral component is termed a "progressive" side shift. The direction of the Bennett movement depends on joint structures and the contraction of the lateral pterygoid muscles, whose origin is medial as well as anterior to its insertion, thus accounting for the lateral and anterior shift. The amount of lateral movement as measured in the horizontal plane averages approximately 0.75 mm, with 80% of all patients having a Bennett movement of 1.5 mm or less (Lundeen et al., 1978).

Functional movements

Except for an area near centric occlusion, border movements are seldom used. As seen in Fig. 9-6, most mandibular movements take place within a reasonably limited three-dimensional space, within the broader border movements. During speech, fewer vertical and lateral movements are used than during chewing. Also, although intercuspal position is commonly used during chewing, occlusal contact does not typically occur during speech. Most individuals swallow with the jaw brought into intercuspal position by contracting the mandibular elevator muscles.

When not chewing, speaking, or swallowing, the mandible is most often held in clinical, or postural, rest position. In this position the mandible is open from 1 to 3 mm and is approximately 2 mm protrusive from a most retruded border position (see Figs. 9-2a and b). Originally it was believed that the muscles that position the mandible were at rest in this position; thus it was termed *rest position*. It was assumed that the mandible "rested" in this position due to an equilibrium between the inferior pull of gravity and the natural elasticity of the muscle and other soft tissue. We now know that when the muscles are truly relaxed the mandible opens to approximately 8 mm. To raise the mandible to postural rest position, the masseter, temporalis, and, probably, medial pterygoid muscles must contract slightly. The vertical opening where the

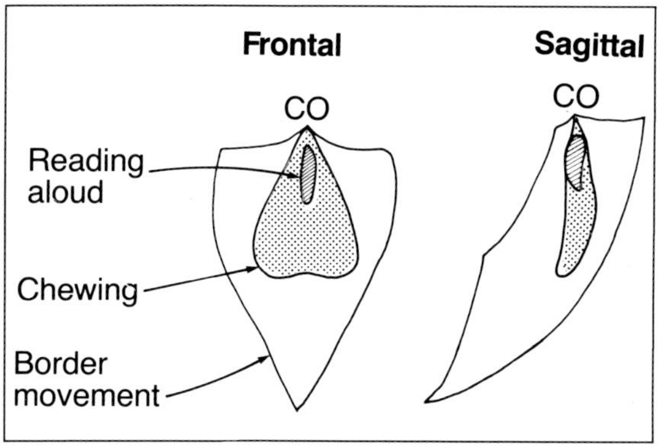

Fig. 9-6 Functional movements of the mandible, such as chewing *(dotted area)* and speaking *(hatched area)*, take place in a relatively small area within the border tracings *(outer solid lines)*. Border positions are used only within a few millimeters of centric occlusion during chewing. (Modified from Gibbs and Messerman, 1972.)

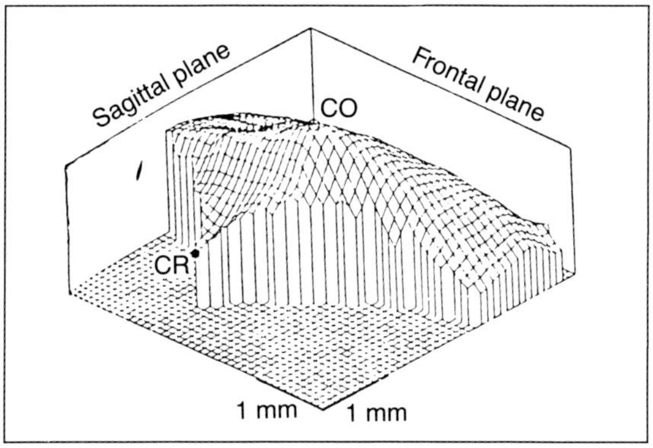

Fig. 9-7 Contour map of the coronal aspects of the border movement; see text for discussion. Centric occlusion *(CO)*; centric relation *(CR)*. (Modified from Graf, 1981.)

muscles are most relaxed (~8 mm) is referred to as *electromyographic rest position* to distinguish it from clinical rest position (Rugh and Drago, 1981). The two rest positions should not be confused clinically. Postural rest position is important because it is commonly used as a reference point for establishing the vertical dimension of occlusion.

Unfortunately, both postural rest position and electromyographic rest position vary widely among and within patients. Factors such as head posture, physical exercise, pain, age, loss of teeth, use of drugs, and emotional tension affect the resting position of the mandible (Mohl, 1984; Rugh and Johnson, 1984). In an upright position, the mandible is usually held at clinical rest position (1 to 3 mm), with the jaw elevator muscles slightly contracted. It is uncommon for individuals to let the mandible drop to electromyographic rest position (~8 mm) unless they have been taught deep-muscle relaxation or have fallen asleep while sitting upright. The term *interocclusal distance* or *freeway space* refers to the separation between the mandible and maxilla at postural rest position, that is, 1 to 3 mm.

Of particular interest in restorative dentistry is what has been termed the *occlusal interface* (Storey, 1975). If the teeth are lightly held together and the jaw is moved in multiple directions laterally and protrusively, a topographic map of the jaw's vertical placement at different tooth-to-tooth positions can be made (Fig. 9-7). Centric occlusion, where the teeth intercuspate best, is easily recognized as a peak in elevation. In centric occlusion the mandible reaches its most superior position with respect to the maxilla because of the fit of the cusps into the fossae of the opposing teeth. It is this difference in vertical and the cuspal inclines that guides the mandible into centric occlusion during chewing.

Clinical significance of tooth and joint morphology

As discussed above, the coronal aspects of mandibular movement are limited primarily by the teeth and joint morphology. The movements that the mandible may make are determined by the

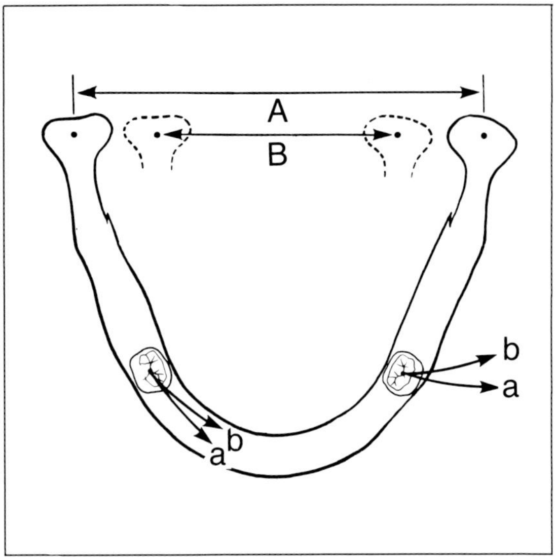

Fig. 9-8 The trajectory of the mandibular first molars (horizontal view) during a left lateral movement depends on intercondylar distance. The wider intercondylar distance *(A)* results in a more anterior movement *(a)* during lateral excursion. Shorter intercondylar distance *(B)* results in a more posterior movement trajectory *(b)*.

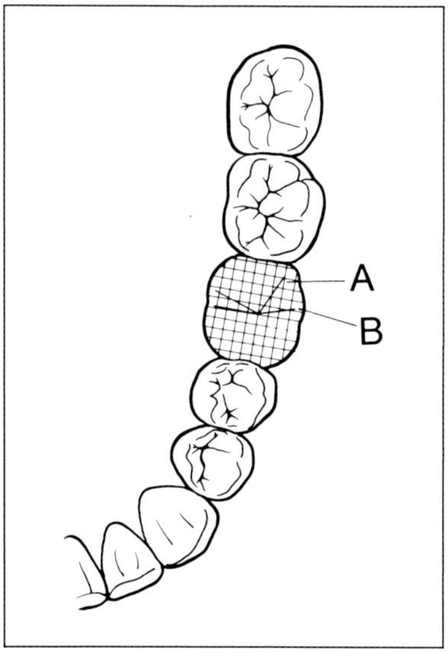

Fig. 9-9 Horizontal plane recordings of lateral jaw movement at the left first molar showing the effects of Bennett movement. Tracing *A* is with no Bennett movement, and tracing *B* is with excessive Bennett movement of 3.5 mm. (Modified from Lundeen et al., 1978.)

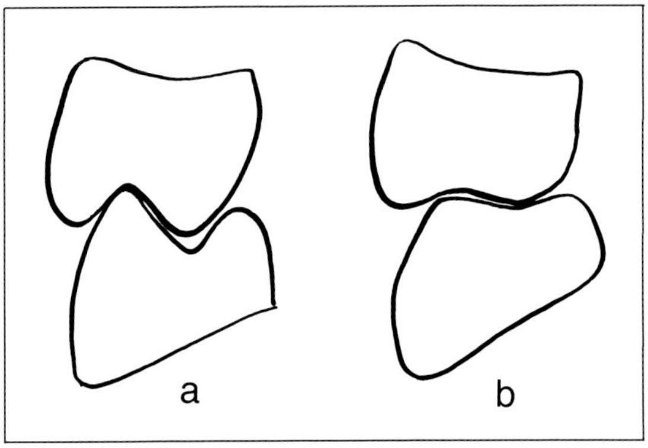

Fig. 9-10 Effect of Bennett movement on height of cuspal inclines: steep cuspal inclines are found with an inferior and late lateral shift *(a)*; shallow cuspal inclines are necessary with a superior and early lateral shift *(b)*.

shape, relative position, and anatomy of the teeth and joint. Familiarity with jaw movements and their relation to occlusal and joint anatomy is very important clinically because they are interdependent. For example, a left lateral excursion of the mandible as viewed from the first molar is analyzed in Fig. 9-8. As the (right) nonworking side condyle translates inferiorly, anteriorly, and lingually on its articular eminence, the right mandibular molar moves anteriorly and to the subject's left, while the left mandibular molar moves almost directly laterally toward the working side. Remember that the mesiolingual supporting cusp of the maxillary first molar, which remains stationary during this movement and usually occludes in the central fossa of the mandibular first molar. Thus, on the right side, this cusp would travel through the distobuccal groove of the mandibular right first molar. On the working side, it would pass through the lingual groove of the mandibular left first molar as the mandible moves left.

The distobuccal supporting cusp of the mandibular first molar, which ordinarily occludes with the central fossa of the maxillary first molar, would traverse between the mesiobuccal and distobuccal cusps of the maxillary first molar during lateral excursion to the working side. The trajectories of these cusp-to-groove movements are dependent on the radius formed by the mandibular tooth and the rotating working side condyle. If the intercondylar distance were less and the radius were shorter, as in Fig. 9-8*B*, the arc of movement of the mandibular working side cusps and fossae would occur in a more distal direction compared with the arc that takes place with the longer radius associated with a wider intercondylar distance, as in Fig. 9-8*A*. The effect on the working side is particularly important in restorative dentistry because it is this side that is most often in occlusal contact during lateral excursion. The nonworking side teeth usually disclude.

It is useful to study these movements in one's own mouth and on an articulator. In restoring the dentition, if the intercondylar distance of the articulator is significantly different from that of the patient, a possibly detectable impingement of the mandibular working side cusps may occur as they attempt to move laterally past and through the maxillary cusps and grooves. Thus, the relationship among intercondylar distance, movement radii, and occlusal form and position is relevant to clinical, and especially restorative, dentistry. This does not imply, however, that mandibular movement is so rigid that it cannot adapt to minor and subtle differences imposed by an articulator-fabricated occlusion.

The Bennett shift described previously also has important implications for occlusal morphology and restorative dentistry. First, it is important to note that the amount of side shift of the mandible affects the path the mandibular cusps follow in relation to the maxillary cusps, fossae, and grooves. The greater the Bennett shift, the more distally the mandibular cusps will pass in relation to the maxillary cusps as they move to the working side during lateral excursion. Figure 9-9 shows the different trajectories the mandible may follow with and without the Bennett side shift. The importance of these different movement patterns is for the correct placement of the maxillary and mandibular supporting cusps and their opposing fossae, cusps, and grooves when restoring these teeth. Note the location and potential movement trajectories of the mesiolingual cusp of the maxillary first molar and opposing central fossa of the mandibular first molar in Fig. 9-9. Some clinicians feel that if the side shift of the articulator is much different from that of the patient, restorations fabricated on that articulator have the potential to "bind" during working side excursion when placed in the patient's mouth.

The nature of the Bennett movement may also be important for the height of the cusp and depth of the fossa. When the mandible moves laterally, and canine guidance exists, the canines will contact and slide over each other. This canine guidance, in turn, will either separate the posterior teeth or allow them to travel over each other in a functioning relationship. If, during lateral movement, the condylar shift on the working side is in an inferior direction, then the cusp and fossa inclines on the working side posterior teeth may be steeper. If, however, the shift is in a superior direction, then the cusp-fossa angles on this side must be flatter (Fig. 9-10). Some clinicians think that failure to accommodate these relationships may result in time-consuming adjustments of restorations after placement in a patient's mouth. This, however, has not been verified in clinical research.

Articulators and study casts

Early dental investigators and clinicians realized the need to study the relationship of the teeth to the TMJ in an extraoral setting. Articulators pro-

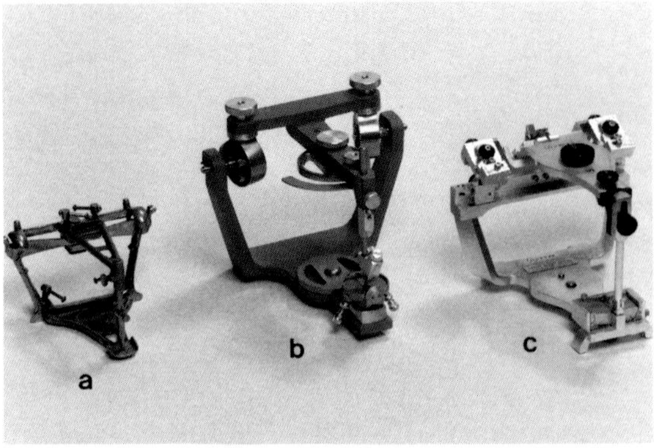

Fig. 9-11 Three types of articulators: simple hinge *(a)*, semiadjustable *(b)*, and fully adjustable *(c)*.

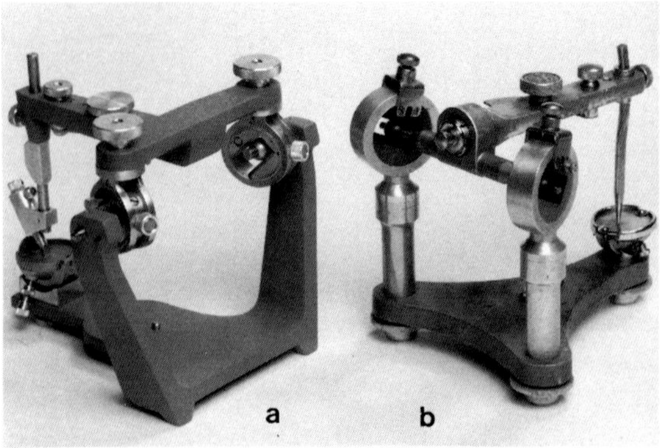

Fig. 9-12 Arcon *(a)* and nonarcon *(b)* type semiadjustable articulators.

vide this capability. Modern articulators are mechanical devices representing the TMJ, the maxilla, and the mandible, to which casts may be attached and observed in some functional relationship.

Early articulators were simple hinge devices (Fig. 9-11). Later attempts simulated protrusive and lateral movements; from these attempts evolved the semiadjustable articulators that allow study of morphologic differences between patients. More recently, fully adjustable articulators have been available that more accurately reproduce mandibular border movements.

It must be emphasized that even the most sophisticated articulator systems do not truly reproduce all of the complex movements available to a biological entity such as the masticatory system. Furthermore, as a mechanical device, articulator movement is rigid and unyielding in contrast to the innumerable movement accommodations made by the mandible during all of its functional and parafunctional activities. Nevertheless, the use of articulators is important in aspects of clinical dentistry that involve restoration or replacement of occlusal surfaces.

It is important that the clinician understand the strengths and weaknesses of any articulator system to be used in the fabrication of restorations or prostheses that involve occlusal position, form, and function. See chapter 12 for a historical review of concepts of occlusion and associated articulators.

Articulator classifications

Historically, articulators have been divided into three categories: simple hinge, semiadjustable, and fully adjustable. The hinge-type articulator (Fig. 9-11), as previously mentioned, is the simplest. It generally consists of a hinge that allows the casts to be disarticulated. The hinge-type articulator also usually has an adjustable vertical stop, to prevent damage to the casts and rough changes in occlusal vertical dimension. The physical limitations of this device preclude its use in the more complicated restorative or diagnostic procedures. For instance, if the position of the articular hinge produces a closing trajectory different than that of the patient, binding of cusp inclines may occur on restorations placed in a patient's mouth. Another inherent weakness is that lateral movements cannot be examined on such a device.

Semiadjustable articulators have multiple advantages over the hinge types. Most of these instruments allow for a face-bow transfer in order to mount the maxillary cast at the appropri-

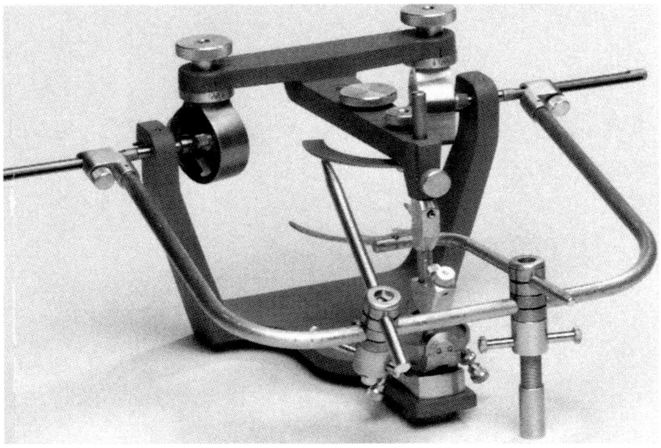

Fig. 9-13a *(above)* Face-bow used to align the maxillary cast to the condylar rotational axis.

Fig. 9-13b *(right)* Face-bow in use.

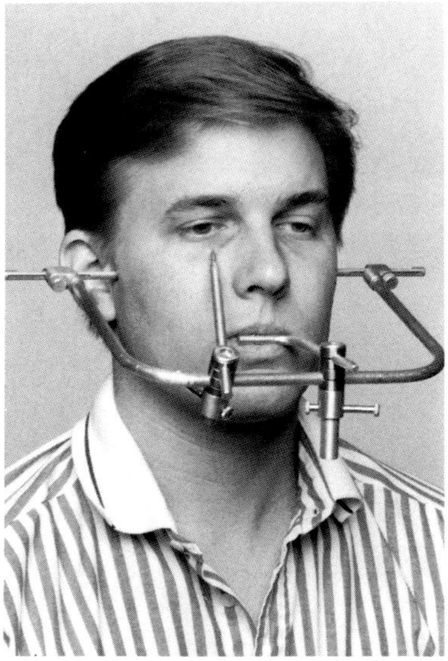

ate relationship to the condylar hinge axis. They will accept protrusive interocclusal bite registrations in order to allow adjustment of the condylar inclination to roughly simulate the anterior and inferior movement of the patient's condylar translation.

Such articulators will also accept lateral interocclusal bite registrations to permit adjustment of the condylar angulation, as well as the condylar inclination, on the instrument. In some cases, these variables often are locked into standard positions representing the average adult morphology, and interocclusal bite registrations are not specifically recorded. The latter method is obviously less accurate than actual registrations recorded from an individual patient. But the individual registrations may be associated with relatively great errors. In some centers, therefore, the advantages of individual registrations are questioned, and average settings are used (even when semiadjustable articulators are employed).

The semiadjustable articulators are further subdivided into the *arcon* (*ar*ticulator-*con*dyle) and the *nonarcon* types (Fig. 9-12). The arcon types have the condylar path attached to the upper member of the articulator; the nonarcon types have the condylar path attached to the lower member. The arcon corresponds most closely to the patient's situation. Although these instruments are much more sophisticated than the hinge types, they still fall short of replicating true mandibular movements: most have flat condylar guides and so cannot replicate true anatomic contours, which are curvilinear. Despite these shortcomings, when it is properly used and its limitations are recognized, the semiadjustable articulator can give valuable information to aid in the construction of dental restorations.

The fully adjustable articulators reproduce mandibular border movements more accurately. They are not, however, required in treatment of all patients but are limited to more complicated restorative cases and research. To use a fully adjustable articulator, special training, more time, and considerable expense are required.

Face-bows

The face-bow (Figs. 9-13a and b) is used with the articulator to allow the operator to align the maxillary cast properly with the condylar rotational, or hinge, axis. This relationship is important when altering the patient's vertical occlusal relationship.

Also, in the event that this relationship is not recorded properly, the arc of closure will be incorrect. For example, if the arc of closure is too low compared with that of the patient, cusp inclines on restorations in the posterior region will bind or contact first when the patient attempts to close on them. Use of the face-bow also prevents rotational inaccuracies in the horizontal plane, which may cause incorrect occlusal relationships.

There is controversy as to whether the hinge axis should be located specifically (by using a kinematic face-bow) or arbitrarily. Arbitrary selection will suffice for most purposes when used with the semiadjustable articulator. The use of anatomical averages (e.g., 13 mm along the tragus-canthus line) is certainly more accurate than the arbitrary mounting of casts on an articulator without the use of a face-bow.

Following the mounting of the maxillary cast into the correct relationship on the articulator with the face-bow transfer, proper occlusal registrations must be taken in order to properly relate the mandibular cast to the maxillary cast. Historically, the casts are commonly mounted in centric relation, particularly for diagnostic purposes. Recently, several other relationships have been suggested, including a voluntary relaxed muscular closure, a "power bite," and intercuspal position.

Mounting casts on articulators

Mounting the casts in centric relation is done in several steps. First, the operator guides the mandible into centric relation several times when nothing is in the patient's mouth. This is to ensure that the proper relationship can be obtained once the wax bite record is inserted. Next, a strip of baseplate wax is cut to cover the occlusal surfaces of all the teeth. The wax is heated to a dead soft stage and placed over either of the dental arches. Then the mandible is guided into centric relation and closed into the wax without perforating the wax or having the teeth contact. The wax is allowed to cool, checked for thickness, and reinserted into the mouth for verification. The thickness of the wax is important, because if it is too thick it will give incorrect occlusal contacts once the casts are brought into occlusion. The wax should be as thin as possible without perforating. Any slight discrepancy in the hinge axis—as is often the case when using an arbitrary hinge axis—can cause occlusal contacts to be recorded incorrectly.

If the teeth are allowed to contact when obtaining a bite registration, the mandible may be deflected, resulting in a bite relation that will not fit the cast. Any soft tissue impressions on the bite registration should be removed because they may not allow the wax bite record to fit the cast.

Next, the wax bite record is used to mount the mandibular cast in relation to the previously mounted maxillary cast. Following mounting, the first occlusal contact in centric relation in the subject's mouth should be compared to the first contact on the mounted casts to ensure a comparable jaw relationship. The articulator is now ready to have the condylar inclination set. This can be performed by means of an average setting (30° to 40°), or from an individual registration.

To set an individual condylar inclination, or the angle at which the condyles translate down their eminences, a symmetrical protrusive wax bite record is needed. Have the subject bite into softened wax at approximately 4 mm anterior to centric relation. Insufficient anterior movement will provide an inaccurate setting, while excess anterior movement will be outside the necessary functional range. The bite relation is taken to the mounted casts, the condylar locks are opened on the articulator, and the casts are occluded into the wax bite optimally by adjusting the condylar guidance. While there is often a 2° to 5° difference between the two sides, the difference can be even greater (Isaacson, 1959). Other studies have shown that precision and accuracy of such protrusive wax registrations are poor, and in general "everyday" dentistry, the method is often replaced by average settings. It must be remembered that condyles undergo curvilinear translation during protrusion, but that most articulators allow for rectilinear translation only. These and other constraints mean that the use of intraoral protrusive bite registrations for condylar inclination settings are very rough estimates at best. The same can be said for lateral records used to record condylar angulation.

These mounting procedures will suffice in most types of restorative or prosthetic work. Some practitioners believe more accurate articulators and mounting techniques should be used for extensive rehabilitative work or research. In these situations, casts may be mounted on a fully adjustable articulator following use of a kinematic face-bow recording. Articulator settings are obtained from extraoral tracing devices that record condylar movement (pantography). Such procedures are long and involved and will not be discussed here. No data show clinical superiority of the more complicated registration methods over simpler ones.

Summary

Movement of the mandible is limited by teeth, joints, and ligaments to a certain three-dimensional space. This three-dimensional space is described through drawings of mandibular border movements or "Posselt diagrams." The most superior movements of the jaw are determined by the teeth. Protrusive, retrusive, lateral, and opening movements are limited by the TMJ structures, the ligaments, and muscle. Typically, movement of the jaw for purposes of speech and chewing occurs within a small area within these extreme border positions. During chewing and swallowing the most superior or coronal aspects of the border movement are used, and these are determined by the topography of the teeth. One should be able to visualize the frontal, sagittal, and horizontal border movements from the point of view of the mandibular central incisors. Also, one should be able to picture the inferior and anterior movement of the condyles as the mandible is opened. On lateral jaw movements, the lateral shift of the condyle, known as "Bennett movement," and the distance between the two condyles are clinically important when restoring proper anatomy on the teeth, particularly on the working side.

Articulators are designed to simulate the joint mechanism and hold study casts of the teeth such that functional relationships of the joint and teeth can be studied outside the mouth. Articulators vary in complexity with respect to how well they are able to simulate jaw movement. Considerable skill is required to accurately mount study casts. Even when study casts are accurately mounted on the most elaborate articulators, articulators only approximate the dynamic characteristics of functional jaw movements.

Chapter 10

Mastication

John D. Rugh and Brian R. Smith

Mastication, or chewing, is one of the most important functions of the stomatognathic system. Knowledge of how the mandible moves during mastication has greatly influenced procedures in clinical dentistry. Historically, an understanding of mandibular movement was considered important in removable prosthodontics so that dentures could be constructed to be compatible with the patient's own jaw movements. Later, information gathered from studies of jaw motion was used in the design and setting of articulators, and in the design of the dentures and denture teeth themselves. Today the importance of jaw movements has become apparent in fixed prosthodontics, periodontics, orthodontics, and in the diagnosis and treatment of pain disorders of the masticatory system.

Mandibular movement

The mandible is capable of very complex movements and is thus difficult to study. Six degrees of freedom are required to fully describe the motion of the mandible in the three planes of space (frontal, sagittal, and horizontal). It is difficult to make measurements of mastication. A number of techniques for studying mastication have been used, including cinematography, electromyography, cineradiography, electromagnetic inductive devices, and photoelectric techniques. Useful information has also been gathered by the study of wear facets on natural teeth. Researchers have even studied wear facets on teeth in anthropologic skull samples.

The basic jaw movement during mastication is more than a rhythmic up and down motion. A closer look shows that there is also protrusive-retrusive movement, rotation in the horizontal plane, and a lateral shifting of the mandible. From plots of chewing strokes in the sagittal plane (Fig. 10-1) it can be seen that the opening and closing paths are all anterior to the terminal hinge position. From these tracings it is also apparent that there is seldom a pure hinge movement during mastication. Instead, it is a complex movement involving simultaneous hinge, sliding, and rotary motion at the condyles (Gibbs and Lundeen, 1982).

Gliding contacts create curved wear patterns on the teeth that are concentric with the condyles (Fig. 10-2). Wear facet studies have indicated that mastication involves gliding contacts with lingual and buccal phases, then intercuspation. These phases correspond to opening of the jaws, closure, and centric occlusion, respectively. Wear patterns are unique to each individual and are changed by extraction of teeth or restorations that alter the occlusion, indicating that the chewing pattern is determined to some extent by the occlusion.

The typical adult chewing pattern as represented in the frontal plane is a teardrop shape with the opening phase medial to a more lateral closing phase (Fig. 10-3). The maximum extent of vertical and lateral movement in normal mastication is about half of the maximum vertical and lateral movements possible, as shown in Fig. 10-4. This figure shows the jaw movement patterns of two individuals with different occlusal

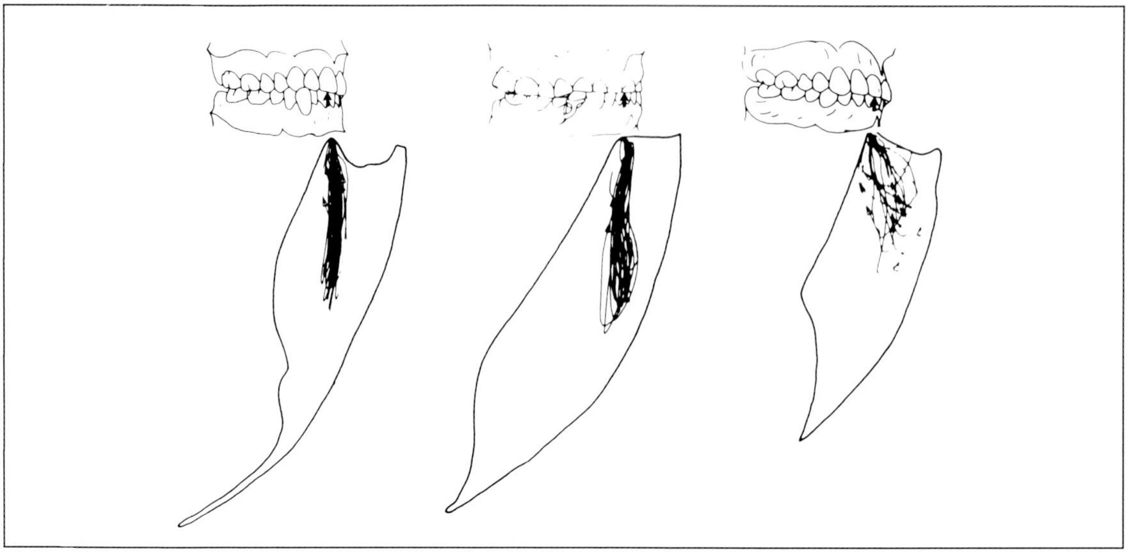

Fig. 10-1 Mastication and border movements recorded in the sagittal planes of three adults. (Modified from Gibbs and Lundeen, 1982.)

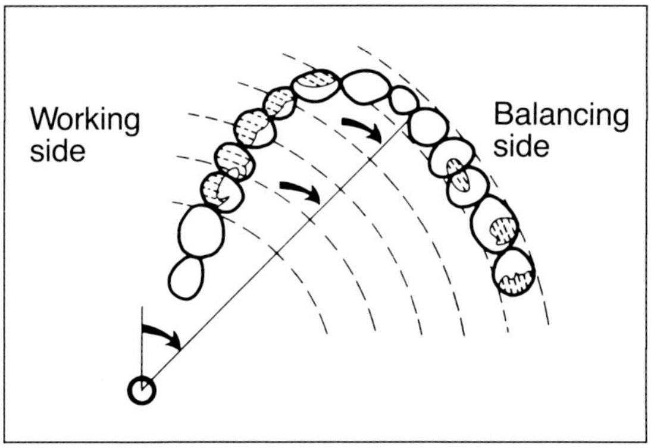

Fig. 10-2 Wear patterns on the maxillary teeth are often concentric to the condyles. (Modified from Murphy, 1964.)

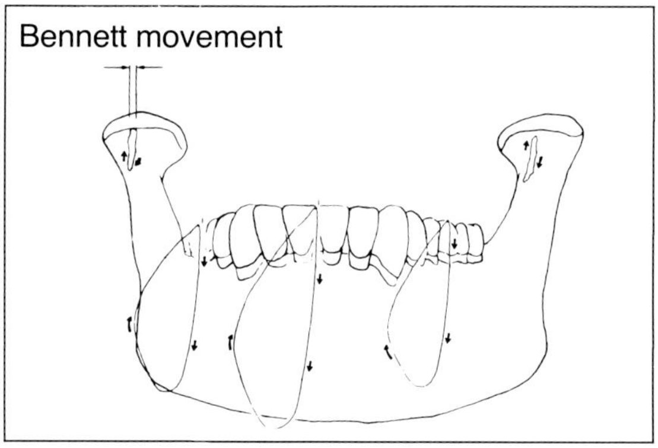

Fig. 10-3 Movement patterns of the mandible during a right-sided chewing cycle. This frontal view shows movement as viewed from the central incisor, first molar, and condyle. (Modifed from Gibbs and Lundeen, 1982.)

characteristics. The chewing pattern is relatively consistent for each individual; however, it is affected by the nature of the food being chewed, the bolus size (Gibbs et al., 1981c), and changes in the occlusion (Wood et al., 1981) or number of teeth (Bates et al., 1975a).

From Fig. 10-4, it can be seen that the closing movements often coincide with the border movements in the vicinity of intercuspal position. From this it is inferred that there is gliding contact between the teeth as they are guided into intercuspal position (Gibbs et al., 1981a). The teeth are often separated by a thin layer of the bolus. It is generally agreed that there are frequent gliding contacts as the jaws are closed into intercuspal position, and that these contacts are greater when lateral movement is larger, which is common when chewing tough, resistant foods. The angle between the closing path and opening path (vertex at intercuspal position) is always less than or equal to the angle formed by the cuspal inclines.

There is less agreement on the extent of gliding tooth contacts in the opening phase. It is certain, however, that they are less frequent and less extensive. Lateral movements with gliding contacts appear to occur in most patients, yet there have been reports that vertical jaw movements are more frequent in Angle Class III prognathic malocclusions and in complete denture wearers (Ahlgren, 1966; Atkinson and Shepherd, 1967; Gibbs and Lundeen, 1982).

Mastication can be unilateral, bilateral, or bilaterally alternating (Dubner et al., 1978). The patient will commonly chew on the side with the most teeth in contact during lateral excursions (Bates et al., 1975a). This side is also likely to be the most efficient side to chew on; it is often called the preferred side. Unilateral preference patterns in mastication have recently been associated with increased muscle spindle sensitivity on the preferred side (Hoogmartems et al., 1980). In patients whose occlusion is very similar on both sides, there is a tendency to regularly alternate the bolus from side to side (bilateral alternating mastication). Some patients chew on both sides at the same time. This is reported to be more common in complete-denture wearers.

Persons with severely worn occlusions, such as those with a bruxing habit or from a primitive culture with a very abrasive diet, tend to exhibit wider lateral chewing movements with longer glide lengths, as shown in Fig. 10-4. The average glide length of Australian aborigines, who have a diet consisting of very tough meat contaminated with abrasive sand and ashes, is about 2.8 mm (Beyron, 1964). These people exhibit generalized occlusal wear that is progressive throughout their lives. People in modern societies who have a nonabrasive diet and do not brux have an average glide length of about 1 mm (Gibbs and Lundeen, 1982).

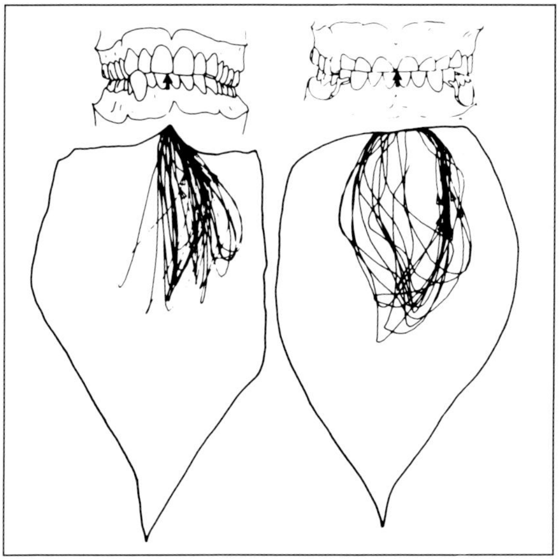

Fig. 10-4 Mastication and border movements recorded in the frontal view for two adults with different occlusal characteristics. (Modified from Gibbs and Lundeen, 1982.)

Condylar movement

From Fig. 10-3 it can be seen that both condyles move inferiorly and toward the working side during opening, then superiorly and toward the nonworking side during closure. It should be noted that the working side condyle reaches its highest position at the same time the teeth reach intercuspal position.

The sagittal view (Fig. 10-5) indicates that the working side condyle moves inferiorly and anteriorly on opening, and then posteriorly and superiorly on closing, with a slight anterior movement on final closure. In this sagittal view the opening and closing paths of the working side condyle do not coincide.

The nonworking sagittal view of normal chewing movements is illustrated in Fig. 10-6. Notice that the opening and closing paths of the nonworking side condyle are longer than the movement of the working condyle. The movement patterns nearly coincide on opening and closing.

The motion of the mandible during normal chewing in the horizontal plane is shown in Fig.

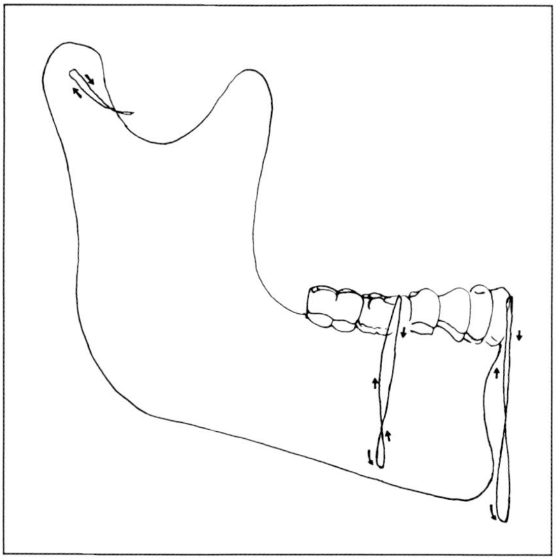

Fig. 10-5 Mandibular movement pattern on the working side during one chewing stroke; sagittal view. (Modified from Gibbs and Lundeen, 1982.)

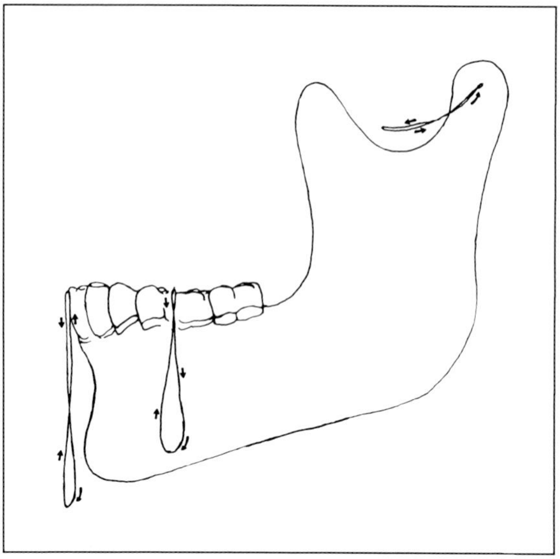

Fig. 10-6 Mandibular movement patterns on the nonworking side during one chewing stroke; sagittal view. (Modified from Gibbs and Lundeen, 1982.)

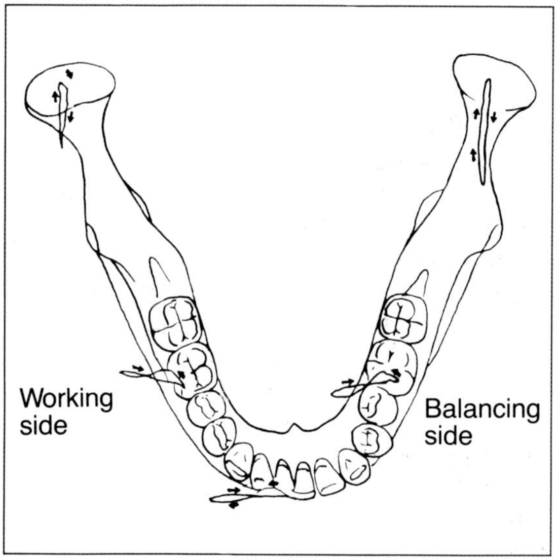

Fig. 10-7 Mandibular movement patterns from a horizontal perspective during one chewing stroke on the right side. (Modified from Gibbs and Lundeen, 1982.)

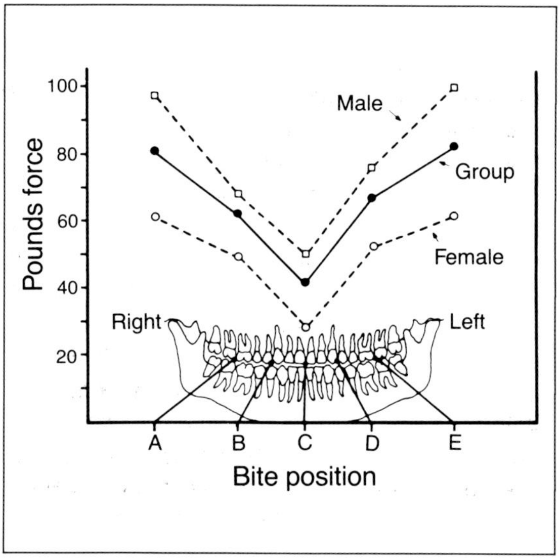

Fig. 10-8 Mean adult bite forces at different positions (*A* through *E*) of the jaw. (Modified from Rugh and Solberg, 1972.)

10-7. The distance traced by the working condyle is less. Also, notice that the working side condyle and first molar make a slight anterior movement on final closure. The nonworking side condyle, in contrast, does not make an anterior movement on final closure. The working side anterior and medial movements on final closure are important because they show the likelihood of retrusive range contacts (posterior to intercuspal position) on the working side. The medial movement represents the Bennett shift occurring when the working side moves from a lateral to a medial position during final closure. It has been shown that there are no terminal hinge contacts in normal mastication (Haddad, 1974); however, there are retrusive range contacts. Because of this, lateral retruded border registrations for articulator settings have been recommended in restorative dental procedures.

To summarize, mastication involves very complex movements of the mandible. In addition to up and down movement there is also protrusive-retrusive rotation in the horizontal plane and bodily lateral shifting of the mandible. Mastication is never a pure hinge movement but involves simultaneous sliding and rotary movement at the temporomandibular joints (TMJs). Six degrees of freedom are required to fully describe the motion of the mandible.

Masticatory forces

Several facts about biting force are important to the dentist attempting to restore chewing capabilities for patients. Maximum biting forces generally vary from about 20.5 to 104.4 kg (244 to 1,245 N), although forces greater than 363.7 kg (4,339 N) have been reported in some individuals (Gibbs et al., 1986). Maximum biting force appears to be slightly higher in males and is highest when measured in the molar area and lowest when measured at the incisors (Fig. 10-8). Bite force is highest when the teeth are separated by 9 to 10 mm.

Bite force can be increased by practice. An exercise experiment showed that chewing of paraffin wax for 1 hour per day for 30 days increased the maximum bite force by 20% to 25%. However, most of the increase was lost by 2 weeks after the training ended (Brekhus et al., 1941). Bite force during chewing is not well correlated with maximal strength of the masticatory muscles and is probably controlled by other factors such as pain thresholds, sensitivity of mucosal and periodontal receptors, emotional status, and area of distribution of force. If the force is distributed over only a few teeth, the forces tend to be lower.

In complete-denture patients, maximum biting forces are much lower than for patients with a full natural dentition. Measurements of forces in patients with teeth are five to six times greater than in denture wearers (Haraldson et al., 1979). This has been attributed to the fact that denture patients have a much lower area for distributing the forces (Zarb, 1982). It has been shown that anesthesia of the supporting mucosa will increase the maximum biting force recorded in full-denture patients, which suggests that pain is the limiting factor. After rehabilitation with osseointegrated implant fixed partial dentures in edentulous people, a substantial increase of the bite force had been achieved (Lindqvist and Carlsson, 1985).

However, studies on subjects with natural teeth have indicated that anesthesia of the periodontal ligaments of the teeth decreases maximal biting force. This decrease has been attributed to blockage of a positive feedback loop involving the periodontal mechanoreceptors (Lund and Olsson, 1983). Apparently, there is more than one mechanism that can limit maximal bite force. What actually limits force in a given patient is probably affected by a variety of factors. To be safe, the dentist generally must plan for the worst case when considering the strength of dental materials and design of the prosthesis.

A new system recently has been developed that measures total interocclusal forces during mastication. The system measures low-frequency sound transmission through occlusal contacts between the teeth (Gibbs et al., 1981b).

This system has the advantage of measuring total interocclusal force in eccentric positions, as well as in intercuspal position. In studies using this new method, it was found that interocclusal force levels are relatively high; the average maximal force in chewing is about 40% of the maximal biting force. Chewing forces are highest at the intercuspal position, about 22.4 kg (267 N), and second highest during terminal closure contacts just before reaching the intercuspal position. The high level of force at the intercuspal position suggests that this position is significant in mastication, probably for the completion of food grinding. Occlusal forces in eccentric positions are also significant, and although their level is lower and duration shorter than the force in intercuspal position, they may be more significant with regard to periodontal trauma.

Chewing speeds range from 49 to 120 cycles per minute. The usual rate of chewing is 70 to 80 chews per minute. The speed of the mandible is higher in the opening phase than in the closing phase. The closing speed decreases as the teeth contact the bolus of food and just before the teeth contact each other. Mandibular movement speeds are generally in the range of 64 to 135 mm per second (Bates et al., 1975b). There appears to be little change in the chewing rate when teeth are lost or when full dentures are worn. However, if the stability and fit of dentures are not good, the chewing rate can be decreased.

The number of chews before swallowing varies with the individual and can be altered if there is a cause to hurry through a meal (Rugh, 1972). The chewing rate (mandibular velocity), force of chewing, and duration of pauses between bursts of chewing can also be altered by the individual.

Masticatory efficiency

One of the main functions of mastication is to break down food so that it can be swallowed and digested. Masticatory efficiency is a measure of how well a person can break down food. It is usually measured by sieving a sample of food expectorated by a subject after the person has chewed but not swallowed it. Masticatory efficiency decreases with loss of teeth and is generally lower in complete-denture patients. However, it is interesting to note that older men have better chewing performance than younger men with teeth in similar condition. This is most likely caused by improvements in the contact areas due to abrasion of the teeth (Dahlberg, 1943).

As teeth are lost, efficiency decreases if the teeth are not replaced (Carlsson, 1984). It is interesting to note that when occlusal surfaces are lost, patients do not tend to compensate by chewing longer, but instead swallow larger particles. Fortunately, there is little effect of decreased efficiency on food digestion. Probably a more significant factor is the avoidance of certain tough or hard foods by denture wearers and people with multiple missing teeth. Usually tough foods are avoided by these patients because they are difficult or uncomfortable to chew. However, such avoidance can lead to malnutrition (Österberg and Steen, 1982).

It is not clear whether there is any difference in chewing efficiency between anatomic and nonanatomic denture tooth forms. However, it is clear that occlusal markings or grooves improve masticatory performance. A well-fitting, stable denture base with accurate peripheral extensions is essential to obtaining good chewing efficiency with complete dentures. Also, it is reported that denture patients generally improve their masticatory performance after wearing and adapting to their dentures for a period of time (Bates et al., 1976).

A number of factors, in addition to the teeth, influence masticatory efficiency. Among these is the coordination of tongue, jaw, and facial movements to accurately maintain the bolus between the teeth. The tongue is also important in the wetting of the bolus and in detecting when it is ready to swallow. There are also fairly large differences among individuals of equivalent masticatory efficiency in the extent to which they grind up their food; some chew it until it is very finely ground, while others prefer to chew it just enough so that it can be swallowed (Carlsson, 1974).

Development and learning of mastication

The development and learning of mastication is an area of great interest. One theory suggests that mastication develops as an extension and modification of suckling. Suckling is the first feeding experience of the newborn. The newborn has available at birth all of the neuromuscular mechanisms necessary for suckling. Like mastication, suckling involves rhythmic up and down jaw movements coordinated with tongue and facial movements and swallowing. The tongue and jaw are used to compress the nipple against the palate and to create suction that aids in expressing milk. Suction probably plays a minor role, as milk is actively delivered from the mammary ducts by contraction of the myoepithelial cells in response to stimulation of the nipple (Jenkins, 1966).

Proponents of the theory that chewing is an extension of suckling note the cyclic nature of suckling and the coordination of tongue, facial, and jaw movements. They suggest that the central pattern generator begins its activity by providing the timing for suckling jaw and tongue movements, and that later, with the eruption of teeth and the appearance of the sensory feedback (such as putting hard food in the mouth), mastication develops. Observations of infants' uncoordinated first attempts at chewing tend to support this theory.

The eruption and occlusion of teeth is said to be an important prerequisite for the learning of mastication. However, children that lack teeth congenitally also learn to chew, indicating that teeth are not absolutely necessary.

Others theorize that mastication is a fundamentally different behavior that develops separately from suckling. There is some support for this view in studies that show that certain electromyographic (EMG) patterns are linked to specific stages of eruption of teeth (Dubner et al., 1978). Also, it is noted that infants are able to suckle long after they learn to chew. Adults also maintain the capacity to suckle, suggesting that these are two related but independent behaviors.

Chewing movements in young children with primary dentitions differ from the typical adult pattern; young children utilize wide lateral gliding movements on opening toward the working side. This pattern changes to the typical adult pattern when the child reaches 10 to 12 years (Wickwire et al., 1981). The eruption of the adult anterior teeth, which occurs in this time period, has been suggested as a reason for the adoption of the adult chewing pattern. In contrast to the relatively shallow anterior guidance of the primary teeth, the anterior guidance is usually much steeper in the permanent dentition. It is believed that this steeper anterior guidance reduces the lateral movement component. This is supported by measurements of chewing patterns of adults with anterior open-bite occlusion (and hence lack of anterior occlusal guidance). Patterns in these individuals were found to be very similar to those in children with primary dentitions (Gibbs and Lundeen, 1982).

When the natural teeth are replaced by complete dentures, a great number of new factors are brought into play that may have profound influences upon mastication. Among these are loss of periodontal mechanoreceptors, mucosal displaceability, movement of the denture bases, involvement of the tongue and facial musculature in stabilizing the dentures, a decrease in the area of support of chewing forces, and changes in vertical dimension. With these changes, one would expect significant differences in the chewing behavior of complete-denture patients. In fact, the chewing patterns of complete-denture wearers appear to be more irregular on the average than those in patients with natural teeth. This is likely a result of the movement of the denture bases and the displacement of the mucosa on which they rest, as well as preoccupation of the tongue and perioral muscles with denture base retention. The form of the chewing cycle in complete-denture patients does not seem to be influenced by the cuspal inclinations (Drago, 1981). This is fundamentally different from patients with natural teeth, whose final mandibular closures are guided by occlusal surfaces of the posterior teeth.

Rates of chewing for patients with complete dentures are about the same as for those with natural teeth, averaging about 80 chewing cycles per minute (Bates et al., 1975b). Chewing forces and chewing efficiency are much lower with complete dentures than with a good natural occlusion.

Neurological control of mastication

Early physiologists who studied mastication proposed control mechanisms based on reflexes. The early reflex theory by Sherrington (1917) was based on the jaw opening reflex that he had demonstrated to follow intraoral stimulation in decerebrate cats. He suggested that the jaw-opening reflex coupled with rebound closure would maintain mastication after voluntary closure. Later, workers added the jaw-closing reflex to the theory to account for the "rebound closure" of Sherrington's mechanism. Also, it was shown that electrical stimulation of the cortex could initiate chewing. In its simplest form, a reflex mechanism of mastication would include initiation via cortical influence resulting in jaw opening, stretching of masticatory muscle spindles, reflex jaw closure, reflex jaw opening, and so on, until swallowing.

A newer and now more generally accepted theory of the control of mastication suggests that the cyclic pattern of mastication is provided by a central neural program located in the brain stem and can operate in absence of afferent information from intraoral sites (Lund, 1976). Similar pattern generators are known to control cyclic processes in a wide variety of animals.

Support for a central pattern generator comes from studies where rhythmic chewing has been shown in animals and humans who have undergone anesthesia of the gingiva, periodontium, and TMJ. Anesthesia decreases the ability to control the food bolus, but the cyclical chewing movements are not affected. Other experiments have shown that rhythmic bursts of activity in the digastric and masseter motor nerves, which stimulate chewing activity, are not interrupted by complete blockade of muscle activity with the use of a neuromuscular blocker (Dellow and Lund, 1971). Work with monkeys in which the mesencephalic nucleus of the trigeminal nerve was removed showed that rhythmic chewing could still be accomplished. This demonstrates that information from muscle spindles about the stretch of masticatory muscles is not obligatory for mastication (Goodwin and Luschei, 1974). The mesencephalic nucleus receives afferent information from the muscle spindles of the masticatory muscles and some periodontal mechanoreceptors.

Although the concept of the brain-stem pattern generator is generally accepted, it is also known that the peripheral stimuli have considerable influence on natural chewing. It has long been observed that biting on an unexpectedly hard object can interrupt the chewing cycle (the jaw-opening reflex). This reflex is commonly thought of as a quick, reflexive opening of the jaws in response to a painful stimuli; but more recent studies suggest that, although the jaw-closing muscle activity is interrupted, reflexive jaw opening does not occur (Gibbs and Suit, 1973). Many receptors are implicated in feedback to the masticatory pattern generator, including periodontal mechanoreceptors, bare pain receptors in numerous intraoral locations, TMJ receptors, Golgi tendon organs, and muscle spindles.

There is evidence for a positive feedback loop that adjusts the chewing pattern and force level depending on the consistency of the food being chewed. As the jaws begin to close on a hard type of food, EMG levels are low. As the teeth contact the food and the crushing phase begins, closing muscle EMG levels rise sharply. As mastication progresses and the food is softened, the high-amplitude EMG activity during the closing phase is reduced.

Although the central pattern generator has been shown to be able to produce cyclic mastication in the absence of sensory feedback and in decerebrate animals, during normal mastication there is a great deal of interaction between peripheral inputs, the cerebral cortex, and the brain stem pattern generator to produce the complex behavior of mastication. It is likely that the more variable aspects of mastication, such as tongue movements and lateral jaw movements, are more susceptible to peripheral modification than are the basic jaw opening and closing movements.

Very little is known at this time about the exact nature or location of the masticatory pattern generator. It is thought to be located in the reticular formation of the pons, which is very near the trigeminal sensorimotor complex (Hannam, 1979).

Descending central nervous system influences are very important in determining how much effect a particular peripheral stimulus will have. The brain apparently leaves gates open for nociceptive information, yet closes off, through presynaptic inhibition, pathways carrying other sensory information. Öwall and Møller (1974) report that tactile sensitivity of teeth is markedly reduced during mastication in humans. The ability of a stimulus to cause a change in masticatory behavior depends on the appropriateness of the stimulus for the phase of the masticatory cycle (Lund and Olsson, 1983).

To summarize, mastication is a complex neurophysiological activity thought to be dependent on a central neural pattern generator that programs much of the activity. Chewing is initiated and modified by cortical influence. Peripheral feedback is important in modification and coordination of chewing activity. The effects of peripheral feedback depend on the phase of the chewing stroke.

Muscle activity associated with mastication

Muscle activity during mastication has been studied most successfully by use of electromyography (see chapter 7). Typically, electrodes are mounted on several muscles of mastication, and recordings of these muscles are made simultaneously (Møller, 1966). It is important to note that EMG measures electrical activity associated with contraction only. Motion cannot be inferred from the recordings because the muscles undergo both isometric (no change in length) and isotonic (no change in tension) contractions during a single chew. Also, there are often antagonistic muscles working together to increase control and provide stabilization, which clouds the interpretation of motion from EMG recordings. However, simultaneous recordings of jaw motion and muscle activity have been made that can be used to determine the roles played by the individual muscles during mastication. The jaw-opening muscles are the mylohyoid, anterior digastric, and lateral pterygoid. These muscles tend to be recruited in the order listed. Also, the infrahyoid muscles must be active in order to stabilize the hyoid bone, which is necessary for the jaw-opening muscles to be effective. The lateral pterygoid muscle has other activities as well and has been reported to take part in jaw closure, lateral movements, and protrusive movements. The two heads of the lateral pterygoid muscle have been shown to act independently, which accounts for the multiple activities of this muscle.

The time relationship of jaw-muscle EMG activity during a chewing cycle is shown in Fig. 7-12b. The anterior temporalis on the working side becomes active slightly before the muscles on the nonworking side. Because activity is about the same on both sides, it is thought that anterior temporalis muscle is concerned more with elevating the jaw. The posterior temporalis muscle is thought to be important in lateral movement of the mandible, as well as in mandibular closure. The nonworking side posterior temporalis muscle is involved in the movement of the mandible medially during the closing phase. The masseter muscle is considered to be primarily involved with force development during mastication. The activity level is much higher on the working side, yet the nonworking side muscle begins activity earlier and maintains it longer than on the working side. The medial pterygoid muscles initiate jaw closure. Their activity closely parallels that of the masseter muscles, and outlasts the activity of the anterior temporalis by about 100 ms.

The working side lateral pterygoid muscle predominates in early jaw opening, but later the nonworking side muscle dominates, first moving the mandible toward the working side, and then assisting in jaw closure. After initial tooth contact, the working side muscle also assists in jaw closure and in bringing the mandible medially toward intercuspal position.

The anterior digastric muscle is active during jaw opening; however, it sometimes appears to be active during the entire masticatory cycle. The mylohyoid muscle has activity similar to that of the digastric muscle, but also has frequent irregular bursts of activity that may be associated with tongue movement. The tongue muscles are very active and of obvious importance in coordination of the bolus, teeth, and jaw muscles. Little is known about tongue muscle activities at this time, however.

Summary and clinical implications

Perhaps the most important reason the dentist maintains and/or replaces missing teeth is to provide patients with good masticatory abilities. As discussed in this chapter, mastication is affected by the position and anatomy of the teeth, which are often modified by dental procedures. It is thus imperative that dentists know how mastication normally occurs and understand how it is influenced by the position and anatomy of the teeth. This understanding is necessary to ensure that dental procedures improve, rather than reduce, the patient's ability to eat.

Important characteristics of mastication are that

1. The typical adult chewing pattern, as viewed from the frontal plane, is teardrop shaped. The most superior aspects of the movement are determined by the teeth. Closing into intercuspal position results in the mandibular buccal cusps on the working side gliding along the lingual inclines of the maxillary buccal (guiding) cusps. Similarly, retrusive and protrusive inclines guide the mandible into intercuspal position in the anteroposterior dimension.

2. Chewing efficiency is related to the number of teeth and number of contacts. Of concern is that patients do not tend to compensate for loss of occlusal surface by chewing longer. Maintenance of teeth is thus important.

3. Most patients tend to chew bilaterally; however, if patients are missing teeth, they will chew more on the side that has the greater number of teeth and occlusal contacts.

4. It is important to remember that the mandible moves not only vertically during mastication but also anteroposteriorly and laterally. It is this horizontal movement that is most important to restorative efforts. For example, lateral retruded border registrations for articulator settings have been suggested because the working side condyle moves retrusively during mastication.

5. In restoring the teeth it is also important to remember that, although forces during chewing average about 22 kg, some individuals have been found to bite as high as 360 kg. The implication of these forces for restorative materials and the design of prostheses is obvious.

6. Forces used by complete-denture patients are about five times less than patients with natural teeth. However, the dentist must plan for the worst case when considering the strength and design of prostheses.

7. Finally, regarding the control of masticatory movements, it is believed that mastication is learned early in life, then controlled primarily by a central pattern generator. Although masticatory movement can be altered by changes in the occlusion, these patterns are relatively automatic and resistant to change, particularly in patients with complete dentures. It is for this reason that it is usually considered wise to make restorations compatible with the functional movement patterns of the patient rather than expect the patterns to adapt to fit the restorations.

Chapter 11

Deglutition, Respiration, and Speech

George A. Zarb, Norman D. Mohl, and Hugh F. MacKay

Deglutition

The mastication of food results in the preparation of a solid or liquid bolus for *deglutition,* or swallowing. Simply stated, the function of deglutition is one whereby the bolus is propelled from the mouth into the esophagus, and eventually the stomach, without endangering the airway. Although some modern diets could actually preclude the need for an adequate dentition for preswallowing preparation, the teeth are probably indirectly involved in deglutition nonetheless. The swallowing of a nonpulpy or hard bolus necessitates contraction of the closing muscles of mastication and tooth contact, and it is believed that a relatively intact dentition, without gross occlusal discrepancies, facilitates such reflex muscular activity (Dubner et al., 1978).

Deglutition is a complex reflex that serves the upper airway and the alimentary tract. Its functional designation is both supportive and protective. Effector sites in the mouth, pharynx, and esophagus elicit the supportive reflex when exposed to air and food intake. On the other hand, deglutition initiated from the larynx protects the larynx from invasion by saliva, liquid bolus residues, esophageal regurgitation, and nasopharyngeal and tracheal secretions (Dellow, 1976).

Deglutition may be initiated voluntarily or by reflex. It appears to be regulated by a "swallow center" in the caudal brain stem, which organizes and exerts a sequential pattern of excitatory and inhibitory effects on the various motor neuron populations involved in the deglutition act. The tools of cineradiography, pressure transducers, and electromyography (EMG) traditionally have been used to study deglutition. The act of swallowing has been described as consisting of four phases with each phase merging imperceptibly into the next (Bosma, 1957). This act ensures establishment of a pressure gradient, prevention of reflux, and protection of the airway.

The essential features of deglutition are shown in Table 11-1. An intraoral pressure gradient is created through the combined result of a piston-like action of the tongue, the pharyngeal constrictor muscles' activity, and the peristaltic movements of the esophagus. The tongue's activity is accompanied by contraction of muscles of the floor of the mouth, the facial muscles, and/or the mandibular closing muscles (see chapter 7). These combined muscle activities serve to stabilize the base of the tongue. The bolus is contained and reflux prevented by the creation of an anterior oral seal. This results from the contact of lips, the occlusion of teeth with a resultant incisor overbite, or, where required, the thrusting of the tongue into an open bite space. Reflux is prevented by the contact of the base of the tongue with the palate, and subsequently with the posterior pharyngeal wall. The hypopharyngeal sphincter contracts, as does the gastroesophageal sphincter following its initial relaxation, to allow bolus entry into the stomach. Airway protection is achieved by cessation of breathing, contact between the soft palate and the posterior pharyngeal wall, adduction of the vocal folds, and laryngeal elevation.

Table 11-1 Events occurring during deglutition

Pressure gradient
- Piston action of the tongue
- Muscular stabilization of tongue base
- Stuffing action of pharyngeal constrictors
- Peristaltic movements in esophagus

Reflux prevention
- Establishment of an oral seal
- Tongue/palate opposition
- Tongue/pharynx opposition
- Hypopharyngeal sphincter contracts
- Gastroesophageal sphincter contracts

Airway protection
- Opposition of palate and pharyngeal cord
- Laryngeal elevation
- Adduction of vocal folds
- Cessation of breathing

The muscles responsible for deglutition are the obligate muscles, and they are characterized by a rigid activity pattern. Muscles sharing these characteristics include the mylohyoid, geniohyoid, posterior tongue, palatopharyngeus, pharyngeal constrictors, thyrohyoid, thyroarytenoid, cricothyroid, and the striated musculature of the esophagus.

In contrast to the obligate muscles, which participate rigidly in the synergy of deglutition, facultative muscles participate to a variable extent. Their role is particularly interesting from a clinical standpoint. Facultative muscles are the extrinsic tongue muscles, the facial muscles (especially the orbicularis oris), and the mandibular closing muscles. They may or may not participate in deglutition; but, when they do, they do so in a graded fashion which, in contrast to obligate muscles, is very sensitive to neurosensory feedback.

The degree of participation of facultative muscles depends on individual demands for tongue base stabilization and the adequacy of anterior mouth structures to effect an anterior oral seal. The obligate muscles of swallowing appear to be programmed before birth, and their action persists (Bosma, 1973). Facultative muscles, on the other hand, undergo developmental changes.

A newborn's swallow—the *infantile* or *visceral* swallow—is characterized by orbicularis oris and buccinator muscle activity, tongue thrusting, and an absence of activity in the closing muscles of the mandible. In the newborn, the maxillary and mandibular gum pads do not contact during deglutition. The relatively large tongue is thrust between the gum pads in order to stabilize the mandible. This transient bracing of the mandible permits the suprahyoid muscles to act more efficiently as they contract to raise the hyoid bone and larynx during deglutition.

With the eruption of teeth, the pattern of previously used facultative muscles changes: the circumoral musculature demonstrates minimal activity, tongue thrusting is significantly reduced, and the closing muscles become dominant, particularly during deglutition of a solid bolus. This is referred to as an *adult* or *somatic* swallow. Even with a fully developed dentition, varying evidence of facultative muscle involvement becomes apparent. When liquids (e.g., saliva) are swallowed, the tongue requires less stabilization than when swallowing a resistant bolus, and minimal contraction of facial and mandibular closing muscles can be observed. It appears that the swallowing of a resistant bolus may require not only tongue stabilization, but mandibular stabilization as well.

If an acceptable occlusion is present, the teeth are brought together by contraction of the closing muscles, bracing the mandible against the maxilla. Electromyography of this activity may be seen in Figs. 7-13a and b. Again, this mandibular stabilization appears to be important for the efficiency of the suprahyoid muscles as they act to elevate the hyoid bone during deglutition. If the patient is edentulous, or has severe occlusal discrepancies or a skeletal open bite, mandibular stabilization may be brought about via activity of the facial musculature (Dubner et al., 1978).

The characteristic tooth-apart infantile deglutition is quite normal for the adult when liquids or soft boluses are swallowed. It can be concluded that in the dentate individual both the tooth-apart and the tooth-together swallow of saliva and liquids are normal. However, a tooth-apart swallow for a solid bolus would be indicative of an abnormality.

Deglutition occurs several hundred times a day (saliva and food-related), and far less frequently during the night, probably as a result of a decrease in salivary secretion. The total time of tooth contacts that may occur in association with deglutition is only a few minutes per day. The axially directed forces appear to be similar to those of mastication, and, although fleeting in nature, last somewhat longer than masticatory occlusal contacts. These contacts occur at, or very near to, the intercuspal position of the mandible. It has been estimated that deglutition forces during occlusal contact are in the range of 6 to 8 kg, as recorded by strain gauges placed in a tooth inlay (Anderson and Picton, 1958; Carlsson, 1974).

Lip and tongue forces can also be concentrated on the teeth during deglutition. Consequently, the tongue-thrust swallow is considered to be of importance by the dentist and the speech pathologist, who cite it as a cause of anterior open bites. However, because the duration of tongue forces during deglutition is very brief, it is unlikely that a simple cause-and-effect relationship could be regarded as compelling. Dubner et al. (1978) suggest that if the role of the genioglossus is a facultative one, then it should be possible to alter the muscle's participation by altering feedback (e.g., orthodontic correction of an open bite). If, on the other hand, the participating role of the genioglossus muscle is that of an obligate muscle, the prognosis for such an open bite would be a poor one. The popular dental theory, which presumes an equilibrium of forces among lips, cheeks, and tongue, is supported by clinical examples of the effects of large hyperactive tongues and small or absent ones. However, some investigators suspect that the equilibrium must also involve the postural forces of tongue and lips, because these forces are longer lasting, although smaller in force than those of deglutition. Current clinical wisdom suggests that the horizontal imbalance of swallowing forces has little significance in the determination of normal or abnormal tooth position (Dubner et al., 1978).

Respiration

The relationship between respiration, deglutition, and occlusion is largely one of coordinating these functions with mastication. Respiration continues during mastication, but once food has been chewed, softened, and molded by the tongue into a bolus, breathing is interrupted to allow the bolus to be swallowed. This is the only time respiration needs to be stopped during mastication. The vestibular folds and vocal cords are brought together, while the larynx elevates and the epiglottis is pressed down over it. The larynx has been lifted, moved forward, and covered, to be out of the way of the bolus as it is swallowed. It is shielded by the epiglottis and, as a second line of defense, by the vestibular folds.

There is presumed to be a relationship between the inherent functional efficiency of the dentition—numbers of effective teeth in occlusion—and the time required to triturate and soften a bolus of food so that it can be swallowed easily without any of it being aspirated. Any full account of the chewing-swallowing-breathing interaction must consider sensory awareness, muscle strength and coordination, rates of reflex responses, rate of stimulated salivary flow, taste, strength and promptness of the coughing response, and, probably, much more. But one item of paramount importance dominates: *respiration is never interrupted for long, and the patency of the airway is always protected.* Coughing is regarded as the best defensive reflex in the upper airway. It can be elicited from the larynx, large bronchi, and trachea, as well as from nonairway sites.

Dental aspects of respiration

Some considerations of a specifically related dental nature that are relevant to this brief discussion are as follows:

1. Patients are frequently referred to dentists after an episode of choking or near aspiration. The assumption in this case is that a better chewed bolus would have been less likely to

have caused uncertainty in swallowing. And it is not illogical to assume that a bolus is easier to swallow if a good occlusion is present. However, no restoration of the dentition can ensure that a patient will chew a food bolus to a consistency that will be swallowed easily. Nor will a good occlusion guarantee coordinated swallowing-breathing alternation. Nevertheless, an adequate occlusion is an important element for efficiency of bolus preparation. Affecting as it does most coordinated neuromuscular actions, old age can weaken the synchrony of the oropharyngeal reflexes. The only element in the whole array of mechanisms that could possibly be modified and improved for the elderly is the occlusion itself. Maintaining and, where necessary, restoring the best efficiency of the occlusion is a matter of considerable importance in geriatric dentistry, particularly because the strength and response time of the cough reflex is often diminished in old age.

2. Obstructions of the nasopharynx (e.g., adenoids) may lead to a reflex response to ensure the patency of the airway. The mandible assumes a dropped or open position, and mouth-breathing results. This chain of events does not have a direct bearing on the already developed occlusion, but it may be associated with a gingivitis as a result of dehydration of the gingival tissues.

3. The tongue space and its relationship to airway patency can be crowded or distorted by natural causes such as enlarged or inflamed tonsils, a large tongue, or small maxillary or mandibular arches. Jaw opening and tongue protrusion are conjoint responses to an infringement (i.e., reduced diameter) of the pharyngeal airway. Dental appliances such as biteplanes, or monoblocs and palatal cribs used in orthodontics, may elicit a similar response. It may very well be that the response to any interocclusal appliance involves a specific lingual response. Consequently, by virtue of its associated tongue crowding, such an appliance elicits a jaw-opening response. This may, in turn, counter the jaw-closing muscle activities associated with occlusal parafunction and account, at least in part, for the efficacy of interocclusal appliance therapy for patients with tonic muscle hyperactivity or overt bruxing habits. It should be emphasized that this is speculation, and is not as yet supported by experimental evidence.

Speech

Speech is the most complicated of human learned responses. It is so frequently and spontaneously used that its complexities are rarely apparent. A brief outline of normal speech underscores the fascinating aspects of the mechanism of speech sound production.

Natural speech

Speech development starts with the infant's first cries, which are reflex responses to any form of discomfort or fear. The baby enjoys vocal play before he or she is 8 weeks old, and this babbling stage will soon stop if the various produced sounds are not used in the language around the baby. At about 6 months, the infant is aware of the sounds he or she makes and deliberately imitates them. In so doing, the infant begins to learn to articulate and to vary his or her expressions to indicate pleasure or anger or to gain attention. The association of what the child learns with sound production is an important step in his or her development. By the end of the child's first year, he or she begins to show interest in speech sounds made by others. While meaning is not associated with the sounds, the child is learning to listen and mimic.

Soon a deliberate production of an appropriate word becomes evident, an effort that is reinforced by parental repetition of the word and association of it with the action or object. Pronunciation of words will gradually develop and improve, particularly as the parent continues to provide the correct pattern for the child to copy.

Auditory and visual images are reinforced when the child is able to feel, taste, or smell the object. Gradually the child's ability to convey meanings by varying intonations increases, and a rapidly developing vocabulary and grammatical construction become apparent. Obviously, this progression requires adequate hearing, guidance, and motivation—these factors influence children's growing ability to understand speech and to express themselves. The mechanics of speech production are usually developed naturally by 7 or 8 years of age (Ross and Johnston, 1972).

Mechanism of speech

All speech sounds are made by controlled air. The source of air is the lungs, which expel the air and pass it through the larynx. Speech sounds need more air than does quiet exhalation, and, consequently, subtle adjustments in air flow contribute to variations of pitch and intensity of the voice. The controls for the speech sounds are the various articulations or "valves" made in the pharynx and the oral and nasal cavities. Each sound is affected by the length and diameter of the vocal tract and by the locations of constrictions along its way.

Because nearly all speech sounds are emitted from the mouth, the nasopharynx (airway into the nose) is closed off from the oropharynx during speech. Closure is affected by an upward lift of the soft palate, which is brought about by the action of the levator palati muscles and the palatopharyngeal constrictor muscle toward the posterior pharyngeal wall. The synchronous action of the superior constrictor muscle narrows the dimension of the pharynx, thereby ensuring complete velopharyngeal closure. Rapid continuous movements of the entire length of the soft palate take place during speech, and the palate is lifted higher for some sounds than others. Intimacy of pharyngeal wall contact by the soft palate varies with the nature and sequence of the speech sounds. As the outgoing air passes through the mouth, it is modified by tongue, lip, and mandible movements. The tongue needs optimal mobility in order to lift, protrude, flatten, and contact adjacent tissues freely, while a normal dental occlusion helps direct the escaping air. Jaw and tooth relationships (if within acceptable limits) enable the tongue to articulate against the maxillary teeth or alveolus, permit the maxillary teeth and lower lip to make easy contact, and allow the lips to touch.

The individual's ability to take fullest advantage of his or her speech mechanism is influenced by learning, intelligence, language aptitude, and environment. An ideal speech mechanism does not guarantee good speech skills. Therefore, many deviations from an ideal mechanism or compensations for an inadequate one are encountered by speech pathologists.

Speech sound production

Speech sounds are described by the manner in which they are produced and by the speech articulators involved. The two main groups of speech sounds are vowels and consonants.

Vowels

Vowels are voiced, or phonated, sounds; that is, the vocal cords vibrate in their production. They are the free emission of a speech sound through the mouth, and require subglottic pressure for their production. The vowel letters in English are *a, e, i, o,* and *u*.

Consonants

Consonants may be either voiced sounds or produced without vocal cord vibration, in which case they are breathed sounds. Consonants are produced as a result of the airstream being impeded, diverted, or interrupted before it is released, such as *p, g, m, b, s, t, r,* and *z*. Most consonants may be classified in pairs that are formed in the same manner, except that one is breathed and the other voiced. For example, *p* is breathed, *b* is voiced; *s* is breathed, *z* is voiced; *t* is breathed, and *d* is voiced.

Table 11-2 shows the six types of English consonants and the structures involved in the different "valves" that modify the flow of air to produce these sounds.

Plosive consonants are produced by the

Table 11-2 Normal English consonants: positions and modes of production

	Mode of production											
	Plosives (stops)		Fricatives		Affricatives		Nasals		Liquids		Glides	
Position	Breathed	Voiced	Breathed	Voiced	Breathed	Voiced	Breathed	Voiced	Breathed	Voiced	Breathed	Voiced
Bilabial	*p* (pay)	*b* (bay)						*m* (man)				*w* (witch)
Labiodental			*f* (fan)	*v* (van)								
Linguodental			*th* (thumb)	*th* (there)								
Linguoalveolar	*t* (to)	*d* (do)	*s* (so)	*z* (zoo)				*n* (name)		*l* (less)		
Linguopalatal			*sh* (shoe)	*z* (vision)	*ch* (chin)	*j* (jar)				*r* (rose)		*y* (you)
Linguovelar	*k* (back)	*g* (bag)	*h* (who)					*ng* (bang)				

buildup of air behind two firmly contacting articulator components. When these articulators part, the air is released in a sudden, quick explosion. The soft palate articulates with the pharyngeal wall to achieve this pressure.

Fricative consonants are produced by air being squeezed out slowly through nearly obstructed articulation between the two structures of the "valve." These sounds require particularly good velopharyngeal closure. Fricatives characterized by a hissing or whistling quality are called sibilants; examples are the sounds "s" or "z."

Affricative sounds "ch" and "j" contain both plosive and fricative elements, and depend on a tight velopharyngeal seal for their articulation.

Nasal consonants comprise the three voiced sounds: "m," "n," and "ng." During their production the pharynx does not contract and the soft palate is not fully extended. As a result, velopharyngeal closure does not occur. Oral exit of air does not occur, because it is prevented by the lips ("m"), the tongue's tip against the maxillary alveolus ("n"), and the back of the tongue touching the palate ("ng").

A liquid consonant is one that is produced without friction and is capable of being prolonged with a vowel, such as *l* and *r*. The glide is a sound characterized by a gliding, or gradually changing, articulator shape. It is always followed by a vowel such as *y* in the word "you" and *w* in "witch."

Speech may also be described by characteristics other than speech sounds. These characteristics include voice quality, pitch, resonance, and rate and rhythm. Emotion can affect articulation, as well as pitch and expression (Mehringer, 1963).

The six consonant positions listed in Table 11-2 denote the component structures involved in providing the necessary valving effect for the consonants' production. To some extent, the first five of these valves can be affected by the positions of the teeth. Consequently, when replacing missing teeth, dentists must understand the relationship of tooth orientation to the different speech valve positions. Three simple examples underscore the importance of this understanding. (More comprehensive discussions can be found in textbooks dealing with the treatment of partially and completely edentulous patients.)

1. *Bilabial sounds.* The sounds "p" and "b" are made as air pressure is built up behind the lips and finally released. Insufficient support of the lips by the teeth and an analogue for a missing or resorbed alveolus (labial flange of a prosthesis) can cause these sounds to be defective. Consequently, the anteroposterior position of the anterior teeth and the thickness of a denture's labial flange can affect the production of these sounds.

2. *Labiodental sounds.* The sounds "f" and "v" are made between the maxillary incisor and the labiolingual center to the posterior one third of the lower lip. If the maxillary anterior teeth are to be replaced and the prosthetic teeth are too

short, or are placed too high up, the "v" sound will be more like an "f" sound. If the prosthetic teeth are too long, or are set too far down, the "f" sound will be more like a "v" sound.

3. *Linguoalveolar and linguopalatal sounds.* Most people produce an "s" sound by placing the tip of the tongue against the anterior palate in the rugal area, with a small space for air escape between the tongue and the alveolar process. The size and shape of this small space will determine the quality of the sound. If the opening is too small a whistle will result. If the space is too broad and thin, the "s" sound will be developed as a "sh" sound, somewhat like a lisp. The frequent cause of undesired whistles with wearing removable maxillary prostheses most often is a posterior dental arch form that is too narrow.

Some people make the "s" sound with the tip of the tongue contacting the lingual side of the anterior mandibular dentition, and arching itself up against the palate to form the desired shape and size of the airway. If artificial mandibular teeth are placed too far back on a prosthesis, the tongue will be forced to arch itself up to a higher position, with a resultant reduction in the airway and a whistling sound. To a very large extent, artificial teeth should be placed in the same position the natural teeth occupied, a clinical decision based on experience and the awareness of tongue position vis-à-vis the dentition when speech sounds are made (Hickey et al., 1985).

Dental irregularities and malocclusion may affect pronunciation. However, the extent and nature of this influence are variable. It has been observed that poor anteroposterior jaw relationships are more frequently detrimental to speech. The associated need for the tongue to overextend in either direction in order to articulate with the maxillary central incisors and alveolus is, of course, frequently adapted to. However, the tongue has to protrude further forward in an Angle Class II jaw relationship, or retract and lift to touch the maxillary teeth in a Class III one. Most consonants may consequently be affected by the distortion in the shape and control of the outgoing airstream. However, these risks of jaw articulation speech defects and similar ones resulting from severe malocclusions usually correct themselves as orthodontic treatment leads to normal jaw relationships. It is logical that any speech defect is easier to correct when the tongue is in as normal a position as possible relative to the jaws and has optimal space during postural rest position and speech.

In general, speech articulation is affected by dental occlusal factors. The dentist, therefore, indirectly plays an invaluable speech role in supervising and guiding a dentition's development. Routine dental and interceptive orthodontic treatment together with tooth replacement procedures, where indicated, ensure the establishment of normal structural landmarks to optimize an individual's scope for maximal speech development. The dentist also utilizes normal speech sounds as an adjunct in clinically determining occlusal vertical dimension. This determination is a very important one, because treatment planning for occlusal rehabilitation depends on an assessment regarding optimal jaw position records. The vertical component is established by using a variety of clinically evolved techniques, one of which is the *closest speaking space* method (Hickey et al., 1985). During speech the teeth are separated by variable distances (Table 11-3). During the pronunciation of the "s" sound, as in counting from 60 to 70, the interincisal separation, or vertical distance, averages 1.0 to 1.5 mm and is referred to as the closest speaking space (Fig. 11-1). This distance is used as a tangible guide to preclude the teeth being placed too far apart vertically (with consequent risk of an esthetic compromise—the face will look overclosed and the patient may appear edentulous). It is also used to ensure that the teeth do not encroach upon this necessary functional space, risking a functional compromise (teeth will click or chatter) or an esthetic compromise (the teeth will appear to be too long or "toothy").

Table 11-3 summarizes vertical jaw position during some important and common speech sounds. It may be noted that occlusal contact does not occur during any speech sound. The sibilants cause the mandible to be elevated to a position just short of tooth contact. The diph-

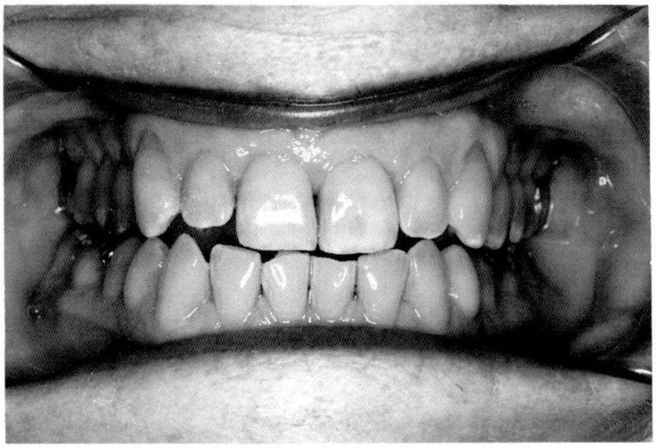

Fig. 11-1 Note position of mandible and approximate incisal separation of 1.0 to 1.5 mm during speech sound "s."

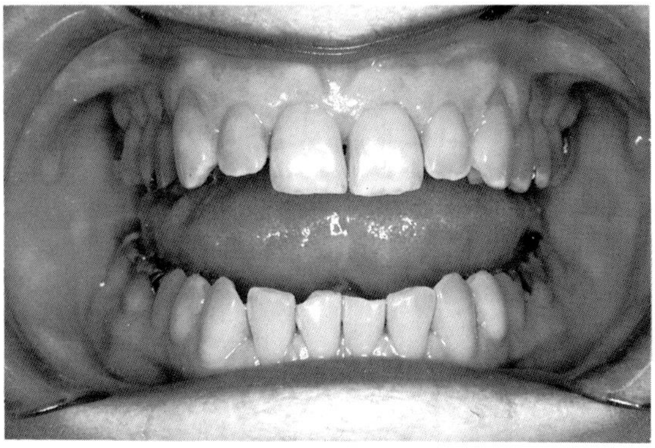

Fig. 11-2 An incisal separation of well over 5 mm while saying the diphthong "ae."

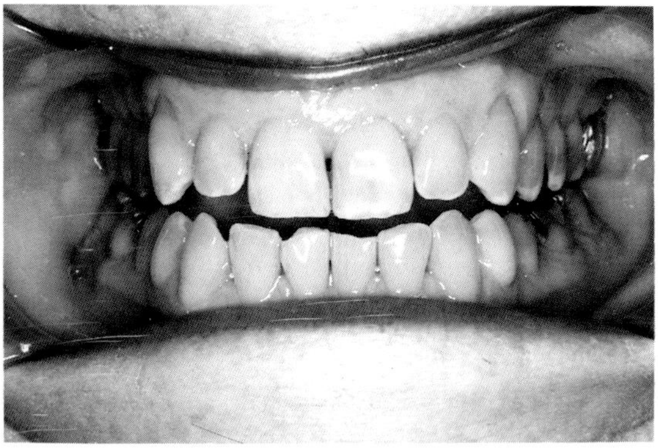

Fig. 11-3 Speaking the nasal sonant "n" with an incisal separation of 2 to 4 mm. This vertical position of the mandible approximates postural rest position.

Table 11-3 Vertical jaw positions during some common speech sounds

Sibilants:

High-frequency fricative sounds made by directing a stream of air through a minimal incisal separation or gap

- "s," "sh," and "ch" are breathed—that is, without laryngeal vibration
- "z," "zh," and "j" are voiced—that is, with laryngeal vibration
- Incisal separation: 1.0 to 1.5 mm

Nasal consonants:

Low-frequency voiced sounds made without an oral exit of air and without velopharyngeal closure

- Examples: "m," "n," and "ng"
- Incisal separation: 2 to 4 mm

Diphthongs:

Sounds made by rapid transition of one vowel to another vowel

- Examples: "ae" and "ie," as in the English words *eight* and *nine*, respectively
- Incisal separation: 5 to 10 mm

thongs result in a mandibular opening well beyond postural rest position (Fig. 11-2). Production of the nasal consonants brings the mandible to a vertical position that approximates postural rest position (Fig. 11-3). Thus, the sibilants are often used to assess occlusal vertical dimension via use of the closest speaking space. The nasal consonants, on the other hand, are frequently used to evaluate and record postural rest position of the mandible.

Summary

The salient features of deglutition, respiration, and speech have been reviewed. Each of these functions has been correlated with mandibular position and movement.

Chapter 12

Concepts of Occlusion

Norman D. Mohl and Robert M. Davidson

It is well recognized that human dentitions vary greatly. However, the question may be asked as to whether certain features exist that are common to most, if not all, occlusal relationships that enhance the function and health of the masticatory system. This question is particularly relevant in therapy when dentists are called upon to modify or create occlusal relationships. For many years, dentists have attempted to identify and define concepts of occlusion that could be applied to the dentition in diagnostic and therapeutic situations. This debate continues today, and the student of Occlusion should be familiar with the history and principal issues involved in it.

Although early anatomists such as Andreas Vesalius and John Hunter described the static relationships of the human natural dentition, these issues were not directly addressed until dentists began to evolve concepts related to the replacement of the natural dentition by artificial complete dentures. The problem of replacing missing teeth has faced dentists since ancient times. However, it was not until the end of the last century that a concerted effort was made to develop concepts of occlusion that could be applied to complete dentures with the view to enhance masticatory efficiency and optimize denture stability, retention, comfort, and esthetics. In 1925, Washburn wrote, "The past seventy-five years have marked the greatest period of advancement in dentistry, due largely to the evolution of ideas pertaining to occlusion." This progress was made by the "prosthetic man," he said (1925). This perception was understandable in an era when loss of the natural teeth was almost to be expected and the construction of functioning artificial dentures was a significant problem (Fig. 12-1).

In an edentulous situation, the dentist must make several determinations when constructing artificial teeth. These include vertical position of the mandible, anteroposterior and lateral relationships of the mandible with respect to the maxilla, occlusal form and position, and occlusal relationships during both "centric" closure and eccentric excursive movements of the mandible. This must all be done without the benefit of existing natural teeth, and it is within this context that the early concepts of occlusion were formulated. Obviously, similar questions can be raised about the natural dentition when it requires restoration, adjustment, orthodontic therapy, or other types of occlusal treatment. Although the same issues may apply to both artificial and natural dentitions, the crucial question is whether the same concepts can, and should, be applied to both clinical situations.

It must be recognized at the outset that complete artificial dentures are placed on a single solid base that covers the mucosa of the edentulous ridges of the maxilla and mandible, whereas the natural dentition contains individual teeth independently anchored to the jaws by roots and periodontal structures. This fact by itself suggests that concepts of occlusion applied to these two therapeutic situations may be somewhat different.

This chapter will consider the foundations of two basic concepts of occlusion: *(1)* balanced

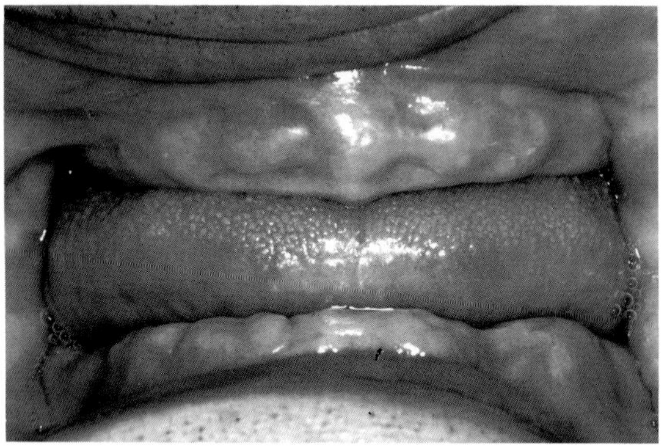

Fig. 12-1 Edentulous mouth.

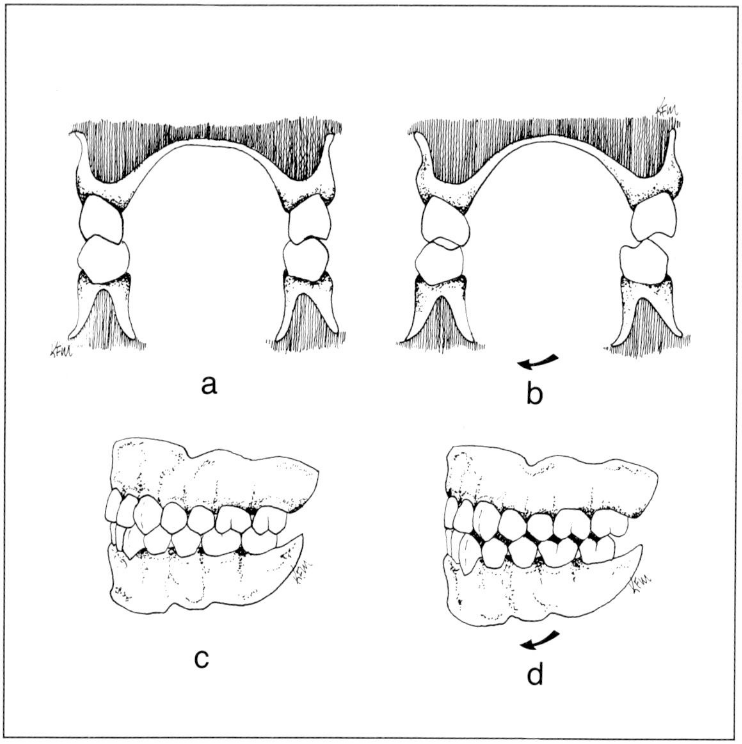

Fig. 12-2 Complete dentures with a fully balanced occlusion. Frontal view with maxillary and mandibular dentures in centric occlusion *(a)*. Movement to lateral excursion with simultaneous buccal-to-buccal and lingual-to-lingual cusp contact on the working side (cross-tooth balance), and maxillary lingual to mandibular buccal cusp contact on the nonworking side (cross-arch balance) *(b)*. Lateral view of dentures in centric occlusion *(c)*. Protrusive movement with simultaneous contact of maxillary and mandibular incisors, as well as maxillary and mandibular posterior teeth (protrusive balance) *(d)*.

occlusion and *(2)* mutual protection. We will trace the evolution of these concepts and consider modern concepts from this historical perspective. Balanced and mutual protection concepts both refer to a functional relationship between the dental arches and describe, respectively, the characteristic lateral and protrusive dynamics embodied in each approach.

A *balanced occlusion* is one in which simultaneous and equal contacts are maintained among opposing tooth surfaces throughout the entire arch and throughout the entire excursion. Lateral excursion in a balanced scheme implies simultaneous working side and nonworking (balancing) side contact (cross-arch balance), while occlusal contacts are maintained on both anterior and posterior teeth as the mandible moves anteriorly into protrusion (Fig. 12-2).

Mutual protection may be defined as a selective pattern of disclusion of nonworking tooth surfaces during similar mandibular excursions. In a sense, by serving to disclude the nonworking side teeth during lateral excursion and the posterior teeth during protrusive incisal contact, the working teeth or inclines "protect" the nonworking teeth or inclines.

Early concepts

Bonwill, a mathematician and dentist, began his studies of the human occlusion around 1850. In 1885, he presented his first paper to a dental society in which he described his "geometric and mechanical laws of articulation." Bonwill's tenets became firmly entrenched, and, for several decades, provided a frame of reference for subsequent hypotheses concerning the nature of the occlusion.

Bonwill analyzed the mandible and described it in terms of an equilateral triangle with 10-cm sides connecting both condyles and the mesioincisal angles of the mandibular central incisors. His concept of a *geometric ideal* was "for the purpose of bringing into contact the largest amount of grinding surface of the bicuspids and molars, and, at the same time, to have the incisors all come into action during lateral movements" (Bonwill, 1885). The resulting balanced occlusion would be for "equalizing the action of muscles on both sides simultaneously, and getting the greatest amount of grinding surface at each movement," and, in addition, "to equalize the pressure and force on both sides or parts of the dental arches." These conditions presumably would help to curtail tipping and dislodgement of the complete dentures when functioning in the mouth.

Prior to Bonwill's "laws," concepts of occlusion were based on the idea of a single, centrally located static hinge. This was embodied in the simple hinged "articulators" of the middle and late 19th century.* In an attempt to more faithfully reproduce mandibular function and anatomy, Bonwill developed an equilateral "anatomical" articulator with two independent condylar elements. This instrument is considered the first example of the application of mathematical principles to problems of occlusion (Butler and Zander, 1968), and served as the model for mechanical instrumentation for many years. Bonwill's instrument was limited insofar as it did not allow for the influence of the articular eminence on the condyle path during protrusion or lateral excursion. As the mandibular member was advanced relative to the maxillary member, there was no inferior component to the path of the condyle, an essential ingredient if one is to accurately create a balanced occlusion. Thus, as noted by Washburn (1925), "One of the phenomena of dental history is that no one for forty years discovered that teeth set up to balance in a Bonwill articulator did not balance in the patient's mouth."

According to Washburn, this inconsistency was first noted in 1893 by Walker, who recognized that the condyle path is inclined inferiorly because of the articular eminence: the so-called *condylar inclination*. He designed an articulator with an adjustable condyle path mechanism and a complex extraoral tracing device to record the inclination of this path for each patient (Walker, 1896). This forerunner of later "gnathological" concepts and instrumentation gave impetus to the idea that the creation of a balanced occlusion required the recording of the patient's condylar inclination during protrusion and lateral excursion.

The concept of a balanced occlusion itself is often credited to Ferdinand Graf Spee, who, quite independently in 1890, presented his observations on the function of the natural teeth of humans. Spee proposed that *(1)* the contacting occlusal surfaces of all natural mandibular teeth "glide" against those of the maxillary teeth, *(2)* these areas of contact lie on the same cylindrical

*Invention of first simple articulator is usually credited to Gariot in 1805.

surface, and *(3)* the horizontal axis of the cylinder's curvature pass through the middle of the medial surface of the orbit behind the lacrimal duct.

Spee suggested that the occlusion functions like "grinding millstones" and that mandibular movement occurs in "circular paths just as a pendulum moves around an axis." The term *curve of Spee* derives from his observation that, when viewed laterally, "the masticatory surfaces of the molars are aligned in a downward convex curve along the upper jaw and in an upward concave curve along the lower jaw" (Spee, 1890). He also believed that a posterior continuation of this curvature would pass along the anterior surface of the condyle, which "also moves on a circular path with the same length of radius on the occlusal surfaces of the molars," that is, "on the same cylindrical surface." Spee concluded that

> As forward and backward gliding of the mandible takes place in a path of circular motion, such displacements can occur over longer distances without any need for the arches to separate from each other. Thus, masticatory efficiency is guaranteed. A separation of the occlusal surfaces is only inevitable in order to overcome the contact of strongly protruding upper and lower canines. But this can also be eliminated by wear. . . . This ought to be considered in the construction of dentures, not only to enable better mastication but also in order to avoid lever effects during chewing.

Thus, the balanced occlusion concept of occlusal organization was born, particularly for complete denture prosthodontics.

During this same period, Edward Hartley Angle was developing his classification of malocclusion, which became known as the *Angle System*. Angle began to describe his concepts in 1887 (Weinberger, 1926), and they have had a profound effect in the field of orthodontics and in dentistry in general. He defined his classification of malocclusion as follows (Angle, 1900):

> **Class I**—Relative positions of jaws and dental arches mesiodistally normal, with first molars usually in normal occlusion, although one or more may be in lingual or buccal occlusion.
>
> **Class II**—Relative mesio-distal relations of jaws and dental arches abnormal, all the lower teeth occluding distally to normal the width of one bicuspid tooth and producing very marked inharmony in the incisive region and in the facial lines.
>
> **Class III**—The relation of the jaws and dental arches is abnormal, the lower being more or less mesial to the upper.

Although this classification, with associated refinements, has proven to be the principal method to diagnose anatomical malocclusions, it must be noted that it only deals with static occlusal relationships in centric occlusion. Thus, Angle's concepts, although very valuable, did not directly deal with the issues of balanced occlusion, mutual protected occlusion, or occlusal organization associated with eccentric positions of the mandible.

The focus on balanced occlusion concepts continued into the 20th century. In 1910, Alfred Gysi criticized the continued use of the simple up-and-down hinged articulator. He recognized the complexity of applying Walker's techniques of recording individual condylar inclinations, and developed simpler methods to more accurately record the pathway of the condyle as it translates anteriorly and inferiorly on the articular eminence. Gysi built several new articulators and extraoral tracing devices during this period, as did many other dentists who wished to record condylar inclinations and other mechanical aspects of jaw movement for the purpose of achieving a balanced occlusion in their patients during complete denture construction. The simplest of the methods had been developed in 1902 by Christensen, who found that he could estimate the condylar inclination of a patient with intraoral wax records, a technique still widely used in restorative dentistry and prosthodontics to this day.

Gysi recognized Bonwill's essential contribution with regard to mandibular function, i.e., the need to incorporate in an instrument excursions on a horizontal plane. He contended, however, that the method of measuring the inferior inclination of the condyle path used by Christensen as well as Walker "is quite incorrect in cases where the condyle path does not form a straight line but follows a more or less curved line or an S-shaped curve, as it most frequently does according to my measurements" (Gysi, 1910). Their measurements, according to Gysi, "register only the direct line between the beginning and the end of the curve." Thus, Gysi discovered that the condyle path does not form a straight line, as believed by Bonwill, but follows a more or less curved line or an S-shaped curve. With this additional information added to Bonwill's equilateral triangle concept, he claimed to be able to "direct the movement of the mandible in all the combinations of the masticatory movements" (Gysi, 1910).

Gysi also took exception to Spee's idea of a true center of rotation of the mandible. He believed that mandibular movement is dependent on incisal as well as condylar inclination. His pioneering work anticipated the gnathological theorists, and he developed techniques to record rotational axes of mandibular movements. However, he did note that "from the position of these rotation points it is plain that they could not be considered as anatomically fixed points . . . [but result] from the diverse contractions of the masticatory muscles, and happens to coincide only now and then with the condyles" (Gysi, 1910).

Gysi understood and accepted the morphological variation later anatomists took for granted, and, unlike Spee, distinguished between the functional and anatomical characteristics of patients with natural teeth and the unique situation of the edentulous patient. Although he predicated his understanding of occlusion on an appreciation of the dentulous state, Gysi understood the biomechanical problems of artificial teeth and proposed a treatment approach to accommodate them into a bilaterally balanced occlusion.

In a direct extension of portions of the work of both Bonwill and Spee, George S. Monson (1920, 1922, 1932) proposed the "spherical principle in the solution of the problem of human occlusion." The problem Monson referred to concerned the hypothetical center of rotation of the mandible with respect to the maxilla.

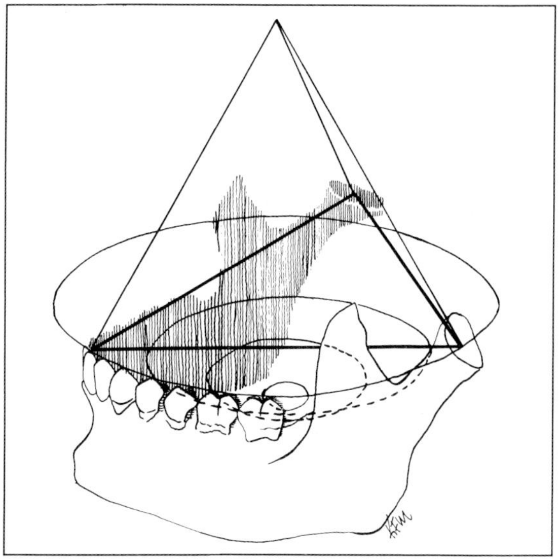

Fig. 12-3 Composite drawing illustrating Bonwill's 10-cm equilateral triangle (heavy lines from central incisors to and between condyles) and Monson's sphere with the equal 10-cm radii converging to a common center of rotation (apex of pyramid), and all mandibular cusp tips and incisal edges contacting the circumference of the sphere. These ideas represent a geometric ideal.

Bonwill had applied a mathematical model in his description of the mandible and understood that translation along a horizontal plane took place during excursions. Spee had considered the axis of rotation in an essentially anteroposterior dimension and described a cylinder, the axis of which formed a transverse line connecting the center of curvature of one side of the occlusion with the other. Monson disregarded the Bonwillian horizontal excursion. However, he adapted the 10-cm equilateral triangle that formed the basis of Bonwill's theory, and added it to the occlusal curvature-fixed central axis of rotation concept of Spee. His conclusions produced the 10-cm radius sphere, a geometric embodiment of the function, form, and "beauty" of the masticatory system (Fig. 12-3).

Monson's theories were readily applied to clinical practice. His concept of occlusion was based on an a priori geometric ideal that presupposed an optimal anatomical configuration and functional occlusal relationships. Whatever component of the natural dentition was at variance with Monson's ideal was made consistent with that ideal or removed. According to Monson,

> Elongated teeth must be reduced in their length and teeth that have been in excessive function built up to their proper occlusion, bringing the occlusion of all teeth to conform to the surface of the sphere having proper interlocking cusps to maintain them in their alignment. The teeth are then ground into the full range of occlusion (1920).

Bilateral balance was a natural consequence of such an approach to occlusion, yet it was incidental to the attempt to make functional activity conform to a geometric ideal. Although the spherical ideal has been shown *not* to be a naturally occurring characteristic (Dempster et al., 1963), it remains today as a concept that is at least partially employed by some dentists in the occlusal rehabilitation of natural dentitions (Mann and Pankey, 1963).

Monson did recognize that two schools of thought regarding movements of the human mandible had evolved. In 1932, he stated, "The first believes that the shape and movement of the condyles govern the occlusion of the teeth, while the second group contends that the occlusion of the teeth is the dominant guiding factor which determines the shape and movements of the condyles in the glenoid fossa" (Monson, 1932). Monson was obviously in the latter group and the articulators he utilized reflected this concept, having a single midline pivot 10 cm above the occlusal plane, and no condylar mechanism whatsoever.

These divergent theoretical approaches to understanding and reproducing mandibular function shared one essential therapeutic objective: a completely balanced occlusion for full-denture prostheses. Denture stability was paramount, and as a result the cross-arch, cross-tooth, and protrusive elements of balance were accepted. In essence, balance mandated continuous contact between multiple surfaces of teeth during eccentric excursions. *Cross-arch balance* referred to the simultaneous contact of working and nonworking teeth, *cross-tooth balance* referred to simultaneous contact of buccal-to-buccal and lingual-to-lingual cusps of working side teeth, while *protrusive balance* provided simultaneously contacting inclines of both anterior and posterior teeth during protrusion. Balance was equated with stability of the artificial denture base and was the accepted approach to restoring function to the edentulous patient. (It should be noted here that this concept has been modified in modern complete denture prosthodontics, particularly with regard to protrusive balance, which often sacrifices esthetics and speech articulation.)

Concepts applied to the natural dentition

Gnathology

In 1926, B. B. McCollum and a group of dental colleagues founded the Gnathological Society of California (McCollum, 1939). They coined the term *gnathology,* which has been defined as the "study of temporomandibular joint movements, their selective measurement, reproduction, and use as determinants in the diagnosis and treatment of occlusion" (Kaplan, 1963).

McCollum and his associates developed their concept of occlusion on what was considered the immutable and ideal nature of the relationship between the condyle and fossa, which in turn was responsible for guiding the mandible in its correct relationship to the maxilla. Convinced that "heredity will for many years leave the greatest majority of humanity the victims of unsound tendencies" (McCollum, 1939), McCollum and others dedicated themselves to restoring "ideal" function and anatomy.

Natural dentitions that did not adhere to their predetermined criteria were considered to be pathological. As McCollum (1938) stated, "There is a subtle pathology of function in every

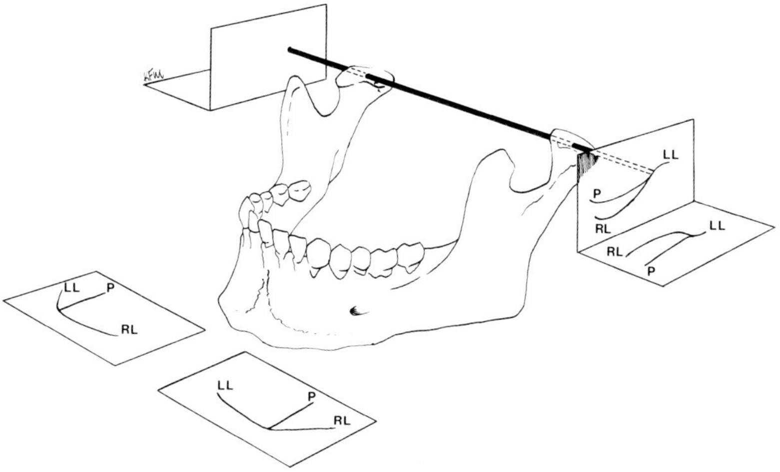

Fig. 12-4 The basis for the gnathological concept of occlusion. Condylar movement is recorded by styli, which make tracings on horizontal and vertical tracing plates. In this figure, the two horizontal tracing plates in front would be attached to and move with the mandible. A symmetrical protrusive movement would trace lines *P*. A right lateral excursion would trace lines *RL*, while a left lateral movement would trace lines *LL*. The terminal hinge axis is represented by the "rod" through the condyles. The "apex" of each gnathological tracing illustrates the location of centric relation.

mouth, due entirely to the malrelation between the opposing teeth themselves and between the interdigitation of the teeth and jaw motions. This pathology has for some time been called *malarticulation*." Thus, deviations from the anatomical and functional ideal were thought to be the result of malpositioned cusps and teeth, which were then altered to conform to the recorded positions and movements of the condyle. Correct occlusion, therefore, could only be approached from an understanding of the relationship between the condyle and its articulation with the temporal bone.

Mechanics of temporomandibular joint (TMJ) function were based on the idea that "the combined joints, in spite of their being biological mechanisms, still provide definite, measurable, recordable movements that can be reproduced in an artificial mechanical contrivance" (McCollum, 1939). The belief was that if an articulator could absolutely duplicate jaw relations and condylar movement, it would be possible to make teeth that occlude ideally. As a result, techniques were developed that embodied these two basic assumptions (McCollum and Stuart, 1955). McCollum modified a Snow face-bow,* attached it to the mandible, and thus created the hinge-axis locator (kinematic face-bow), a device to precisely pinpoint the transverse axis of condylar rotation. A pair of upper and lower face-bows were developed to produce the pantograph, an instrument used to record the three-dimensional movement patterns of the condyles during protrusion and lateral excursion (Fig. 12-4). A fully adjustable articulator was also developed that was capable of following these recorded condylar pathways.

Historically, the development of the modern casting machine, which enabled dentists to accurately reproduce the laboratory ideal for the patient, coupled with the desire to prevent and treat "dental disease," gave these men the impetus to achieve their philosophical and clinical

*George B. Snow invented the face-bow in 1907.

objectives. The gnathological concepts and technology that were developed became, and have remained, very influential in the field of Occlusion.

McCollum embraced the idea of a completely balanced occlusion for the *natural dentition,* the attraction being that it was totally consistent with his notion of an idealized biomechanical mechanism. He used sophisticated techniques to achieve exquisitely balanced occlusal arrangements in the laboratory, which were then transferred to the patient's dentition. The presumed objectives were *(1)* to maintain idealized occlusal contact throughout all excursions, coordinated in function with the stable condyle-fossa relationship, thereby eliminating potential tooth interferences during the ideal condyle positions and movements; and *(2)* to distribute occlusal contacts among as many teeth as possible, resulting in reduced loading to individual teeth and curtailment of periodontal breakdown.

Functionalism

In 1929, Clyde H. Schuyler published his first of many articles on occlusal concepts. Although this paper gave little indication of his influence for the next 50 years in this field, Schuyler did state at the outset that

> This does not mean that all principles of occlusion pertaining to full denture prosthesis are applicable to the natural dentition, nor that it would be possible to obtain in other branches of dentistry the same degree of perfection in occlusal relations as may be produced in full denture restorations. While such perfection might be desirable, it is not altogether essential to the health and maintenance of the supporting structures of the natural teeth. . . . The term "balanced occlusions" is most applicable to restorations supported by soft tissue (1929).

Although, like the gnathologists, Schuyler believed in harmony between centric relation and centric occlusion for the natural dentition, he did not impose a set of rigid standards on the occlusion that, if lacking, was tantamount to pathology. This concept, when applied to the natural teeth, was referred to as *functionalism.* It was defined as "such arrangements of the teeth as will provide the highest efficiency during all the excursions of the mandible which are necessary to the function of mastication." Although this was a very loose definition, it had the effect of recognizing the essential difference between the edentulous and dentulous conditions and, most significantly, did not impose rigid anatomical standards on an idealized relationship between condylar movement and occlusal organization.

In 1935, Schuyler developed the first detailed technique for occlusal adjustment based on the careful grinding of specific inclines in contradistinction to the "ruthless, haphazard manner," sometimes with abrasive pastes, then employed by some dentists, including prosthodontics and periodontists, trying to achieve a "balanced occlusion" (Schuyler, 1935). Like the gnathologists and other dentists of the time, Schuyler believed there was a relationship between functioning occlusal inclines and potential stress to the periodontium, and his occlusal adjustment techniques were meant to ameliorate these stresses. He suggested reducing the contact areas during maximum intercuspation, and described a "division of labor" between inclines, cusps tips, and occluding surfaces of teeth. In anticipation of later "long centric" concepts, Schuyler favored point contacts opposite flat planes during maximum intercuspation, and opposing gliding inclined planes during lateral excursions.

The demise of balanced occlusion

His insights and manuscripts notwithstanding, Schuyler persisted in supporting essentially balanced occlusion during his early clinical years. With time, however, not unlike the gnathologists, Schuyler began to observe clinical failures of balance when applied to the restored natural dentition. In 1953, he stated, "In the natural dentition I fail to see the real value of contacts on the nonfunctioning side, as they do not reduce the application of stress being applied to the teeth on the working side, and their contact may be a contributing factor to traumatic injury" (Schuyler, 1953).

Schuyler later suggested that during function "balancing contacts that may have appeared to be harmless may, with the unilateral application of force, become traumatic, most destructive, and extremely undesirable" (Schuyler, 1961). Two years later, he wrote:

> Balancing contacts of the posterior teeth in either the lateral or the protrusive eccentric functional movements may be desirable or essential for the stability of complete dentures, but they are not essential for the stability of the natural dentition. . . . Their value in distributing functional stress is negative (1963).

His observations and suggestions effectively signaled the end of "balance" as an acceptable treatment approach to the dentulous patient.

Schuyler also emphasized the important influence of incisal guidance as the "predominating factor" determining posterior occlusal morphology (1959). This was consistent with his view that, although the direction of movement of the mandible is controlled by the muscles and TMJs when the dentition is out of occlusion, "when the opposing teeth of the natural dentition come into contact, the guiding inclines of the teeth immediately assume almost complete control of the direction and the extent of movement of the mandible" (Schuyler, 1958). His concepts thus included the importance of canine guidance and the "canine-protected occlusion" that was used for "the desired relief of stress upon the balancing inclines of posterior teeth" (1961).

During this period, many gnathologists were also changing their idea of the balanced occlusion concept as applied to the natural dentition. Several, including some members of McCollum's original group, were "courageous enough to admit that the majority of his cases did not stand the rigid test of time and were failures. This they attributed to the trauma caused by the multitudinous contacts which was and still is part and parcel of their theory" (Schweitzer, 1963). More specifically, Stuart and Stallard (1960) noted, for example, that balanced occlusion in reconstructed natural dentitions *(1)* often required injudicious increases in occlusal vertical dimension to achieve balance, *(2)* often led to instability of the occlusion, *(3)* frequently showed increased wear of the teeth and restorations, and, in addition, *(4)* provided poor group usage of the teeth.

In 1963, Stallard and Stuart wrote:

> Since the rise in favor for balanced occlusion much has been learned about the neuromuscular physiology of the gnathic system. We have learned a little about how mouth automation takes place and how the mouth rests. It seems that balanced occlusion does not insure oral rest and it requires the patient to learn anew how to automate his chewing. The collectivization of teeth into balanced occlusion was held out as a hope that it would spare the periodontium. We have since learned that most periodontal diseases are due to other than maloccluding factors.

The last sentence in the above quote is particularly significant and has been substantiated by subsequent research. Compounding the clinical repercussions of balanced restorations was the extraordinary technical demands implicit in restoring the natural dentition to full balance. In addition, the esthetic character of the restored balanced occlusions, which often required severe reduction of anterior overbite, was found to be far from adequate. It is also significant that these gnathologists also recognized that "former attempts to stereotype patterns" were incompatible with "the necessity for variations," and that "any pattern of occlusion that tolerates no variations in details and relations is impossible" (Stallard and Stuart, 1963).

Thus, some parallel ideas evolved in the concepts of both the gnathologists and the functionalists, and both groups came to speak of the *mutual protection* concept of occlusion. This concept is based on the premise that the teeth should act as specialized groups so that in centric or eccentric positions of the mandible certain teeth or groups of teeth are best able to withstand the occlusal loads and, in doing so, will protect other teeth or groups of teeth from unfavorable forces.

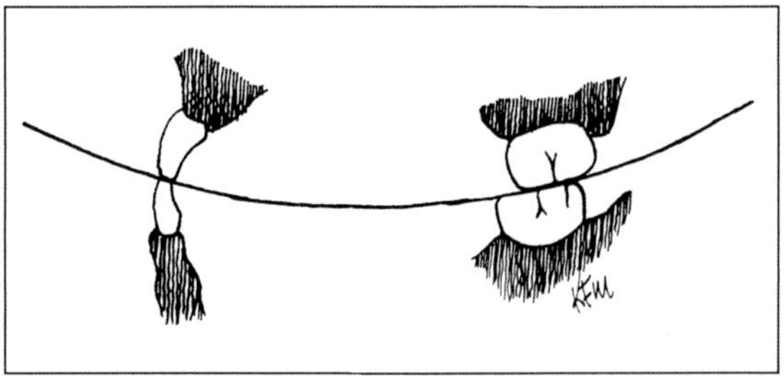

Fig. 12-5a *(above)* Schematic drawing of aboriginal dentition showing flattened edge-to-edge incisors and flattened molars.

Fig. 12-5b *(right)* Reverse curve of Wilson. The reverse curve develops because of the higher relative rate of attrition of the supporting cusps. When present, the Carabelli cusp may come into functional occlusion.

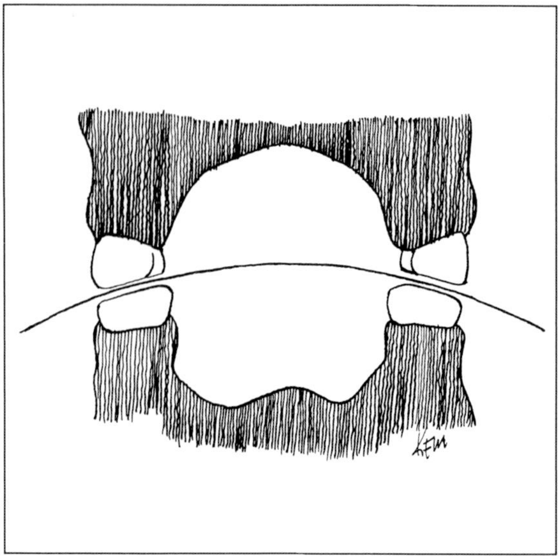

Influence of physical anthropology

The arguments over these concepts were greatly influenced by dental anthropological studies conducted during these years. Spee had emphasized the ruminantlike grinding action of the human dentition, which strongly implied laterally directed excursive-incursive shearing movements of the mandible. Examination of the flattened edge-to-edge occlusions and reverse curve of Wilson found in aboriginal societies (Figs. 12-5a and b) seemed to bear witness to the importance of the lateral component of the chewing cycle and to the maximum shearing of multiple inclined planes—an idea seemingly compatible with both the geometric ideal and early gnathological concepts.

In studies of the dentitions of Australian aborigines, Begg noted severe interproximal and occlusal attrition* and concluded that this attritional process produced the "only anatomically correct occlusion." He continued: "The accepted textbook normal occlusion of civilized man is anatomically incorrect because his food is too soft and concentrated to cause tooth attrition" (Begg, 1954). Begg wrote:

> High unworn cusps are wrongly considered to have evolved to maintain stability of occlusion throughout life, whereas the only advantage of high cusps is that they help to guide the teeth into their occlusal relationships at the time the teeth are erupting and then to hold them only for a short time after eruption (1954).

He concluded that a high rate of attrition is supposed to occur in modern humans and is the result of a natural evolutionary process. Although Begg did not directly refer to the pattern of occlusal contacts in eccentric positions, his implication is that multiple contacts are meant to occur in all excursive movements of the mandible.

Beyron also studied the Australian aborigine dentition and the masticatory movements of live subjects, finding the same severe occlusal and interproximal wear that seems common in primitive cultures with their extremely abrasive diets and more frequent use of the teeth as tools. He

*Begg calculated average loss of more than 1 cm in mesiodistal dimension of the dental arch by age 20 in aborigines. This is in contrast to an estimated loss of 1 cm by age 40 in nonaborigine cultures (Goldman and Cohen, 1968).

also reported, however, that "in only about 10 per cent of the (aboriginal) subjects of the present study did the intercuspal position coincide with the retruded position. The average distance between the two positions was slightly more than one millimetre. This finding is in agreement with the values reported for other (nonaboriginal) groups of people judged to have excellent occlusions" (Beyron, 1964).

Beyron also found that "the occlusal relations of the anterior teeth showed that in the intercuspal position a minute space existed between the upper and lower incisors of most of the subjects"—an observation completely compatible with the mutual protection concept. Because of the degree of attrition, Beyron noted that many of the teeth were in contact on the working side during lateral excursion *(group function)*. Although observing that "this 'group function' was a characteristic feature of Australian aboriginal material," he also found that "another striking feature was the absence of occlusal contact on the nonworking side, a contact that should be present in the 'ideal' occlusion, according to the concept of 'balanced occlusion.'" These findings were reported in spite of the presence of a very wide lateral component to the "tear drop" form of the chewing cycle in the frontal plane (Beyron,1964).

Beyron's findings were consistent with his earlier reports in which he suggested that some attrition of the dentition was natural and desirable and that there is a close reciprocal relationship between occlusion form and direction of the contact gliding movements (Beyron, 1954b). However, "balancing contact on the unengaged side does not contribute to a reduction in the stress applied to the teeth on the working side," and "in this connection the danger of excessive contact of balancing cusps inclines should be emphasized, since such contact obstructs gliding movements" (Beyron, 1954a). These conclusions had also been reached in an anthropological study by Jones, who observed that, in humans, "mastication is from lateral to medial, and is unilateral, the teeth of the opposite side being definitely not in contact" (Jones, 1947).

The work of D'Amico (1958) contrasted sharply with that of Begg. D'Amico's conclusions had a direct impact on the thinking of dentists with regard to concepts of occlusion. He studied the dentitions of pre- and post-European California Indians and concluded that

> The immediate change from their primitive culture to the modern European way of life eliminated the abrasive factors which caused rapid attrition of the teeth and reduction in the vertical relation of the mandible. The result of this sudden change was the development of the overlap relation of the upper incisors and cuspids. Evolutionary or organic changes do not develop in such brief periods (1961).

D'Amico developed the view that *(1)* the flattened edge-to-edge occlusions seen in aboriginal dentitions were due to *excessive* attrition and are abnormal, *(2)* a lateral ruminating type of mandibular function in humans is not typical, *(3)* steeply cusped teeth are entirely appropriate, and *(4)* the maxillary incisors and canines are meant to exhibit overbite so as to disclude the posterior teeth during eccentric positions of the mandible. D'Amico, in particular, emphasized the maxillary canines having the principal occlusal contact in lateral excursion and serving to guide the closing movement of the mandible into centric occlusion. This idea has been termed *canine protection,* and is a modification of the more generalized mutual protection concept of occlusion.

The question of whether attrition, particularly extensive attrition, should be considered physiological or pathological is still being debated (Berry, 1986). This issue will not be further clarified until clinical research data become available that show specific relationships between the *effects* of moderate or extensive attrition on signs, symptoms, or functional efficiency of the masticatory system.

Current concepts

In summarizing the transition to current concepts of occlusion, Stuart and Stallard (1960) stated:

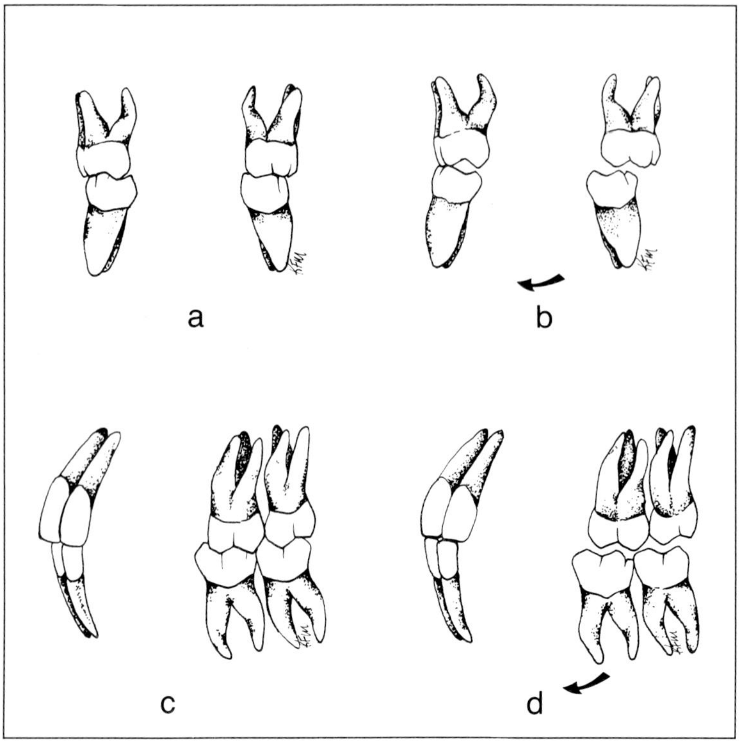

Fig. 12-6 The mutual protection concept of occlusion. Frontal view with molars in centric occlusion *(a)*. In lateral excursion, there is buccal-to-buccal contact on the working side and disclusion on the nonworking side *(b)*. Centric occlusion viewed laterally *(c)*. In protrusion, only maxillary and mandibular incisors are in contact *(d)*. Compare this concept of occlusal organization with that illustrated in Fig. 12-2.

> To many students of occlusion, it seemed logical to assume that the least violent arrangement of oral parts would come from an articulation of cusps in which there would be both bilateral and protrusive balanced occlusion. They held that this classic and revered collective tooth arrangement in which all the teeth were together in nearly every biting station, would afford a stability because the muscles would strain neither the teeth nor the joints and could not overburden teeth singly.

For many years, in fact, this concept of occlusion was adhered to by functionalists as well as gnathologists, even though clinical observations and anthropological studies failed to support such beliefs. Cross-arch, cross-tooth, and protrusive balance as a conscious goal in therapy of the natural dentition has generally been abandoned in favor of an occlusal arrangement that provides for some medium of protection for nonfunctioning teeth and cusps (Fig. 12-6).

In the transition from the theories of balance to those of mutual protection, there arose what may be considered the dual views concerning working side canine protection (D'Amico, 1961) (Figs. 12-7 and 12-8) versus group function (Schuyler, 1961) (Fig. 12-9). In the broadest sense, mutual protection can be applied to anterior teeth with respect to posterior teeth, and to functioning posterior teeth with respect to nonfunctioning posterior teeth. Clinically, distinctions between canine protection and group function are often difficult to make, but the differences in the rationale underlying each is quite clear. The modern gnathological concept of canine protection is based on the assumption that "tooth blades and cusps are arranged for vertical chewing" (Stuart and Stallard, 1960), and that cusp-fossa-groove position and form must be strictly integrated with condylar and mandibular movements so that minimal tooth contacts occur during function. From this perspective, the canines help to prevent the lateral enmeshment of working side posterior teeth, which is considered not only superfluous, but potentially damaging as well.

To functionalists, in contradistinction, "the eccentric movements of the mandible during mastication are extremely varied and follow no specific pattern except when all eccentric movements are restricted by exceedingly steep interlocking inclines of the anterior teeth." When this occurs, the individual "is forced to masticate or cut food with a chopping vertical motion" (Schuyler, 1961). Within this context, canine protection would preclude the engagement of multiple working side cusps and the desired lateral component to the chewing cycle—that is, working side group function.

Studies on the incidence of the canine-protected occlusion have produced equivocal results. This is probably due to the use of different criteria, amounts of lateral excursion, age groups, cultures, and other variables among the studies. Collectively, however, the data tend to support the premise that the relative incidence of canine protection and group function is related to the age of the subject and the amount of attrition on the canines and other teeth, as well as on the basic structural features of the occlusion.

Butler and Zander (1968) conducted a short-term experiment with two subjects, each of whom had two fixed partial dentures constructed, one with a canine-protective occlusal scheme and the other with multiple group function occlusal contacts in lateral excursion. Each fixed partial denture was worn for 1 month, during which electromyographic (EMG) activity and canine contact patterns during mastication were recorded (by intraoral telemetry) on several occasions. No noticeable differences in EMG activity were found between the two occlusal types. Butler and Zander concluded, "Both patients were satisfied and comfortable with either type of working side occlusion and could detect no difference in the functional qualities of the two different reconstructions." However, "there were found to be significantly fewer lateral contacts on the cuspid when each patient was wearing the cuspid-protected type reconstruction"

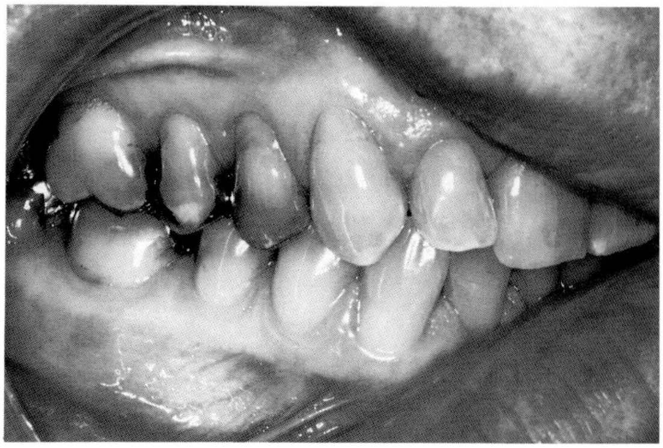

Fig. 12-7 Dentition in centric occlusion of a 52-year-old woman.

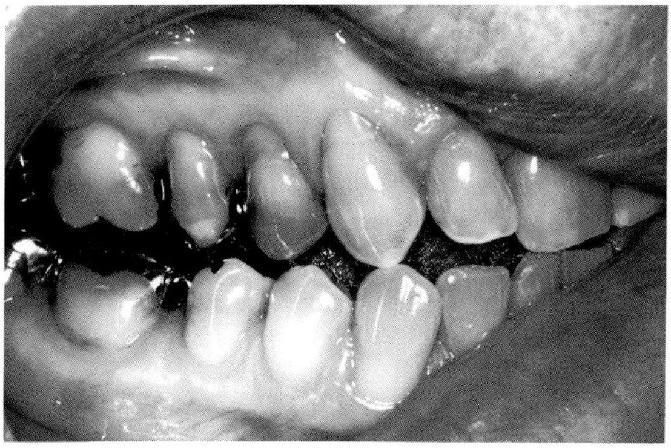

Fig. 12-8 Same dentition shown in Fig. 12-7, demonstrating canine protection in lateral excursion.

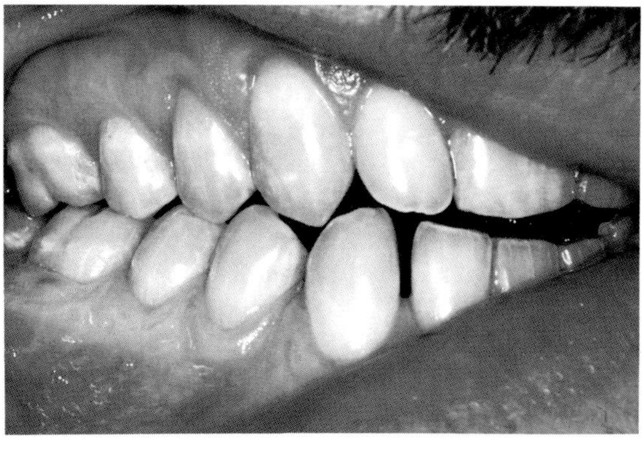

Fig. 12-9 Dentition demonstrating multiple contacts on working side teeth during lateral excursion, that is, group function of a 23-year-old man.

(Butler and Zander, 1968). Their sample is too small to draw generalizations from, but it does suggest that the canine-protected occlusion may lead to a more direct closure into full intercuspation during mastication than does the group function occlusion. More studies of this type are obviously needed.

Despite the continued dual perceptions of canine protection versus group function, the development of the *mutual protection concept* represents an embodiment of both gnathological and functionalist ideas, and is compatible with each. Functionalism's most crucial contribution may have been the understanding of the variability and impreciseness of mandibular function and the intercuspation of teeth. Gnathology has provided a biomechanical model and rationale for understanding TMJ function and occlusal morphology. Mutual protection, in the broadest sense, can embrace both perspectives, and provides a basis for arranging teeth that takes into account these apparently contradictory approaches.

Mutual protection

Organized disclusion, a term coined by Stallard and Stuart (1963), is an apt description of this concept of occlusion, both in maximum intercuspation and in lateral and protrusive excursions of the mandible. Our understanding of mutual protection should be considered in its broadest sense; the following organizational scheme and functional relationships of the natural dentition are derived from such a perspective:

1. In the intercuspal position, primary occlusal loading, axially directed, is absorbed by contact-supporting areas on posterior teeth only. Anterior teeth contact very lightly and should not bear these potentially heavy forces.
2. In protrusion, the overbite-overjet relations of the incisors produce an incisal guidance that is steep enough to cause disclusion of all posterior teeth.
3. In lateral excursion, the overbite-overjet relationship of the contacting teeth on the working side should be sufficiently steep to cause disclusion of all nonworking side teeth. The question of whether the working side canines alone should be in contact (canine protection) (see Fig. 12-8), whether the premolars should also be in contact, or whether all working side posterior teeth should also be in contact (group function) (see Fig. 12-9) is probably best determined on an individual case-by-case basis, depending on such clinical factors as preexisting relationships, root-crown ratios, and the degree of mobility or fremitus of the teeth involved.

Controversies

Vestiges of the dichotomy between the gnathological and functionalist schools still persist. Although mutual protection has become an accepted approach to occlusal organization during therapy, questions still abound regarding working side canine protection versus group function, tripodization of cusps in fossa versus flat areas of contact, the nature and significance of centric relation, coincidence of centric relation, and centric occlusion versus "freedom in centric." In addition, issues regarding diagnostic criteria are still being debated: the significance of tooth mobility; the role, if any, of occlusal factors in the etiology of bruxism; TMJ and muscle problems; criteria for occlusal therapy; and techniques of occlusal adjustment.

One area of continued controversy involves the question of the static relationships of the mandible to the maxilla in centric occlusion. Proponents of the "point centric" feel that the intercuspal position must exactly correspond to the retruded contact position of the mandible. Proponents of the "freedom in centric" concept feel that an area of freedom should exist to allow the mandible to function on a slight anteroposterior flat plane between the intercuspal and retruded contact positions. Both views, however, fall within the general criteria for mutual protection and are not inconsistent with either canine protection or group function. The two interpretations of the optimal intercuspal relationship are intended to provide end-point guidelines for occlusal therapy, and thus should be viewed as therapeutic considerations rather than descriptions of naturally occurring anatomical features.

It must be emphasized that the historical view presented in this chapter deals with concepts of occlusion for the natural dentition that are most appropriately applied *after the decision to commence therapy has been made*. The mere fact that a patient does not exhibit the features to be expected from a dentist's own concept of occlusal organization is not, in itself, a mandate to treat that occlusion. Other diagnostic factors must be present before a decision to initiate therapy—particularly irreversible therapy—is made. These factors will be discussed in chapter 13 and in other parts of this textbook.

Finally, it must also be recognized that past and present concepts of occlusion have been based largely on biomechanical considerations and have been promulgated over the years mostly as a result of empirical clinical observations and interpretations. Such interpretations, when done in an objective and unbiased manner, are not without validity. However, all such concepts deserve to be observed under controlled scientific conditions before conclusions regarding cause-and-effect relationships, diagnostic criteria, and therapeutic efficacy are drawn.

During the past few decades dentistry has developed an intense interest in research involving occlusal and mandibular function and dysfunction. Basic and applied studies have involved most of the biological, behavioral, and clinical disciplines and have included the use of epidemiology, clinical trials, EMG, intraoral telemetry, jaw-tracking techniques, and histopathology, to name a few. While continuing to emphasize the importance of mechanical and biomechanical principles and techniques, we have witnessed an increased interest in a better understanding of the biological and behavioral aspects of this subject. This will certainly continue. New information and insights will require continued analysis of our concepts, which are likely to change over time. This trend, coupled with our knowledge of human anatomical and functional variability and adaptation, requires that we *avoid any unalterable dogma regarding any one concept or therapeutic approach to occlusal problems*.

Summary

This chapter reviewed concepts of occlusal organization and relationships, particularly with regard to the adult natural dentition. Emphasis has been given to the mutual protection concept, as contrasted to that of balanced occlusion. Consideration of these two concepts of occlusion embodies the historical continuity of our present concepts from complete artificial denture construction to the organization of the natural dentition. Thus, a historical review has traced the development of these concepts and some of their corollaries through their several stages of development and modification.

The purpose of this discussion has been to provide perspective to some of the terms, issues, and concepts that have engaged the interest of dentists in the field of Occlusion over the years, and to serve as a frame of reference prior to a consideration of the diagnosis and management of occlusal and dysfunctional problems in the subsequent Parts II and III of this book.

PART II
Occlusal and Dysfunctional Problems of the Masticatory System

This section deals with the definition, etiology, differential diagnosis, pathophysiology, and sequelae of occlusal and dysfunctional problems of the masticatory system. Such problems are related to the structural relationships of the components of the system and/or to mandibular functional or parafunctional activity that adversely affect one or more of these components. Signs and symptoms of these problems may be manifested in the teeth themselves, in the periodontal supporting apparatus, in the temporomandibular joints, in the masticatory muscles and associated nervous system, and in related tissues and systems.

This section provides an essential foundation for understanding the relevant structural and functional problems of the masticatory system prior to a consideration of treatment. Part II includes these chapters:

Diagnostic Rationale: An Overview
Examination and Differential Diagnosis of Occlusal Problems
The Dentition: Occlusal Variations and Problems
The Periodontium: Responses to Occlusal Forces
The Temporomandibular Joint: Problems Related to Occlusal Function
Occlusal Parafunction

Chapter 13

Diagnostic Rationale: An Overview

Norman D. Mohl

An accurate diagnosis based on an adequate history, examination, and utilization of relevant information is fundamental to the treatment of patients. Whenever possible, specific cause-and-effect relationships should be established as a prelude to treatment decisions. These principles apply to the management of patients with occlusal and dysfunctional problems of the masticatory system. Their application, however, can only be accomplished within a conceptual framework that enhances one's ability to make logical and consistent diagnostic and therapeutic judgments.

The critical question faced by all clinicians is not necessarily *how* and *what* to treat, although this is obviously of great importance. The essential question is very often *when* to treat and *when not* to treat. The answer to this question is based on the development of a diagnostic rationale that can be applied to a wide variety of clinical situations.

Thus, a conceptual framework is needed. It is needed because the diagnostic process itself is ambiguous unless comparisons can be made between a concept of "health" or "normality" and that of "disease" or "nonnormality." Since diagnosis is the art of recognizing disease, the diagnostician must have some basis for distinguishing "disease" from "nondisease" or "normality" from "nonnormality." For example, the diagnosis of a "poor" or "abnormal" occlusal relationship implies that the examiner has compared this with a "good" or "normal" occlusal relationship and made a value judgment between them. Furthermore, does the so-called poor occlusal relationship necessarily require treatment? The answer to this question requires a judgment as to whether or not it has or will have a destructive influence on the patient's masticatory system or general well-being.

In addition, a conceptual framework is needed in order to make logical diagnostic and therapeutic decisions in the absence of clearcut etiological factors: a common situation. The medical axiom "remove the cause" is an extremely desirable principle, but it is difficult to apply when problems exist in the absence of readily apparent cause-and-effect relationships. The development of a diagnostic rationale is therefore needed in order to enhance the diagnostic/therapeutic decision-making process, make it more consistent, and improve communication among clinicians.

In developing this rationale, the term "normal" will not be used. The description "normal occlusion," for example, is too vague because to some it implies an occlusion that meets a preestablished norm, and to others it is the one that most often occurs naturally—two incompatible ideas. The conceptual framework to be used is based on the idea that distinctions can be made between occlusions that

1. Adhere to predetermined standards (theoretically ideal occlusion)
2. Show variability from a predetermined standard but do not require treatment (physiologic occlusion)
3. May need treatment (nonphysiologic occlusion)
4. Have been structurally modified for therapeutic reasons (therapeutic occlusion)

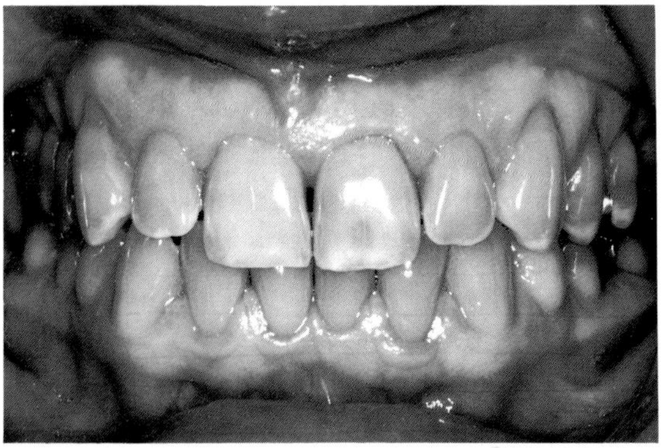

Fig. 13-1 The dentition of a 52-year-old woman with all of the criteria enumerated for a theoretically ideal occlusion.

Theoretically ideal occlusion

The theoretically ideal occlusion is a preconceived view of structural and functional relationships. Such an occlusion does not represent the norm in a statistical sense, and only occasionally represents the characteristics of a given individual. The concept is used as a series of idealized parameters against which variations may be compared. It goes well beyond a consideration of lack of pathological sequelae. According to this concept, an occlusion and the masticatory system should ideally (Fig. 13-1) be such that

1. All components of the masticatory system are present.
2. "Classical" anatomical relationships exist among all maxillary and mandibular teeth.
3. In centric occlusion, the supporting cusps of all posterior teeth occlude with marginal ridges, except for the distal buccal cusps of mandibular molars and the mesial lingual cusps of maxillary molars, which occlude with central fossae of their opposing teeth. The anterior teeth are in contact, but the major support of occlusal vertical dimension is by the posterior teeth.
4. The dentition is in harmony with its basal bone and with other craniofacial structures.
5. The long axes of teeth are aligned so that functional occlusal forces act through, or close to, these axes.
6. The periodontium is intact and there is no clinically detectable fremitus or tooth mobility.
7. The occlusion is stable—teeth do not migrate or otherwise change position other than slow physiological compensatory movements.
8. The teeth do not exhibit attritional wear beyond what would be expected for the age of the individual.
9. The muscular contact position is coincident with the intercuspal position; that is, the individual can voluntarily close the mandible into centric occlusion accurately and consistently with the head erect.
10. Centric occlusion is in harmony with centric relation; that is, the two positions are coincident, or centric occlusion is a short distance (within 1 mm) to the anterior of centric relation in the mid-sagittal plane.
11. During protrusion, the posterior teeth disclude so as not to interfere with the ability of the opposing incisor teeth to occlude and function properly.
12. During lateral movements, the teeth on the nonworking side disclude so as not to interfere with the ability of the opposing working side teeth to contact and function properly.
13. During lateral movements, there is occlusal contact between the opposing canines on the working side, either alone or together with one or more pair of adjacent posterior teeth.
14. A postural rest position that provides for an adequate interocclusal distance.
15. All masticatory, deglutition, speech articulation, esthetic, and respiratory requirements are met and are satisfactory to the patient.
16. Tonic activity of the masticatory muscles can be reduced to low levels at times of repose.
17. Minimal parafunctional activity, that is, little phasic muscle activity, occurs.
18. Self-perpetuating structural and functional

adaptation to aging and to altered conditions can be achieved.
19. Multidirectional masticatory function can be accomplished satisfactorily with a wide variety of food.
20. No signs or symptoms of pain or dysfunction from any component of the masticatory system can be detected.
21. The patient has an aura of unawareness of the occlusion and masticatory system.

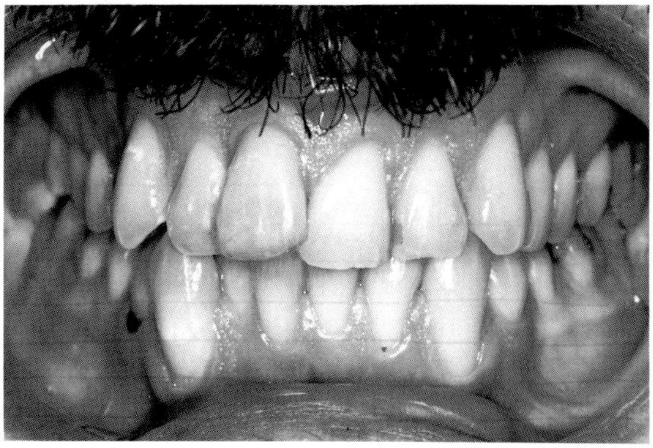

Fig. 13-2 The dentition of a 45-year-old man with malocclusion, but with all of the criteria of a physiologic occlusion.

Physiologic occlusion

Physiologic occlusion, usually found in adults, deviates in one or more ways from the theoretically ideal yet is well adapted to its particular environment, is esthetically satisfactory to the patient, and has no pathological manifestations or dysfunctional problems. It represents a state of harmony, and does not require therapeutic intervention.

In physiologic occlusion, either static or functional occlusal relationships may be at variance from the classical characteristics of an occlusion. Although it may be a malocclusion, it is a malocclusion in a state of health. It may demonstrate maxillomandibular relationships different from theoretical criteria, but no untoward effects are observed. Parafunctional activity may be present, but all components of the masticatory system are responding well, and no pain or dysfunctional signs or symptoms can be demonstrated. The system has adapted and continues to adapt to the unique structural and functional circumstances of that individual. Other criteria enumerated for the theoretical ideal may fall short of the hypothetical standards, but no evidence of problems exist (Fig. 13-2).

If one were to apply the strict criteria of the theoretical ideal to therapeutic decisions with no regard for signs and symptoms of disease or for problems involving a lack of adaptation, the overwhelming majority of the population would require treatment—a clearly untenable proposition. *The amount of variation from a preconceived ideal is enormous among human beings, particularly with regard to the masticatory system.* One cannot, and should not, expect patients to conform to preconceived idealized concepts, particularly when so few healthy people exhibit all of them.

Variations from the ideal, by themselves, do not warrant treatment. It may be argued that therapeutic intervention under such circumstances should be done for presumably prophylactic reasons. However, this rationale is also untenable when applied to adults. Preventive therapy implies that specific cause-and-effect relationships are consistently observed and well understood. The prophylactic removal of plaque from teeth, for example, is indicated because its role in the production of dental caries and periodontal disease is clearly documented and recognized. The same cannot be said for occlusal variability, particularly in adults who have had a chance to demonstrate adaptation to their particular occlusal situation.

The treatment of a gross malocclusion in a child or adolescent is justified because the physiologic outcome at the end of the growth period is not predictable. Likewise, a strategic tooth that has recently been lost should be replaced, as it is highly unlikely that a physiological outcome will result if it is not replaced. However, the same tooth that has been missing for 40 years without consequence and with complete adaptation need not be replaced because a physiological result has already been demonstrated. Therapy for presumably preventive reasons must also be based on some knowledge of the predictability of an eventual unfavorable or nonphysiological outcome, that is, reasonable certainty of cause and effect.

Therapy should not be instituted unless either the situation does not meet the criteria of a physiologic occlusion or it can be reasonably predicted that nonphysiological conditions will result if the situation is not treated.

The critera for a physiologic occlusion are

1. Occlusal stability: teeth should stay in position without a tendency to extrude, drift, rotate, or otherwise migrate within a dentition. The slow, compensatory, *physiological* movement or adaptation that accompanies wear at contact areas in order to maintain the continuity of the arch, or passive eruption to maintain occlusal contact in the presence of a normal rate of attrition, are to be expected and are acceptable. Migration beyond this (i.e., occlusal instability) is not acceptable.

2. Masticatory function is satisfactory to the patient. This is a subjective assessment on the part of the patient. If a patient can meet his or her own masticatory and dietary needs, the situation is considered physiological. The replacement of a missing tooth only because the dentist thinks that mastication will be improved, despite the patient's lack of concern, is unwarranted.

3. Speech articulation is acceptable to the patient. This is also a subjective assessment. An impaired speech sound resulting from a malocclusion may be considered physiological if the patient has no concern about this situation. An anterior open bite accompanied by faulty sibilants, for example, need not be treated if the patient's assessment is neutral and no other unfavorable conditions exist.

4. Esthetic considerations are acceptable to the patient. This is obviously a completely subjective assessment and must be left entirely to the patient. For example, a diastema between the maxillary central incisors may be absolutely unacceptable to one patient and completely acceptable to another. The clinician should not impose his or her esthetic value system on the patient except to advise the individual of therapeutic possibilities once the patient has expressed concern.

5. Freedom from signs or symptoms involving the periodontal attachment apparatus that are related to functional loading. Clinically detectable fremitus or mobility of teeth not directly attributable to the inflammatory process resulting from periodontal disease should be regarded as functional in nature. A physiologic occlusion precludes this phenomenon, particularly if such fremitus or mobility are progressive.

6. Freedom from signs and symptoms of conditions involving the teeth themselves that are attributable to functional activity. Thus, a physiologic occlusion would preclude such conditions as excessive attritional patterns from parafunctional activities or from a very abrasive diet.

7. Freedom from signs and symptoms involving the temporomandibular joint or the musculature associated with mandibular function. Although a physiologic occlusion, by definition, may not exhibit such signs or symptoms, their presence *does not necessarily imply that the cause is in faulty occlusal or maxillomandibular relationships.* It merely suggests that the overall situation is not physiological, and that some type of therapy may be indicated.

Nonphysiologic occlusion

A nonphysiologic occlusion is one in which there are signs or symptoms of pathology, dysfunction, or inadequate adaptation of one or more components of the masticatory system that can be attributed to faulty structural relationships or to mandibular functional or parafunctional activity. The concept also includes *patient nonacceptance of occlusally related esthetics, speech articulation, or masticatory function parameters.* A nonphysiologic occlusion does not necessarily imply that the existing occlusal or maxillomandibular relationships are the cause of signs or symptoms. Such signs and symptoms may be the result of how the patient uses the occlusion, and not a result of its structural features. Thus, the term *nonphysiologic occlusion* does not imply cause and effect. It merely suggests that a problem already exists, or that a physiological outcome is doubtful, and that treatment may be indicated.

In addition to the *subjective* criteria for treatment as expressed by the patient's concerns over esthetics, speech articulation, or masticatory function, there are *objective* criteria. These are signs or symptoms of *(1)* periodontal conditions attributable to functional loading, *(2)* pathological conditions of the teeth that can be attributed to mandibular functional or parafunctional activity, and *(3)* temporomandibular disorders.

Periodontal conditions attributable to functional loading

The evidence is quite clear that, although occlusal forces do not cause or influence the development of gingivitis, periodontitis, or pocket formation, they do play a role in the repair process, the width of the periodontal ligament space, and the qualitative characteristics of the periodontal ligament. Functional loading, therefore, has a great influence on the degree of fremitus or mobility of any tooth. In the absence of overt inflammation and systemic factors, clinically detectable tooth fremitus or mobility may be attributable to loading forces. In the presence of an essentially intact periodontium, fremitus or mobility is ordinarily caused by excessive occlusal forces and is termed *primary occlusal trauma.* Teeth may also be loose because of previous periodontitis that has destroyed a significant amount of the supporting apparatus. Under these conditions, even normal functional forces may keep these teeth mobile. This situation is referred to as *secondary occlusal trauma.*

Clinically detectable fremitus or mobility in the absence of periodontitis and systemic factors are not pathological but merely expected adaptation to functional forces. The displacing forces being exerted have led to qualitative and/or quantitative remodeling changes of the periodontal ligament and its alveolar bone attachments. However, it may be argued that loose teeth are not conducive to optimal function and comfort and that, under these conditions, treatment may be warranted in an effort to reduce the mobility or, at the least, to curtail additional or increased fremitus or mobility of teeth over time. Such therapy would be directed at reducing the functional activity that is causing the excessive loading and/or making the direction of loading on a loose tooth more favorable or distributing the loading to more teeth so as to reduce unfavorable effects on any one tooth. See chapter 16 for a more detailed discussion of periodontal responses to occlusal forces.

Pathological conditions of the teeth due to mandibular functional or parafunctional activity

Among the conditions attributed to excessive occlusal loading are root resorption, cemental tears, tooth fracture, pericementitis, pulpal hyperemia, pulpitis, and excessive or retrograde attrition of the teeth. The latter deserves some additional remarks because it is so common and because it so obviously is caused by excessive functional activity, not to mention the character of the diet. There can be little question that tooth wear is an adaptive physiological process provided that the rate of attrition is not too great. In aboriginal societies, because of extremely coarse diets and the greater use of the dentition as tools, wear occurs at a very rapid rate. Such wear, when seen in a modern society with its "civilized" diet, must be attributed to excessive functional activity, which is acting as a destructive process. The age of the patient must obviously be considered. For example, a worn, seemingly 70-year-old dentition seen in a 30-year-old person is a strong indication that tooth structure is being lost at a rapid rate, and efforts to reduce the functional activity is warranted. See chapter 18 for a detailed discussion of occlusal parafunction.

Temporomandibular disorders

Signs and symptoms of temporomandibular joint or masticatory muscle problems most often involve pain, tenderness in one or more of the muscles of mastication, restricted mandibular movement, and/or joint sounds. Current knowledge suggests that many of these problems have a multifactorial etiology. *In any given patient, the existing occlusal or maxillomandibular relationship may not necessarily be an etiological factor.* Indeed, such relationships may be the result of the problem, rather than the cause. It is important, therefore, that the clinician not draw immediate conclusions regarding specific cause and effect, and that treatment for most of these disorders be initiated by completely reversible modes of therapy. See chapters 17 and 18 for detailed discussions.

Therapeutic occlusion

A therapeutic occlusion is one that has been modified by appropriate therapeutic modalities in order to change a nonphysiologic occlusion to one that, at the least, falls within the parameters of a physiologic occlusion, if not the theoretically ideal. Such an occlusion may contain structural modifications not necessarily found in nature in order to optimize the health and adaptative potential of the masticatory system. Examples include the creation of a "freedom in centric" concept of occlusion, and cusp-to-fossae posterior occlusal relationships instead of cusp-to-marginal ridge relationships.

Summary

The concepts of theoretically ideal, physiologic, and nonphysiologic occlusions form a conceptual framework in an attempt to develop a more consistent rationale for the diagnosis of structural and functional problems of the masticatory system. Without such a framework, diagnosis tends to be arbitrary, inconsistent, and prone to highly subjective assessments on the part of and among clinicians. Because diagnosis must precede therapeutic decisions, such a framework has a direct relationship to this decision-making process.

Chapter 14

Examination and Differential Diagnosis of Occlusal Problems

George A. Zarb and Gunnar E. Carlsson

The examination of a patient's masticatory system should be carried out in an organized fashion. Several component examinations are involved that, when considered together, enable the dentist to comprehensively evaluate a patient's oral health. The procedure to be presented in this chapter forms an integral part of a more generalized format that includes information about the patient's systemic health history, previous dental conditions and experiences, history of pain or dysfunction, and psychosocial history. Any chief complaint should be noted and discussed with the patient.

The clinical examination itself includes a soft tissue evaluation to detect the presence of abnormalities, the charting of missing teeth, dental caries, and periodontal disease, and an adjunctive radiographic examination. This procedure can be applied in a short or long appointment depending upon the patient's oral health status. Clearly, the examination requirements of a healthy, well-maintained, intact dentition at a recall appointment will involve less time and effort than those of a new patient with a longstanding history of partial edentulism, masticatory difficulties, and periodontal disease. The clinical examination format for occlusal problems comprises the following:

1. An examination of the masticatory system to evaluate the signs and symptoms of mandibular mobility, joint sounds, muscle pain, joint pain, and pain on movement of the mandible
2. An examination of the occlusion

These items are listed in the sequence in which they should be carried out in a clinical setting. However, because this is a textbook on occlusion, the related aspects of an occlusal examination will be discussed first and at some length. Later, some of the salient features of temporomandibular (TM) disorders, their clinical examination, and issues related to their differential diagnosis will be briefly discussed.

Examination of the occlusion

The occlusal examination should include an evaluation of the clinical signs and symptoms, an evaluation of radiographic signs, and an analysis of occlusal contacts. The examination assesses dental, periodontal, or other conditions that may be related to occlusal functional activity.

Clinical signs and symptoms

Clinical signs that may contribute to an overall understanding of the state of health of a dentition (other than the presence of caries or periodontal disease) include tooth mobility, open contacts (including diastemata), tilting or drifting of teeth, changes in percussive sounds, atypical occlusal wear, and the presence of adjacent soft tissue changes that may be caused by occlusal parafunctional habits.

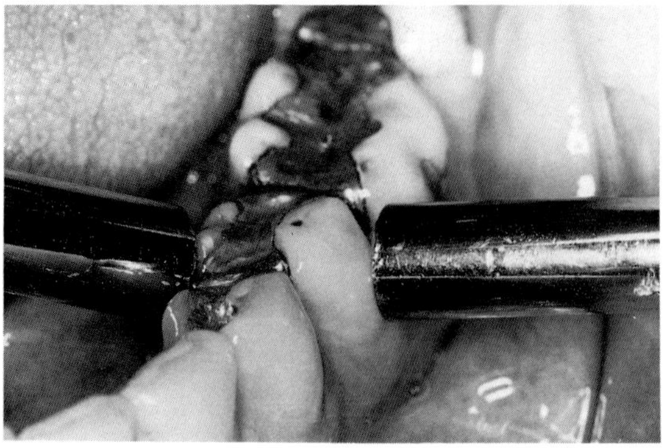

Fig. 14-1 Mouth mirror handles are placed on either side of the tooth being tested in order to subjectively determine the tooth's mobility.

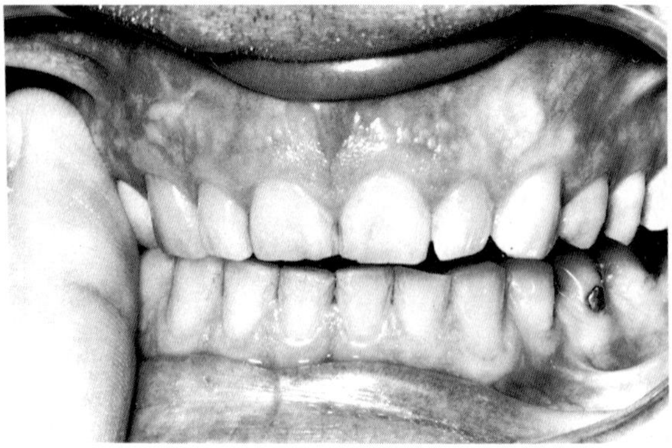

Fig. 14-2 A useful test for checking fremitus involves placing the forefinger on the facial surface of the teeth while the patient is asked to "tap the teeth in an up and down movement of the mandible."

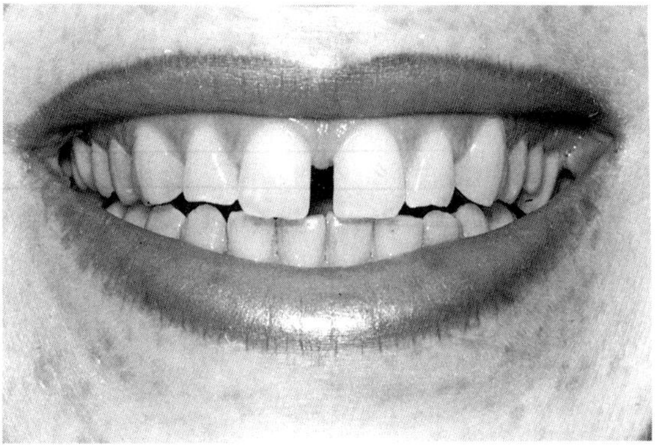

Fig. 14-3a A naturally occurring imbalance between tooth and arch size is associated with space(s) between teeth. In this patient, the diastema is limited to the maxillary midline, but spaces between other teeth, particularly anterior teeth, are frequently observed.

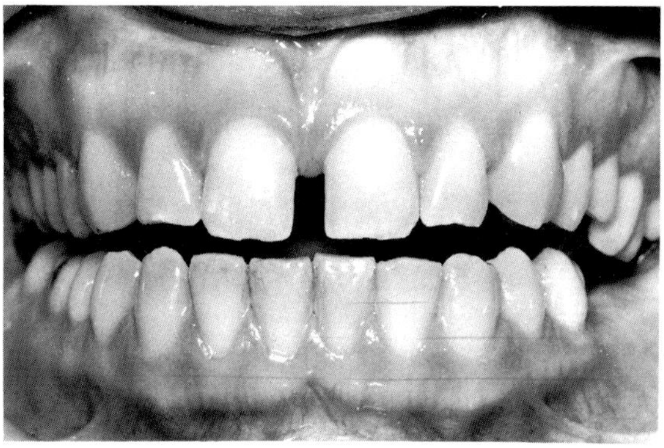

Fig. 14-3b Close-up view of same patient in Fig. 14-3a.

1. *Mobility and fremitus*

Each tooth should be tested for mobility. A subjective assessment can be readily carried out by testing the tooth between mirror handles placed lingually and facially (Fig. 14-1). Although debate still exists about both the recording method and relative significance of tooth mobility, a useful recording method (Schluger et al., 1977) enables the dentist to record whether tooth mobility is increasing or decreasing. In this method, movement is scored from 1 to 3 with half increments marked as (+). The values are interpreted as follows:

Mobility Scores —

0 Normal (i.e., less than 1 mm) mobility
1 Approximate mobility of 1 mm faciolingually
2 Mobility of 2 mm faciolingually but nil in an apical direction (+ = ½)
3 Mobility of greater than 2 mm faciolingually and evident in an apical direction

It should be noted that a mobile tooth may actually move out of the way when a patient brings the teeth together. The test for fremitus can be readily carried out (Fig. 14-2). It involves placing the forefinger on the labial or buccal surfaces of the teeth and guiding the patient to tap the teeth together. Any tooth movement can then be detected by the palpating finger. The same can be done during excursive movements of the mandible.

Increased tooth mobility, with or without attendant evidence of bone loss, is often regarded as the only clinical indicator for occlusal trauma. Current wisdom suggests, however, that it is a mistake to necessarily equate tooth hypermobility with trauma from occlusion (Ramfjord and Ash, 1979). The diagnosis of occlusal trauma is probably impossible to make on the basis of a single examination. This is because diagnosis requires that ongoing progressive injury be demonstrated. Adaptation in tooth position (i.e., a combination of tooth movement and compensatory tissue changes) will frequently neutralize the consequences of the occlusal trauma. Therefore trauma from occlusion is frequently self-limiting. Because the physiological adaptation to function and the pathologic response to excessive function may be manifested as increased tooth mobility, a separation of the two processes is really not feasible. Therefore, a diagnosis of the significance of recorded tooth mobility is based upon continued or increasing hypermobility, persistent discomfort or tenderness, and radiographic evidence of bone and/or root resorption or a widening periodontal space.

↑M ≠ occlusal trauma.

2. *Open interproximal contacts*

Spaces between the teeth may occur naturally or develop as a result of dental arch alterations such as tooth loss and subsequent drifting. The presence of diastemata, particularly of anterior teeth, should be recorded. Careful analysis and questioning of the patient should readily reveal whether the observed spaces or diastemata are *(1)* the result of a naturally occurring imbalance between teeth and arch size (Figs. 14-3a and b) or *(2)* the result of teeth (usually the maxillary ones) that have "flared" as a result of a decrease in occlusal vertical dimension and an increase in

Figs. 14-4a to c Collapse in vertical dimension of occlusion due to premature loss of an already depleted number of posterior occlusal units has led to adverse stress concentration on the maxillary anterior teeth. Resultant openings of interproximal tooth contacts and posterior teeth intrusion are evident.

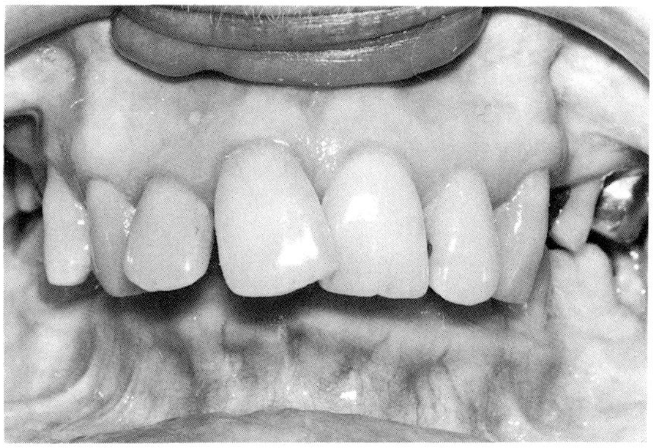

Fig. 14-4a Frontal view.

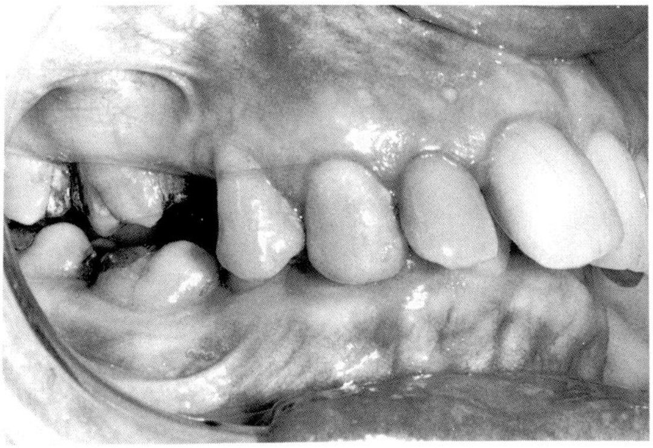

Fig. 14-4b Right lateral view.

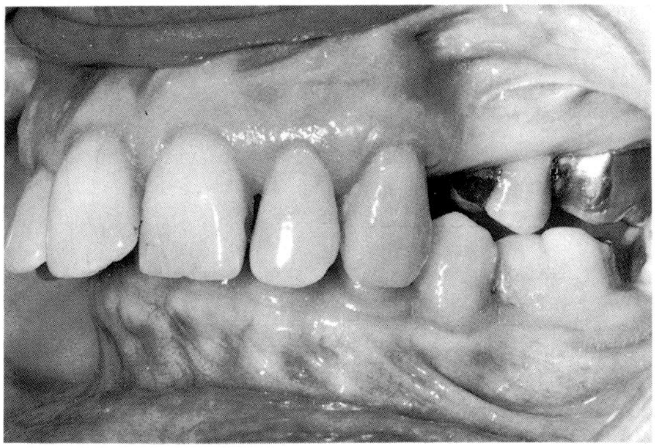

Fig. 14-4c Left lateral view.

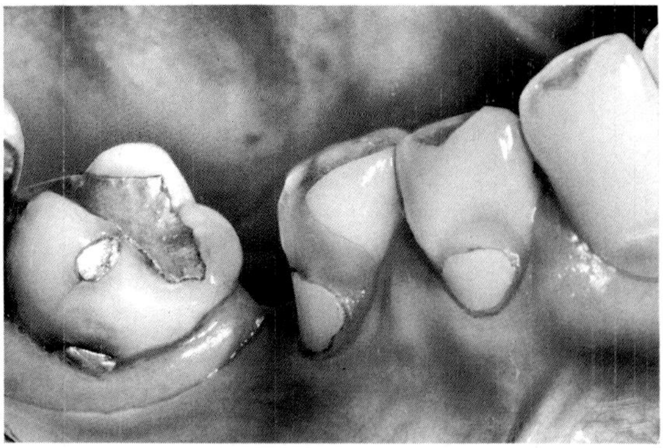

Fig. 14-5a Premature loss of the permanent maxillary first molar was followed by a tilting and drifting of the second molar.

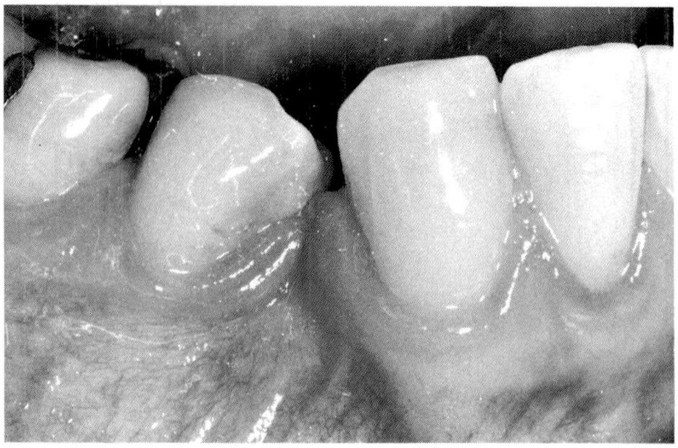

Fig. 14-5b The changes that ensue from the premature loss of a maxillary first premolar. The interproximal spaces anterior and posterior to the second premolar are similar to open contacts associated with faulty restorations.

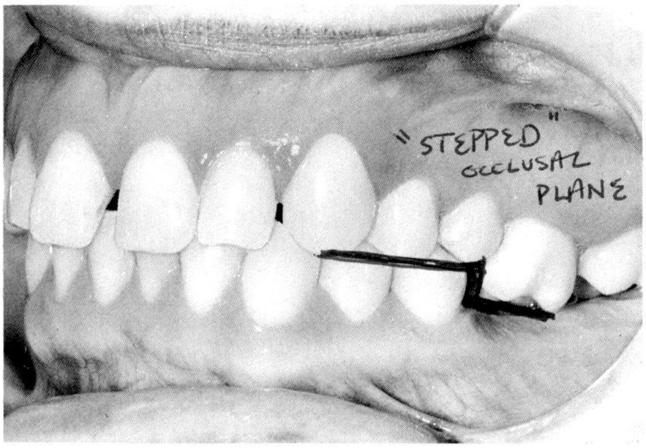

Fig. 14-5c When several posterior teeth are missing, changes in the opposing dentition—extrusion, a "stepped" occlusion—are a frequent consequence. These changes may be accompanied by occlusal vertical dimensional changes if molar loss is bilateral (see Figs. 14-4a to c).

stress concentration on the lingual surfaces of the maxillary anterior teeth (Figs. 14-4a to c).

The extent and rapidity of opening up of interproximal tooth contacts is usually augmented by the presence of periodontal disease around the involved teeth. Generally speaking, spaces between teeth that are 2 mm or wider are self-cleaning. On occasion, however, food impaction may be a problem and orthodontic treatment may be indicated. Closure of diastemata is frequently prescribed for esthetic purposes. Faulty dental restorations may also result in open contacts (Figs. 14-5a to c), which, in turn, could lead to food impaction and the risk of gingival and periodontal inflammation.

In some instances, a supporting cusp occluding with a pair of improperly formed marginal ridges can have a wedging effect and cause transient separation of the opposing teeth with resultant food impaction. Such a cusp is called a "plunger cusp." Meticulous operative and prosthetic procedures can preclude such occurrences.

Tilting or drifting of teeth

The relationship of teeth to each other in both arches should be recorded. A general classification of arch relations can then be noted (see chapter 15) and observations regarding tooth position and orientation can be scrutinized.

The presence of missing teeth in either arch very often leads to occlusal alterations in dental arch morphology. Tilting and drifting of adjacent or opposing teeth frequently result, perhaps leading to functional and/or esthetic problems. Although the relationship of such malocclusions to the development of both periodontal disease and TM disorders is far from compelling, tilted or drifted teeth are often treated orthodontically to enhance the quality of a prescribed restorative treatment plan. For example, mandibular second molars often need uprighting because they tilt and drift into the space left by the extraction of a first molar (see Fig. 14-5a). This may be associated with one or more of the following: the second molar tips and rotates lingually; the unopposed maxillary molar extrudes; the occlusal plane may become "stepped" (i.e., the anterior plane of occlusion is not continuous with the posterior one); occlusal interferences may develop. When more than one posterior tooth is missing bilaterally, the above noted structural features are accompanied by changes in occlusal vertical dimension, increased occlusal loading on anterior teeth, and a risk of a chain reaction of events that upsets occlusal arch form integrity.

Changes in percussive sounds

A tooth with a healthy periodontal ligament produces a sharp sound when percussed. By contrast, a tooth in traumatic occlusion often produces a dull sound. The change is probably the result of the altered width of the periodontal ligament, as well as its consistency. It may also be influenced by the partial resorption of the lamina dura.

Atypical occlusal wear

Occlusal wear reflects functional and parafunctional tooth contact activity. Although it is unlikely that modern civilized diets should be associated with extensive tooth wear, examples of such wear are frequently encountered in routine clinical practice (Figs. 14-6a to f).

Occlusal wear is believed to be compensated for by adaptive mechanisms (Berry and Poole, 1976), but such compensation may be incomplete and severe attrition may be associated with a decrease in the occlusal vertical dimension. The observed and recorded tooth wear facets should be matched on opposing teeth even if this involves asking the patient to move the jaw into unexpected positions. The eccentric location of such matched facets should then be pointed out to the (frequently incredulous) patient. These facets are usually the result of parafunctional activity. Their occurrence and appearance may be augmented by the differential wear rate of currently used restorative materials that may be used for different tooth surfaces.

Parafunction, especially bruxism, is generally believed to be the most significant cause of tooth wear in modern humans. Other contributing factors must also be considered. Aging, for example, correlates strongly with dental attrition. Therefore, a gradual increase of occlusal wear with increased age is considered physiological.

In a numerically reduced dentition the remaining teeth can be expected to wear more rapidly and extensively than in a complete dentition because of more concentrated loading. Dietary and salivary factors may also be contributory. Abrasive and acid components of the diet, as well as in a patient's environment, and a reduced salivary flow should also be considered in the diagnosis of extensive dental wear. Acid regurgitation, which can accompany some gastric and behavioral problems, may lead to enamel erosion, especially on palatal and lingual tooth surfaces. These localized areas of erosion can further enhance the effects of bruxism.

Soft tissue changes

Parafunctional mandibular movements frequently result in tooth tissue changes, yet adjacent soft tissues may also be involved. The most common examples are ridging or scalloping of the tongue or the cheeks. Such observed signs are almost invariably asymptomatic; they may provide useful clues about a patient's unperceived parafunctional habit of tongue-thrusting or cheek-sucking. Either habit may exist on its own or be accompanied by tooth clenching or grinding.

Radiographic signs

A radiographic examination of the dentition is

Figs. 14-6a to f Occlusal wear may vary from mild to severe with different morphologic, esthetic, and functional consequences.

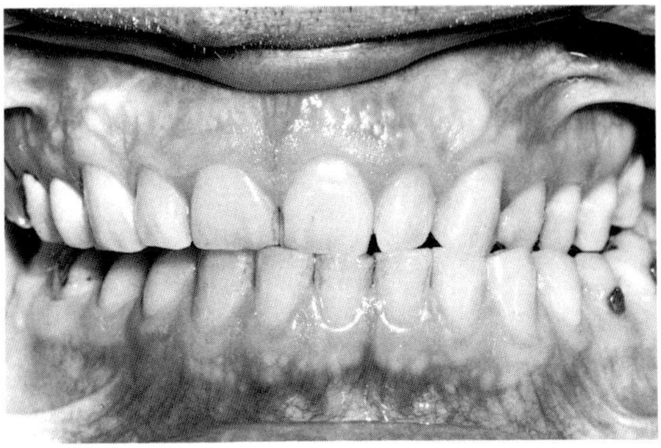

Fig. 14-6a The intact dentition of a middle-aged man is demonstrated in a left lateral contact gliding excursion. Moderate wear has resulted in a multidirectional freedom of contact movement of the mandible in all horizontal directions. The wear pattern on the occlusal surfaces of all teeth is evenly distributed.

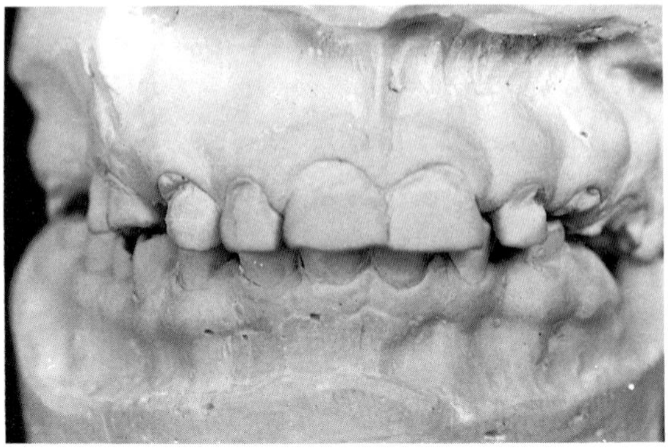

Fig. 14-6b Articulated diagnostic casts, from a patient similar in age to the one in Fig. 14-6a, illustrate severe wear that was influenced and magnified because of morphologic consequences secondary to loss of posterior teeth.

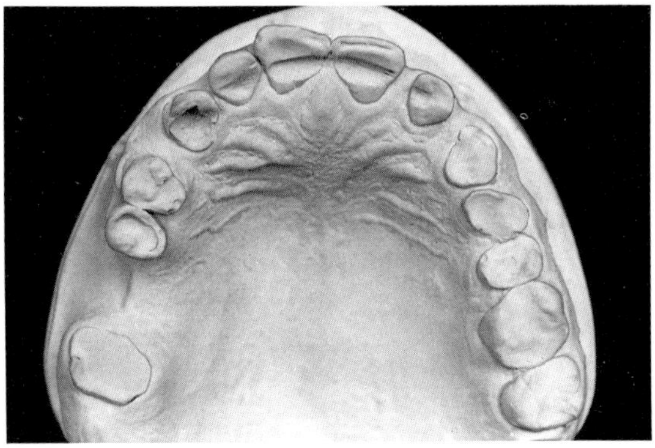

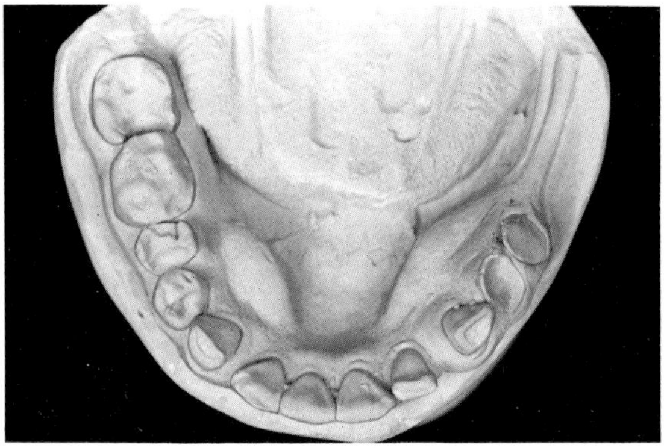

Figs. 14-6c and d Individual tooth changes are conspicuous in occlusal views.

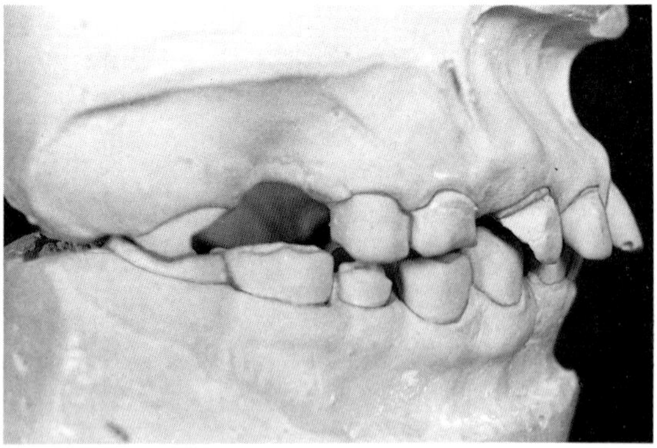

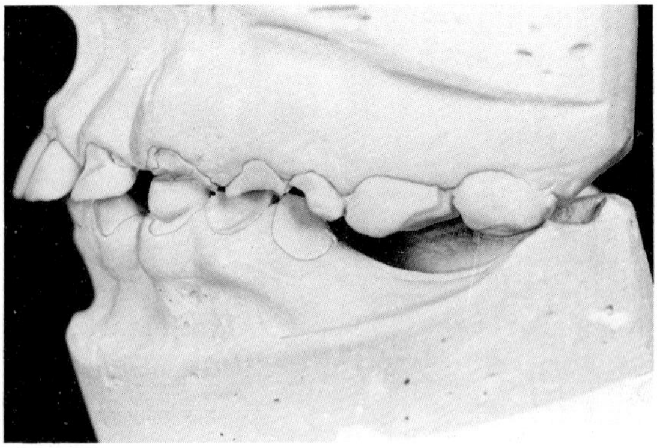

Figs. 14-6e and f Lateral views.

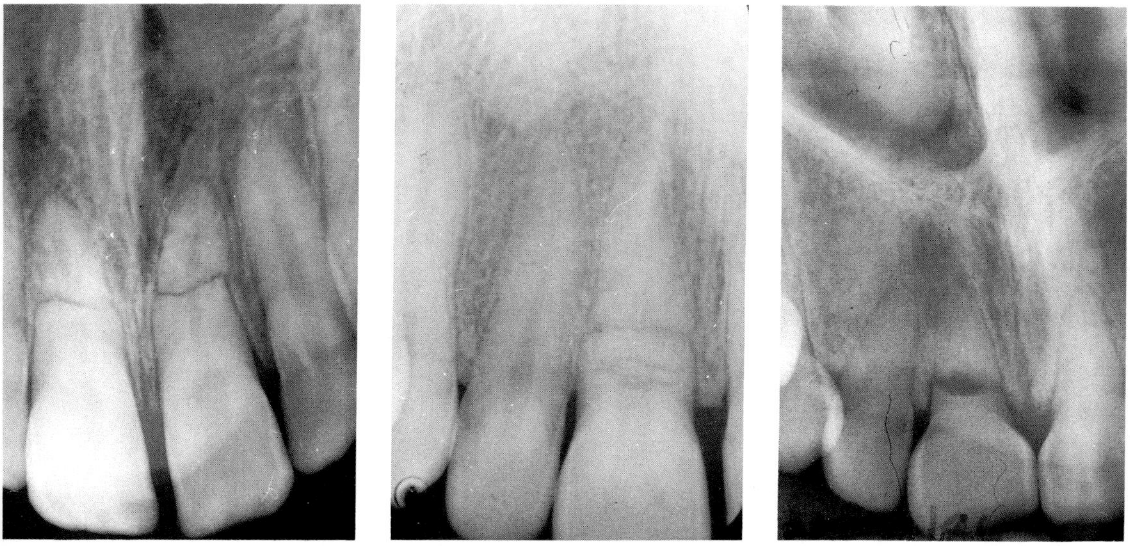

Figs. 14-7a to c Three different examples of tooth root fractures. Although these teeth may be retained for varying periods of time, their prognosis is dubious and certainly poor if the teeth are ever needed for extra loading service (i.e., as fixed partial denture abutments).

integral and routine to a thorough oral examination. The radiographic signs that may be relevant to an examination of the occlusion include

1. *Alteration of the lamina dura*. An increased density of the lamina dura is believed to result from bone sclerosis, which is probably an adaptive bony response to localized occlusal loading. Thickness of the lamina dura is frequently an unreliable sign, however, because it may result from superimposition of the buccolingual aspects of the lamina dura due to concave mesial or distal root surfaces. Loss of continuity of the lamina dura is more important. This indicates that a resorptive process is occurring, which may be a sign of traumatic occlusion.

2. *Alteration of the periodontal space*. An increase in the width of the periodontal space is commonly caused by periodontitis. However, trauma from occlusion may also cause a widening of the periodontal ligament space. Again it must be emphasized that a widened periodontal space in a radiograph *does not* necessarily indicate hypermobility of the tooth due to occlusal trauma. It may mean that trauma has occurred in the past and the tooth has now adapted to it (i.e., become self-limiting). It may also mean that trauma is currently present and additional evidence, such as recent tenderness or subsequent progressive changes, will be needed to confirm a diagnosis of ongoing injury to the supporting tissues.

3. *Evidence of root fracture*. Root fractures may be detected radiographically and the prognosis of such teeth as abutments for fixed partial dentures is dubious (Figs. 14-7a to c).

4. *Evidence of root resorption*. Preliminary evidence of root resorption usually takes the form of fuzziness of the root outline or a slight erosion of the surface. Eventually an actual shortening of the root is visible. Extensive root resorption is rarely seen in cases of traumatic occlusion, but it may result from traumatic orthodontic therapy (Figs. 14-8a to d). When observed, root resorption must be differentiated from hypoplasia or inadequate development of root structures.

5. *Hypercementosis*. This is sometimes asso-

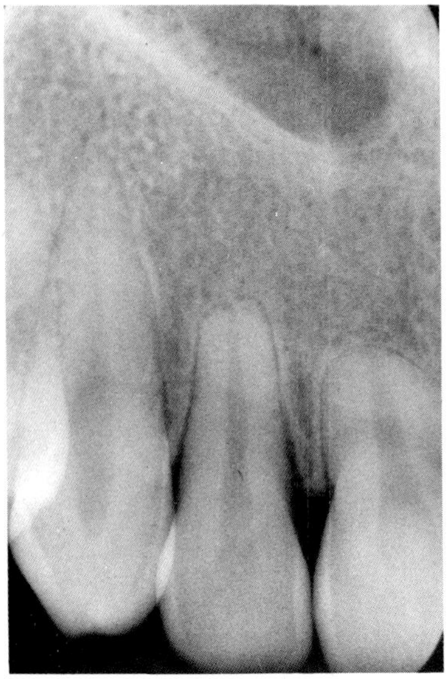

Fig. 14-8a

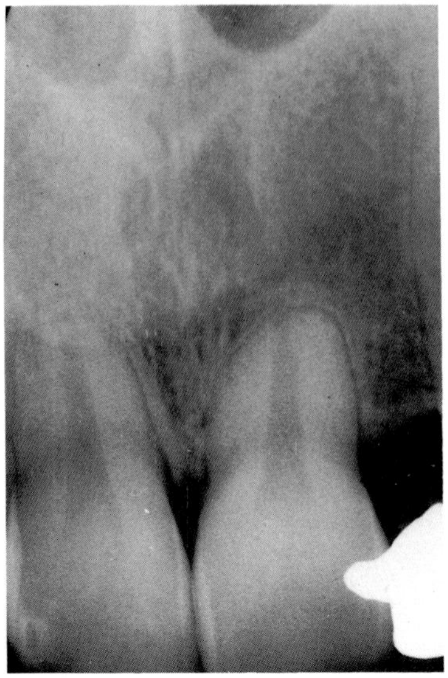

Fig. 14-8b

Figs. 14-8a to d Variable degrees of root resorption in different teeth. The clinical diagnosis in each case was rapidly induced orthodontic forces.

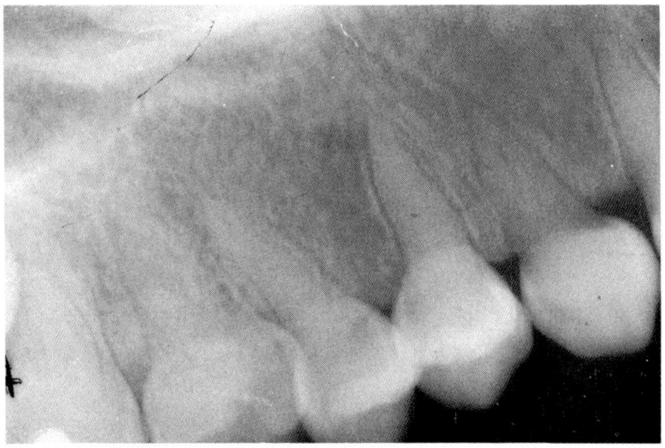

Fig. 14-8c

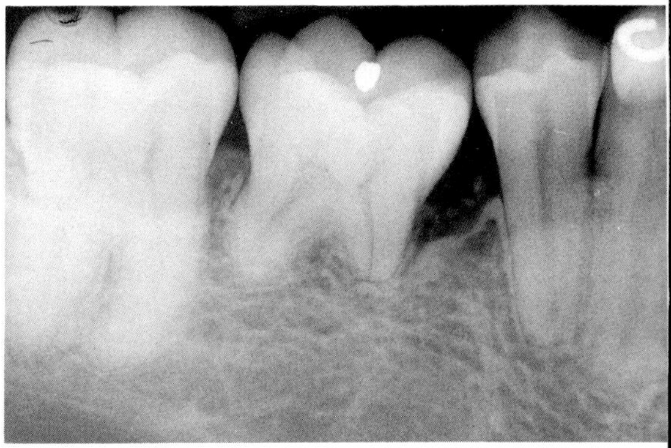

Fig. 14-8d

ciated with teeth that have sustained chronic and severe occlusal loading. It is seen radiographically as a "clubbing" of the apical area of the root (Fig. 14-9).

6. *Pulpal calcifications*. These may be partial or total. They are believed to result from circulatory disturbances of the pulp with dystrophic calcification of pulpal tissues and may be associated with isolated incidents of macrotrauma or with chronic microtraumatic loading activity.

Occlusal contacts

The way the teeth contact—individually and collectively—with their antagonists in the opposite arch should be examined next. This is easily carried out by means of visual inspection and with the help of the contents of an occlusal examination tray setup (Table 14-1). This examination is facilitated and aided by the availability of articulated study casts (Fig. 14-10).

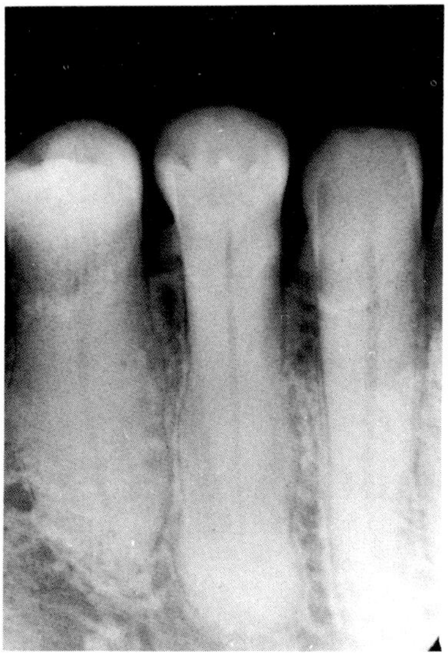

Fig. 14-9 Chronic "heavy" loading of these mandibular teeth led to hypercementosis, particularly in the apical root areas.

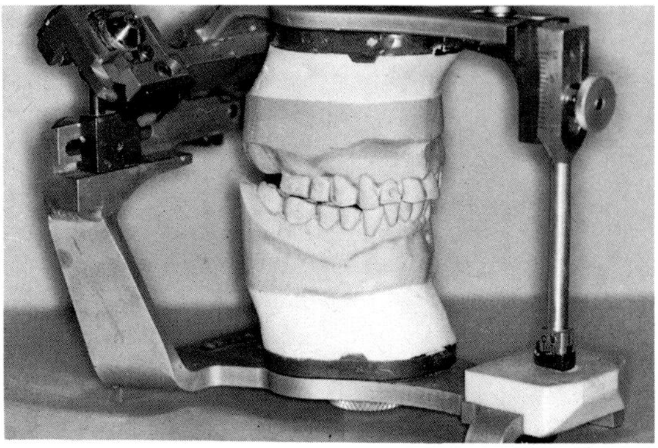

Fig. 14-10 Study or diagnostic casts mounted on an articulator allow for a useful and adjunctive analysis of any occlusion. This analytical step is not necessary for each patient, but it is particularly recommended for patients whose dental therapeutic needs will entail moderate to advanced restorative treatment. Virtually any type of articulator will suffice.

The first items that should be recorded are the number of teeth present and the number of occluding teeth (Table 14-2). The patient should be asked to bring his or her teeth together in the position of "best fit." This is the intercuspal position or centric occlusion and is the relationship of the mandible to the maxilla when the teeth are meshed maximally together (Figs. 14-11a to f). Overall arch relationships should be noted (e.g., Angle classification) along with details of arch irregularity such as crossbites, overerupted teeth, steps in the occlusion, and open bites (Figs. 14-12a to c). Horizontal overlap (overjet) and vertical overlap (overbite) are also measured and recorded.

The number of occluding teeth may play an important role in diagnosing a patient's complaint of inadequate chewing efficiency or of tooth wear or tooth mobility due to excessive loading of remaining teeth. Although a specific correlation between maximal number of occluding teeth and optimal masticatory musculoskeletal health has not been shown, except perhaps for TMJ osteoarthrosis, circumstantial evidence

Table 14-1 Requirements for an occlusal examination

Patient chart

Any system will do as long as it allows for the accurate and complete recording of history, extraoral and intraoral examinations, a radiographic report, and other diagnostic reports.

Instruments or tray setup

- Mouth mirrors
- Periodontal probe
- Articulating paper and tape plus forceps
- Shimstock foil (12 μm) plus forceps
- 2 in. × 2 in. gauze squares (wipes)
- Face mirror for patients
- Plastic ruler

Articulated study casts

These will facilitate evaluation of static intercuspal relationships (also done with hand-held casts) plus simulated movement contact relationships (e.g., lateral and protrusive excursions).

Table 14-2 Examination sequence for occlusal contacts*

Number of teeth

1. 28 – 32
2. 20 – 27
3. 20

Number of occluding teeth

1. 24 – 32
2. 16 – 23
3. 2 – 15

Occlusal interferences between RCP and ICP

1. No interferences; a straight, symmetric anterior slide from RCP to ICP, the distance less than 2 mm
2. Mild interferences with one or both of the following findings:
   a. Unilateral contact in RCP and, during the slide to ICP, the distance less than 2 mm
   b. Lateral deviation of the mandible less than 0.5 mm during the slide from RCP to ICP
3. Severe interferences with one or both of the following findings:
   a. Lateral deviation of the mandible more than 0.5 mm during the slide from RCP to ICP
   b. The distance between RCP and ICP is greater than 2 mm

Occlusal interferences during excursive movements

1. No interferences
2. Mild interferences with one or both of the following findings:
   a. Interferences (single tooth contact) on the working side distal to the maxillary canines
   b. Unilateral contact on posterior tooth or incisor in protrusion
3. Severe interferences with contacts on the nonworking side (uni- or bilaterally) that interfere with the ability to bring the working side teeth into contact

*In Helkimo's 1974 original occlusal index, each of the three items in each general group was assigned a numerical value. The premise, not proven, was that a high total score (e.g., scores of *2* or *3* in several groups) would be associated with a higher risk of TM disorder.

suggests that a fewer number of occluding teeth or only unilateral centric stops may be associated with a higher risk of masticatory pain or dysfunction (see Table 14-2).

Clinical experience suggests that while it may be tempting to automatically correlate a decreased number of occluding teeth with an increased risk of signs or symptoms associated with TM disorders, the prudent dentist should not lose sight of the extensive biological range of adaptability of the masticatory system. Over the years, vast numbers of patients with quantitatively depleted dentitions have been examined and treated, but they seemed to suffer little, if any, undermining of the quality of their masticatory function.

The presence or absence of occlusal interferences should be recorded next. Such interferences can be encountered between the retruded contact position (RCP) and the intercuspal position (ICP) and when the mandible carries out horizontal "teeth contacting" movements during lateral or protrusive excursions (see Table 14-2).

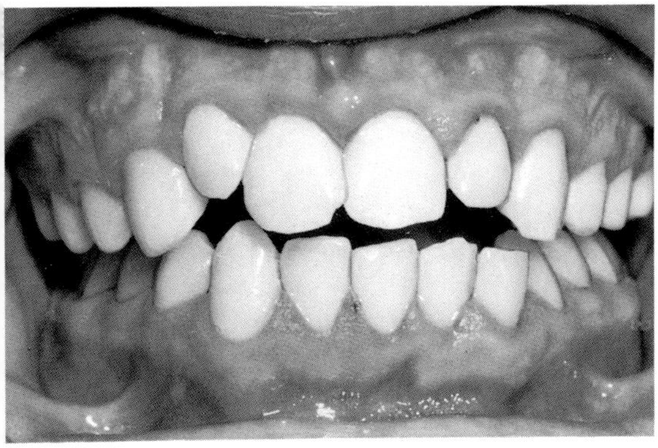

Fig. 14-11a Tooth contacts are assessed in both the retruded contact position (RCP) and the intercuspal position (ICP). Frontal view RCP.

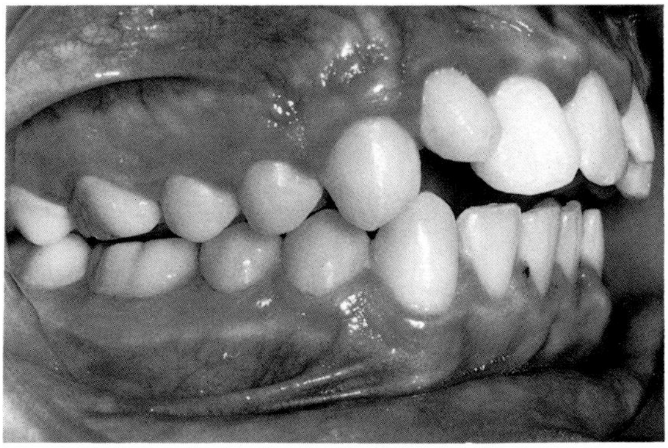

Fig. 14-11b Right lateral view RCP.

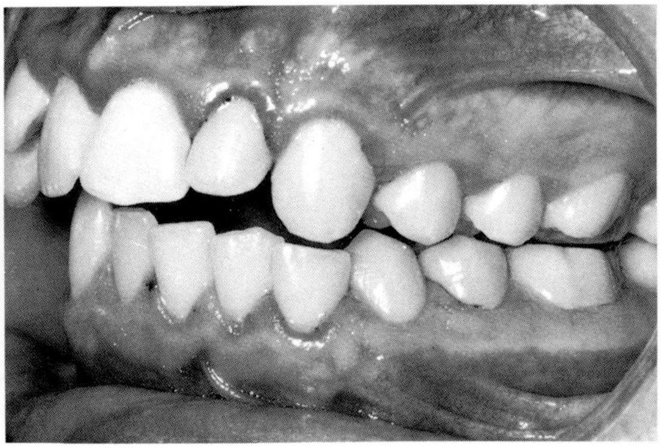

Fig. 14-11c Left lateral view RCP. Note that the initial contact occurs in the second premolar areas exclusively. When the teeth are pressed together, the mandible slides forward into ICP.

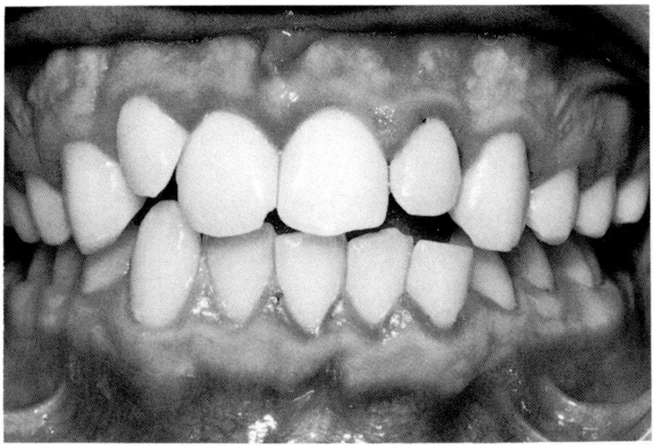

Fig. 14-11d Frontal view of the teeth meshed maximally together. In this particular patient, the measured anteroposterior difference exceeds 2 mm, and because the two positions are easily assumed by the patient, this is referred to as a dual bite.

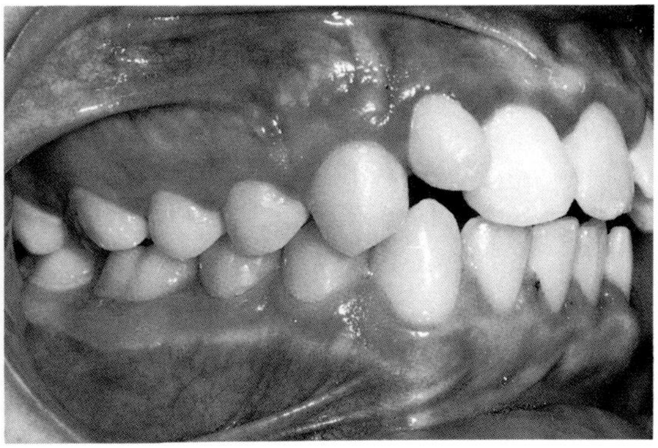

Fig. 14-11e Right lateral view ICP.

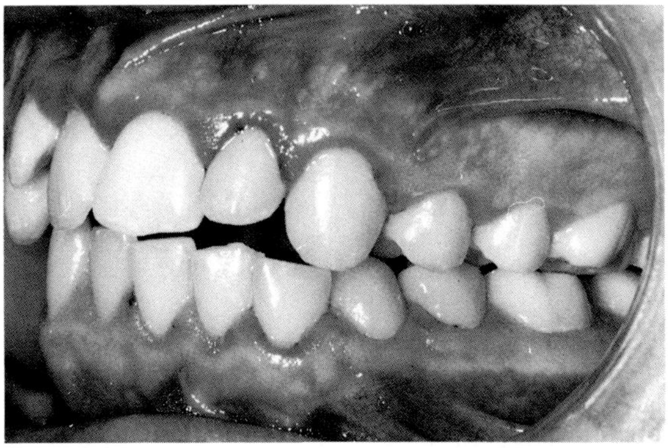

Fig. 14-11f Left lateral view ICP.

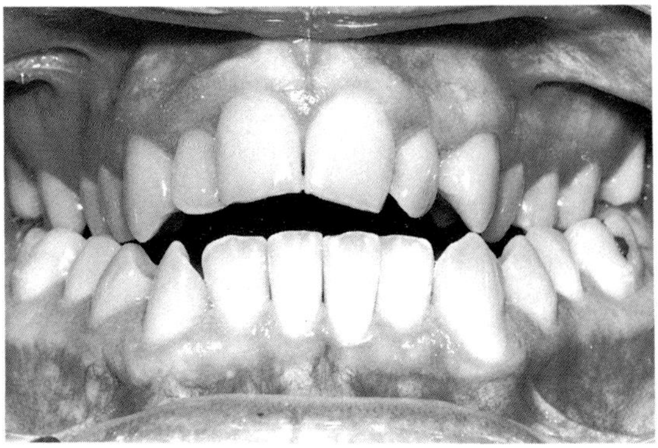

Fig. 14-12a An open bite in ICP. Bilateral posterior crossbites are present. Frontal view.

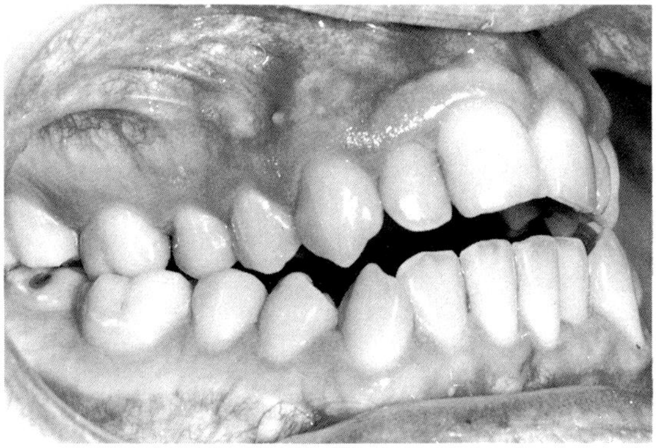

Fig. 14-12b Right lateral view.

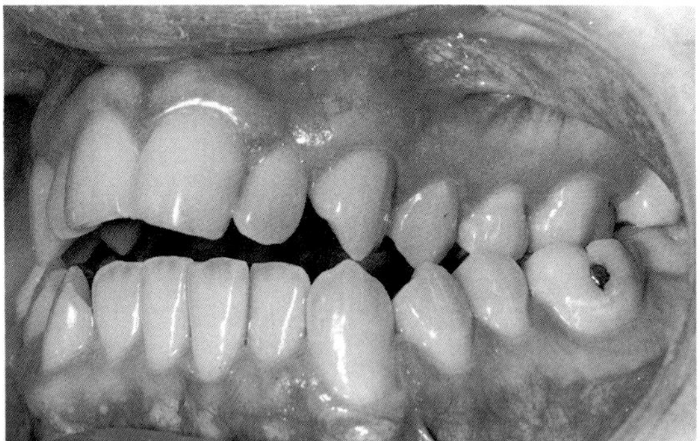

Fig. 14-12c Left lateral view.

Interferences between retruded contact position and intercuspal position

The patient should be seated comfortably in a reclining or semireclining position and be spoken to calmly and confidently; the objective is a relaxed patient. The mandible should be manipulated gently to a position that is just short of occlusal contact. Shaking the mandible vigorously in order to "loosen" the jaw muscles, or pushing the mandible back to get maximum retrusion, may be counterproductive; these can elicit a "muscle tightening" response in a patient.

Some patients may be difficult to manipulate into RCP. Gentle reassurance and considerable patience are mandatory to assist such patients. Various techniques have been proposed, such as fabricating an anterior acrylic resin jig (Fig. 14-13a) or placing a tongue spatula (Fig. 14-13b) between the teeth for 2 to 3 minutes (in the case of the jig, even longer) to enable the muscles to "forget" the mandible's habitual position or to "neutralize" proprioceptive reflexes (see chapter 20). Some patients are so resistant to mandibular manipulation that an acrylic resin interocclusal appliance must be fabricated and worn for a short time before an accurate and reproducible RCP record is feasible. This is certainly more necessary when signs and symptoms of a TM disorder exist. Such an appliance is sometimes referred to as a "disclusion splint."

When the mandible is manipulated to a position of initial tooth contact, the dentist should observe where the contact(s) occur, with or without articulating paper, as well as seek confirmation of the contact locations from the patient. The latter information may not always be reliable but it should not be overlooked.

The dimensions and directions of any observed slides should be noted. The vertical and horizontal components of the slide should also be noted (i.e., the change in distance between maxillary and mandibular incisors in both vertical and horizontal planes) (see Figs. 14-11a to f).

The "ease" of both mandibular manipulation and the slide should be recorded. The degree of freedom involved in achieving either may pro-

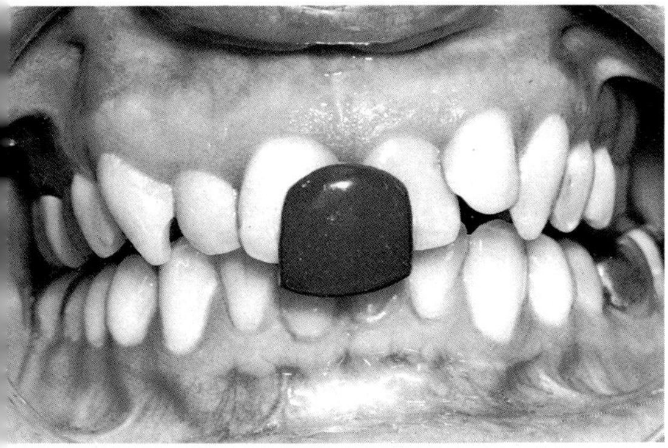

Fig. 14-13a A customized acrylic resin jig can be placed between the anterior teeth to "deprogram" the mandible's habitual position. This technique is popular with many dentists, and its use precludes contact of the occluding surfaces of the teeth.

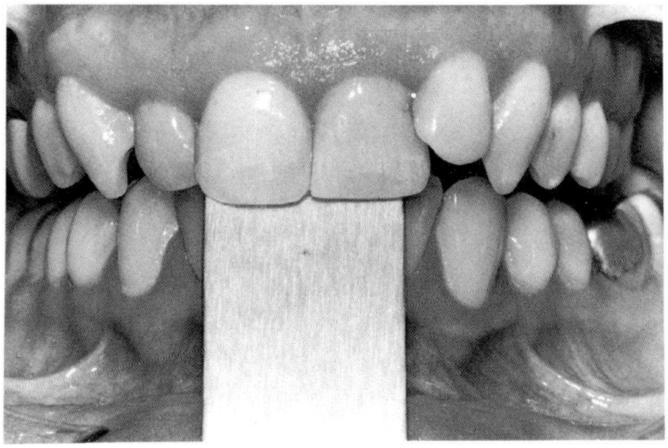

Fig. 14-13b The same effect can be achieved by placing a disposable tongue blade between the teeth in a manner similar to the resin jig. Both techniques necessitate an interval of several minutes for the desired effect to take place.

vide useful clinical information, because "forced" movements suggest muscle tightness or tooth morphology obstruction.

Interferences during excursive movements

Occlusal contacts during movements of the mandible that block optimal occlusal function are known as interferences. These may involve working side, nonworking side, or protrusive contacts.

Working side contacts refer to those contacts made on the side of the dentition to which the mandible moves. The patient should be instructed to close into ICP and move toward the directed side. If the patient experiences difficulty carrying out this movement, the use of a face mirror may help if it is accompanied by a careful and relaxed explanation. When the patient's teeth are in contact during either a right or left mandibular excursion, the dentist should note the following: *(1)* the presence of canine guidance (i.e., contact between the canine exclusively with disclusion of the other teeth), *(2)* the presence of group function or contact of multiple teeth on the working side, and *(3)* the presence of combinations of *(1)* and *(2)*, which is a frequent occurrence.

In the latter situation, initial group function is present, but as the lateral contact excursion is carried through, only the canines will contact. Smooth movements associated with either of the above contact patterns and that do not produce fremitus of working side teeth are regarded as favorable nondisturbances in the articulation.

A single tooth contact distal to the maxillary canines is frequently regarded as a mild interference and may need to be modified to "convert" the excursion into one of the above three described ones.

On the nonworking side, only those contacts that interfere with the ability of the teeth on the working side to achieve optimal contact are regarded as nonworking side interferences (see chapter 4). The dentist should record the presence or absence of nonworking side interferences and any attendant movement of contacted teeth (fremitus). Careful patient guidance and visual inspection, plus use of articulating paper and shimstock, are necessary in this procedure because patients may try to bypass nonworking side interferences. Such interferences (see Table 14-2) are not considered to be beneficial to a dentition's long-term health. They are thus regarded as severe interferences and are frequently removed by occlusal adjustment therapy (see chapter 21).

The patient should next be instructed to close

into ICP and to protrude the mandible until the incisors contact in an edge-to-edge position. Here again the use of a hand mirror may be beneficial to guide the patient. The dentist should record the ease and direction of the mandibular movement, the presence or absence of contacting posterior teeth, and which anterior teeth are in contact during the protrusive excursion. Fremitus of any of the contacting teeth should also be noted.

Dual bite and open bite

This short section on patient examination for occlusal contacts and/or interferences would be incomplete if some emphasis were not placed on dual bite and open bite. These are two occlusal contact positions that are infrequently encountered but are significant enough to deserve individual mention.

Dual bite. A dual bite (see Fig. 14-11d) is considered to be present if the anteroposterior difference between the RCP and ICP exceeds 2 mm and if the two occlusal positions can be easily assumed (Egermark-Eriksson et al., 1979). It is a rare condition in the natural dentition and found in 1% to 3% of studied patient samples. Dual bite is of clinical interest because it is often associated with extensive occlusal wear and symptoms of uncomfortable chewing. It is also considered by some dentists to involve a long-term risk of a TM disorder.

The etiology of dual bite is multifactorial. A list of possible causes includes chronic protrusion in angle Class II postnormal jaw relationship ("Sunday bite"), unbalanced development of the mandible and TMJs, unsuccessful orthodontic or prosthodontic treatment (unfinished activator treatment, "bite jumping"), condylar fractures, and diseases of the TMJ (e.g., rheumatoid arthritis).

A diagnosis of dual bite is usually not difficult. It might, however, be difficult to establish the cause, which is important to know in order to manage the condition. The management may require a range of therapies, from little or no therapeutic intervention in adult subjects who are well adapted to the condition, to extensive occlusal, prosthodontic, and surgical therapy in those with functional difficulties. In children and young people, orthodontic treatment to create a stable occlusion in or close to the retruded position is often justified.

Open bite. A lack of occlusal contacts in any part of the dentition may be caused by a variety of conditions (e.g., developmental problems, oral habits, or diseases of the TMJ). Long-standing finger-sucking habits in childhood may result in an anterior open bite (see Fig. 14-12a), which can be maintained into adult age. A persistent tongue-thrust habit may also move the anterior teeth labially and result in an open bite. It is probable, however, that in many cases the tongue-thrust habit started as a consequence of an open bite, which itself resulted from other causes. The latter condition usually has a good prognosis for reduction or elimination of the open bite (e.g., by occlusal adjustment or prosthodontic treatment). If, on the other hand, the tongue habit is causative, the prognosis is guarded because there is a risk that the bite might open again after treatment.

If there is a gradual development of an open bite in an adolescent or adult patient, a disease of the TMJ should be suspected, such as unilateral condylar hyperplasia or tumor of the condyle leading to unilateral posterior open bite, and rheumatoid arthritis producing a bilateral anterior open bite (see chapter 17). In such situations, TMJ imaging is usually of significant diagnostic value.

History and clinical examination of the masticatory system

Because the subject of Occlusion encompasses most of the structural and functional components of the masticatory system, the entire system needs to be included to some extent when an examination is undertaken. More specifically, an examination of the masticatory and associated musculature as well as TMJ function is essential for a thorough evaluation of the masticatory system. As a health care professional, a dentist should assume the responsibility of being knowledgeable about the entire masticatory system, particularly in relation to laypeople, patients, physicians, and other health care providers.

Patient history of pain-dysfunction

A patient's history can be recorded by means of a self-administered questionnaire, but it is always recommended that information gathered in this way be reviewed and completed by direct interview of the patient. The answers to the questionnaire make a valuable basis for a dialogue between dentist and patient. It is extremely important to listen carefully and try to understand the patient's message. As Sir William Osler once said, "Listen to the patient; he is giving you the diagnosis." An understanding attitude from the dentist and enough time for the patient to elaborate on the current complaints will help establish a good doctor-patient relationship. This will be of great value during subsequent treatment.

It is advisable to start with the present complaint and then ask about its onset and further development, including possible changes over time, their probable causes, and previous treatments and their effect.

Another important part of the history taking is the *general past history,* which should include medical, occupational, emotional, social, and family factors. The patient's answers to questions of what condition they think they have, what they think is the cause of their complaint, and how they evaluate its severity, might be valuable for the choice of therapy and further clinical management. For example, many individuals are worried that they are afflicted by a serious disease. Such patients are often helped by reassurance that their disorder is a benign one.

The necessity of taking a careful history in patients with pain and dysfunction in the masticatory system is evident. Even with routine dental patients, it is desirable to inquire about symptoms of TM disorders. A pain-dysfunction history index, comprising answers to a questionnaire and a clinical assessment has been developed by Helkimo (1974). The index uses a three-point scale based on answers to a few questions related to pain and dysfunction (Table 14-3).

Table 14-3 Pain-dysfunction history index*

0	Absence of symptoms
I	Mild symptoms including feeling of fatigue (tired jaws); jaw stiffness (in the morning or with jaw movement); TMJ sounds (clicking or crepitation)
II	Severe symptoms including one or more of the following: difficulty in opening wide; jaw locking or dislocation; pain on movement of the mandible; pain in TMJ region and/or masticatory muscles

*Modified from Helkimo, 1974.

The classification indicates appropriate questions to ask verbally or in a questionnaire. Helkimo's original index has been widely used in epidemiological and clinical research during the last decade. Although this index has been criticized, largely because it is quite obviously not complete, it is clearly of value for a rapid and efficient preliminary screening of the functional state of the masticatory system. For example, dental patients classified in category I or II should be given a more detailed clinical examination than those in category 0. This index is discussed later, in more detail, under the section, "Clinical pain-dysfunction index."

Clinical examination

Although the clinical examination is obviously concentrated on the components of the masticatory system, observation of the *entire body* might be helpful for a correct diagnosis. This refers especially to muscle and joint diseases. Inspection of the hands, gait, and posture, for instance, may yield information about various rheumatic diseases. Observation of involuntary body movements may reveal the presence of a disease of the nervous system or suggest a psychological disturbance.

During the recording of the history, it is often possible to scrutinize the entire head and face for any detail deviating from a normal appearance, such as swellings, obvious asymmetries, skin changes (e.g., erythema, rash, scars), tics, and some parafunctional activities.

Examination of the masticatory system

The examination should follow a routine and standardized procedure in order to minimize the risk of overlooking some relevant details and to permit comparison with subsequent reexaminations. The examination of various structures should include the TMJs, masticatory and associated muscles, mandibular mobility, oral tissues, the dentition and occlusion, and other structures of the head and face related to the function of the masticatory system. The order they are examined in may vary. In this section a relatively brief description of the structures will be presented. More extensive reviews have been published elsewhere (Schwartz and Chayes, 1969; Carlsson and Helkimo, 1972; Bohl and Knap, 1974; Krogh-Poulsen, 1974).

Temporomandibular joint

Examination of the TMJ comprises inspection, auscultation, palpation, and evaluation of jaw movements. It may include radiography or other imaging techniques.

Direct *inspection* of the joint areas might reveal asymmetries in size or function or scars from previous trauma or surgery.

Auscultation of joint sounds can be performed with a stethoscope, but the combination of listening and palpation is usually sufficient to characterize the sound (i.e., as in clicking or crepitation). The character of the sound and the timing of its occurrence during jaw movements may be significant in explaining the presence of such conditions as osteoarthrosis, condyle-disk incoordination, anatomical impediments, internal derangements, etc. For example, the presence of reciprocal clicking (occurring both in opening and closing of the mouth but at different stages) is probably associated with an internal derangement of the disk, whereas crepitation is indicative of osteoarthrosis.

The most important part of the examination of the TMJ is *palpation,* which can give information on tenderness and on condylar movements. The lateral poles of the condyles can easily be palpated through the skin while the mandible is in the intercuspal position and during various jaw movements. In this way the range and any asymmetry of movements can be observed. For evaluation of joint tenderness, more of the surrounding area and the external auditory meatus should also be palpated. A comparison between the findings in the right and left joint should always be included, keeping in mind that absolute anatomical or functional symmetry rarely exists.

An indirect evaluation of joint function is possible by observing and measuring various *jaw movements* (e.g., opening, closing, lateral, protrusive, and retrusive movements). Deviations from a straight line, sounds and pain, passive and active movement capacity, and differences between right and left excursion should all be noted. Later these will be evaluated in relation to other clinical findings.

Masticatory and associated muscles

The musculature can best be examined by palpation. However, inspection of the face and head can give some information on the superficial muscles. For example, masseter hypertrophy is easily observed and is usually an indication of chronic bruxism. "Muscle play," seen during the history taking, indicates occlusal or oral parafunctions. By palpation, the tenderness, size, consistency, and rigidity of muscles can be assessed. Typically, the left and right sides are compared during the palpation of each muscle pair.

The origin of the *temporalis muscle* can be examined by palpation on the side of the head.

Most interesting is its anterior part over the front of the temple (temporal fossa). This is a location often tender to palpation in patients complaining of headache. The insertion on the coronoid process requires an intraoral approach, with the finger passing from the retromolar fossa upward along the anterior part of the ramus.

The superficial part of the *masseter muscle* can be examined extraorally. However, one very good method entails gently pressing the muscle between the thumb and forefinger (on the right side, the thumb is placed outside and the forefinger inside the mouth; on the left side, the placing of fingers is the opposite). To clearly disclose the outline of the anterior border of the masseter, the patient is asked to clench his or her teeth. The most frequent location of tender spots in the masseter is in the anterosuperior part of the origin, near the zygomatic arch. However, the entire muscle should be palpated for tender or otherwise changed areas. The deep portion of the masseter is palpated extraorally just in front of the TMJ. It is certainly difficult to know if tenderness in this area comes from articular or muscular structures because fibers from the deep masseter muscle join the capsule of the TMJ in many individuals.

The insertion of the *lateral pterygoid muscle* to the condyle is inaccessible to digital palpation. It has been assumed that the inferior part of the origin on the lateral side of the lateral pterygoid plate can be palpated by placing a finger behind the tuberosity of the maxilla and pressing superiorly-posteriorly-medially. This procedure is facilitated if the patient does not open the mouth widely and moves the mandible toward the side that is to be examined. It has been routinely used in many TMJ clinics and in private dental offices. However, an anatomic investigation has indicated that it is not possible to palpate the lateral pterygoid muscle directly without applying pressure through an overlying portion of the medial pterygoid muscle (Johnstone and Templeton, 1980). It is quite probable that the response elicited by such palpation originates from structures other than the lateral pterygoid muscle. For example, a positive response may be due to pressure from the back of the palpating finger against the tendinous attachment of the temporalis muscle on the coronoid process. Tenderness in this region, especially unilaterally, is common in patients with TM disorders, and the palpation behind the maxillary tuberosity is therefore important. To know exactly from which site the positive response is elicited is less significant than assessing whether the response is normal or indicates some disorder.

The *medial pterygoid muscle* can be palpated extraorally at the inner aspect of the angle of the mandible, but then only the most inferior part of its attachment is reached. The main approach is intraoral, pressing the examining finger against the lingual side of the angle of the mandible and following the muscle upward until the hamulus is felt. As already noted, palpation behind the maxillary tuberosity may also involve part of the medial pterygoid muscle.

The digastric and other suprahyoid and neck muscles should also be examined for tenderness to palpation, especially if the patient is reporting pain and dysfunction in the neck regions. Such palpation may also be indicated because pain can be referred from trigger points in some muscles in the neck to the face (e.g., the sternocleidomastoid and trapezius muscles) (Travell and Simons, 1983).

Mandibular mobility

The range of movement of the mandible is an important guide in evaluating the functional capacity of the masticatory system. Measurements of maximal vertical and horizontal movements (i.e., opening, lateral, and protrusive movements) should be performed. Maximal values, regardless of symptoms, as well as the points when pain or discomfort is first experienced, are both recorded. It is also recommended that any difference between an active and passive movement (i.e., one performed voluntarily by the patient and one attained after stretching by the examiner) be examined. Opening and protrusive movements are also observed for irregularities and deviation and any differences between movements to the right and left sides are noted.

Table 14-4 Clinical pain-dysfunction index*

	Criteria		
Symptom	Normal	Slight	Severe
Impaired range of movement/ mobility index	Opening > 39 mm, lateral > 6 mm	Opening 30–39 mm, lateral 4–6 mm	Opening < 30 mm, lateral < 4 mm
Impaired TMJ function	Smooth movement without TMJ sounds and deviation on opening or closing movements < 2 mm	TMJ sounds in one or both joints and/or deviation of ≥ 2 mm on opening or closing movements	Locking and/or dislocation of the TMJ
Pain on movement of the mandible	No pain on movement	Pain on 1 movement	Pain on 2 or more movements
Muscle pain	No tenderness to palpation of masticatory muscles	Tenderness to palpation in 1–3 sites	Tenderness to palpation in 4 or more sites
TMJ pain	No pain	Pain on lateral pressure (either or both sides)	Pain on posterior intrameatal pressure (either or both sides)

*Modified from Helkimo, 1974.

Clinical pain-dysfunction index

Based on evaluation of five clinical signs and symptoms, Helkimo (1974) proposed an index system for the severity of masticatory pain-dysfunction (Table 14-4). These include impaired range of movement, impaired TMJ function, muscle pain, TMJ pain, and pain on movement of the mandible.

Each clinical observation is assessed on a three-point scale: *(0)* normal, *(3)* slight disturbance or pain, *(5)* severe disturbance or pain. For example, opening values of 30 to 39 mm, or horizontal movements of 4 to 6 mm, are classified as slightly impaired mobility. The scores awarded the five groups of signs and symptoms are added together and each examined individual can thus be given a total pain-dysfunction score of 0 to 25 points. As seen in Table 14-4, a clinical pain-dysfunction index can then be assigned to each examination of the patient's masticatory system. This method allows some degree of quantification of an otherwise subjective assessment.

The quantifying attempt of this classification is vulnerable to criticism (Farrar, 1982). Nevertheless, it has been used extensively in various investigations and in clinical work in many centers. Its value lies in its ease of describing the severity of clinical findings of pain and dysfunction and the possible relationship of such a classification to treatment needs and to treatment results. Furthermore, it has been shown to be closely correlated to patients' reported symptoms and to their severity (Mejersjö and Carlsson, 1984).

Differential diagnosis of pain and dysfunctional problems

Pain is often associated with dysfunction of the masticatory system. It is probably the symptom that most often makes an individual seek dental consultation. Pain is a phenomenon with many confusing qualities because it is subjective and based upon past experiences and psychological and cultural factors. Thus, pain perception is dependent on individual reactions and interpretations. This is especially true for chronic pain, and many patients seeking advice for TM disorders fall into this category.

There are innumerable possible causes and sources of facial pain. All possibilities must be considered in the differential diagnosis of pain-dysfunction of the masticatory system.

In this section, no attempt will be made to cover all aspects of orofacial pain and dysfunction, a large and detailed subject in its own right. The intention is merely to emphasize some conditions of importance for differential diagnosis. For further information the reader is encouraged to refer to more extensive surveys (e.g., Dalessio, 1972; Sternbach, 1974; Alling and Mahan, 1977; Lance, 1978; Seltzer, 1978; Block, 1979). The following description will include some aspects of TMJ and muscle pain and dysfunction, diseases of the teeth, diseases of jaws and neighboring structures, neuralgias, and headaches.

Temporomandibular joint and muscle pain and dysfunction

The TMJ may be affected by a wide variety of diseases (see chapter 17). Most of them are capable of creating symptoms of pain and dysfunction. Such symptoms may be similar to those attributed to primary masticatory muscle problems, often called myofascial pain-dysfunction. One explanation for this observation is that pathologic conditions in the TMJ often result in hyperactivity of associated muscles, which eventually leads to muscular tenderness and pain. Another is that overloading of the TMJ caused by masticatory muscle hyperactivity (bruxism) may also elicit tenderness of the joint proper.

A complicating factor adding to the diagnostic problem of differentiation between muscular and articular origin of pain and dysfunction is the obvious shortcomings of TMJ radiography. Lesions limited to the articular soft tissues, which are common in the early phases of many TMJ diseases, cannot be seen in ordinary radiographs. It is also frequently impossible to differentiate radiographically between osteoarthrosis and mere joint remodeling without surface lesions. Therefore, pain and tenderness in the masticatory muscles and the TMJ may well be a consequence of lesions of the TMJ proper, without the TMJ showing any signs of radiographic changes.

Osteoarthrosis. The signs and symptoms of osteoarthrosis of the TMJ are not specific (Zarb, 1983) but may, if present, include pain in the TMJ region radiating to or including the temples and cheeks, joint sounds, and difficulty in opening the mouth. Often, the TMJ region is particularly tender to palpation and seems to be the center of the disorder. In the later stages of the disease crepitation is the dominating joint sound and radiography is more likely to reveal structural changes in the TMJ.

Rheumatoid arthritis. Temporomandibular joint involvement usually occurs late in the course of rheumatoid arthritis when a diagnosis of the systemic disease is already established. In rare cases the TMJ may be the first, or among the first joints, to be affected. The signs and symptoms of pain and dysfunction are then similar to those in other TMJ and neuromuscular disorders. A thorough history will usually disclose symptoms from other joints (e.g., in the fingers and hands), a general malaise and/or fatigue, or perhaps a low grade fever. Such findings indicate the necessity to refer the patient for medical examination and laboratory tests.

There are several other systemic inflammatory joint diseases that can affect the TMJ (gout, ankylosing spondylitis, and psoriatic arthritis), but their occurrence is infrequent and will not be discussed here.

Traumatic injuries. External major trauma, including fractures in the TMJ region, seldom offer diagnostic problems. However, radiography should always be performed for evaluating the effects of the injury. In minor traumatic damage to the TMJ there may be swelling, limitation of movement, and occlusal changes (e.g., loss of contact on the side of the traumatized joint), besides pain. If the edema of the joint is minimal, there will be little, if any, detectable radiographic changes. The history and clinical findings should provide the diagnosis. Occasionally, the patient may at first be unaware of any obvious trauma because it was not severe and/or occurred in the middle of hectic activities such as games and sports or during sleep.

Dental disease

The most common source of orofacial pain is dental disease or its sequelae. While pulpal or periapical changes as sources of pain may sometimes be difficult to detect, a systematic examination that combines a careful history with clinical and radiographic observations will usually reveal the cause. Pulpitis will hardly ever, and periapical lesions only rarely, give rise to myofascial pain-dysfunction. However, with long-standing pain, the masticatory muscles may become secondarily involved, resulting in muscle hyperactivity. Subsequent muscle pain may then occur simultaneously with dental pain, which will easily cause confusion. As always when two or more different disorders overlap, each in turn has to be diagnosed and treated. An important diagnostic adjunct in these situations is the use of local anesthesia.

A complicating factor with prolonged dental pain is that it may radiate to other structures or refer to remote sites. Cases of pulpitis simulating myofascial pain-dysfunction, for example, have been reported (Duquette and Goebel, 1973).

Myofascial pain-dysfunction as a secondary phenomenon, because of reflex muscle hyperactivity or direct involvement of masticatory muscles, may be found in many inflammatory conditions of the jaws related to dental diseases (e.g., impacted mandibular third molars with acute pericoronitis, acute and chronic osteomyelitis, lateral periodontal abcesses, fractures or other lesions of the jaws with secondary infection, etc.). In all of these conditions, a careful history and clinical/radiographic examination will usually identify the cause(s) of the pain.

Pathologic conditions of the ears and sinuses

Patients often think TM disorder pain is caused by an ear disorder and may then first consult an ear, nose, and throat physician. Ear disease is, therefore, frequently excluded when a patient comes from the ear, nose, and throat specialist for consultation or examination of TM disorder pain and dysfunction. But if there is any doubt of differential diagnosis of TM disorder pain, a primary ear disease should be considered. These are usually otitis externa or otitis media. Otitis externa is easily diagnosed because touching or pulling on the earlobe or meatal entrance will be extremely painful.

Although ear and sinus pathology are not primarily associated with masticatory muscle problems, they may become so following long-standing disease with accompanying pain. As in chronic oral pain, the phenomenon may involve reflex hyperactivity of masticatory and associated muscles with ensuing pain, tenderness, and dysfunction. As in all situations with differential diagnostic problems, it is imperative to know the characteristics of the disease and carefully determine the history of onset. Both ear and sinus disease generally follow an upper respiratory tract infection and the patient may have elevated temperature and experience a general malaise. Sinus pain, in particular, is often dull or throbbing and may be exacerbated by rapidly bending or turning the head. This is not the case with myofascial pain-dysfunction or other types of TM disorders.

Disease of the parotid gland

Both inflammatory, obstructive, and neoplastic conditions of the parotid gland may resemble TM disorder pain and dysfunction, especially in the early stages. However, salivary secretion is often affected, pain generally increases with the thought, sight, or intake of food, swelling is usually present and much more extended than with TMJ arthritis, and the earlobe may appear swollen or elevated. Obstruction of the parotid duct, which may give rise to similar pain and swelling, is usually caused by sialolithiasis. In rare cases, masseter hyperactivity has been reported to block the duct, perhaps because the duct passes through a portion of the masseter in some individuals.

Differentiation of parotid problems from TM disorders can usually be made by history taking or by palpation and sialography, but it may occasionally need support by biopsy. Differential diagnostic problems in cases with symptoms involving some atypical features have been described in the dental literature (Jagger and Carlsson, 1978).

Temporal arteritis

Temporal arteritis (also called giant cell arteritis or cranial arteritis) is a systemic disease. It is part of a polyarteritis with varying clinical manifestations, including general symptoms such as fatigue, weight loss, and moderate fever. Local symptoms of pain and dysfunction in the TMJ region may lead to confusion in its diagnosis. Pain is predominantly found in the area of the tender and inflamed superficial temporal artery, but it may radiate to the masseter and temporal muscles due to reflex hyperactivity. Stiffness and painful limitation of mandibular movement may, therefore, be concomitant findings.

The combination of general symptoms, an elevated erythrocyte sedimentation rate, and changes along the superficial temporal arteries (e.g., tenderness, enlargement, absence of pulsation) should lead to a suspicion of temporal arteritis, especially in elderly female patients. At medical examination, the diagnosis is generally confirmed by biopsy of this artery. A description of two patients illustrating clinical features, therapy, and differential diagnostic problems in connection with temporal arteritis is worth perusing (Haraldson and Mejersjö, 1982).

Styloid-stylohyoid syndrome

Pain and functional discomfort related to the throat, occurring together with an anomaly consisting of an elongated styloid process or ossification of the stylohyoid ligament, have been known as *Eagle's syndrome* (Breault, 1986). It has usually been attributed to post-tonsillectomy sequelae (scarring of the tonsillar fossa). Sometimes it is described in connection with the differential diagnosis of TM disorders because a small portion of the patients with a diagnosis of styloid-stylohyoid syndrome has experienced pain in the TMJ and facial areas.

The prevalence of anomalies of the styloid process and stylohyoid ligament have been estimated by anatomists to affect approximately 4% of the population. Little or no correlation between clinical symptoms and the length of the styloid processes, as evaluated from panoramic radiographs, has been found in epidemiological and clinical studies (Gossman and Tarsitano, 1977; Breault, 1986).

From clinical experiences involving thousands of patients over many years, the conclusion can be drawn that Eagle's syndrome is an extremely rare alternative in differential diagnosis of TM disorders. If the styloid process is palpable in the tonsillar fossa and the palpation elicits the type of pain that prompted the examination, the diagnosis is possible. This can usually be confirmed by the use of local anesthesia and, of course, by radiographs.

Enlarged coronoid process

Enlargement or hyperplasia of the coronoid process may influence mandibular mobility. When the limitation of movement is combined with pain and discomfort, which may be a consequence of the process making contact with the maxilla (and possibly getting caught), differentiation from other types of TM disorders may be difficult. However, radiological examination will usually reveal an elongation of the coronoid process (Worth, 1979).

Postinjection trismus

A severe limitation of mouth opening developing a day or two after an inferior alveolar injection is occasionally seen without evidence of needle track infection and swelling. Spontaneous pain is unusual but forced opening of the mouth causes pain and discomfort. The mechanism of this condition is not entirely understood but it has been suggested that the injection needle pierced a small artery, which produced a hematoma that organized into a fibrous band in, or in the vicinity of, the medial pterygoid muscle. The trismus might be a form of guarding of the damaged structure (Brooke, 1979). Treatment should be conservative (e.g., heat and jaw exercises) because forcible opening under general anesthesia does not seem to secure a more predictable and rapid recovery. Most patients will have unrestricted mouth opening within 4 months but the condition will seldom resolve in less than 4 weeks. The patient will need some reassurance that this will eventually occur.

Neuralgias

The best known of the major neuralgias is trigeminal neuralgia, or tic doloureux. It is a strictly unilateral, recurrent paroxysmal facial pain that occurs along one or more of the branches of the trigeminal nerve (most frequently the second and third divisions). There are some characteristics that enable one to diagnose the condition from the patient's description only: *(1)* there are transient jabs of intense, lancinating pain that last only for seconds; *(2)* the pain may be provoked by stimulation of so-called trigger zones, often on some part of the skin of the face but sometimes on mucosal areas in the mouth; *(3)* there is a short refractory period after each paroxysm when a new pain attack cannot be stimulated; *(4)* a period of pain attacks may last for months; and *(5)* there is a tendency to spontaneous remissions for months or years between such periods of pain. Furthermore, the onset of the neuralgia is usually in individuals over 50 years of age, and it occurs somewhat more commonly in women than in men.

It has been suggested by a few authors that trigeminal neuralgia may be associated with myofascial pain-dysfunction or other TM disorders, and that occlusal and functional dental treatment might be able to reduce the pain. The documentation for this relationship is, however, very poor. It is highly probable that these reports were based on patients who did not have genuine trigeminal neuralgia, or if so, had an overlapping TM disorder that was successfully treated with or without a spontaneous remission of the neurologic pain. Nevertheless, if patients with trigeminal neuralgia are also found to have pain and dysfunction in the masticatory system, they should, of course, be treated with adequate methods to resolve these problems along with the appropriate therapy for the neuralgia. The neuralgic pain usually responds to the administration of carbamazepine, which has greatly reduced the necessity for neurosurgical intervention.

Headaches

There are many types of headaches. They have different causes and vary in severity from a lack of sleep, to a hangover, to a fatal brain tumor. There is a growing knowledge of relationships between some types of headaches and myofascial pain-dysfunction, which makes the diagnosis and management of patients with recurrent headaches of interest to dentists (Dawson, 1974; Heløe and Heiberg, 1980; Magnusson, 1981; Forssell, 1985; Wänman and Agerberg, 1986). Headaches of the tension or muscle-contraction type are particularly relevant to dentistry because the precipitating factor to such headaches appears to be muscular hyperactivity. Hyperactivity of the masticatory muscles is closely related to that of other muscle groups in the face and head.

Without going into details of differential diagnosis of headaches (see surveys by Dalessio, 1972; Lance, 1978), it is certainly reasonable for the dentist to start treatment of patients with recurrent tension headaches who also have tender masticatory muscles. This should only be initiated, however, after more serious conditions such as intracranial pathology have been excluded. The reason for this recommendation is that several studies have shown that a large proportion of patients with muscular hyperactivity related to tension headache along with masticatory myofascial pain-dysfunction experience a reduction in frequency and severity of their recurrent headaches after therapy for the myofascial pain-dysfunction (Magnusson and Carlsson, 1980a, 1983a).

Summary

There are numerous conditions that may cause occlusal and dysfunctional problems of the masticatory system. Some of these have been reviewed in this chapter but it is important to realize that there are other possibilities as well. If a patient does not respond to the recommended course of therapy, the initial diagnosis should be reevaluated. A possibility that should not be overlooked is that two or more conditions or disorders may exist at the same time which evidently will give differential diagnostic problems. For example, a chronic pulpitis can cause pain with vague localization or distant referral pattern. Simultaneously there may be a TM disorder such as osteoarthrosis. One of the conditions may be more acute and/or its diagnosis easier to make; it would then be managed first.

Signs and symptoms that remain after the first condition has been resolved will usually allow a much easier second diagnosis. If the symptoms persist and the diagnostic problems remain unsolved, the patient should be referred to appropriate health care specialists. This chapter has outlined a systematic approach to the dentist's examination of the patient's masticatory system.

Chapter 15

The Dentition: Occlusal Variations and Problems

Gunnar E. Carlsson and Bengt Ingervall

As described in chapters 3 and 4, a theoretically ideal occlusion is seldom found. Most patients have, to varying degrees, deviations from "ideal" conditions according to prevailing definitions. The term *normal occlusion* is often used instead, indicating the occlusal situation found most frequently or implying a state commonly found in the absence of disease.

Even if normality is difficult to define correctly, it is obvious that normal occlusion includes deviations to some degree from the "ideal" situation, because malocclusions of different types are more commonly found in the population than are ideal occlusions. The concept of normal occlusion should, therefore, include the functional capability of the masticatory system to adapt and tolerate some deviations from the ideal occlusion. Every dental student can get an idea of the great variation of "normality of occlusion" by looking at the dentitions of a group of fellow students. One way of avoiding the difficulty of defining normality would be to use the term *anatomic occlusion* instead, as suggested by Berkowitz et al. (1978), or *physiologic occlusion,* as used in this book. These definitional problems have been further discussed in chapter 13.

It is not only the morphology of the dentition that varies greatly between individuals. Occlusal contacts during functions such as mastication and deglutition are also extremely variable, as shown in a survey of relevant literature (Woda et al., 1979). If the still greater variability of contacts during parafunctional activity is added, it is not difficult to understand that there is no general agreement on which contacts represent "normal" or "good" occlusion. With respect to the great diversity of occlusal conditions found even in individuals with a well-functioning masticatory system, it is obvious that small deviations from an ideal occlusion in a patient with a natural dentition should not be dramatized.

However, some deviations from normal occlusion have to be more closely considered in relation to diagnosis and treatment of occlusal problems. These are *(1)* physiological tooth wear and loss of tooth substance, *(2)* loss of teeth, *(3)* morphological and functional malocclusions, *(4)* trauma and diseases affecting the occlusion, and *(5)* effects of prior dental treatment.

Loss of tooth substance

Loss of tooth substance can occur in different ways related to function and wear. The most common of these are attrition, abrasion, and erosion, with the following definitions:

Attrition. The physiologic wearing away of tooth substance as a result of tooth-to-tooth contact, as in mastication. Attrition is most obvious on occlusal and incisal surfaces, first as small polished facets, and later as flattening of occlusal surfaces (Figs. 15-1a and b). It may also occur on interproximal surfaces as a consequence of the small horizontal and vertical movements of the teeth during function.

Abrasion. Pathological wear of tooth sub-

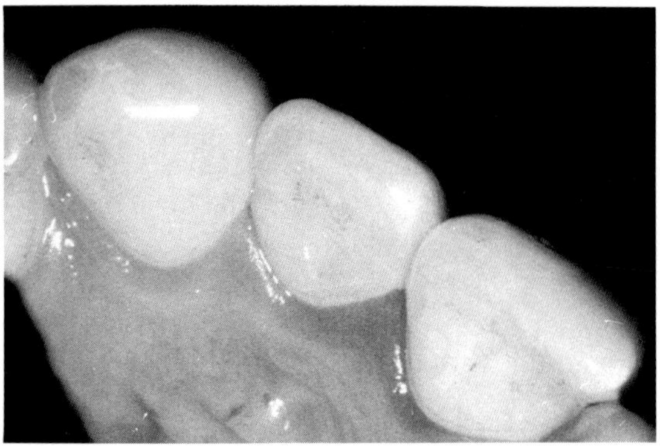

Fig. 15-1a Attrition. Facet covering the lingual and buccal sides of the tip of a maxillary canine in a young man.

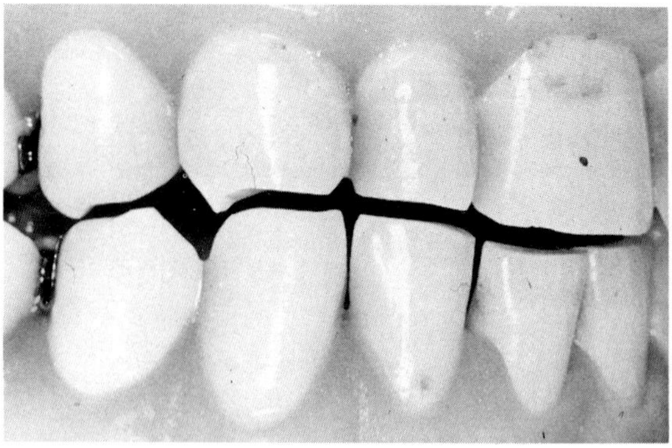

Fig. 15-1b Extensive incisal wear in a young bruxist.

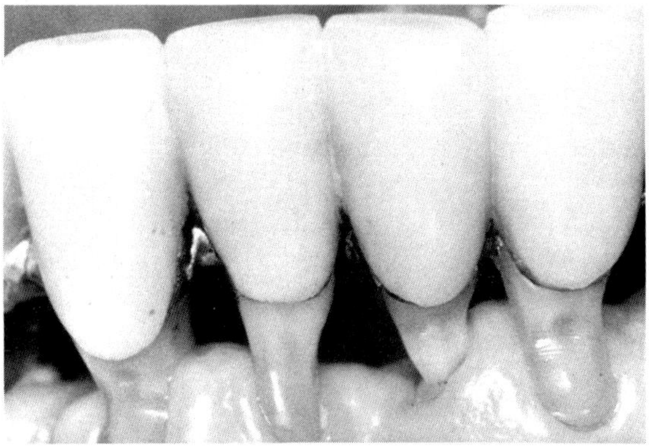

Fig. 15-2 Abrasion of roots of mandibular incisors caused by excessive toothbrushing.

stance through (abnormal) mechanical processes. Examples of causes of abrasion are improper or excessive toothbrushing, mainly affecting exposed root surfaces (Fig. 15-2), and oral habits, such as keeping a pipe stem, nails, or pins in a specific position between a few teeth. In some factories (foundry, stonemasonry, and mines) abrasive components in the air may come between the teeth of workers without a mask and cause abrasion, especially if they clench or grind their teeth.

Erosion. Chemically induced loss of tooth substance, mainly through an acid. The erosive acid may have an extrinsic or intrinsic origin: the former through diet (e.g., citrus fruits or juices) or air (in some chemical plants), the latter through regurgitation of gastric acids (habitual vomiting, as in anorexia nervosa) (Figs. 15-3a and b).

Tooth wear

All teeth taking part in mastication and other functions of the masticatory system will gradually show some attrition in spite of the enamel being extremely resistant to wear. Loss of tooth substance is, in general, associated with aging or, more strictly speaking, with the length of time the teeth have been exposed to occlusal functions. Thus the third molars show less wear in a middle-aged person with normal jaw relationships than do the incisors and first molars. This correlation of dental wear with age is almost linear in individuals living on an abrasive diet (Beyron, 1964; Molnar, 1971). Progressive dental wear can, therefore, be used for age determination in anthropological materials and in primitive cultures with abrasive diets.

In modern society the association between dental wear and age is not as obvious, because the food we eat today is so refined and nonabra-

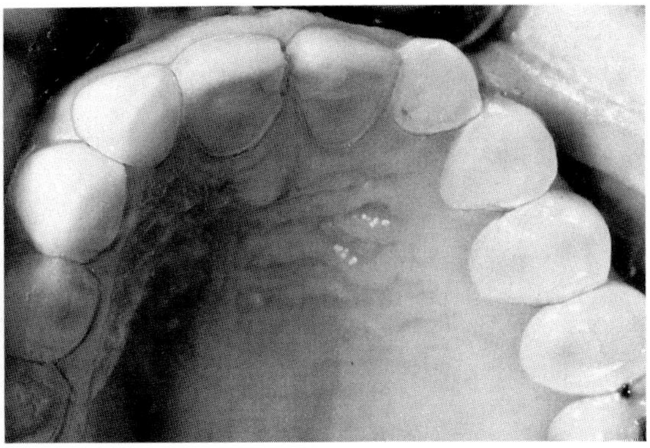

Fig. 15-3a Erosion caused by frequent vomiting in a 30-year-old woman. She suffered from anorexia nervosa from age 18 to 23. In the maxilla, the loss of tooth substance is extremely marked on the lingual side of the teeth.

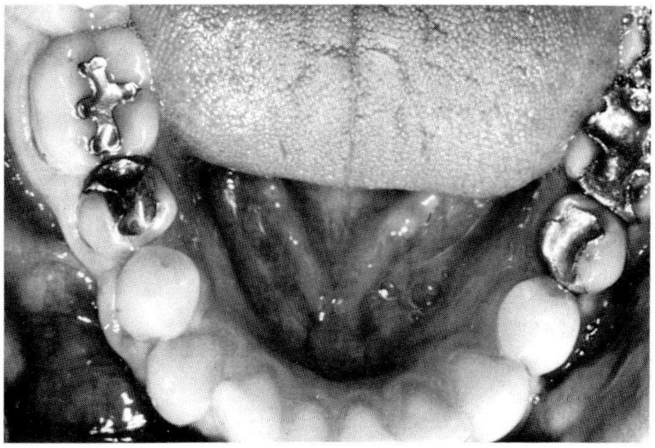

Fig. 15-3b Loss of tooth substance is more uniform in the mandible. Note that the amalgam fillings protrude above the eroded tooth surfaces.

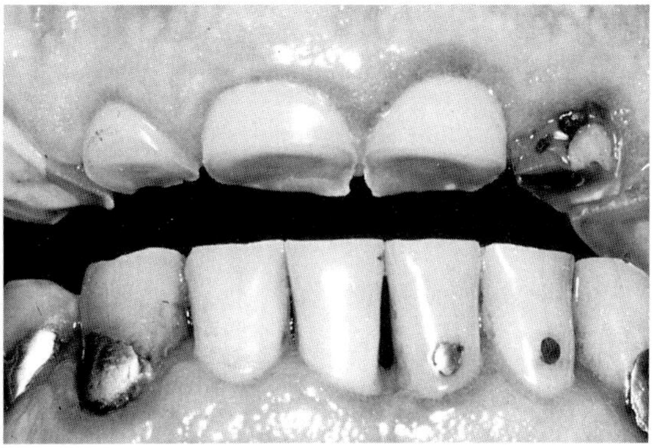

Fig. 15-4a Dental wear in a person with occluding teeth only in the anterior region during the last several years. Anterior view.

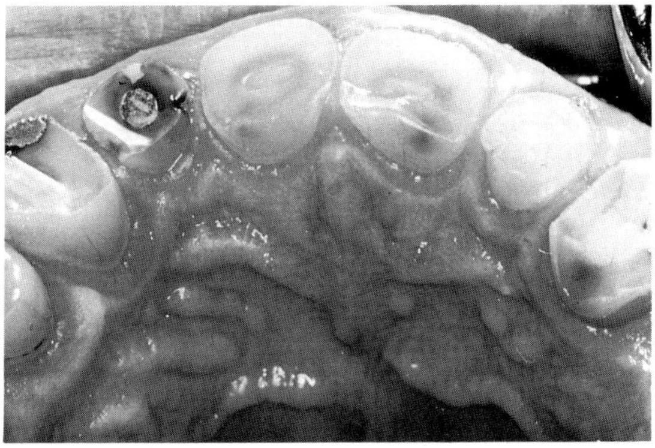

Fig. 15-4b Occlusal view of maxillary anterior teeth (reversed, taken in a mirror). Because of lack of posterior support, all functional and parafunctional activity is taken up by the incisors.

sive. The age dependence is therefore obscured; other factors gain in importance. In diagnosis of extensive tooth wear, it is thus necessary to also consider other conditions, such as quantity and quality of contacts between opposing teeth (e.g., numbers of teeth and their hardnesses and degrees of calcification, location and alignment of teeth and jaw relationships, cusp height and angulation, mobility of teeth and periodontal conditions, bite force and bruxing habits, amount and quality of saliva, chemical and mechanical factors of the diet, and the oral milieu).

It is often difficult to see the borderline between physiological and pathological conditions for many of these factors.

Diagnosis of tooth wear

It is often impossible to differentiate in a patient among *attrition, abrasion,* and *erosion*. In extensive cases of tooth wear there are, in fact, often combinations of causes, as exemplified in Figs. 15-4 to 15-8.

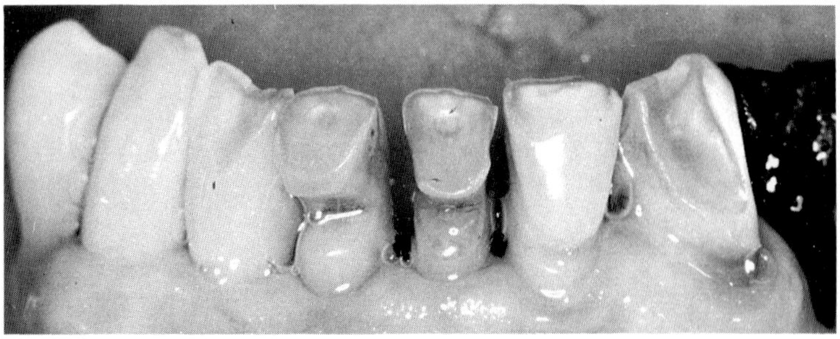

Fig. 15-5a Loss of tooth substance caused by a combination of factors. Anterior view of mandibular incisors in a man who worked for 7 years in a citrus plantation where he ate many acid fruits every day. Besides erosion, abrasion through toothbrushing and attrition through masticatory function has added to the loss of tooth substance.

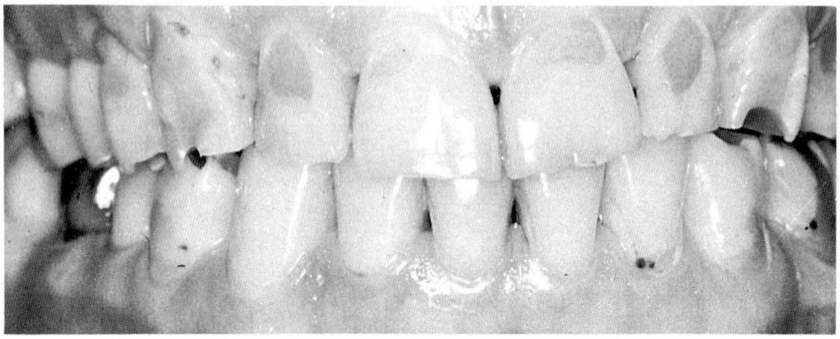

Fig. 15-5b Extensive fruit juice consumption, toothbrushing, and bruxism have contributed to the loss of tooth substance in this 35-year-old man.

In patients with one or more prosthetic reconstructions, diagnosis is complicated by the varying abrasive qualities of restorative materials (see Fig. 15-7). Furthermore, all teeth do not have enamel of the same resistance to wear. Special oral habits might also have odd effects and confuse diagnosis (see Figs. 15-8a and b).

It is often said that extensive tooth wear in modern humans is indicative of parafunctional activities, mainly bruxism. The previous discussion and listing of possible etiologic factors show, however, that diagnosis may not be so straightforward. For instance, it is extremely difficult to say with certainty when the loss of tooth substance happened, if it is a continuing process, or if it stopped long ago (Figs. 15-9a and b). It is usually necessary to make repeated observations using casts or photographs at reasonable intervals (several months to a year) to evaluate the *rate* of continuing wear before treatment begins. A careful search for the main cause(s) should be followed by a well-planned course of therapy. Such therapy usually involves an interim phase and an assessment of the results of temporary measures prior to the initiation of major definitive reconstructive procedures. An occlusal splint used for long periods of time can often eliminate the need for occlusal reconstruction, even in extensively worn dentitions (Figs. 15-10a and b).

Tooth loss

The loss of teeth is the most common cause of a

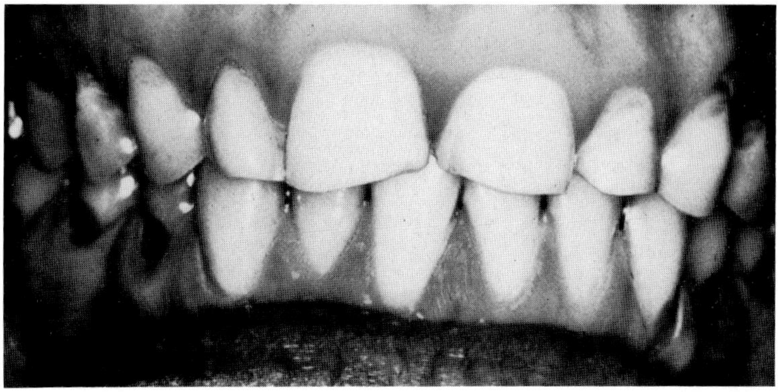

Figs. 15-6a and b Combination of regurgitation of a gastric acid and bruxism has caused severe destruction of tooth substance in this 22-year-old woman. The cervical lesions are probably due to abrasion and erosion.

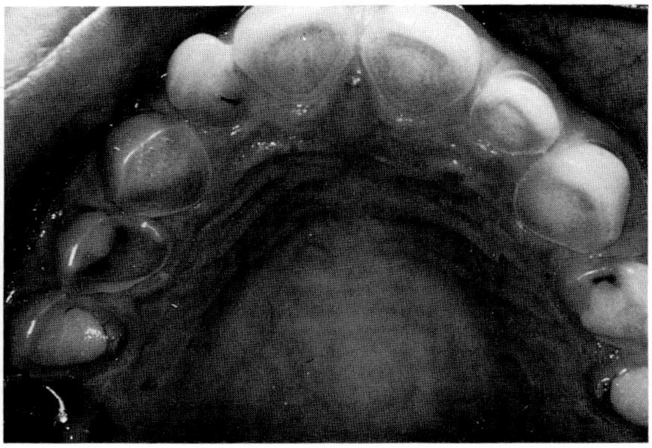

Fig. 15-6b

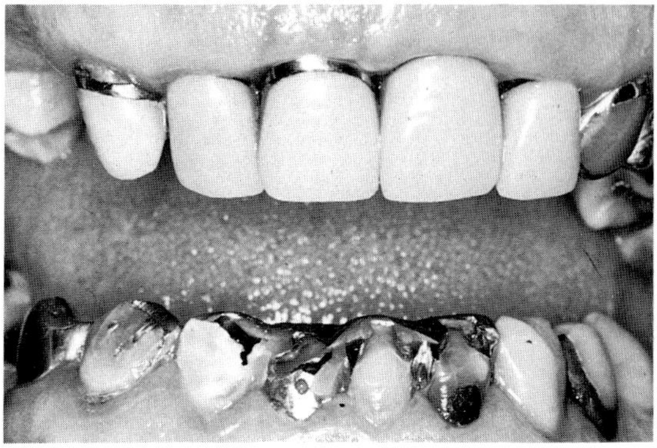

Fig. 15-7 Wear on gold restorations, acrylic facings, and natural tooth substances in mandibular incisors occluding against porcelain crowns.

physiologic occlusion developing into a nonphysiologic occlusion. In a healthy, complete dentition, there is an equilibrium of forces from lips, cheeks, tongue, neighboring teeth, and normal function that help to maintain a relative stability of individual teeth and of the occlusion. The loss of a single tooth may lead to drifting, tipping, rotation of neighboring teeth, and extrusion of opposing teeth (Fig. 15-11).

Migration of teeth

In a classic paper, Hirschfeld (1937) presented a lengthy list of undesirable sequelae to the dentition and the whole masticatory system following the loss of one tooth. Some of the potential consequences of the loss of the mandibular first molar, for example, include the mesial tipping of the mandibular second and third molars and the extrusion of the maxillary first molar. This situation, which is often observed in clinical practice, may lead to functional problems through the creation of occlusal interferences, especially on the nonworking side. Other sequelae may occur, such as loss of occlusal vertical dimension, opening of proximal contacts, uneven adjacent marginal ridges, development of "plunger" cusps, food impaction, and lack of functional cleansing of teeth. However, these are even less predictable because of great individual variation, for example—depending on age at the time of tooth loss—periodontal conditions, and the intercuspation of the teeth adjacent to the lost tooth and their antagonists. An epidemiologic study showed that 20% of patients with tooth

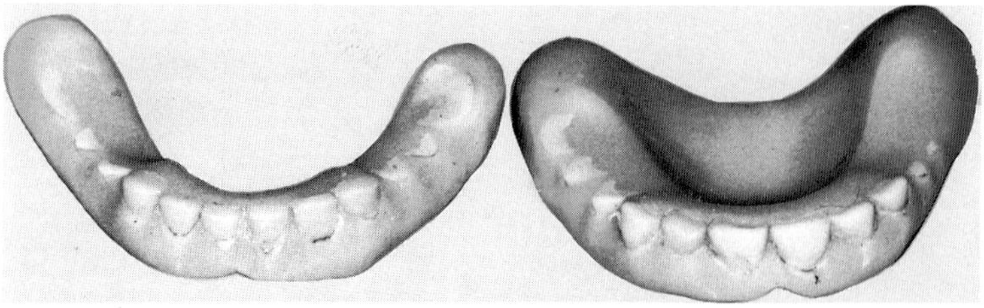

Figs. 15-8a and b Complete dentures with unusual wear caused by strong tongue activity.

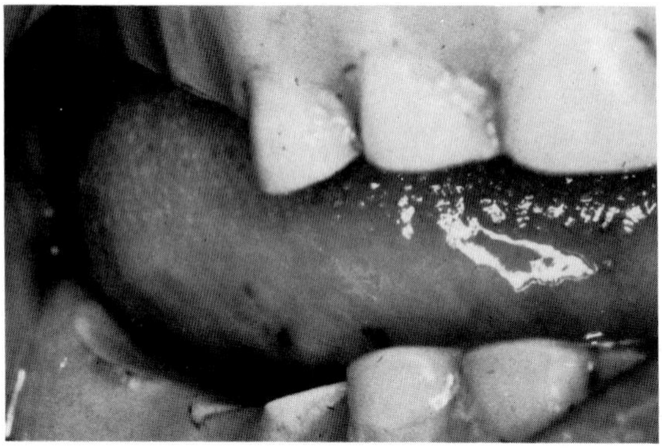

Fig. 15-8b

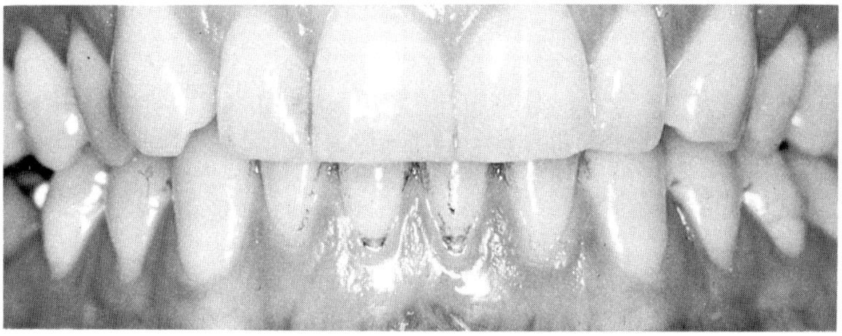

Fig. 15-9a Anterior view of a 25-year-old woman with advanced attrition of incisors.

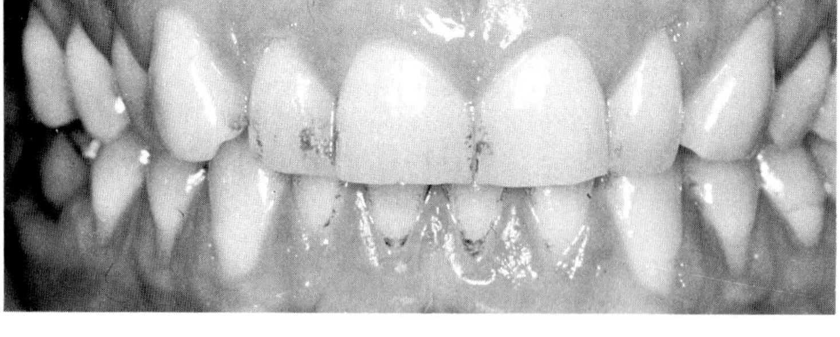

Fig. 15-9b The same patient 8 years later—only a small change has occurred.

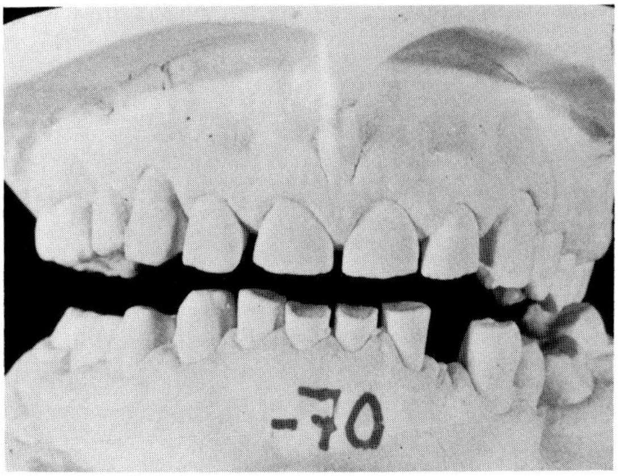

Fig. 15-10a A 55-year-old man with severe attrition (1970) received an occlusal splint for use at night.

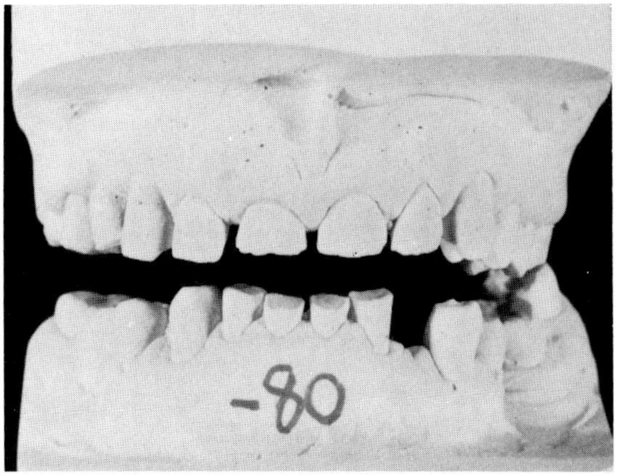

Fig. 15-10b Ten years later the maxillary central incisors have additional wear, but other teeth have changed remarkably little. The patient used the splint for about 5 years. He does not wish to have any reconstructions.

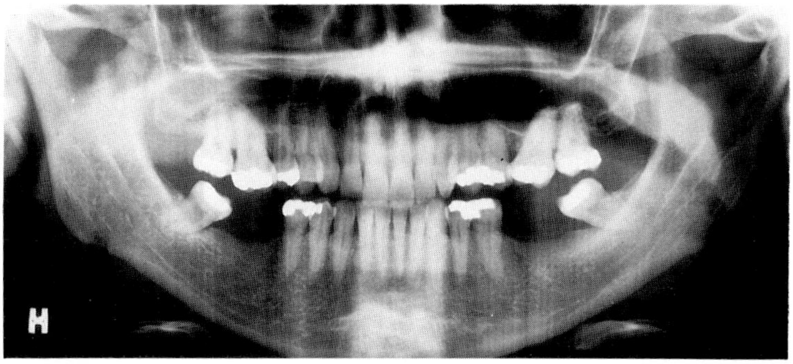

Fig. 15-11 Elongation of maxillary antagonists and tipping of remaining mandibular third molars after loss of mandibular first and second molars (orthopantomogram).

loss at an early age had subsequent closure of the ensuing space (Zarb et al., 1978).

There is almost a total lack of longitudinal, well-controlled studies of changes in the dentition after loss of a single tooth. The classic investigation of Beyron (1954b), however, emphasized the changes of masticatory habits as a consequence of the development of interferences preventing comfortable bilateral function. The resulting pattern of unilateral function often led to unfavorable long-term development of the dentition and to additional occlusal conditions, for example, uneven attrition creating steep facets or oblique planes on occlusal surfaces, overeruption and labial tilting of anterior teeth opposite the area of interference, and opening of proximal contacts with consequent food impaction.

Occlusal conditions leading to, or resulting from, unilateral function represent significant deviations from the criteria of the "optimal occlusion" described later by Beyron (1969). An optimal occlusion is characterized by, among other things, chewing performed with equal ease on both sides, bilateral stable occlusal contacts on most of the teeth in the intercuspal position, bilateral stable contacts on posterior teeth in the retrusive range in the retruded contact position, and a small distance between intercuspal position and retruded contact position in the midsagittal plane.

Even though the ability to adapt within the masticatory system is great, the loss of even a single tooth may lead to occlusal instability and interferences, with unfavorable consequences for occlusal function, chewing habits, and oral hygiene.

Other consequences of tooth loss

Most dentists anticipate that the loss of several teeth will naturally lead to more severe problems. According to available research, as the dentition deteriorates, so does masticatory efficiency and performance (Carlsson, 1974; Bates et al., 1976). But the other consequences of tooth loss are not as evident, mainly because of the wide range of adaptive processes among individuals. In general, the more teeth that are lost, the greater the risk of tipping, migration, extrusion, and attrition of remaining teeth, and of loss of alveolar bone and occlusal vertical dimension.

It is usually said that the more depleted the periodontal support, the greater the risk of trauma from occlusion. According to current knowledge, however, inflammation has a dominating influence on periodontal health, and trauma from occlusion, except for its increasing tooth mobility, is of limited importance (Polson and Heijl, 1980). Even in teeth with markedly reduced periodontal support, occlusal trauma (of the jiggling type) will not cause further destruction of the attachment apparatus, provided the plaque-induced periodontal disease has been cured (Lindhe and Nyman, 1977). In a reduced dentition with healthy periodontal tissues, therefore, the occlusal forces hardly involve a risk of periodontal breakdown. This is verified by excellent long-term results with extensive fixed prostheses in patients with advanced periodontal disease (in which 50% or more of the periodontal tissue support of their dentitions were lost) when inflammation was resolved (Nyman and Lindhe, 1979) (see chapter 16).

Temporomandibular disorders and tooth loss

It is possible that loss of posterior teeth may predispose one to temporomandibular (TM) disorders. Autopsy studies have revealed a correlation between tooth loss and osteoarthrosis of the TMJ (Öberg et al., 1971; Carlsson et al., 1979); this correlation has been verified in at least one clinical study (Kopp, 1977c) (see chapter 17). One explanation may be that the functional load on the TMJ, according to theoretical calculations, is greater when pressure is applied to anterior teeth than to the molars (Hekneby, 1974) (see chapter 6). In an epidemological study by questionnaire, the fewer the residual teeth respondents had, the more impaired mandibular mobility and other dysfunctional symptoms they reported (Agerberg and Carlsson, 1973). In another investigation, which combined history and clinical examination, both the anamnestic (recalled symptoms) and the clinical dysfunction indexes (Helkimo, 1974) increased with decreasing number of residual teeth. And Franks (1967) found unrestored and unevenly distributed loss of teeth bilaterally and unilateral masticatory function to be more common in a group of TM disorder patients than in a control group. On the other hand, Thomson (1971) could not reveal any significant differences in posterior tooth support or other dental parameters between a group of 100 TM disorder patients and a control group of 100. Also, in a comparison of two similar groups of 80 patients each, no correlation between state of dentition and clinical dysfunction was found (Magnusson and Carlsson, 1978).

The diverging opinions about the influence of a reduced dentition on the masticatory system prompted Käyser (1981) to perform a study on the relationship between shortened dental arches and oral function. The results showed two patterns of change in oral function: *(1)* slow change until four occlusal units are left (i.e., pairs of occluding posterior teeth, one molar unit equal to two premolar units), and then rapid change; and *(2)* progressive change without sudden change.

Adaptation to tooth loss was also evident in a

questionnaire study that showed that a loss of up to seven teeth did not seem to impair chewing ability (Agerberg and Carlsson, 1981). In an investigation of people between 25 and 55 years of age, tooth loss and function/dysfunction of the masticatory system was studied (Battistuzzi, 1982). No relationship could be shown between the number of missing teeth and the functioning quality of the masticatory system. In an epidemiological sample of 70-year-olds, the correlation between mandibular dysfunction and dental status recorded with the Eichner index (based on the number of supporting zones in the dentition) was analyzed (Österberg and Carlsson, 1979). Eichner's index showed no certain correlation or only weak correlation with reported and clinical dysfunction of the masticatory system. These findings show that the capacity of the masticatory system to adapt to tooth loss, on the average, is extremely great. It implies that extensive oral rehabilitation is not a necessity for all patients with reduced dentitions. Fish's observation (1970) that prosthetic intervention often means more to the dentist than to the patient is worth considering in all treatment planning.

Tooth loss and neuromuscular changes

The loss of posterior teeth and, thereby, of occlusal support, is often, in a very mechanical way, thought by some to lead to loss of vertical dimension, bite collapse, superior and posterior displacement of the condyles, and eventually to pain and dysfunction, according to concepts first promulgated by Costen in the 1930s and long since repudiated. It is probably more accurate to emphasize the neuromuscular and functional sequelae of loss of posterior teeth. In some individuals, posterior tooth loss is well compensated for by adaptive processes, while in others, it may contribute to functional disturbances. Of particular and controversial interest in the etiology of TM disorders are the often small disturbances of occlusion called *occlusal interferences*. These are often related to loss of teeth, but they may have other origins. This subject is discussed in more detail in the next section.

Morphological malocclusion

The importance of occlusal factors in the etiology of pain or dysfunction of the masticatory system has been extensively discussed in the dental literature. It has been, and remains, an extremely controversial subject. Even in the middle 1980s there are those who maintain there is a close correlation between occlusal "disturbances" and TM disorders and others who believe there is no such association at all. In the following review of these issues, a distinction will be made between morphological and functional malocclusion.

In chapter 3, variations in the development of the permanent dentition were emphasized. Deviations from an ideal occlusion were grouped into dentitional, occlusal, and space anomalies.

Dentitional anomalies include aberrations in the formation, eruption, and alignment of individual teeth as well as in tooth form. A common anomaly regarding tooth formation is hypodontia (partial anodontia)—where one or more teeth are congenitally absent. For the permanent dentition, this occurs in about 7% of the population (the third molars not taken into consideration). The absence of one or more third molars is still more frequent, occurring in about 25% of the population. The consequences of congenital absence of teeth may, if untreated, be migration and tipping of neighboring teeth and extrusion of antagonistic teeth comparable to the sequelae of loss of teeth. In extreme cases with many teeth missing, the occlusal stability may also be jeopardized.

Anomalies of eruption may, among other things, include tooth retention, meaning that the tooth remains nonerupted or the teeth erupt outside of their proper positions in the dental arch. From the occlusal point of view, the former condition is comparable to hypodontia, whereas tooth eruption outside of normal position means a faulty tooth alignment that may give rise to *occlusal interference* (discussed later in this chapter).

Anomalies in tooth alignment may occur as isolated malocclusion traits but are more common in connection with crowding, the most frequent type of space anomaly. In crowding, the teeth are forced to take up positions buccal or lingual to their normal positions in the dental arch, or in a rotated position in the arch, due to lack of space. Occlusal interferences are thus often found in crowded dentitions. The other type of space anomaly, spacing, is less apt to give rise to occlusal problems.

Malformation of individual teeth can create an occlusal disturbance if the morphology of the occlusal surface is involved. Such malformations are, however, more rare than malposition of the teeth.

Morphological occlusal anomalies in the anteroposterior direction are of two main types: postnormal malocclusions (Angle Class II) and prenormal malocclusions (Angle Class III). The Class II, postnormal malocclusion can be divided into two categories, one with proclined maxillary incisors and a large overjet (with or without deep overbite; Class II, division 1), and one with retroclined maxillary incisors, usually associated with a marked deep overbite (Class II, division 2).

Functionally, the Class II, division 2 malocclusion is characterized by very steep incisal guidance during gliding movements due to the deep overbite and retroclined position of the incisors. The Class III malocclusion is usually combined with crossbite of the anterior teeth, and often also with anterior open bite; the overjet and overbite are then negative. Besides possible occlusal interferences, this situation may often lead to a lack of sufficient occlusal support. Thus, Ingervall et al. (1979), in a sample of adults with Class II malocclusions being treated surgically, found that, on the average, only 11 teeth were in antagonistic contact before the operation, compared with 16 after surgical correction of the malocclusion.

Lingual and buccal crossbite can occur as isolated traits but are also seen combined with other occlusal anomalies. Thus, lingual crossbite of posterior teeth often occurs in Class II, division 1 and Class III malocclusions, whereas buccal crossbite often is seen in Class II, division 2 malocclusion.

A lateral open bite is a rare anomaly, while an anterior open bite occurs with a moderate frequency (2% to 4%). There are two types of anterior open bites. One is a result of a sucking habit in childhood and tends to improve after the abolition of the habit. The other is of skeletal origin, developing as a consequence of a posterior mandibular growth rotation and bringing about serious orthodontic treatment problems (see chapter 3). Both types may be combined with lingual crossbite of posterior teeth. Anterior open bite, probably of skeletal origin, has been a relatively frequent finding in subjects with amelogenesis imperfecta, adding an occlusal problem to the hereditary enamel defect (Persson and Sundell, 1982).

Due to the negative overbite in anterior open bite, there is no anterior guidance during gliding movements. This often leads to a nonworking side occlusal interference, especially when combined with crossbite of posterior teeth.

The importance of a morphologic malocclusion predisposing to a functional malocclusion is discussed below.

Functional malocclusion

Functional malocclusion is another term for the concept of occlusal interference. This has been defined as "cuspal contacts forcing the mandible to deviate from a normal pattern of movement" (Posselt, 1968), "occlusal contacts hampering or hindering smooth, gliding harmonious jaw movements with the teeth maintaining contact" (Ramfjord and Ash, 1983), or, simply, "part of tooth structure that is in the way of harmonious jaw function" (Dawson, 1974). All of these definitions lead to the question of what is a normal or harmonious pattern of movement of the mandible.

Mandibular movements are largely guided by neuromuscular control mechanisms. In a functionally optimal occlusion the types of tooth contacts should be such that the muscles are not required to perform unnecessary activity.

According to some authors, there are specific types of tooth contacts that may predispose to unfavorable muscular activity. For example, Posselt (1968) noted the following as the most severe "occlusal disharmonies":

1. A large difference or a lateral slide between the retruded contact position (RCP) and the intercuspal position (ICP) of the mandible, as well as unilateral contact in RCP—collectively called an *interference in RCP.*
2. Tooth contacts on the nonworking side that prevent contact on the working side—a *nonworking side interference.*
3. Steep cuspal inclines on the working side that hinder working side movement—a *working side interference.*

Occlusal interference in retruded contact position

In habitual closure into occlusion the neuromuscular system strives to achieve a position with the mandibular condyles more or less centered in the joint fossae. This corresponds to a position close to the retruded contact position, because in this position the condyles are also more or less centered in the fossae (Posselt, 1952; Hickey et al., 1963; Ingervall, 1968).

This has led to the hypothesis that, if the mandibular condyles, because of unfavorable intercuspation upon closure, are deflected from their "centered" positions, symptoms of a TM disorder may arise. This type of occlusal interference is often associated with a clinically detectable large anteroposterior distance between RCP and ICP, or a lateral component of the slide between the two mandibular positions (Fig. 15-12).

Most children as well as adults have a small difference between RCP and ICP, the mean value as measured at the incisors being about 0.9 mm (Posselt, 1952; Ingervall, 1968). According to the above hypothesis, the larger the difference between RCP and ICP, the more the condyles in ICP are forced out of their "centered" positions in the fossae (Fig. 15-13). Thus, a large anteroposterior difference between the mandibular positions in RCP and ICP implies that both condyles are not "centered" in ICP, whereas a lateral discrepancy between RCP and ICP means that one of the condyles in ICP is not "centered" (Fig. 15-14). In other words, in this type of interference the intercuspation may deflect the condyles bilaterally when the RCP–ICP difference is large, or unilaterally when a lateral RCP–ICP discrepancy is present. Even though some authors such as Weinberg (1975, 1977) have emphasized concentricity of the condyles in the fossae as essential for the health of the masticatory system, conflicting findings have been reported in patient and nonpatient samples. Tomographic surveys of nonsymptomatic subjects have shown great variation of condyle positions among asymptomatic subjects (Blaschke and Blaschke, 1981; Pullinger et al., 1985, 1986). Also, in epidemiological samples of both children and adults, and in clinical series of patients with TM disorders, only small proportions of individuals with large mandibular displacements between RCP and ICP have been observed. An example of the distribution of these distances in 402 children is shown in Fig. 15-15 (Egermark-Eriksson, 1982). The literature is not conclusive regarding the importance of the relationship between RCP and ICP, although there has been a tendency to associate more problems to larger distances.

A situation where the RCP-ICP distance is more than 2 mm, particularly if two occlusal positions can easily be taken up, is sometimes referred to as a *dual bite.* The etiology of this condition is not fully known, but it may be caused by mandibular fractures, unsuccessful orthodontic or prosthetic treatment ("bite-jumping" or mandibular repositioning), or, most particularly, it may be developmental in origin. Treating dual bite with any type of occlusal therapy is usually thought to present considerable diagnostic and technical problems. However, a study of 12 subjects with dual bite showed that most would not be undergoing any complicated treatment, as they had no, or only mild, subjective symptoms (Egermark-Eriksson et al., 1979). Thus, the contribution of a dual bite to TM disorders is questionable.

It is not known to what extent occlusal interference in RCP mechanically deflects the mandible

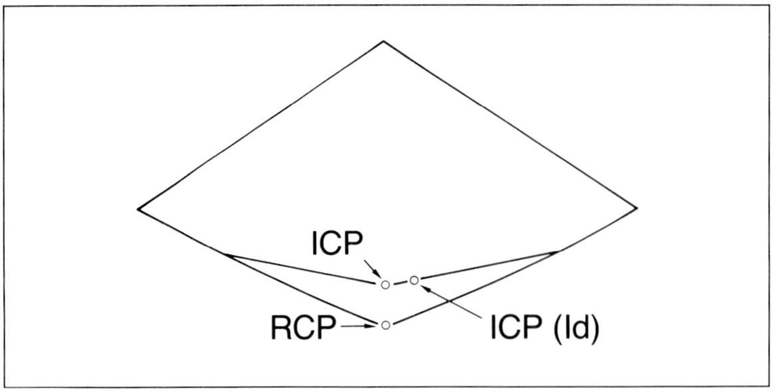

Fig. 15-12 Upper area of movement space of mandibular incisors. *RCP* and *ICP*: retruded and intercuspal positions of mandible, respectively. *ICP (Id)*: intercuspal position characterized by lateral deviation between *RCP* and *ICP*.

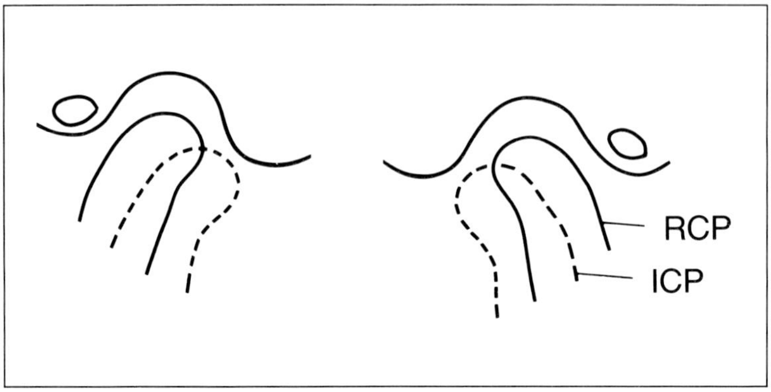

Fig. 15-13 Schematized condyle positions in case of large anteroposterior difference between retruded *(RCP)* and intercuspal *(ICP)* mandibular positions.

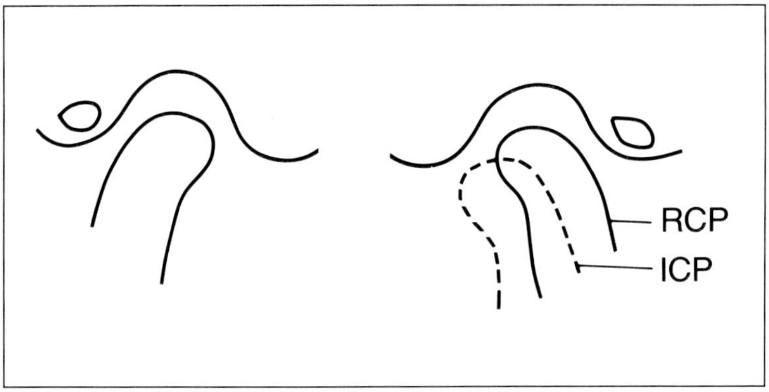

Fig. 15-14 Schematized condyle positions in case of lateral deviation between retruded *(RCP)* and intercuspal *(ICP)* mandibular positions.

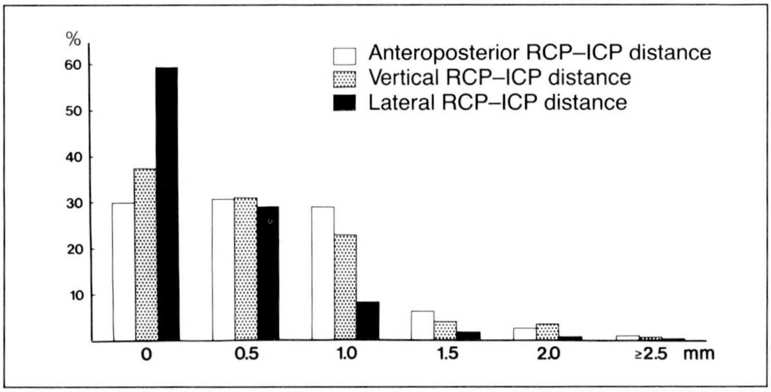

Fig. 15-15 Distribution of clinically measured distances from RCP to ICP in 402 children 7 to 15 years of age.

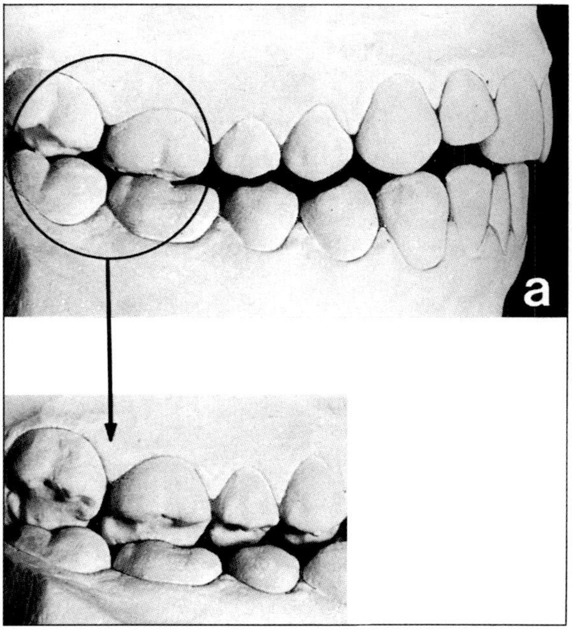

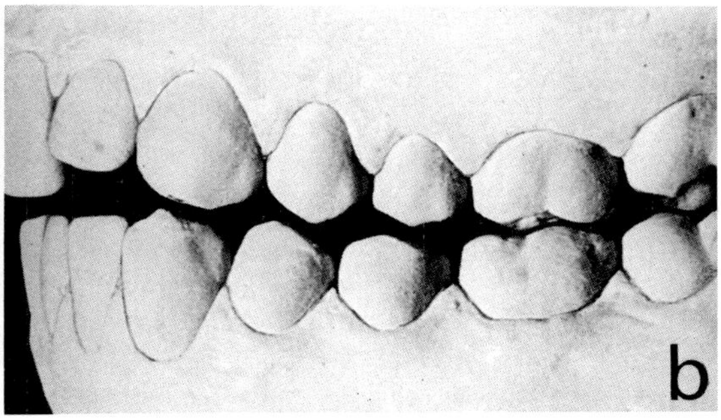

Fig. 15-16a *(left)* Case with nonworking side interference. Tooth contacts only on the nonworking side.

Fig. 15-16b *(above)* No tooth contact on the working side.

during closure, and to what extent the neuromuscular pattern is modified to avoid mechanical interference. That a muscular avoidance pattern exists is evident from studies of children with a lateral deviation between RCP and ICP (Troelstrup and Møller, 1970; Ingervall and Thilander, 1975). In such children, the muscular contraction pattern, including that seen in postural position of the mandible, was found to deviate from the normal. This was interpreted as an adaptation in order to avoid mechanical interference upon closure.

Nonworking side interference

In epidemiologic studies of adults, a nonworking side interference (i.e., tooth contact on the nonworking side preventing contact on the working side) has been found to occur in 8% to 10% of the sample (Figs. 15-16a and b) (Ingervall, 1972; Ingervall et al., 1980; Mohlin, 1983). Figures 15-16a and b are correct for lateral gliding up to 3 mm from ICP (measured at the mandibular midline), approximately corresponding to an edge-to-edge position of the working side teeth.

If the lateral gliding movement is examined in greater detail, prevalences of nonworking side interferences are found: 26% in adult women (Mohlin, 1983) and 18% to 40% in 7- to 15-year-old children (Egermark-Eriksson et al., 1981).

In children, there seems to be a reduction in nonworking side interferences from 7 to 15 years of age (Egermark-Eriksson et al., 1981). This reduction is probably due to the full development of an articular eminence in the TMJ, and to development of anterior guidance in the dentition, which usually awaits eruption of the permanent incisors and canines. Both of these factors strongly influence nonworking side disclusion during lateral excursion. The reduced presence in 7-year-olds, as compared with 15-year-olds, accounts for the higher incidence of nonworking side interferences at the earlier age.

In patient samples from TMJ clinics (Mohlin and Kopp, 1978), considerably higher prevalences of nonworking side interferences than in

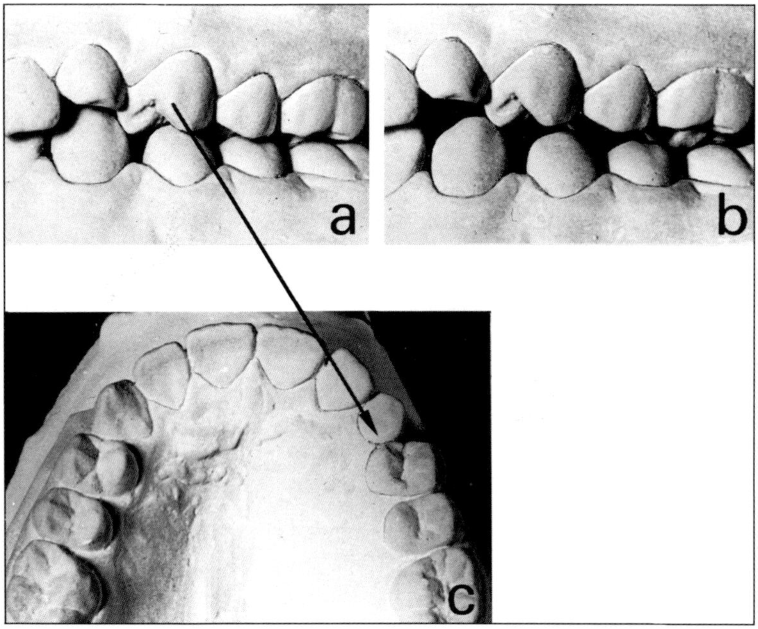

Fig. 15-17 Child with hampered lateral guiding movement related to steep cuspal inclines on the working side *(a)*, and malposition of left maxillary first premolar *(c)* with lingual crossbite *(b)*.

the unselected population samples have been found. This has been interpreted as evidence that this type of interference is an important factor in the etiology of some TM disorders. However, it is common to adapt to occlusal interferences. In a sample consisting of young adults with nonworking side interferences without marked symptoms of a TM disorder, the functional pattern of the masticatory muscles had modified to adapt to the occlusal interference (Ingervall and Carlsson, 1982). No dramatic changes in muscular activity could be demonstrated upon elimination of nonworking side interferences in this group.

Experimental studies of nonworking side interferences have also given conflicting results. Thus, DeBoever (1969) found no significant alteration in EMG pattern after the insertion of a nonworking side interference, while Schärer et al. (1967), on the other hand, found such interferences to result in a high percentage of inhibitory pauses (silent periods) during chewing. More recently it was shown that psychological factors may affect the experience of occlusal interferences. Magnusson and Enbom (1984) told 24 volunteers that occlusal interferences would be inserted, with possible effects on the masticatory system. In 12 subjects, nonworking side interferences were inserted bilaterally with composite resin restorations; the other 12 acted as controls—the insertions were only simulated and no permanent changes in the occlusion were performed. In the interference group, ten individuals reported one or more subjective symptoms during the 2-week experimental period, and seven exhibited clinical signs of dysfunction. In the control group, three experienced subjective symptoms and three clinical signs of dysfunction. One week after the experimental period, signs and symptoms had disappeared in all subjects but two, one from each group. The authors concluded that there is no simple relationship between occlusal interferences and signs and symptoms of TM disorders.

It is important to distinguish between a nonworking side interference and tooth contact on the nonworking side. In the natural dentition, many individuals on lateral gliding have tooth contact both on the working and nonworking sides (balancing contacts) (Ingervall, 1972a; Sadowsky and BeGole, 1980). Only when the tooth contact(s) on the nonworking side hamper(s) contacts on the working side is the term *nonworking side interference* justified.

Working side interference

There is no general agreement regarding the desirable type of tooth contact on the working side (see chapter 12). Although some authors favor a so-called canine-protected occlusion, others prefer an occlusion with many contacts on the working side, that is, "group function." Some authors stress that lateral excursion should be possible as a smooth gliding occlusal contact movement (Ramfjord and Ash, 1983). Beyron (1954a) found the most favorable long-term occlusal development in adults who could perform multidirectional gliding movements along shallow paths of movement. Individuals with a steep cuspal guidance when gliding toward one side, and a shallow one when gliding to the other side, often avoided chewing on the side with steep cusps. The attrition developed asymmetrically, with an even more pronounced unilateral movement pattern with time.

In an epidemiologic study of middle-aged men (Ingervall et al., 1980), antagonistic contact between only one molar or premolar tooth pair on the working side was called "single-tooth contact on the working side." A less-than-desirable number of contacts was found to be positively correlated with both subjective symptoms and clinical signs of dysfunction. These results have to be verified in further studies aimed at determining the most favorable type of tooth contact on the working side.

In two more recent studies, one on a group of 50 patients with TM disorders and one on a nonpatient group of 48 young adults, the relationships between many of the above-mentioned occlusal variables and signs and symptoms of pain and dysfunction of the masticatory system were analyzed (Droukas et al., 1984, 1985). The occlusal conditions varied considerably, but did not show significant correlations with signs and symptoms of TM disorders in any of the groups.

Obviously, canine-protected occlusion and group function occurring in the natural dentition can function well. However, in individuals with hampered lateral gliding movement, due, for example, to steep cuspal inclines in buccal crossbite, the suspicion of a working side interference may sometimes be justified (Fig. 15-17). The clinician should not adopt a single unalterable concept of working side contact that will be applied to all patients. The unique conditions of each dentition must be considered. For example, a patient with a canine-protected occlusion whose canines show no fremitus or mobility and whose occlusion functions well, should not have the canine relationships in working side excursions altered.

Morphological malocclusion predisposing to functional malocclusion

Morphological malocclusion, per se, does not give rise to TM disorders. However, certain types of morphological malocclusion predispose to occlusal interferences and these, according to some, may contribute to their etiology (Ramfjord and Ash, 1983).

Mohlin and Kopp (1978) found a higher prevalence of crossbite and anterior open bite in patients of a TMJ clinic than would be expected from their incidence in the general population. A relationship was demonstrated between crossbite of posterior teeth (both unilateral and bilateral) and occlusal interference in RCP, and between crossbite and working side interference. Working side interference was also related to tipped mandibular molars, mostly due to loss of neighboring teeth.

Some epidemiologic studies (Egermark-Eriksson, 1982; Mohlin, 1983) point to an increased risk for occlusal interference and TM disorders with Class II and III malocclusions, anterior and posterior crossbites, and anterior open bite. The studies uniformly point to the relationship between anterior open bite and

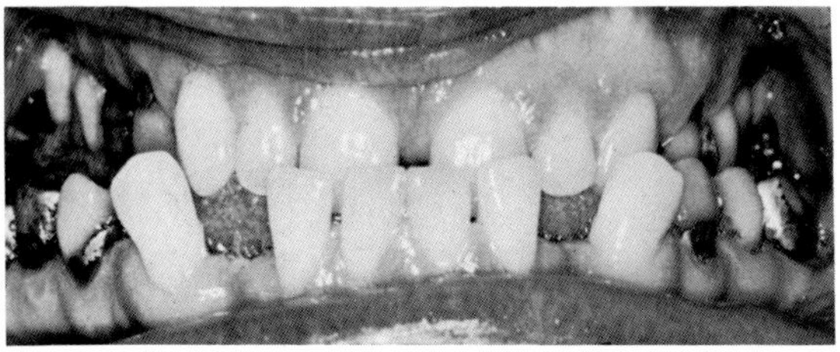

Fig. 15-18 Acromegaly. Enlargement of the mandible with loss of occlusal contacts.

nonworking side interferences, and the negative correlation between deep overbite and the same type of occlusal interference. In none of the studies referred to has deep overbite been found to involve the risk of disorder or occlusal interference. The positive and negative correlations between anterior open bite and deep overbite, respectively, on nonworking side interferences emphasize the importance of anterior guidance to disclusion of posterior teeth during gliding movements. The potential for occlusal interference both in RCP and on the nonworking side in cases with lingual crossbite is also documented in the above-mentioned studies.

The relation between postnormal occlusion and occlusal interference in RCP is further substantiated by studies in children showing that individuals with this type of malocclusion have a greater-than-average anteroposterior distance between RCP and ICP (Ingervall, 1968; Malmgren, 1980).

Although statistically significant correlations can be demonstrated between certain types of morphological and functional malocclusions, the correlation coefficients are numerically weak. All individuals with these types of morphological malocclusions do not have occlusal interferences, and all individuals with occlusal interferences do not develop symptoms of TM disorders. *This strongly suggests that other factors must be present to bring about signs and symptoms of such disorders.*

In the American Dental Association President's Conference on TM disorders (1982) the following statement was made: "Although the scientific literature has not shown that occlusal problems cause temporomandibular disorders, clinical data do confirm the two conditions frequently coexist, but the nature of the relationship between them is unclear at this time."

Diseases and trauma affecting the dentition

Deviations from normal occlusal conditions may be seen in several diseases affecting different components of the masticatory system. The most prevalent are found in the embryologic, developmental, and traumatic categories. Among the congenital anomalies contributing to malocclusion, the cleft lip and palate deformities are the most common. Also, developmental anomalies of the TMJ must be remembered as possible causes of malocclusion, as they "are probably far more common than is realized" (Ross, 1979). The dentitional disturbances that accompany such anomalies fall outside the scope of this book.

Diseases affecting the TMJ may cause occlusal disturbances. For example, unilateral condylar hyperplasia and growing tumors in the condyle will lead to an open bite on the involved side due to the rapid inferior growth of the mandible on that side. Rheumatoid arthritis involving destruction of the condyles will inevitably lead to changes in the occlusion, the most striking sign being a progressive opening of the bite (Carlsson et al., 1979). Acromegaly, when associated with enlargement of the TMJ and the whole mandible, will lead to mandibular prognathism and, in extreme cases, to loss of occlusal stability (Fig. 15-18).

Trauma to different components of the masticatory system may frequently contribute to disturbances in occlusion as well (Harrigan, 1981). Trauma may be limited to only one tooth, or may involve several teeth, an alveolar segment, the TMJ, or fractures of the mandible or maxilla. Each of these conditions is associated with evident changes in the occlusion. Of particular interest are the fairly common mandibular fractures, especially those of the condylar pro-

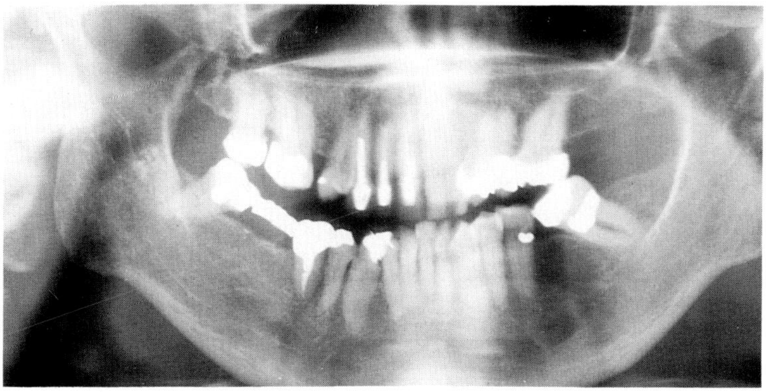

Fig. 15-19a Consequence of condylar fracture. Orthopantomogram after fracture of the left condylar process.

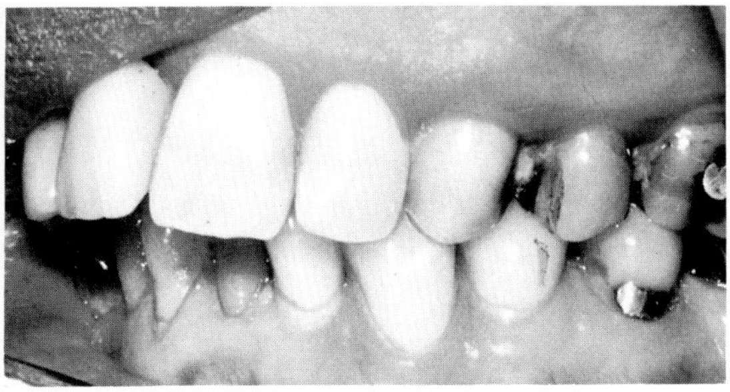

Fig. 15-19b Intercuspal position.

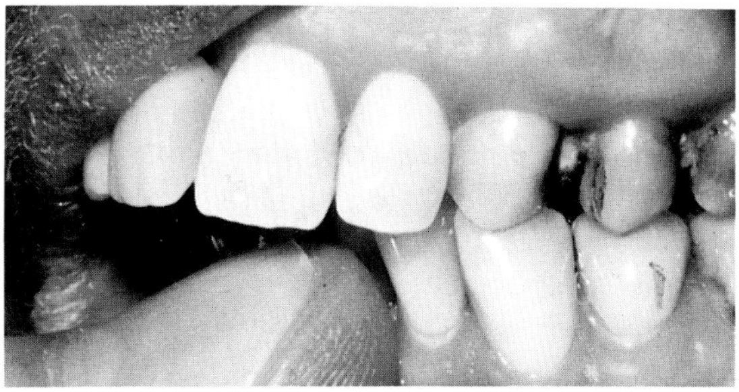

Fig. 15-19c Retruded contact position 3 years after the fracture. Note the large sagittal RCP–ICP distance.

cess, and their consequences for occlusal stability. In most children with condylar fractures, the remodeling capacity of the joint will lead to a normalization of skeletal relations and occlusion. In many adults an abnormal relationship between the retruded and intercuspal positions of the mandible (large RCP-ICP distance; Figs. 15-19a to c) will persist for many years after the fracture (Lindahl, 1977). Mandibular fracture, therefore, is one cause of dual bite (Egermark-Eriksson et al., 1979).

Effects of prior dental treatment

Deviations from the "ideal" dentition previously described can be treated with orthodontics, occlusal adjustment, operative and prosthetic dentistry, and, on occasion, surgery. But when the subject is well adapted to the condition (a physiologic occlusion), the morphological or functional malocclusion is best left untreated. There is very little documentation about long-term effects of different methods of treating—or not treating—occlusal problems. This is not surprising, since it is extremely difficult to perform clinical studies to answer questions about treatment efficacy and make comparisons among treatment methods. A few studies have been successful. Longitudinal studies of orthodontically treated patients 5 to 10 years after termination of treatment have, in general, shown some small relapses but have maintained good function of the masticatory system (Larsson and Ronnerman, 1981). Long term, the signs and symptoms of TM disorders did not differ between orthodontically treated subjects and untreated subjects (Sadowsky and BeGole, 1980; Janson, 1981).

In patients treated with removable partial dentures, the rehabilitative results deteriorated rapidly with poor oral hygiene irrespective of denture design (Carlsson et al., 1965). However, in patients who managed to maintain good plaque control and resolve the marginal inflammation, the partial dentures continued to function well for many years (Bergman et al., 1977). This interplay between occlusion and marginal periodontitis is still more evident in the management of advanced periodontal disease (Polson and Heijl, 1980). Extensive fixed prostheses in patients with reduced periodontal tissue support can function well for many years, provided the marginal inflammation is resolved. They will fail whatever occlusal design is used if treatment is not based on resolution of the inflammation (Lindhe and Nyman, 1977; Nyman and Lindhe, 1979).

Complete dentures can restore good occlusal conditions in edentulous subjects. However, there is often a rapid loss of the initial occlusal stability because of changes in denture-supporting structures, mainly continuing alveolar bone resorption (Bergman et al., 1964). This is probably one of the reasons no superiority in long-term results could be found in patients given complete dentures constructed according to complicated jaw registration and occlusal adjustment procedures, compared with those who were treated in a simpler way (Nicol et al., 1979).

These references should not be interpreted so that occlusion appears to be of little consequence in clinical dentistry. Harmonious occlusal relationships are exceedingly important. Factors such as masticatory function, integrity and stability of the dentition, distribution of forces to withstand bruxism, esthetics, protection of the periodontium from food impaction, relative ease of plaque control, and degree of tooth mobility are some of the factors that are closely related to harmonious jaw relationships. Its importance becomes particularly evident when the need arises to adjust, move, restore, or replace part or all of the occlusion. Here, adherence to basic principles and attention to detail are required. Our understanding and utilization of these structural relationships are greatly enhanced, however, when issues of behavior (e.g., bruxism), cause and effect of nonphysiologic conditions, differential diagnosis, prognosis, treatment efficacy, and the patient's overall well-being are considered. Chapters 21 and 22 will deal with specific treatments of malocclusion.

Summary

This chapter has described and assessed the potential consequences of loss of tooth substance, tooth loss, morphological malocclusion and its relation to functional malocclusion, disease and trauma, and the effects of prior dental treatment. A consistent theme has been proposed, that a great deal of structural and functional variability exists, including local and general responses to such variability. Thus, the diagnosis of occlusal or dysfunctional problems must be done within the context of the unique morphological and functional characteristics possessed by the individual patient.

Chapter 16

The Periodontium: Responses to Occlusal Forces

George A. Zarb and Douglas A. Deporter

Salient features of the normal periodontium, particularly as they relate to occlusion, were described in chapter 5. This chapter will reconcile the implications of occlusal forces and occlusal parafunctions with clinical and research observations on changes in the periodontium.

The point has been made that functional occlusal contacts are of minimal duration and intensity. They are infrequently associated with the development of traumatic forces of any significance, presumably because of proprioceptive input from neurosensory receptors in the periodontal ligament, muscles of mastication, tendons, and temporomandibular joint (TMJ) capsule. Consequently, mastication, deglutition, and speech are unlikely to be associated with damage to the periodontium. Furthermore, these functional activities tend to generate primarily vertical forces in the direction of the long axes of the teeth. Clinical experience suggests that these forces are well tolerated, even in teeth with compromised periodontal support.

It is therefore tempting to conclude that occlusal parafunction has the potential to compromise the integrity of the periodontium. The effects of parafunctional activity can be recognized clinically as a series of adaptive tissue changes (Table 16-1). If the stimulus that provokes the adaptive change(s) persists, there is the risk of exceeding the tissues' capacity for adaptive change, and possible irreversible damage to the periodontium may ensue. However, although this "linear" relationship between trauma and periodontal damage is attractive and appears logical from a theoretical aspect, it has not been substantiated by adequate clinical research.

Occlusal trauma

Occlusal trauma (trauma from occlusion) can be classified as either primary or secondary. *Primary occlusal trauma* refers to the effect of abnormal forces acting upon the normal periodontium. *Secondary occlusal trauma* refers to the effect of occlusal forces that may or may not be excessive in relation to the normal periodontium on an already reduced or weakened periodontium.

The periodontal tissues respond to the stresses of occlusal forces by means of adaptive changes. If this adaptive process is exceeded as a result of increased stresses of varying magnitude, frequency, or duration, a traumatic injury in the tooth's attachment apparatus may occur: occlusal trauma has taken place, with rather specific microscopic and clinical sequelae.

The ensuing microscopic changes have been comprehensively investigated, and they affect both the periodontal ligament and alveolar bone (Svanberg, 1974; Svanberg and Lindhe, 1974). The lesions in the periodontal ligament may range from a slight derangement of normal ligament architecture to an area of frank necrosis, whereas the lesions in alveolar bone may also involve necrosis but always include resorption and new bone formation. These changes, however, are largely reversible when the tooth moves away from the influence of the force (Polson et al., 1976) or when the force is discontinued. The obvious example of primary occlusal trauma is that which follows placement of a "high" restoration (one that is larger or taller than the tooth tissue it replaces), and the histologic changes

Table 16-1 Range of clinical responses and therapeutic outcomes from traumatic occlusal forces

Traumatic stimulus →	Acts on →	Elicits range of changes →	Therapeutic outcomes
Occlusal parafunction: mainly bruxism of the grinding variety with its implied horizontal force components. Effects of such forces will depend on their magnitude, frequency, and duration as well as their direction.	A Limited area of periodontium: reduced number of residual teeth	1. No clinical response: adaptation	1a. None
		2. Clinical response: mild pain or discomfort, mobility, or fremitus	2a. Usually self-limiting, but should be treated if iatrogenically caused
		3. Overt clinical response: increasing mobility or fremitus, undermined function or comfort	3a. Optimization of stress distribution: • occlusal adjustment therapy • interocclusal appliance therapy • prosthodontic therapy • minor orthodontic therapy
	B Large area of periodontium: intact or quasiintact dentition	1. No clinical response: adaptation	1a. None
		2. Mild clinical signs or symptoms	2a. Optimization of force distribution
	C Limited to large area of periodontal support that has been compromised by the effects of periodontitis	1. Mobility response magnified; increasing mobility or fremitus	1a. Control of inflammatory process resulting from the periodontitis
		2. Other sequelae of periodontitis are not enhanced	2a. Stabilization of occlusion and optimization of force distribution with least possible interference to plaque control and periodontal maintenance

are not unlike those seen following orthodontic tooth movement.

Apparently, both microscopic and macroscopic changes can occur following occlusal trauma *without* any effect on the level of connective tissue attachment as determined clinically, provided that the gingival tissues are free of inflammation. In other words, periodontal pocket formation is *not* initiated by occlusal forces. It has been reported (Waerhaug, 1979a, 1979b) that prolonged and repeated occlusal stresses do not of themselves undermine the attachment of the supracrestal gingival fibers to the cementum surface. This stability of the attachment apparatus is probably due to the fact that tissue damage is confined to the subcrestal periodontal tissues, that is, to the periodontal ligament and alveolar bone.

Although trauma may be caused by biting down on a hard object (e.g., food) or else on the tooth itself (e.g., a high restoration), it more frequently results from occlusal parafunctional loading. Single teeth appear to be more vulnerable (increased force concentration on a limited area), particularly if their morphologic position fits into the so-called discrepancy category, for example, a nonworking side interference (see chapter 14), but groups of teeth may also be affected. The teeth may be overloaded simply because they are in the way of the parafunctional movements—they impede multidirectional freedom of tooth contact movements.

Based upon a 1961 study, Ramfjord concluded that, in the presence of psychological tension, occlusal interferences could precipitate bruxism (1961b). More specifically, an asymmetric shift between retruded contact position and intercuspal position would be the primary occlusal trigger for bruxism, while a nonworking side interference would be the next most common occlusal trigger for this type of oral habit (Ramfjord, 1961a). Because occlusal parafunction appears to be very important in the etiology of some types of TM disorders, it would therefore follow that these occlusal interferences are important predisposing factors in these disorders. This theory has been very popular and widely disseminated. It has led many educators and practitioners to regard the routine and even prophylactic elimination of so-called occlusal discrepancies by occlusal adjustment as being essential to treat or prevent bruxism and as a principal therapy for the pain and dysfunction elicited by some TM disorders (Dawson, 1974). Unfortunately, the experimental evidence that this theory is based upon has never been examined by means of a well-controlled clinical trial. Moreover, current research suggests that bruxism is brought about by central—not peripheral—intraoral factors (see chapter 18).

Clinical diagnosis of occlusal trauma

Clinical evidence of occlusal trauma includes pain and discomfort from damaged supporting tissues, tooth mobility, fremitus, and even tooth migration. All of these may be self-limiting, because movement of teeth, repair, and compensatory changes can eliminate the occlusal factor, thus reducing the trauma as well as the clinical signs and symptoms. A clinical diagnosis of trauma from occlusion, according to Ramfjord and Ash (1981), requires evidence of active injury. Significant radiographic evidence is loss of continuity of the lamina dura, which may or may not be associated with a widened periodontal ligament space. It should be remembered that tooth mobility usually occurs buccolingually, whereas radiographs only demonstrate the periodontal ligament space on mesial and distal aspects of the roots. It must also be emphasized that radiographic evidence of a widened periodontal space is a nonspecific change and does not in itself indicate trauma from occlusion. Likewise, tooth mobility may be caused by active periodontitis and by certain systemic factors such as hormonal changes during pregnancy.

Some authors (Burch, 1975) list the following clinical and radiographic changes as sequelae of occlusal trauma:

1. Funnel-like changes of periodontal ligament space adjacent to the alveolar crest

2. Furcation rarefaction
3. Vertical bone loss
4. Hypercementosis
5. Pulp stones
6. Root resorption
7. Condensation of trabecular bone
8. Gingival recession

Although these changes are frequently encountered in dental practice, a clear association with occlusal trauma is far from compelling. Some of these changes certainly appear to be adaptive responses to force magnitudes and frequencies that are excessive, but this is educated speculation and not supported by scientific data at the present time.

Occlusal trauma in the presence of periodontitis

Good data exist to document the fact that gingivitis and the various forms of periodontitis have a bacterial origin and that the composition of the pocket flora differs significantly between gingivitis and periodontitis, and from one form of periodontitis to another (Slots, 1979). Furthermore, it appears that host defense mechanisms determine host susceptibility to periodontal disease and its pattern of destruction. As mentioned earlier, it is clear that traumatic lesions superimposed upon normal periodontal structures do not initiate periodontitis, that is, loss of attachment. It has, however, been proposed that the progression of existing periodontal pockets can be accelerated when occlusal trauma is present (Polson et al., 1976). This superimposition of an increase in magnitude, duration, or frequency of occlusal stress (or stresses) upon periodontally compromised teeth is thought to include angular bone loss and the formation of infrabony pockets. Several investigators have sought to confirm this proposed "codestructive" relationship, but they have provided inconclusive results. Although experiments and observations on both humans and animals have been ongoing for almost half a century, the nature of this relationship still remains controversial.

Current research suggests agreement on the induction of specific histologic alterations in the periodontium as a result of occlusal trauma. But while these changes can result in increased tooth mobility that varies with the status of periodontal support, this may be reversible and does not lead to pocket formation in the absence of plaque-induced periodontal disease. The notion that imposition of occlusal trauma on an already existing periodontitis will enhance the rate of periodontal breakdown (i.e., loss of attachment) is still scientifically untenable.

Occlusal trauma and inflammation caused by local irritants are not necessarily codestructive. Waerhaug's work (1979a, 1979b) indicates that the apical progress of microbial plaque along the root surface, and the associated loss of attachment, are responsible for the morphology of the observed lesions. Trauma from occlusion does not appear to be the culprit.

It should be emphasized that the animal experiments of Lindhe and Svenberg (1974) (with beagle dogs) and Polson et al. (1976) (with squirrel monkeys) have had a profound influence on the practicing dentist's increased understanding of the relationship between periodontal disease and occlusal trauma. It is tempting to extrapolate these researchers' work to humans, but prudence must be a consideration at all times. Clearly, the popular dental strategy of splinting mobile, periodontally involved teeth as an integral part of periodontal therapy is no longer tenable. On the other hand, splinting of teeth to optimize stress distribution, when the teeth are to be used as abutments for fixed, or less frequently removable, prostheses is still an acceptable clinical objective.

Therapeutic considerations

It is not clinically possible to judge the histologic response to current or past occlusal trauma in the periodontium. The presence of tooth mobility and radiographic evidence of a widened periodontal ligament space and/or loss of continuity of the lamina dura suggest the presence of occlu-

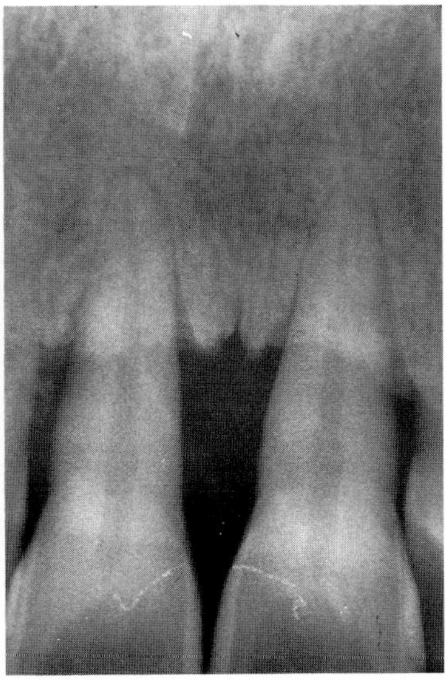

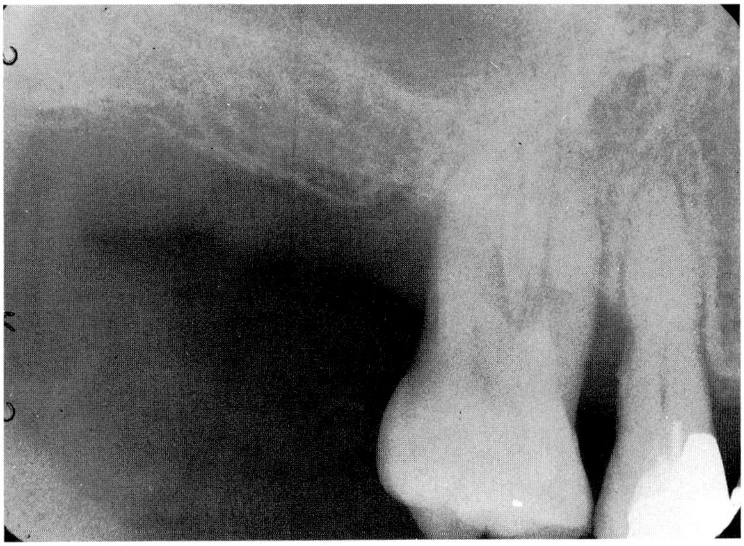

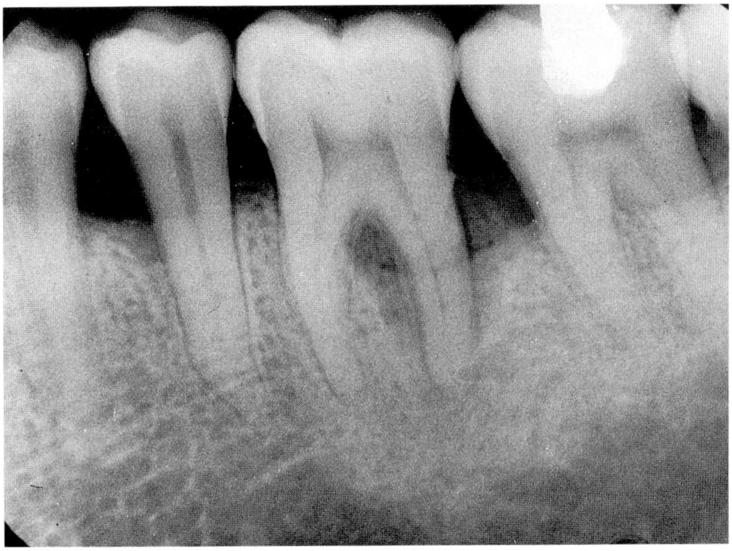

Figs. 16-1a to c Radiographic evidence of periodontal disease is characterized by different degrees of alveolar bone loss, loss of continuity of the lamina dura, and a widened periodontal space. These changes do not appear to be initiated by occlusal forces but result from a bacterial etiology and are influenced by host defence mechanisms. The superimposition of functional forces on the depleted periodontium, however, may exacerbate the degree of mobility.

sal trauma. However, the cause-and-effect relationships can only be established in the context of careful scrutiny of functional and parafunctional contact movements of the mandible. Other considerations include the adverse stress that may be induced by components from a restoration, a removable prosthesis, or an orthodontic appliance. The observed mobility or fremitus should be regarded as an adaptive response. The mobility and fremitus will probably be reduced if the force is eliminated, particularly in primary occlusal trauma. The periodontium can continue to adapt or remodel in its efforts to cope with even large displacing forces with

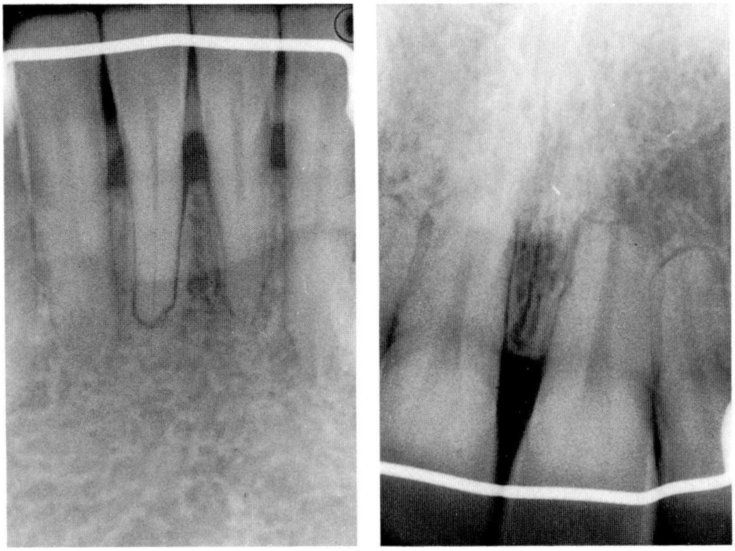

Figs. 16-2a and b Some of the radiographic changes associated with trauma from occlusion may range from the subtle to the extensive. These radiographs demonstrate widened periodontal ligament, increased lamina dura thickness, and even some degree of apical root resorption, which are consequences of traumatic occlusion in both patients. The shadow over the superior parts of the crowns of the teeth is a splinting wire that was bonded on the compromised, mobile teeth for patient comfort purposes.

resultant increasing mobility. The latter should be avoided if patient function and comfort are undermined. Therefore, patient-tolerated mobility can be adapted to, both biologically and subjectively, without the necessity of dental intervention.

Increasing mobility or fremitus, on the other hand, almost invariably demands a clinical intervention (occlusal adjustment, prosthodontic rehabilitation, interocclusal appliance therapy, etc.). This need can only be determined if the mobility response is monitored over a period of time. It deserves to be noted that occlusal adjustment therapy remains a viable procedure. However, its intent is *not* to curtail parafunctional habits, such as bruxism, but to ameliorate their effects by a redistribution of occlusal forces (see chapter 21).

Patients with advanced periodontitis frequently present for treatment with overt evidence of periodontal destruction and tooth mobility. As a result of this compromised support, the increased clinical tooth mobility is understandable, and it may be quite independent of any occlusal traumatic influences (Figs. 16-1a to c). The superimposition of parafunctional trauma on this structurally depleted milieu should elicit more adaptive changes in the periodontium, leading to increased or increasing mobility. The presence of both destructive periodontal changes and increased tooth/teeth mobility will then preclude definite clinical decisions about the relative influence of the traumatic and inflammatory contributions to the hypermobility (Zander and Polson, 1977). *However, lack of this information does not require that the therapy should be simultaneous aggressive management of the inflammatory and hypermobility conditions.* Current knowledge about the management of this clinical predicament strongly suggests that the therapeutic priority is resolution of the inflammatory condition (Slots, 1979). This resolution frequently leads to a significant decrease in tooth mobility. This clinical experience suggests that aggressive mechanical/prosthetic efforts to stabilize the occlusion (e.g., splinting) may not be necessary. The so-called technique of periodontal prosthesis appears, therefore, to be based on dubious scientific information, and therapy may be regarded as palliative at best. The splinting of mobile teeth does not necessarily cause those teeth to tighten; they are only *held* tightly (Figs. 16-2a and b). Thus, management (rather than treatment) of residual mobility or fremitus should be undertaken in the context of the patient's functional and comfort responses.

Summary

The normal periodontium appears to be capable of adapting to occlusal forces. This is usually seen as increased tooth mobility, which is usually reversible and should be managed clinically only if patient comfort is undermined.

The compromised periodontium may also be accompanied by tooth mobility. Hypermobility is certainly more overt if occlusal parafunction is also present. Increasing hypermobility may demand clinical intervention, but only after the periodontitis has been resolved.

Active clinical management methods of the perceived effects of occlusal trauma are probably elective initiatives. When undertaken, they should follow an aggressive, ongoing commitment to controlling and avoiding marginal inflammatory activity and an effort to reduce the amount of occlusal parafunctional activity. This chapter has reviewed the nature of occlusal trauma, its clinical diagnosis, and its therapeutic considerations.

Chapter 17

The Temporomandibular Joint: Problems Related to Occlusal Function

Sigvard Kopp and Gunnar E. Carlsson

The role played by problems of the temporomandibular joint (TMJ) in producing pain and dysfunction of the masticatory system has been much discussed in the literature. A great diversity of opinion still exists about clinical diagnosis, concepts of etiology, and methods of treatment for TMJ problems. However, like other joints of the body, the TMJ may be affected by a wide variety of diseases. The pathological changes of the joint tissues are capable of causing a number of signs and symptoms similar to those found in neuromuscular disturbances of the masticatory system, especially sounds and pain on movement of the joint, and limitation of mandibular mobility. Although many problems may afflict the TMJ, only six main types are introduced in this chapter. Emphasis is given to those conditions most commonly related to the occlusion. For a more definitive discussion of TMJ problems the reader is encouraged to consult textbooks that specifically deal with this subject.

Degenerative joint disease

There are several synonymous terms used for degenerative joint disease: arthrosis, osteoarthrosis, osteoarthritis, and degenerative arthritis, among them. We prefer *osteoarthrosis,* defined as a primarily noninflammatory disease of synovial joints characterized by deterioration and abrasion of the articular soft tissue surface, and by simultaneous remodeling processes in the underlying bone (Sokoloff, 1969). It generally produces symptoms in single joints of the body, including the TMJ, although generalized involvement may occur. The general state of physical health is seldom affected in this disease.

The frequency of osteoarthrosis in the TMJ increases with age (Carlsson et al., 1979). Seldom, however, does it develop in its primary form before the age of 40. Several autopsy, clinical, and radiological studies have revealed a higher frequency of females with osteoarthrosis of the TMJ (Ericson and Lundbergh, 1968; Öberg et al., 1971).

Temporomandibular joint crepitation, the single most reliable clinical sign of osteoarthrosis, has been found in about 25% of populations studied in Sweden (Hansson and Milner, 1975). This figure is in agreement with the frequency of osteoarthrosis of the TMJ found at autopsy (Öberg et al., 1971). The frequency of radiographic signs of osteoarthrosis of the TMJ has been investigated in many clinical series, and figures ranging from very low up to near 50% have been presented. The criteria of the radiographic signs differ among studies, which explains some of the variation in frequency (Kopp and Rockler, 1978). Nor is it possible to detect incipient changes in the mineralized tissues of the joint, which makes underdiagnosis common (Carlsson, 1980). On the other hand, rather extensive destruction of the subarticular compact bone may occur in spite of an intact articulating surface. This can lead to overdiagnosis.

Etiology

The etiology of osteoarthrosis is not yet entirely understood. It probably embraces both local and systemic factors. Age is a predisposing factor, but there is no evidence of any functionally important age-dependent alteration in the joint tissues to indicate that aging plays a primary etiologic role. The most important single etiologic factor known is mechanical overloading of the joint. There are strong indications that the TMJ is exposed to load during masticatory function, the contralateral side probably receiving larger forces than the ipsilateral (Hylander, 1979a, 1979b).

Research data also suggest differences in loading within the TMJ. The lateral part seems to experience more stress and, therefore, more wear and tear than the medial part (see chapter 6). In skull material, a correlation has been found between dental attrition and form and surface changes of the bony, mineralized TMJ components, indicating a relationship among heavy masticatory function, loading, and changes of the TMJ. Autopsy studies have revealed a correlation between tooth loss and macroscopic lesions of the TMJ. Loss of molar support has also been found to be associated with TMJ crepitation and osteoarthrosis in patients with TMJ pain and dysfunction.

These findings indicate that an increased functional load caused by loss of molar support is one of the factors responsible for the development of osteoarthrosis of the TMJ. Other factors that also may increase the load carried by the TMJ are heavy masticatory function, muscular hyperactivity (bruxism), chronic unilateral chewing, deformity following trauma, and congenital defects. The local mechanical factors are also influenced by largely unknown systemic factors. A combination of local and systemic factors seems to determine the development and progression of osteoarthrosis of the TMJ, as in other joints.

It is widely accepted that osteoarthrosis begins in the articular soft tissue surface. The earliest macroscopic change at the joint surface is *fibrillation,* a condition in which the surface assumes a matte instead of a glossy appearance. This is probably due to the loss of glycosaminoglycans in the articular tissues, as a result of mechanical failure of the collagen fiber component of the articular tissues because of persistent loading. This early change does not necessarily proceed to overt osteoarthrosis, but the process may progress and in rare cases end up with complete denudation of the articular soft tissue surface, which results in eburnation of the underlying bone. The release of necrotic articular tissues may elicit a low-grade round cell synovitis, which may elicit pain and may eventually lead to fibrosis and capsular contraction.

The degenerative development in the articular soft tissue lining is followed by remodeling in the underlying bone. The shapes of the bony tissues are changed as a result. The articular eminence and the condyle are thereby flattened and the marginal peripheral areas of the condyle is hypervascularized leading to bony outgrowths (osteophytes).

Osteoarthrosis of the TMJ probably begins in its articular disk. Long-standing compressive overload here results in thinning, cell necrosis, intercellular matrix degradation, and, eventually, perforation. There is an increased vascularization in the damaged disks, which has been interpreted as a sign of repair. The thinning or perforation of the disk increases the strain on the other opposing joint components, and if their adaptability is exceeded, osteoarthrotic changes develop here, too. In severe cases, the combined effect of osteoarthrosis and remodeling results in a highly deformed joint (Figs. 17-1a to d).

Symptoms of osteoarthrosis, such as pain, stiffness, and reduced mobility, can often be attributed to secondary inflammation of the synovial membrane (synovitis): hence the term *osteoarthritis*. Inflammatory response can also be elicited in osteoarthrosis of the TMJ. Pyrophosphate has been found in high concentrations in the synovial fluid from joints with osteoarthrosis. Free crystals of pyrophosphate in the synovial fluid elicit an acute inflammatory response in the synovial membrane.

Figs. 17-1a to d Temporomandibular joints with osteoarthrotic lesions.

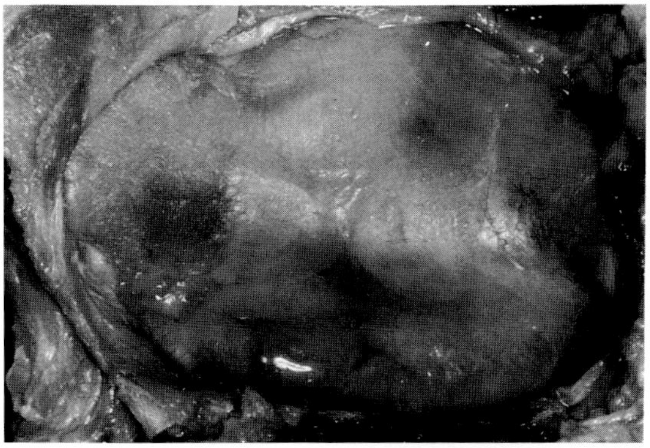

Fig. 17-1a On the lateral aspect of the remodeled eminence, the articular surface is matte and uneven.

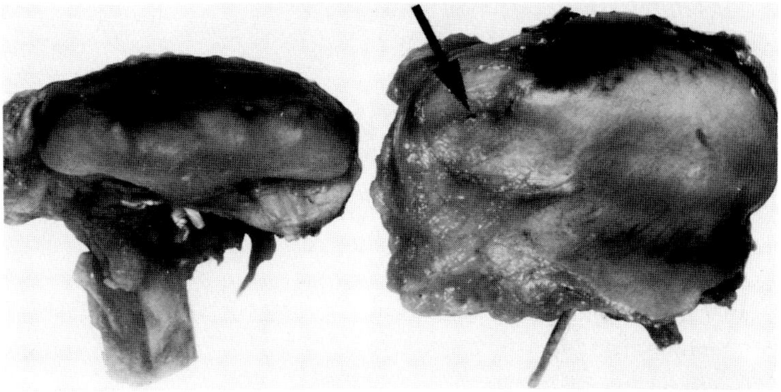

Fig. 17-1b The condyle is changed in shape, but without surface lesion, while the disk is thinned in the lateral aspect, with a small perforation *(arrow)* opposite the surface change on the eminence.

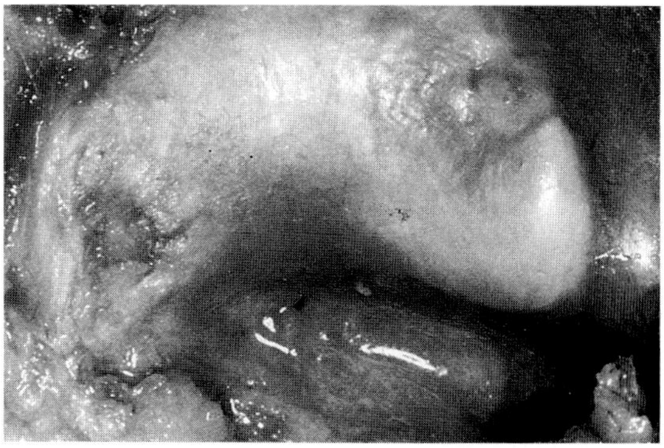

Figs. 17-1c and d Similar but more extensive changes, including a surface lesion on the condyle (which is less common than in the other components).

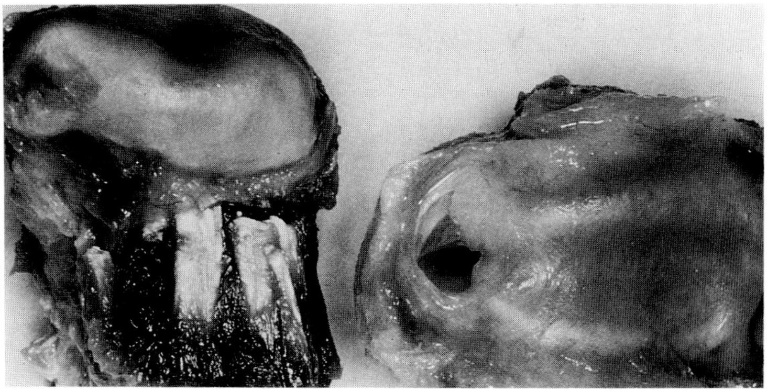

Fig. 17-1d

Signs and symptoms

The *subjective symptoms* associated with osteoarthrosis of the TMJ resemble those of other forms of TM disorders (Kopp, 1982), and include pain referable to the TMJ and masticatory muscles, stiffness, and difficulties in opening the mouth widely. Sounds of the TMJ on mandibular movement is a common symptom, often described by patients as a grating noise. It develops relatively late in the progress of the disease.

The *clinical signs* in osteoarthrosis of the TMJ also resemble those of other forms of TM disorders (i.e., tenderness to palpation of the TMJ and masticatory muscles, reduced mobility of the TMJ, reduced range of movement of the mandible, and pain and deviations on mandibular movement). More specific for structural lesions of the TMJ is a palpable or audible coarse type of crepitation (equivalent to the grating sound observed by the patient) accompanying joint movement. Crepitation of the TMJ is often correlated to radiographic signs of osteoarthrosis. Weakness and tenderness to palpation of the masticatory muscles are common sequelae in painful phases of the disease, and the bite force is reduced as a result.

Radiographic findings

Radiography is the most common means of diagnosing osteoarthrosis of the TMJ. Interpretation of the radiographs, however, offers difficulties, especially the differentiation between degenerative changes and merely deviation in form. The radiographic signs of reduced joint space, subcortical sclerosis, and flattening of the lateral parts of the joint (Figs. 17-2a to d) are associated with each other and are characteristic of osteoarthrosis of the TMJ. The conventional transcranial radiographic methods pose problems in the interpretation of joint form and joint space; tomography should, therefore, be used when possible to give the most accurate information about the status of the TMJ. Marginal osseous outgrowths, known as osteophytes, are common as a sequela to both remodeling and degenerative processes, as is flattening of both joint osseous components. This makes the differentiation between remodeling and osteoarthrosis by means of radiography difficult and sometimes impossible.

Intraosseous destructions (cysts) can develop in severe cases of osteoarthrosis, especially in the condyle. Erosive (osteolytic) lesions of the cortical bone plate can be seen in both the condyle and the articular eminence, but they are much more conspicuous in inflammatory joint disease such as rheumatoid arthritis.

Arthrography* may be used for evaluation of disk perforation and structural damage to the soft tissue articular surface (Westesson, 1982). This examination is only indicated in patients with severe pain and local clinical symptoms from the TMJ and in whom conventional radiography has revealed nothing pathological.

Treatment

Functional overloading during mastication or during occlusal parafunction such as bruxism most probably plays a role in the cause and progression of osteoarthrosis of the TMJ. Any treatment capable of reducing the strain on the TMJ is indicated. This means that habitual grinding/clenching of the teeth should be minimized. A most effective and simple treatment is a full-coverage interocclusal appliance. The role played by specific occlusal interferences in the etiology of bruxism and TMJ osteoarthrosis is uncertain, but gross interferences should be eliminated.

Loss of molar support is probably a common cause of TMJ overloading. Replacement of lost molar support is, therefore, a primary objective in patients in painful phases of TMJ osteoarthrosis. Patients with chronic unilateral mastication should be taught to switch the bolus in order to achieve multidirectional chewing. Physical exercise is a good supplementary form of treatment when pain has subsided. It prevents muscular atrophy, diminishes the risk of capsular contrac-

*Injection of a radiopaque dye into one or both joint compartments.

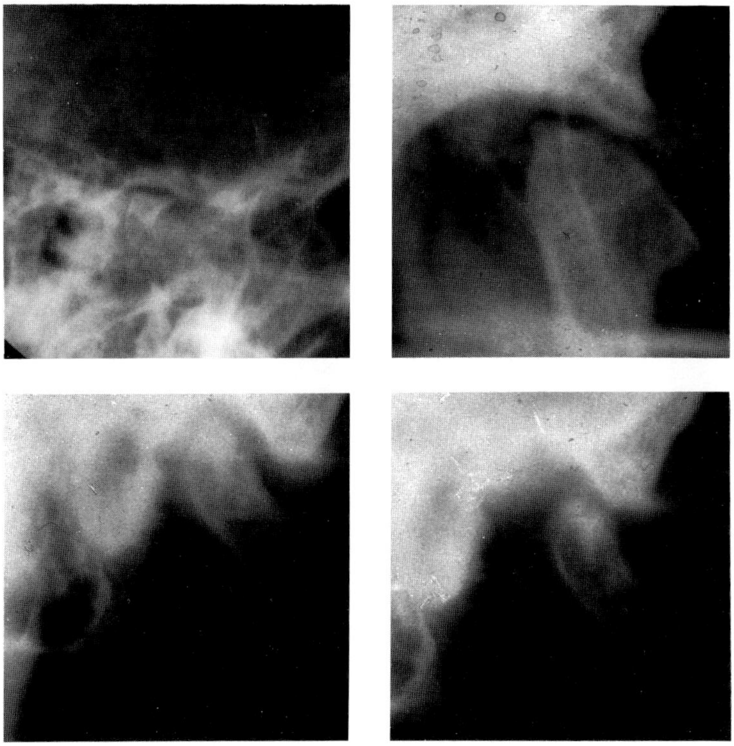

Figs. 17-2a to d Radiographic findings in TMJ osteoarthrosis.

Fig. 17-2a *(left)* Lateral oblique transcranial projection of TMJ showing flattening and irregularity of the cortical lining.

Fig. 17-2b *(right)* Transmaxillary projection of TMJ showing flattening and cortical sclerosis of the laterosuperior part of the condyle.

Fig. 17-2c *(left)* Tomogram of TMJ in intercuspal position showing a normal joint space.

Fig. 17-2d *(right)* Tomogram of TMJ in protruded position showing a reduced space between the condyle and the eminence, suggesting a disk perforation. Observe the sclerosed and irregular/eroded condyle.

tion, and restores the mandibular mobility. Rest, heat, and soft food may mitigate pain and supplement other treatments. Infrared light, shortwave diathermy, and ultrasound have beneficial short-term effects in some patients. The palliative effect is ascribed to muscular relaxation and increased blood supply to the joints and muscles. The best effect is obtained by a combination of heat and physical exercise, because heat increases the elasticity of the tissues and makes the exercises more effective.

In patients with moderate to severe pain it is often useful to prescribe an analgesic drug initially to make the patient more comfortable until further treatment can be given. Pain in osteoarthrotic joints often has an inflammatory component, for which reason a drug with both analgesic and anti-inflammatory properties should be used. Intraarticular injection of corticosteroid sometimes is indicated in patients with severe pain caused by secondary synovitis. It can often be used successfully as short-term treatment of patients with persistent TMJ pain in whom conventional therapy has failed. Surgical treatment is only indicated in very few patients with long-standing severe local pain in the TMJ with both clinical (palpatory tenderness or crepitation) and radiographic evidence of osteoarthrosis that does not respond to other treatment.

Rheumatoid arthritis

The most important of the inflammatory joint diseases that may afflict the TMJ is rheumatoid arthritis (RA), a systemic connective tissue disease of inflammatory nature. The disease may involve any joint of the body, but often starts in peripheral joints, like finger and toe joints, spreading proximally eventually to involve large joints, such as the knee and shoulder. The extent of joint involvement and the severity of the inflammatory process can vary considerably, but often the disease turns a slow, chronic course with progressive destruction of cartilage, bone, and other joint tissues and weakening of the nearby muscles. This process often results in a stiff and deformed joint.

The occurrence of TMJ symptoms caused by RA involvement depends on the severity of the systemic disease, but according to several clinical investigations, it can be expected that approximately every second patient with RA will also experience symptoms from the TMJ. The occurrence of radiographic signs of RA in the TMJ is more frequent than subjective and clinical symptoms—around 70%. In Stockholm, Sweden, 2.5% of the population above 20 years of age has been reported to have RA, women being affected three times as often as men. The disease often starts in the mid-30s. Severe forms of the disease, with great functional disability, occur in about 10% to 15% of the patients.

Etiology

The etiology of RA is still largely unknown, but there is substantial evidence that immunological mechanisms play an important part. The development in the joint of immune (antigen/antibody) complexes elicits synovitis. Cell-mediated immunity reactions (lymphocytes) are also able to mediate synovitis. The etiology appears to be complex, and several other factors, among them genetic factors and stress, also play roles.

The rheumatoid process starts as an inflammatory reaction in the synovial membrane (synovitis) and surrounding connective tissue (capsulitis). The synovial membrane becomes hyperplastic and granulomatous (rich in blood vessels) and grows to extend over the articular surfaces. This phenomenon is called pannus formation. The pannus erodes the underlying articular soft tissues and may cause destruction of the bone.

The inflammatory process in RA is not confined to the joint tissues proper, but also affects the tendons, ligaments, and nearby muscle attachments, which, in addition to articular soft tissue and bone destruction, impairs function and weakens the muscles. The maturation of the granulation tissue (healing) may result in adhesion or ankylosis of the joint surfaces and contraction of the joint capsule, with serious deleterious effects on joint mobility.

Signs and symptoms

Rheumatoid arthritis usually starts in joints other than the TMJ, even though the symptoms in the TMJ may be what leads to the diagnosis of RA. The patient must be questioned about the existence of general joint symptoms when organic disease of the TMJ is suspected. Symptoms in the TMJ include pain at rest and on mandibular movement, stiffness in the morning, difficulty opening the mouth, and, sometimes, swelling. In the later phases of the disease, the patient also often experiences a grating noise in the joint.

The most specific clinical signs in the TMJ are palpatory tenderness of the joint (laterally and/or posteriorly) and crepitation (palpable or audible) from the joint. These signs are not specific, however, and may occur in osteoarthrosis as well. Pain confined to the joint during mandibular movements is also a valuable sign, although it depends more on the patient's subjective judgment. A characteristic feature of severe RA in the TMJ is a progressive anterior bite opening due to bilateral destruction of the mandibular condyles (Figs. 17-3a to f). Due to the superior pull of the powerful jaw-closing muscles, the mandible is rotated posterosuperiorly around the last molar teeth, creating an anterior open bite. This may interfere with mastication, particularly incisal function, as well as speech articulation and esthetic difficulties. The open bite may be created in a couple of months during an acute episode of the general disease. The amount of joint destruction and the degree of resulting bite opening depends on the severity of the underlying systemic disease and varies considerably among

Figs. 17-3a to f Rheumatoid arthritis involving the TMJ in a patient with a 10-year duration of RA.

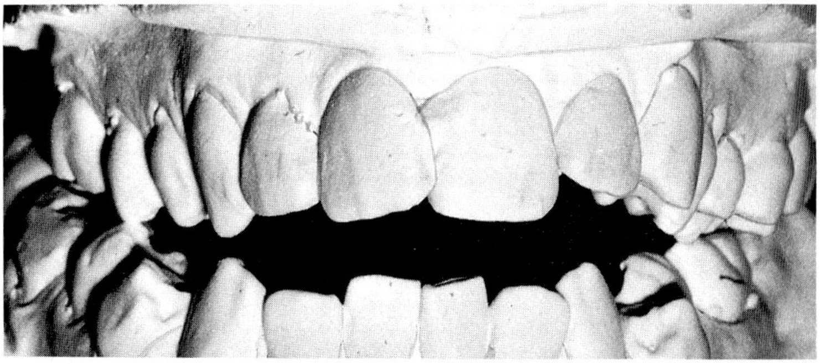

Fig. 17-3a Anterior open bite. There was a normal overbite and overjet up to 8 years ago.

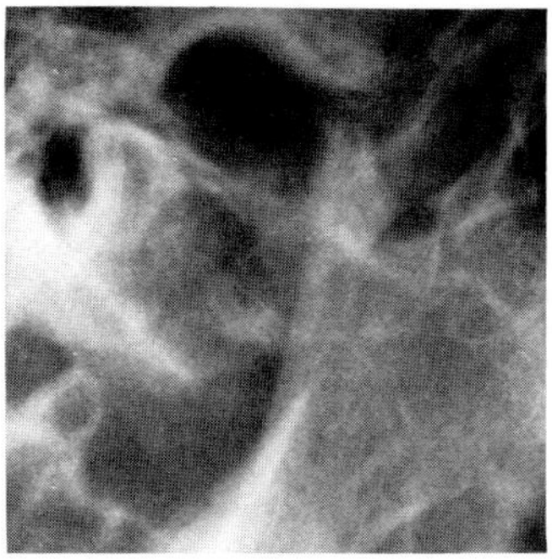

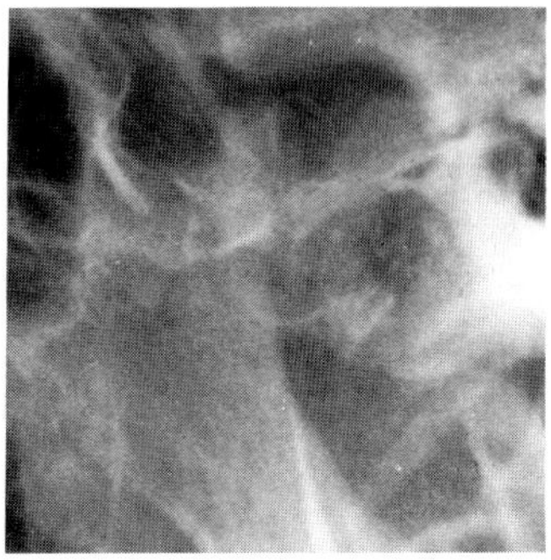

Figs. 17-3b and c Lateral oblique transcranial radiographs of the TMJs in maximal opening. Severe destruction of the condyles but relatively good mobility; the patient is in a chronic phase with low disease activity.

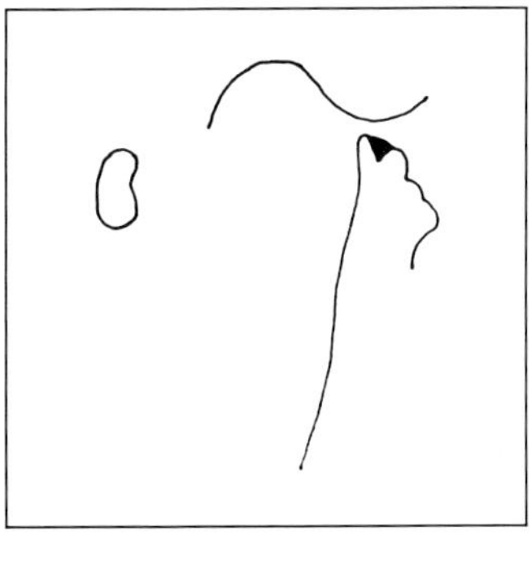

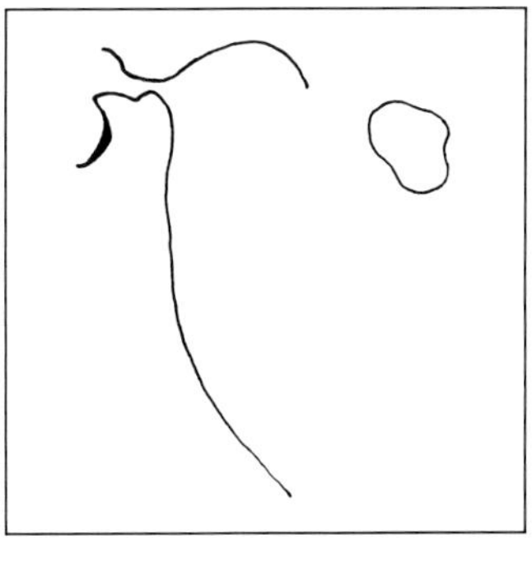

Figs. 17-3d and e Tracings of radiographs shown in Figs. 17-3b and c.

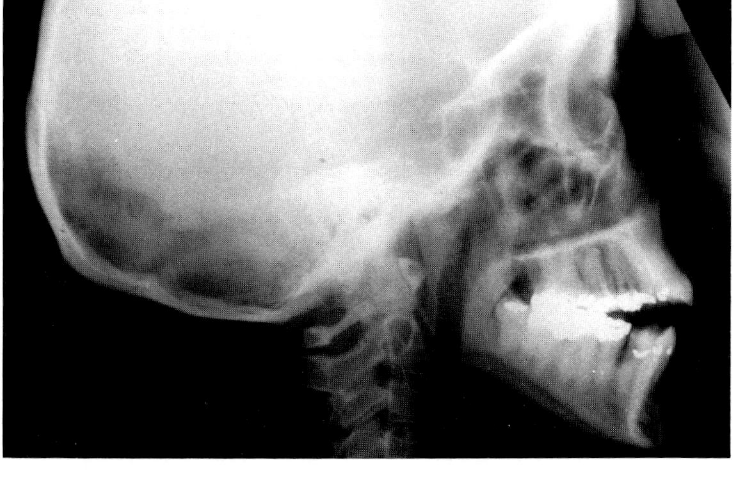

Fig. 17-3f Profile radiograph showing the anterior open bite.

patients. Unspecific findings like tenderness to palpation of the masticatory muscles, reduced mandibular mobility, and irregular mandibular movement patterns complete the clinical picture.

Radiographic findings

The most characteristic radiographic signs of RA in the TMJ are reduced joint space* and marginal erosion of the cortical lining. Later, subchondral cystic destructions and severe destruction of the subcortical bone can eventually lead to almost complete loss of the condyle (see Figs. 17-3a to f).

The reduced joint space is caused by destruction of the articular soft tissues, which results in a narrowing of the mineralized joint surfaces. Bone sclerosis and bony outgrowths (osteophytes) may also occur, but they are more characteristic of osteoarthrosis. A specific radiographic diagnosis of RA in the TMJ is, therefore, uncertain, especially in the early phase. In addition, there is a time lag in the development of radiographic changes as compared with the clinical symptoms.

Laboratory findings

There are several laboratory tests that are significant for the diagnosis of RA. They are of value when a patient with TMJ pain and dysfunction is suspected of having systemic joint disease such as RA. The blood plasma can be examined for the presence of rheumatoid factor, which is an antibody (usually IgM) against the patient's own IgG that is present in 60% to 80% of patients with RA. The test is not specific for RA, however, in that other inflammatory diseases also show a high frequency of positive rheumatoid factor tests. This and other tests, such as the erythrocyte sedimentation rate, give information only about the possibility of a systemic etiology of the TMJ disorder rather than being an account of inflammatory joint disease activity.

**Joint space* is a radiographic term meaning distance between bony components of a joint. It is not a true space.

Treatment

Generally, treatment for rheumatoid arthritis aims to alleviate pain, reduce inflammation, restore and maintain function, and, if possible, prevent further destruction of the joint. This usually requires a comprehensive treatment program consisting of information, medication, physical and occupational therapy, and adequate diet. Because this is a systemic problem, primary care must be rendered by a physician. However, the dentist has a role to play in management of the local TMJ signs and symptoms. This usually involves supportive therapy to reduce pain, inflammation, and excessive joint loading.

When the pain has subsided, or in patients with low-grade symptoms, physical exercises are indicated to improve joint-muscle function and strength. The effect of heat and short-wave diathermy is unpredictable, but could be beneficial before the start of physical exercises.

The role played by occlusion is controversial, but the general opinion is that the occlusion should be stable and free from gross interferences to exclude the possibility of aggravating the condition in the joint. Open bite caused by RA is an occlusal problem that should be solved according to the common principles of selective grinding and prosthetic rehabilitation. However, *the patient's physician should be consulted before any irreversible prosthetic treatment begins* in order to obtain information about the disease activity. It is not advisable to begin any extensive irreversible prosthetic treatment on a patient with "uncontrolled" RA. The treatment of patients with RA involving the TMJ is thus the task of both the dentist (local treatment) and the physician (systemic treatment).

Traumatic joint disease

Traumatic arthritis is an inflammatory response to excessive external trauma to the joint tissues. In the TMJ, it may be complicated by condylar fractures (subcondylar or intracapsular fracture of the condyle). External facial trauma often oc-

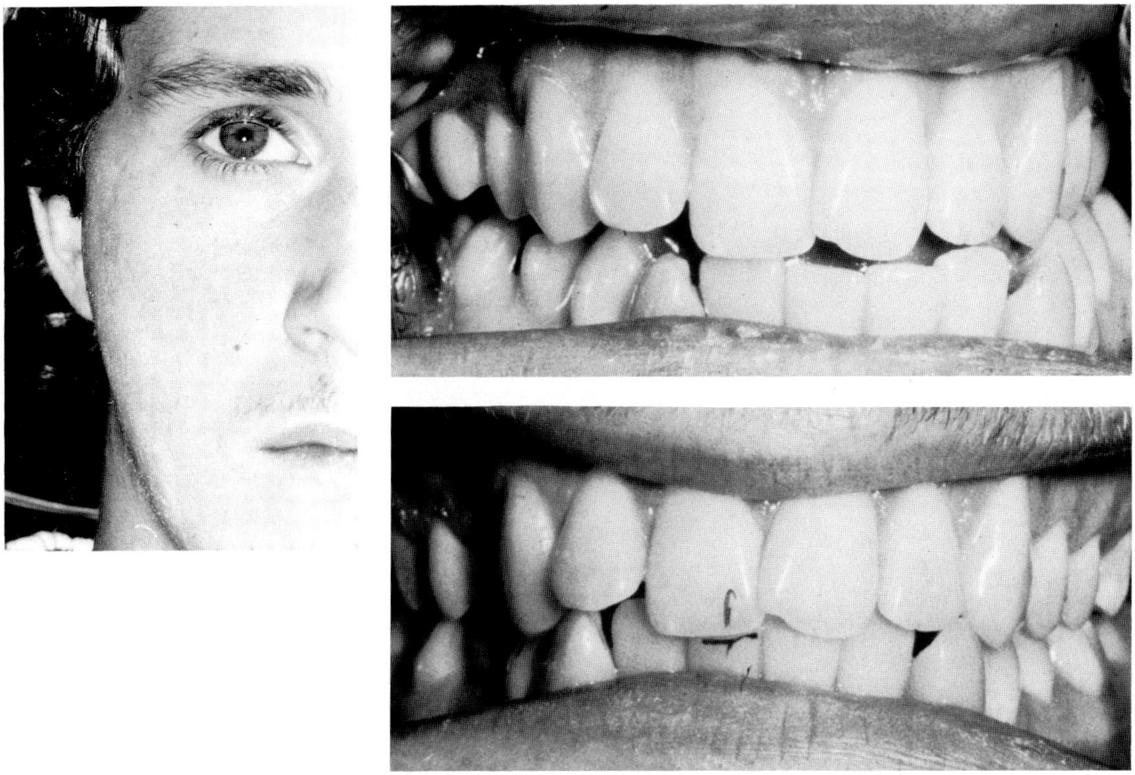

Figs. 17-4a to c Traumatic arthritis of the right TMJ.

Fig. 17-4a *(above left)* Swelling of the lateral part of the face, especially of the TMJ region, which is extremely painful.

Fig. 17-4b *(above right)* Loss of normal occlusal contacts in the acute situation.

Fig. 17-4c *(lower right)* Normalized occlusion after 1 week.

curs to the mandible in the chin area, whereupon forces are transmitted to one or both of the TMJs. The posteriorly directed forces result in a compression of the posterior, highly innervated, and vascularized parts of the disk and capsule. Depending on the magnitude of the forces, the soft tissues may be torn, and intracapsular bleeding may ensue. The capsule and ligaments are subjected to a pull that may tear the capsule and loosen the ligament attachments. The inflammatory response develops shortly after the trauma and is characterized by increased vascular permeability leading to edema with joint effusion.

The clinical picture is dominated by painful limitation of movement and joint swelling caused by the effusion. The condition is usually unilateral in the TMJ. The swollen joint is very tender, and the intraarticular effusion often displaces the mandible (the chin) to the contralateral side—which means the occlusion does not fit (Figs. 17-4a to c). The occlusion can, however, be forced into its normal state by backward pressure on the chin as a part of the examination. However, this is a painful procedure. The radiographic picture of the joint is normal, except for a possible widening of the joint space. The radiographic examination is important to rule out associated mandibular fractures. The diagnosis is thus based on the clinical signs *and* a recent history of trauma.

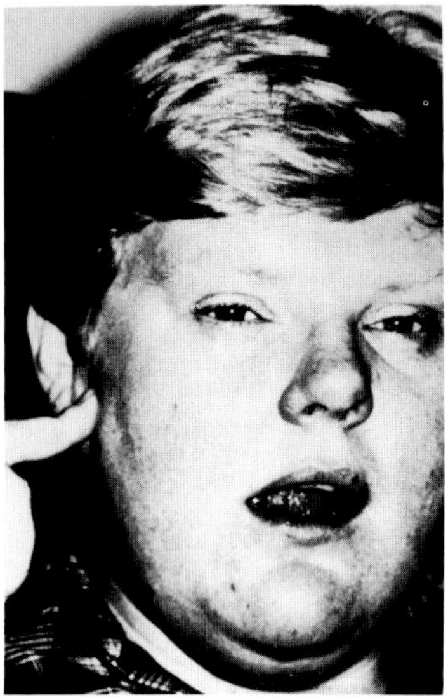

Fig. 17-5a Patient with pain on mandibular movement, reduced mobility of the right TMJ, a maximal mouth opening of 24 mm, and a deviation of the chin to the right, indicating a "closed lock."

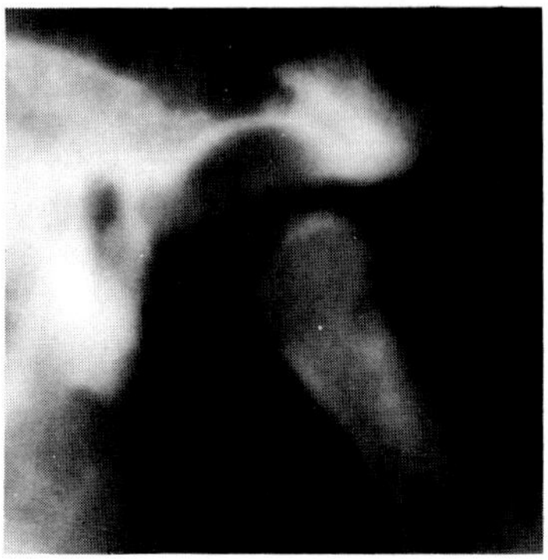

Fig. 17-5b Tomogram of the right TMJ in painful maximal mouth opening, showing an increased joint space, and indicating a locked articular disk.

Treatment

Treatment for traumatic joint disease is conservative and includes rest, soft food, an analgesic, and anti-inflammatory drugs in the acute stage. Because occlusal changes are the result of the traumatic joint problem, the occlusion should not be altered irreversibly. The acute symptoms often subside within a week. Physical exercises may be indicated after the acute stage to restore mandibular mobility and muscle power. The gradual recovery after mild injury is usually completed within a month, leaving no residual signs and symptoms of dysfunction. When the damage has been severe, however, the joint may not recover so rapidly, degenerative changes may develop, and surgical intervention may sometimes be indicated.

Internal derangement

The term *internal derangement of the TMJ* alludes to disturbances between the articulating components within the joint proper. The term has come to be used mainly for changes in the normal disk-condyle relationship. The disk can be displaced either anteriorly or posteriorly in relation to the condyle. Both conditions may cause pain and functional disturbances of the masticatory system. The anterior displacement is the most common of these derangements and is the only one discussed here.

Anterior dislocation of the disk

An acute anteriorly displaced disk with ruptured or stretched posterior attachment may be a permanent obstacle to anterior translation of the mandibular condyle. It may cause a marked reduction (to 25 to 30 mm) of the mouth-opening capacity (closed lock), as well as joint pain (McCarty, 1980). Lateral excursion of the mandible to the opposite side is limited. The condition most often develops insidiously—chronic reciprocal joint clicking (i.e., clicking on both opening and closing) may be the first and only symptom.

The cause of acute anterior disk displacement may be a sudden trauma to the mandible (e.g., by an accident, extraction of teeth, or intubation), or it may develop gradually from the chronic phase of clicking. It has been suggested

Figs. 17-6a to d Double-contrast arthrography of the TMJ. *Arrows* indicate posterior band of articular disk. (Courtesy of P.-L. Westesson, D.D.S., Ph.D.)

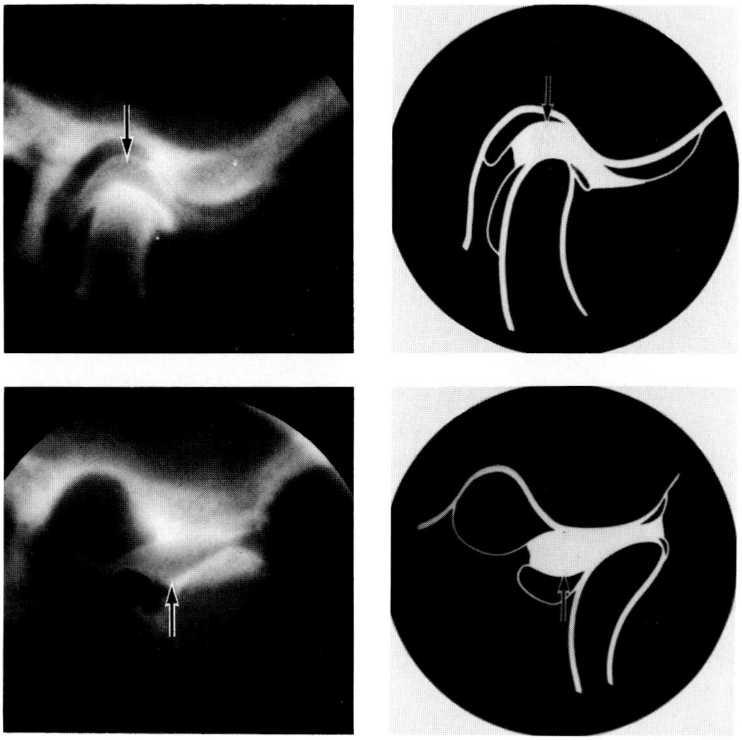

Fig. 17-6a *(left)* Normal joint with mandible closed.

Fig. 17-6b *(right)* Drawing of radiograph shown in Fig. 17-6a.

Fig. 17-6c *(left)* Normal joint with mandible open.

Fig. 17-6d *(right)* Drawing of radiograph shown in Fig. 17-6c.

that chronic disk displacement may be caused by microtrauma such as that resulting from loss of posterior teeth; chronic muscular hyperactivity in various parafunctions; or occlusal interferences resulting in posterior displacement of the mandible. However, there is no evidence to support any of these hypotheses. Very little is known about the prevalence of disk displacement. Some authors maintain it is extremely common, whereas others believe it is a rare condition. More research is needed in disk displacement, a field that has received much speculative interest in the last few years.

Diagnosis

The diagnosis of closed lock due to an unreduced anterior disk displacement is derived from *(1)* a history of clicking that suddenly disappears and changes to severe difficulty in opening the mouth widely; *(2)* clinical examination that finds reduced mouth opening due to reduced mobility of one or both joints, deviation of the mandible during mouth opening, or pain from the TMJ when passive opening is tried; and *(3)* radiographic examination that shows increased space between the articular eminence and the condyle in maximal opening position (which results in reduced anterior mobility of the condyle) (Figs. 17-5a and b).

A more accurate diagnosis may be secured by arthrography, an old technique that has met with new and extensive interest in the last few years (Murphy, 1981). A promising improvement for better diagnosis of internal derangements is double-contrast arthrotomography (Westesson, 1982). A comparatively small

Figs. 17-7a to d Double-contrast arthrography of the TMJ. Note location of posterior band of articular disk *(arrows)* as compared with Figs. 17-6a to d. (Courtesy of P.-L. Westesson, D.D.S., Ph.D.)

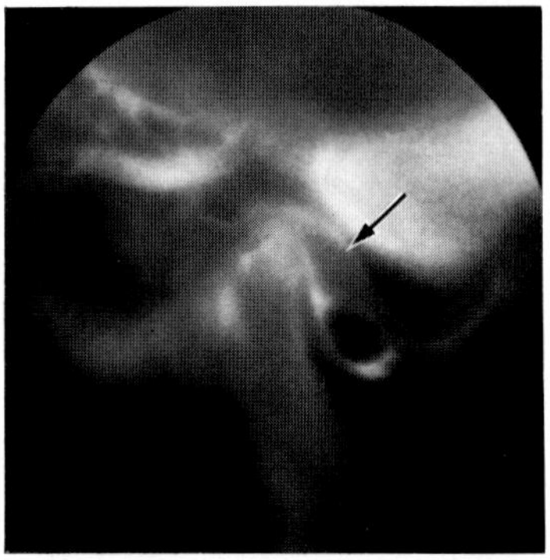

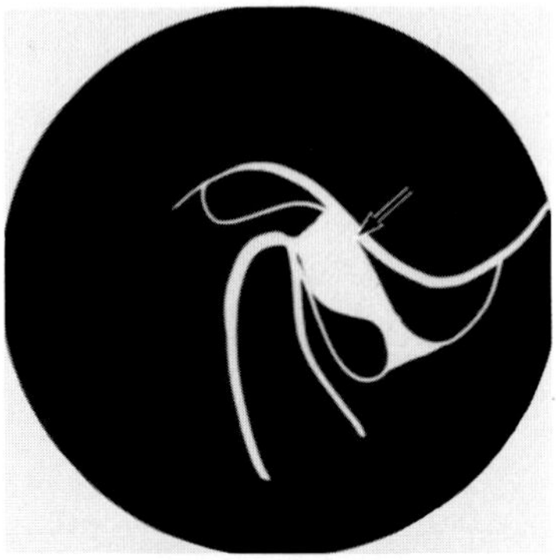

Fig. 17-7a *(left)* Closed lock with mandible closed.

Fig. 17-7b *(right)* Drawing of radiograph shown in Fig. 17-7a.

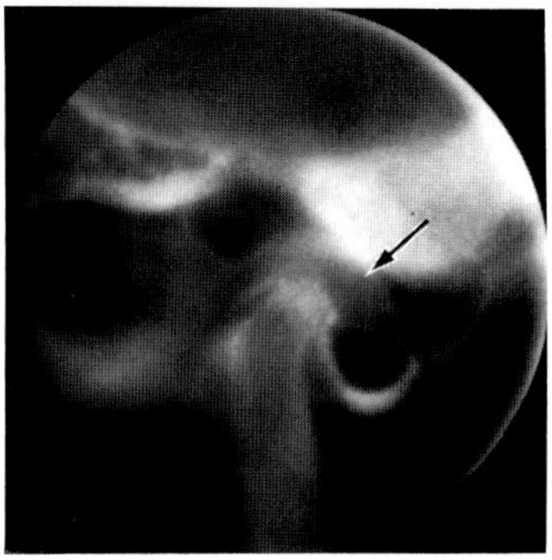

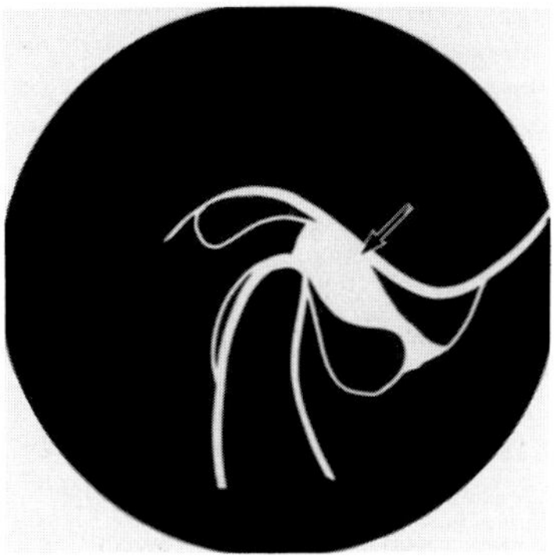

Fig. 17-7c *(left)* Closed lock with mandible open.

Fig. 17-7d *(right)* Drawing of radiograph shown in Fig. 17-7c.

amount of radiopaque contrast medium is placed in both joint compartments. Air is then injected to coat the articular surfaces with the contrast medium. The soft tissue articular surfaces of the disk, articular eminence, and condyle are thereby discernable, and a disk dislocation can be observed (Figs. 17-6a to d and 17-7a to d). The same radiographic techniques can be used as diagnostic tools for self-reducing anterior disk displacements that produce reciprocal clicking.

Treatment

An anterior dislocation of the disk (closed lock) that has occurred within 3 to 4 weeks may sometimes be repositioned by manipulation of the mandible—the condyle is distracted and pulled inferiorly and anteriorly to reposition the mandibular condyle into the central portion of the disk. The joint will then make a snapping sound and the full range of movement is often restored. It has been suggested that the normal position of the condyle thus obtained should be retained by an interocclusal appliance (splint) that gives an anterior shift of the mandible of around 2 to 4 mm, thereby preventing a new anterior displacement of the disk. The main objective of a repositioning splint is to shift the mandible anteriorly enough to make clicking impossible (McCarty, 1980). The same may be achieved in some patients with a conventional stabilization splint, preventing closure into the existing intercuspal position (see chapter 20).

Jaw exercises, perhaps in combination with a

splint, have been recommended for patients with internal derangements of the TMJ. However, all patients have not responded to such treatment. An explanation can be that the exercises may lead to stretching and possibly traumatization of retrodiscal structures with resultant pain. When conservative measures fail and the symptoms are still severe, surgical treatment can be considered (see chapter 23). In most cases, nonsurgical treatment is effective from a long-term perspective (Mejersjo and Carlsson, 1983).

Congenital anomalies

The TMJ can be affected by several developmental anomalies, embryonic and postembryonic. In extensive surveys, these anomalies have been classified in different ways (Poswillo, 1979; Ross, 1979). A simple (but not complete) classification is congenital anomalies and postnatal growth disturbances.

Congenital anomalies of the TMJ are rare. The most common malformations are partial or complete agenesis of the mandibular condyle (Poswillo, 1979). Most are associated with other facial defects, as in facial microsomia or lateral facial dysplasia. The most frequently affected structures are the TMJ, external and middle ear, zygoma, parotid gland, and muscles of mastication. Despite these often severe anomalies of many facial structures, mandibular function can be surprisingly good.

Postnatal growth disturbances

Postnatal growth disturbances of the TMJ are much more common than congenital anomalies. They may result in underdevelopment or overdevelopment, and can either affect the TMJ only or include a greater part of the face. The disturbances with local cause are most often unilateral, whereas those with systemic (general) etiology are bilateral. The resulting deformity depends both on the severity and duration of the injury and on the age of the individual when it occurs. Any local lesion of the condyle during the growth period will result in TMJ and mandibular deformity, with associated occlusal changes.

Underdevelopment

Underdevelopment due to reduced growth of mainly the condyle may be caused by such things as trauma directly to or transmitted to the TMJ; inflammatory processes, as in juvenile rheumatoid arthritis; local or systemic infections; and radiation. Such changes may influence the development of the occlusion, and thus have an effect on occlusal relationships.

Overdevelopment

Overdevelopment of the TMJ and the mandible can be seen as a sequel to acromegaly (hyperpituitarism), which results in a characteristic enlargement of the mandible with spacing of the teeth, mandibular prognathism, and an increased gonial angle. These changes often affect occlusal relationships (see Fig. 15-18).

Unilateral hyperplasia

Unilateral hyperplasia of the mandibular condyle is relatively rare and is of unknown etiology. It is usually—perhaps always—congenital, but is often not noticed until adolescence, when the condylar growth is increased and the mandibular neck is elongated. The articular eminence and fossa accommodate to the changed shape of the condyle by remodeling. The increased growth usually starts in the teenage years and causes a gradually increased asymmetry of the face. The chin is displaced toward the unaffected side, often resulting in a crossbite malocclusion. Tooth contacts are often lost on the affected side, and in a slowly progressing case a compensatory eruption of the teeth may occur in an attempt to restore occlusal contact.

All of the anomalies and growth disturbances

described result in occlusal disturbances, reduced joint and mandibular mobility, reduced bite force, and impaired chewing efficiency. The treatment of unilateral condylar hyperplasia is often surgical, including complete condylectomy or a less radical condylotomy. The postoperative mandibular function is most often acceptable, although the bite force is reduced on the side operated on, and there is a deviation toward the side operated on during mouth opening. If the condyle is no longer growing, the facial deformity can be corrected by osteotomy of the ramus to shorten the affected side of the mandible.

Other diseases

There are diseases other than those described that can affect the TMJ. For example, neoplasms are of differential diagnostic importance, but are so rare that they will not be described further in this chapter.

Summary

There are many diseases or disorders that may involve the TMJ. Except for osteoarthrosis, specific evidence of a contributory occlusal etiology is lacking. Occlusal form and function may, however, be strongly influenced by these TMJ conditions. Thus, this chapter has reviewed such problems as osteoarthrosis, rheumatoid arthritis, traumatic joint disease, internal derangement, congenital anomalies, and postnatal growth disturbances.

Chapter 18

Occlusal Parafunction

John D. Rugh and Richard Ohrbach

Occlusal parafunctions include bruxism (teeth grinding or clenching), lip-biting, thumb-sucking, and abnormal posturing of the jaw. These behaviors have historically been called parafunction because, in contrast to functional behaviors such as mastication, deglutition, or speaking, these behaviors appear to have no functional purpose.

Parafunctional activities are common and usually do not adversely affect the structures of the mouth. However, in some patients these parafunctional habits are extremely destructive and result in some of the most frustrating problems for the dentist. Oral parafunctional behaviors can result in excessive tooth wear, muscular pain, severe malocclusion, degenerative joint conditions, temporomandibular joint (TMJ) disk derangements, muscular hypertrophy, headache, and periodontal tissue injury (Fig. 18-1). Expensive fixed prostheses can be destroyed within 6 to 9 months by a heavy bruxist. Uncontrolled oral parafunctional behaviors are responsible for a large percentage of the dentist's "problem cases." Because of the seriousness of these conditions in terms of suffering, economic cost, and personal frustration, it is essential that the dentist have an understanding of the etiology, diagnosis, and management of oral parafunctional behaviors.

Several in-depth reviews have been published discussing oral motor behaviors (Nadler, 1960; Olkinuora, 1969; Schärer, 1974; Glaros and Rao, 1977; Mikami, 1977; Bryant et al., 1979; Rugh and Robbins, 1982) and functional oral disorders in general (Laskin, 1969; Bell, 1979; Rugh and Solberg, 1979; Storey, 1979; Yemm, 1979; Sarnat and Laskin, 1980; Malow et al., 1981; Rugh and Lemke, 1984; Rugh et al., 1984). The purpose of this chapter is to discuss the more common and most problematic oral parafunctional behaviors and to review the nature of the various parafunctions, discuss their prevalence and their effects, and present current theories of etiology. This will prepare the reader to identify these problem behaviors in patients. Methods for management of these problems are discussed in chapters 20 and 24.

Nocturnal bruxism

One of the most problematic parafunctional behaviors is clenching and grinding of the teeth during sleep. For most patients, periodic nocturnal bruxism will have no serious consequences. Most have only mild tooth wear, some minor bone remodeling, and/or perhaps slight muscular aching and stiffness upon rising. These symptoms are usually self-limiting. Some tooth wear and joint remodeling is adaptive and may be viewed as an accepted aspect of aging. In extreme cases, nocturnal bruxism has very serious consequences for the patient (Glaros and Rao, 1977; Xhonga, 1977). The most commonly observed consequence of nocturnal bruxism is abnormal wear of the teeth. Wear may be observed on a single tooth or in the entire arch. Tooth wear is often first noticed as a flattening of the maxillary canines, as shown in Fig. 18-2. Notice that

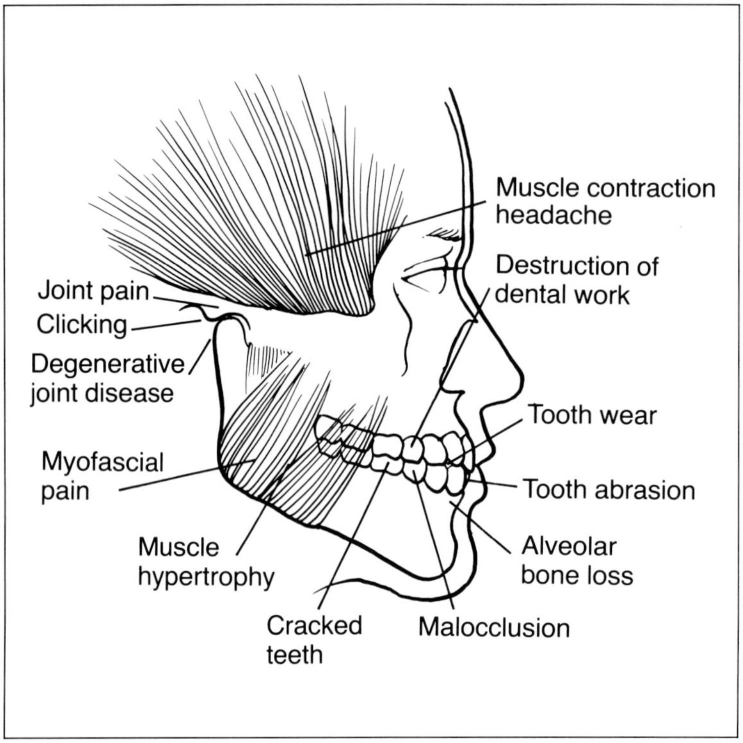

Fig. 18-1 Parafunctional behaviors can result in several serious problems for the patient and considerable frustration for the dentist. (Modified from Rugh and Lemke, 1984.)

in this patient the wear patterns indicate that bruxism occurs with the mandible held in a right lateral position. In more severe cases the wear will be observed on several teeth, as in Fig. 18-3.

Tooth wear from bruxism can be found in both the primary and permanent dentitions. During grinding some forces are directed laterally, thus loading the tooth horizontally rather than axially. This encourages cusp fracture and tooth mobility. The occlusal surfaces of the posterior teeth may be worn to a level below the interproximal contact area, creating spacing problems and resulting in food impaction. Also, sharp edges of flattened teeth are often irritating to the cheek, lips, and tongue. It has been reported that the attrition process is accompanied by compensatory eruption of the teeth, thus maintaining the vertical morphological height of the face. However, it is likely that in some individuals the rate of tooth wear and the vertical pressures of clenching have reduced the vertical dimension of occlusion and thus the facial height.

The excessive tooth wear associated with bruxism may result in pulpal problems. Tooth wear from chewing normally occurs gradually. Under these conditions the pulp recedes and secondary dentin is deposited, thus protecting the pulp. With extreme cases of bruxism, tooth wear may progress more rapidly than the rate of deposition of secondary dentin. This may result in pain and hypersensitivity to temperature changes, pain on percussion, and even pulpal exposure resulting in pulpitis and pulpal death (Ingle, 1960).

The effects of bruxism on the teeth are usually visible to the patient and dentist. The effects of bruxism on the muscles, ligaments, and joints of the masticatory system are not so easily identified, but they are often painful for the patient and have serious long-term consequence. Nocturnal bruxism is considered an important etiological factor in several muscular and TMJ conditions. These include muscular pain, tightness and fatigue upon rising, muscular incoordination, os-

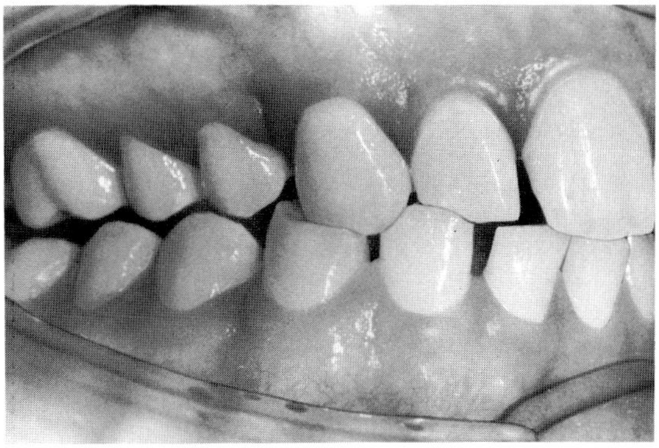

Fig. 18-2 Tooth wear from bruxism in a lateral excursive position in an 18-year-old woman. Historically it was believed that canine guidance occlusion such as that exhibited by this patient would prevent bruxism and the destructive wear shown.

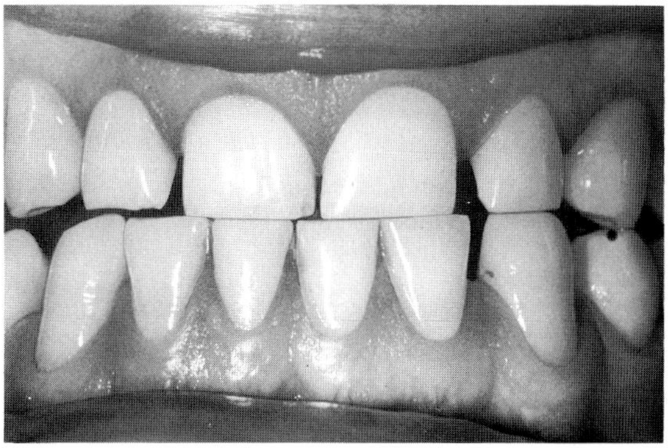

Fig. 18-3 The patterns of tooth wear in this patient suggest bruxism in lateral and protrusive positions, resulting in wear to the canines and central incisors.

teoarthrosis, crepitus, limitations of jaw movements, and, possibly, TMJ clicking and locking of the jaw. The severity of these symptoms in patients has been correlated with their levels of nocturnal bruxism (Clark et al., 1981). The disk may become worn or perforated, and wear patterns of the teeth are often correlated with condylar remodeling. Extreme wear of the posterior teeth has been correlated with severe flattening of the condylar articular surfaces (Mongini, 1975). In some cases, the long-term result is painful degenerative changes that seriously compromise the normal functional capabilities of the masticatory system (Glaros and Rao, 1977).

Nocturnal bruxism may also be an important etiological factor in certain types of muscle contraction headaches (Berlin and Dessner, 1960; Magnusson, 1982). Several studies have found associations between symptoms of mandibular dysfunction and recurrent headaches (Berlin et al., 1956; Berry, 1969; Agerberg and Carlsson, 1975; Lous, 1976; Magnusson and Carlsson, 1978; Kaye et al., 1979). The temporalis muscle, which fans out across the side of the cranium, contracts heavily during episodes of bruxism and may be a source of pain upon rising as well as later in the day. A study of 62 headache patients reported that 87% of the patients were successfully treated using an interocclusal appliance, which was believed to have its effect by reducing jaw muscle hyperactivity (Berlin and Dessner, 1960) (see chapter 20).

Bruxism may also be related to TMJ clicking in some patients. Clicking appears to be most often related to morphological changes in the joint and/or to dislocation of the disk. Some clicking is transient, however, and has been assumed to be related to muscular hyperactivity or incoordination. Some bruxist patients report periodic clicking following nights of heavy bruxism. The transient nature of the clicking suggests a muscular origin of clicking in these patients. Parafunction should be suspected in cases of periodic clicking.

Although not usually painful, jaw muscle hypertrophy may also be a result of chronic bruxism. This condition of enlarged, overdeveloped muscles is usually most noticeable in the masseter muscles and is usually observed bilaterally (Ahlgren et al., 1969). Hypertrophy of the masseter muscle may cause obstruction of the parotid duct and result in symptoms that mimic a parotiditis or sialolithitis. This has been termed parotid-masseter syndrome. Although muscle hypertrophy conditions are usually not painful, they can be an esthetic problem for some patients (Oppenheim and Wing, 1959).

Previously it was believed that bruxism may

cause periodontal disease. This theory has not been supported, and it is now generally felt that bruxism does not cause periodontal disease. However, the heavy forces of bruxism may influence the course of the periodontal condition, increase bone loss, and cause tooth mobility and fremitus (see chapter 16).

The nature of nocturnal bruxism

Knowledge of how bruxism occurs during sleep provides insight into its damaging effects. Bruxism often involves both intense rhythmic grinding patterns and periods of sustained forceful clenching (Fig. 18-4). Bruxist events are scattered throughout the night's sleep but often occur at approximately 90-minute intervals. Bruxism episodes have been found to last as long as 5 minutes. Total tooth contact during sleep totaled 162 minutes in one reported case (Trenouth, 1979).

The forces of nocturnal bruxism may be more harmful than the equivalent forces during mastication because the contractions are often isometric, the intervals are longer, and the teeth contact in an eccentric, unstable jaw position. Bruxism often involves bilateral contractile patterns, that is, jaw-closing muscles on the left and right sides are simultaneously active for extended periods (as shown in Fig. 18-4). During these massive bilateral contraction periods, the mandible is often positioned laterally such that occlusal support is provided only by the canine on one side. There is often no tooth contact or support for the closing forces on the nonworking side. This allows a torquing of the mandible, with adverse pressures being applied to tissues of the joint. Damage to the joint is thus often on the side opposite to that where the most wear is found on the canine (see chapter 6).

In patients with a long history of bruxism, considerable adaptation takes place. Canine wear progresses until nonworking side contacts develop and provide support for the mandible during bruxism. It is theorized that these posterior contacts in long-term bruxists provide balancing support for the forces, and thus protect the joints. Also in patients with a long history of bruxism, the muscles are relatively strong and can withstand clenching without pain or fatigue.

Bruxism episodes have been found during all stages of sleep; however, the majority occurs during stage 2 sleep (Reding et al., 1968; Fuchs, 1975). Bruxism is sometimes found during dream sleep (rapid eye movement: REM), but most often occurs as the sleeper goes from a deeper stage of sleep to a lighter stage. Patients who brux during REM sleep seem to have more symptoms. Bruxism is often accompanied by a change in sympathetic activity of the autonomic nervous system, further suggesting that it is related to arousal or lightening of sleep. The most likely sites for central nervous system control of bruxism are the cortical and limbic areas involved with mandibular movement. The sleep electroencephalogram patterns of bruxers are normal, with no indication of cortical or brain stem lesions. Reports from bruxers on awakening indicate there is no simultaneous emotional mental activity during the clenching or grinding.

The occurrence of nocturnal bruxism during a patient's life is highly variable. Bruxism is found to fluctuate from night to night, from month to month, and from year to year. As discussed later in this chapter, bruxism seems related to stressful life events or periods in a patient's life that are physically or emotionally difficult. The periodic nature of nocturnal bruxism and its relationship to daily activities are shown in Fig. 18-5. Some patients exhibit a weekly cycle of bruxism related to their work. Others demonstrate a monthly cycle of bruxism related to the menstrual cycle, while others exhibit no identifiable periodicity.

Prevalence of nocturnal bruxism

Approximately 10% of adults and 5% of children are aware of grinding or clenching their teeth during sleep, yet signs or symptoms related to bruxism are observed in 80% to 90% of the population (Reding et al., 1966; Solberg et al., 1979). It is likely that all people have brief periods of nocturnal bruxism at some time during

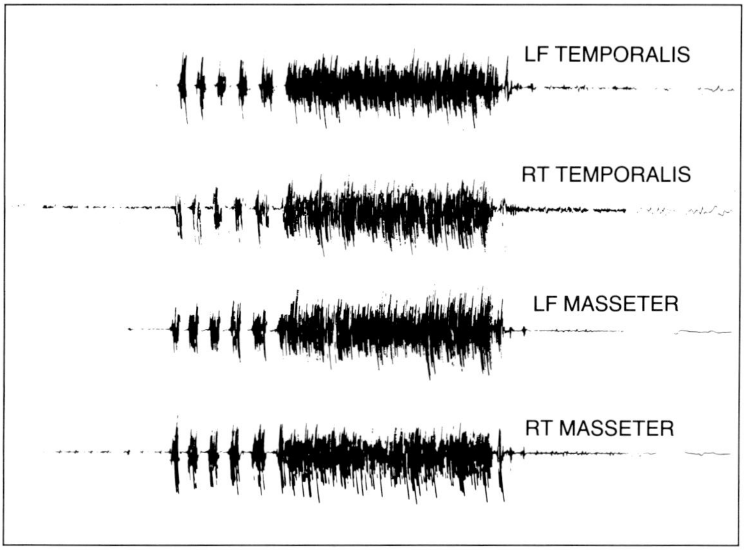

Fig. 18-4 *(right)* Electromyographic recordings of the left and right masseter and temporalis muscles of a bruxist subject during a nocturnal bruxist episode. Bilateral rhythmic bursts similar to mastication are followed by a period of sustained maximal contraction.

Fig. 18-5 *(below)* Long-term EMG monitoring of nocturnal bruxism demonstrates the relationship of stress and nocturnal bruxism and facial pain symptoms. The cyclic character of bruxism and facial pain is a common clinical observation with bruxist patients. (From Rugh, 1983, reprinted with permission from the American Dental Association.)

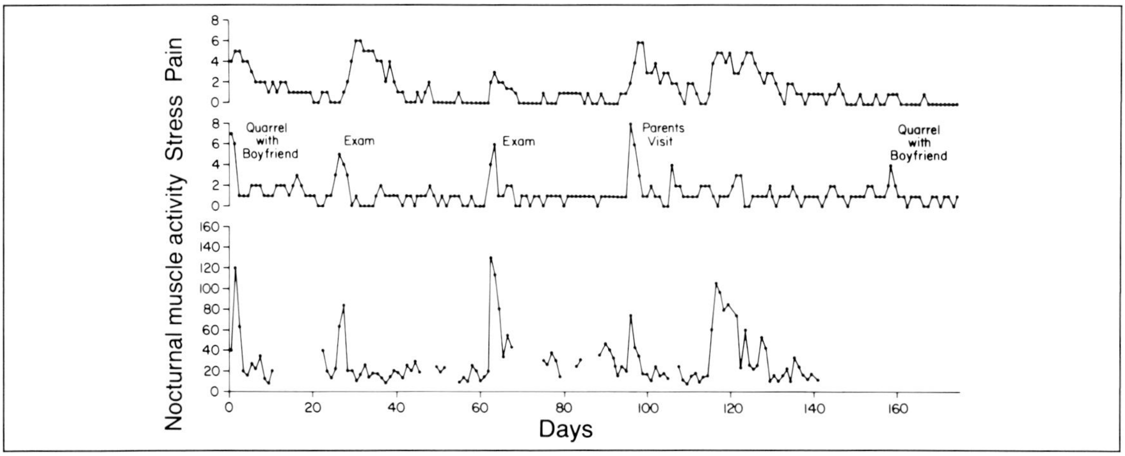

their lives. Most learn of their bruxism only after being told by a sleeping partner, or after their dentist mentions it based on an examination of wear patterns. The prevalence of bruxism is about equal in males and females.

Nocturnal bruxism in children

Little is known about nocturnal bruxism in children. Parents are often alarmed by the very loud noises; however, at this time there is little evidence that permanent damage results from childhood bruxism. Bruxism in children is found less often after age 12 (Reding et al., 1966). It has thus been common to advise the worried parent that the child will probably outgrow the behavior and that it is unlikely that any permanent damage will result. In severe cases, children have been treated with a protective nightguard.

As in adults, the significance of nocturnal bruxism in children may be measured in terms of its possible relationship to muscular pains and TMJ conditions. Symptoms of masticatory pain and dysfunction are relatively common in children (Grosfeld and Czarnecka, 1977). Nocturnal bruxism and tooth wear are greater in children with brain damage and the mentally retarded (Rosenbaum et al., 1966; Lindqvist and Heijbel, 1974; Richmond et al., 1984).

Etiology of nocturnal bruxism

Etiological theories of nocturnal bruxism have been classified as occlusal, psychological, and systemic. Early theories related bruxism to "occlusal triggers." Bruxism was assumed to be elicited by occlusal discrepancies affecting periodontal mechanoreceptors. These afferent inputs stimulated reflex excitation of the jaw-closing muscles. Bruxism was seen as the body's attempt to grind away the offending occlusal irritations. It was thus seen as a symptom of an occlusal problem. Others contended that bruxism was primarily a central nervous system problem related to emotional stress. Some dualist theories proposed that occlusal discrepancies plus emotional stress both were necessary for bruxism. Occlusal theories of nocturnal bruxism persist, although most evidence does not support these theories.

As methods to measure bruxism became available, it was learned that nocturnal bruxism was not related to occlusal discrepancies. It was found that bruxism could not be elicited by experimentally placing an occlusal discrepancy (Rugh et al., 1984) and that occlusal adjustments to eliminate discrepancies did not stop nocturnal bruxism (Kardachi et al., 1978; Bailey and Rugh, 1980). It has also been observed that many people have significant occlusal problems but do not brux, whereas others without occlusal problems have a problem with bruxism (Ingervall et al., 1980; Egermark-Eriksson et al., 1981). In general, there is little evidence to support the theory that nocturnal bruxism is a reaction to occlusal imperfections. As we will discuss later, occlusal features are considered very important in determining how forces of bruxism are distributed in the masticatory system; however, occlusal features are no longer considered an important etiological factor in nocturnal bruxism.

Evidence is mounting that nocturnal bruxism is a sleep disorder related to emotional conditions. Levels of nocturnal bruxism vary greatly from night to night but have been correlated with emotionally stressful days and major life crises such as divorce, loss of job, and major examinations (Rugh and Solberg, 1975; Clark et al., 1981). Anticipation of a stressful event also appears to elicit bruxism (Funch and Gale, 1980). It is known that presleep emotional experiences affect several aspects of sleep; however, it is not clear how these effects are mediated. There is some evidence that nocturnal bruxism is a disorder of arousal since it is usually accompanied by changes in an electroencephalogram, respiration, and heart rate (Satoh and Harada, 1973). It often occurs when the patient is in transition from a deeper to lighter stage of sleep and can often be elicited by calling the patient's name, thus arousing the subject.

It has also been found that bruxist patients differ from nonbruxist patients on several personality and emotional scales. Bruxist patients seldom have major psychopathology, but they often have personality characteristics that increase their general level of stress. Bruxists are found to be more aggressive (Olkinuora, 1972), and tend to be hostile, anxious, and hyperactive (Vernallis, 1955; Thaller, 1960). In addition, bruxist patients often display other symptoms of stress, and have a higher frequency of minor nervous disorders (Olkinuora, 1972).

There are other, less common, causes of bruxism. Nocturnal bruxism has been reported with use of amphetamines (Ashcroft et al., 1965) and with therapeutic doses of L-dopa (Magee, 1970). Fenfluramine, an amphetamine derivative, has also been associated with bruxism (Brandon, 1969). Bruxism is also observed in patients with tardive dyskinesia, which is believed to result from long-term phenothiazine use (Kamen, 1975). There have also been reports that alcohol increases bruxism in certain subjects (Hartmann, 1979). There is also evidence of a genetic predisposition for bruxism (Abe and Shimakawa, 1966; Reding et al., 1966)—children of patients who were bruxists in childhood are more apt to also grind.

Diagnosis of nocturnal bruxism

The ease with which nocturnal tooth clenching or grinding is identified varies among patients. As noted earlier, approximately 10% of the adult population and 5% of children will be aware of their nocturnal bruxism, and thus can be identified simply by questioning them. Their awareness is usually the result of being told by someone who has heard grinding noises. But because only about 20% of bruxist episodes are accompanied by noise, most bruxism will not be identified simply by asking the patient.

Bruxism may be identified in another 40% to 60% by an examination of occlusal wear patterns. Flattening of the cusp tips of the maxillary canines is a frequent sign. Bruxism may also be identified by examining other wear facets. Occlusal facets that appear smooth and shiny often indicate an active bruxist. When bruxism has stopped or the teeth have moved out of contact, these wear facets become dull and appear more like the remaining enamel tooth surfaces. The smooth, shiny, wear facets are usually not the result of normal mastication. Tooth mobility and fractured restorations should also raise suspicion.

In some patients—perhaps the remaining 25% to 45%—whose nocturnal bruxism involves primarily clenching rather than grinding, there is minimal tooth wear. However, the patient may report muscle or joint pain, fatigue, and/or stiffness upon waking. Anterior temporalis headaches are commonly reported. Questioning the patient regarding these symptoms is often useful in identifying bruxism in this population. Muscle hypertrophy is also a helpful clue. A patient's report of muscular tightness or fatigue upon waking is perhaps one of the best aids in identifying nocturnal bruxist patients. These patients may also report a transient hypersensitivity of the teeth. The symptoms are usually more prominent on waking and diminish as the day progresses. With regard to this temporal pattern, it should be remembered that some muscular aches and pains resulting from overuse do not peak until 18 to 24 hours after the strenuous exercise. This delayed muscular soreness is commonly experienced the day after unaccustomed or strenuous physical exercise.

Confirming a diagnosis of nocturnal bruxism

Several methods can be used to confirm a diagnosis of nocturnal bruxism. Often the easiest and most direct method is to perform a *provocation test*. This is accomplished by having the patient move the mandible in lateral and/or protusive positions until the wear facets on the mandibular and maxillary arches correspond, as in Fig. 18-2. With the wear facets matched, the patient is asked to purposely clench or grind maximally until symptoms are noted. If the symptoms produced are similar to the patient's complaints on waking, a relatively strong case can be made for nocturnal bruxism. If a good fit of the wear patterns cannot be found, it is likely that the wear is not due to recent bruxism.

The diagnosis of nocturnal bruxism may also be tested by assessing the impact of short-term treatment on symptoms. One week of 5 mg diazepam given at bedtime temporarily reduces bruxism and symptoms in most patients. Alternatively, bruxism may be temporarily suppressed through sounding an alarm contingent upon the bruxism. A portable electromyogram biofeedback device is used for this purpose (Fig. 18-6). If the diagnosis is sufficiently firm to warrant the expense of constructing a nightguard, success of this treatment will also help confirm the diagnosis.

It is not uncommon for bruxism to spontaneously go into remission. Stress-related bruxism is often cyclic, with painful episodes causing the patient to seek treatment. The symptoms often temporarily resolve, making diagnosis difficult. The clinician must thus be cautious about interpreting the significance of symptomatic relief with treatment.

The presence of wear on a splint that has been airbrushed to a satin finish will also help determine a diagnosis of nocturnal bruxism. However, nocturnal bruxism will be reduced in approximately one half of the patients once a splint is inserted, so the absence of marks on the splint

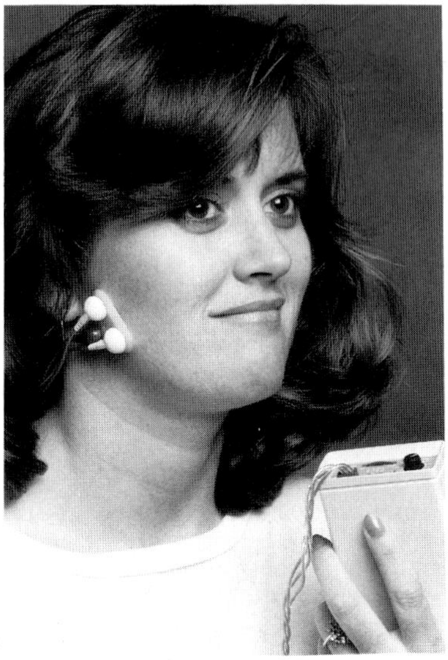

Fig. 18-6 A portable EMG device provides a tone through an earphone to alert patient to bruxism. The alerting device may be used during sleep or waking to signal bruxism.

is not indicative of an absence of preexisting bruxism. Finally, wear of the teeth from parafunctional activities must be differentiated from other sources of wear and erosion. Diet, occupational factors, and gastric acid reflux may each contribute to erosion or abrasion that resembles that of bruxism.

Diagnosis of nocturnal bruxism may require several visits to establish the presence and significance of a parafunctional activity. Identification of nocturnal bruxism is essential for the management of certain TM disorders, and to maintain the integrity of the dentition and its restorations.

Diurnal parafunction

Diurnal (daytime) parafunctional habits include grinding and clenching, thumb- or finger-sucking, lip- or cheek-biting, nail-biting, postural habits, unilateral chewing, and movements associated with musical instruments and other foreign objects. Some are more common in children, such as thumb-sucking, while others are more common in adults, such as postural habits. The effects of the various habits are usually transitory and without clinical significance. The habits usually disappear when the stimulus is no longer active. With reinforcement, however, the habit may become chronic with increased intensity and lead to pathologic sequela.

Habits such as thumb-sucking are relatively common. It has been reported that more than one half of all children suck their thumbs during infancy or childhood (Ayer, 1979). Thumb-sucking usually stops by age 4 or 5 and the effects are generally minimal. If persistent, thumb-sucking may result in changes in the premaxilla, Class II malocclusion, and/or constriction of the maxilla.

Postural habits include bracing the mandible during strenuous physical activities and holding the mandible laterally while engaged in fine, detailed work. Habits of leaning the mandible on the hand when driving, watching television, and reading may induce a mandibular bracing posture or encourage clenching to stabilize the mandible. Bracing forces, such as those induced by rifles placed against the mandible and telephones cradled between the ear and shoulder, could also be considerable.

Unilateral chewing is another habit that may initially be caused by tooth loss or avoidance of pain. It is not known what effect unilateral chewing has on the alterations of skeletal form or development of dysfunctional conditions. However, there may be significant remodeling of the joint with prolonged unilateral chewing. Patients with unilateral internal derangements usually report preferential chewing on one side. Habits of unilateral chewing are difficult to correct and often persist even though the original stimulus (pain, missing teeth) has been corrected.

Oral parafunctional habits during waking hours result in problems similar to nocturnal bruxism. Diurnal parafunctional habits can affect the dentition, periodontium, masticatory muscles, and the TMJ (Glaros and Rao, 1977). Abnormal wear of the teeth may be as extensive from diurnal habits as from nocturnal bruxisms,

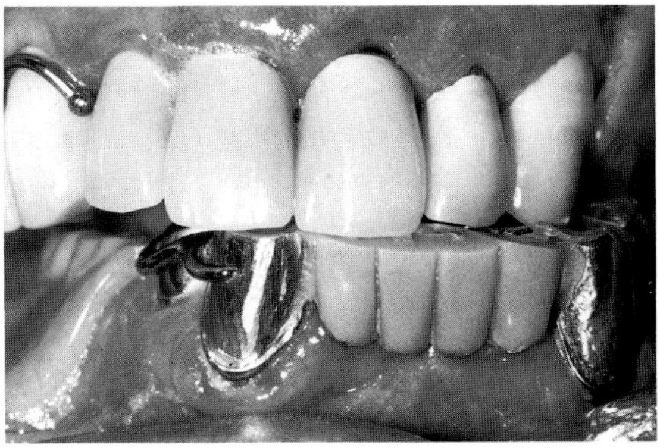

Fig. 18-7 Extensive damage to restorations from recent (2-year) onset of diurnal grinding in an elderly man. Although the patient performed grinding to both sides, he preferentially ground to the left. Maxillary anterior teeth are all porcelain-fused-to-metal, whereas mandibular posterior teeth consist of acrylic resin. The acrylic resin facings on the canine retainers have been fractured off, due to the occlusal parafunction.

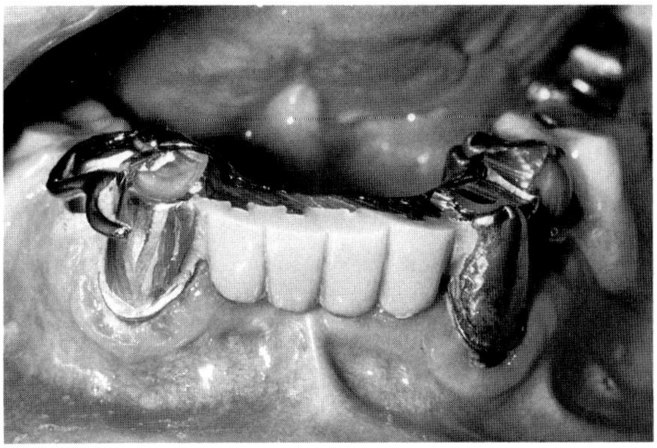

Fig. 18-8 Occlusal view of the same patient seen in Fig. 18-7. Note the grinding marks in the left lateral direction and that both gold retainers have been worn through. The cement seal on the left canine had broken at the gingival margin, resulting in recurrent caries beneath.

as seen in Figs. 18-7 and 18-8. The most common reason people seek care, however, is pain of the face and head. Patients may report a tired or dull aching feeling in the masseter or temporalis muscles as the day progresses. When related to psychological stress, the neck muscles are also often found to be tense. Transient hypersensitivity of the teeth is also frequently reported. The intensity of the pain is variable; it may be dull, mild, moderate, or severe. It may be intermittent or relatively constant. Occasionally, a patient will report that the pain is of a prickly nature. The symptoms are commonly exacerbated by chewing, biting, yawning, or speaking. The pain may cause the person to refrain from normal social activities, thus possibly producing other psychological effects.

There has been considerable research into the relationship between parafunctional habits and pain (Christensen, 1981; Villarosa and Moss, 1985). Pain can be elicited after about 30 minutes of experimental bruxism in healthy subjects. Pain elicited through experimental bruxism occurs bilaterally in the anterior temporalis, TMJ, and teeth. The pain is described as constrictive, oppressive, dull, and, in some cases, as a pricking sensation. Such experimentally induced pain may last for up to 7 days and is found to be exacerbated by cold and more commonly by mandibular movements. The fact that such pain can be experimentally induced provides support for theories that oral parafunctional behaviors can result in significant pain conditions.

Hyperactivity of the musculature through parafunction may result in myalgia, myositis, spontaneous contractions, and trismus. There may be an alteration of the opening or closing patterns and lateral deviation of the mandible.

The hyperactivity of clenching or bruxism may cause painful trigger points in the muscles. In muscle biopsies taken 2 days after exercise, there is a significant amount of disruption of the Z-bands of the striated muscle fibers, called streaming; in places they are totally disrupted. The physical changes are accompanied by symptoms of muscle tenderness, stiffness, and pain (Fridën et al., 1981; Travell and Simons, 1983).

Muscle hyperactivity has been related to certain types of headaches. It is reported that muscle contraction may account for 90% of all headaches (Wolff, 1963). There is evidence that arteries supplying the head and neck muscles respond by vasoconstriction to generalized noxious stimuli, unlike other somatic muscles. It appears that the pain of sustained muscle contraction is augmented by ischemia secondary to the vasoconstriction (Myers and McCall, 1983). Muscle contraction headache is described as an ache or sensation of tightness, pressure, or constriction. Such headaches are associated with sustained muscle contraction usually as a part of the individual reaction during life stress. Clenching and grinding of the teeth are found to be common in migraine, muscle contraction and combination headache patients (Lous and Olesen, 1982). Muscle hyperactivity causing ischemia, tenderness, or pain is thus a possible mechanism in both migraine and the muscle contraction headache.

Joint damage

The effects of diurnal parafunction have also been implicated in damage to the joints. It has been hypothesized that some clicking sounds in the TMJ may come from increased articular pressure or from muscle incoordination, either of which may stem from hyperactivity. This is supported by the disappearance of noises following reduction in hyperactivity. Clinical experience suggests that parafunction exacerbates internal derangements, whatever the cause, and that it interferes with the therapeutic response to therapy for the derangements. Current thinking suggests that diurnal parafunction in the presence of an unstable occlusion can cause excessive loading of the TMJ.

Other sequelae

A number of complete-denture patients have persistent pain and ulceration of the mucous membranes beneath the denture base. These problems may result from diurnal clenching. Clenching may be a habit or the result of a loose denture. There are other etiological factors as well: decreased tissue tolerance, denture design, or occlusion. In an experimental study, a number of these denture-soreness patients were found to have prolonged muscle response to a stress-inducing task (Yemm, 1972b).

Etiology of diurnal parafunction

Until recently, theories of the etiology failed to distinguish nocturnal bruxism from diurnal bruxism. It is now clear that nocturnal bruxism and diurnal bruxism are two distinct problems with different etiologies and probably require different treatments (Ingle, 1952; Reding et al., 1968; Olkinuora, 1969; Robinson et al., 1969).

The causes of diurnal oral parafunctional habits are varied. Some are learned and maintained by internal or external contingencies or reinforcement. The contingencies may be negative or positive. An example of negative contingent reinforcement is the patient who learns to chew exclusively on the left side to avoid pain from a cracked first molar on the right side. An example of an external positive contingent reinforcement is the patient who has learned a habit of chronically protruding the mandible to compensate for a retrognathic mandible. In this case, the learned behavior (parafunction) is maintained through subtle positive feedback from peers regarding improved physical appearance.

The difficulty with learned habits is that the reinforcing contingencies that maintain them are often difficult to identify clinically. It must be noted that oral habits often persist even though

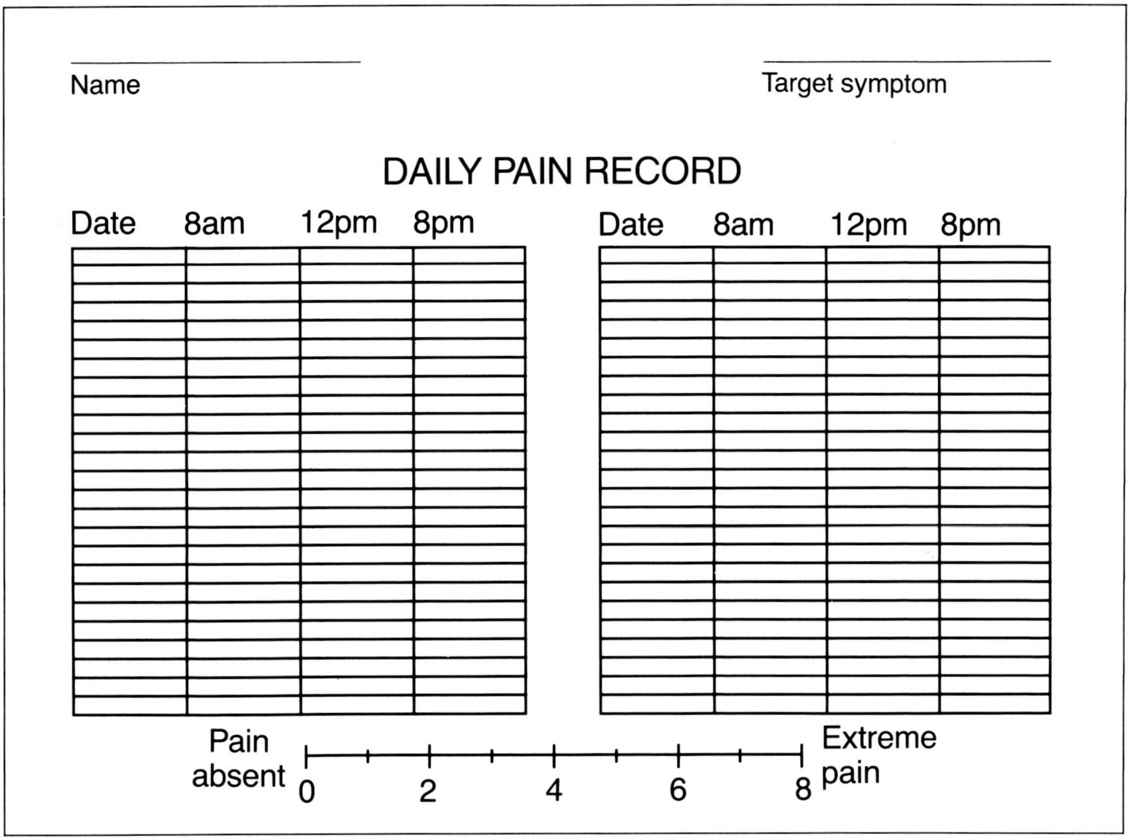

Fig. 18-9 Daily pain charts are often useful in helping to identify and increase patient awareness of parafunctional problems.

the conditions under which the habit originally developed are altered. In the case of unilateral chewing, for example, after the dental problem is rectified, the patient often continues to chew unilaterally. It is thus not always easy to determine the original cause of the parafunctional habit.

Some parafunctions are referred to by psychologists as "superstitious behaviors." This is a behavior pattern that may have initially been reinforced by the chance pairing of a reinforcing event. An example of this is the pencil chewing behavior many students perform during tests. This behavior is often initially reinforced by a solution to a test question. It is maintained by the chance pairing of a solution to a test question.

Other oral habits such as clenching may be linked to nonverbal communication. Clenching is a common expression of anger or threat in many cultures. Laboratory studies demonstrate that various emotional conditions, such as frustration, anxiety, and fear, consistently elicit masticatory muscle tension (Rao and Glaros, 1979). Finally, some jaw-posturing habits are related to occupational factors. Divers and violinists, for example, have been found to suffer muscular and joint problems believed related to chronic posturing of the jaw (Pinto, 1966; Rieder, 1976).

Evaluation of diurnal parafunction

Parafunctional problems may be quite elusive; the clinician needs a thorough history and adequate time to talk with the patient. The identification of diurnal parafunctional habits may require the use of a questionnaire, interviews, and daily pain charts. Pain charts often give insight into the frequency, timing, and the intensity of the symptoms. Cycles in the pain may become apparent. Pain charts often help the patient identify a relationship among stress, specific habits, and their pain symptoms. They also help involve the patient in the management of their problem. A typical pain chart is shown in Fig. 18-9.

If the patient is carefully observed during the interview, many oral habits become evident. It is not unusual for the patient to deny the presence of oral habits while at the same time performing the habit. It is useful to educate the patient about what clenching is and how the masseter muscles feel when the teeth are clenched. The patient will often be more aware of clenching or abnormal posturing by the next appointment. Diurnal electromyographic alerting devices as shown in Fig. 18-6 will help identify hyperactivity of the musculature and educate the patient (Rugh and Solberg, 1975).

All patients with TM disorders should be questioned about the presence of oral habits. A question such as "Are you aware of clenching, grinding, or any other habit during the day, such as when driving or reading?" will open the discussion. Most people will deny having such a habit. Yet, if they observe themselves, they will frequently report at the next clinic visit how they found themselves clenching or performing some other habit. A diary record of the time and activity at every episode often increases the self-awareness. Because of delayed muscle soreness, occurring 18 to 24 hours after exercise, it may be difficult to correlate habits with the symptoms. The pain chart is useful to help establish this relationship.

The patient's occupation may be a factor in certain kinds of damage to the teeth. For example, a carpenter holding nails and a seamstress holding pins, needles, or thread between the teeth may be problematic. Depending on chronicity, this habit may result in unusual notching of the involved teeth. Chronic pressure on an object between the teeth, such as a pipe stem, may lead to abrasion and/or intrusion of the affected teeth. Depending on skeletal form, such as a crossbite or excessive overjet, the specific habit may develop into an occlusal disorder. Ice chewing warrants special mention, as it is quite prevalent in our society. When habitual, the most common sequela from ice chewing is fractured teeth (cracked tooth syndrome) and damaged restorations.

Like nocturnal hyperactivity of the muscles, diurnal hyperactivity may cause hypertrophy of the masseter muscle, either unilaterally or bilaterally. Because this is a gradual process, the patient is usually unaware of the change. Comparison with an old photograph can be helpful in documenting the changes.

Musical instruments may require surprisingly high forces from the muscles of mastication and the cervical musculature. They may be causative factors in the development of a malocclusion or a dysfunctional disorder. This may result from improper handling of the instrument, excessive and/or improper use of the musculature, or a preexisting skeletal problem not conducive to that particular instrument. For example, an individual with excessive overjet who plays an instrument with a small cup mouthpiece (e.g., the trumpet) must protrude the mandible and then brace it into that position in order to establish the proper embouchure. Alternately, playing a reed instrument with a Class III malocclusion may stimulate a tendency to attempt retrusion of the mandible to allow for proper instrument placement. Slight protrusion of the mandible to establish proper placement of the lips for playing a flute, for example, may be a sufficient aggravating factor to cause increased pain in association with a preexisting internal derangement.

Summary

Oral parafunction refers to oral motor behaviors, which appear to have no functional purpose. They include nocturnal bruxism and daytime habits such as thumb-sucking, protrusive posturing of the jaw, and teeth clenching. In the majority of patients, these parafunctional behaviors do not result in clinically important problems. However, in 10% to 15% of patients, these insidious behaviors result in serious destruction of the teeth or dental restorations, muscular pain, or joint pathologies. Nocturnal bruxism, common in both children and adults, is believed to be a stress-related sleep disorder. Diurnal parafunctional behaviors, on the other hand, are most often learned behaviors established through positive or negative reinforcement. Patients should be routinely screened for oral habits that may seriously compromise oral health and the dentist's restorative efforts. An in-depth evaluation for oral habits should be done when signs or symptoms signal a possible problem.

PART III
Management of Occlusal and Dysfunctional Problems

Part III deals with the most relevant treatment modalities related to occlusal and dysfunctional problems of the masticatory system. In the diagnostic rationale used in Part II, we proposed the recognition of four types of occlusions—theoretically ideal, physiologic, nonphysiologic, and therapeutic—with particular reference to the adult natural dentition.

The dentist's professional responsibility is one of nurturing/guiding the developing dentition into a physiologic occlusion. While this can frequently be achieved by preventing and controlling caries and periodontal disease, other dental treatment methods such as orthodontics may be required. This is particularly relevant where esthetic considerations predominate.

The actuality or predictive certainty of a nonphysiologic occlusion demands dental therapeutic intervention(s). It can be argued that the major raison d'être for the dentist is the ability to convert a nonphysiologic occlusion into a physiologic one. Following successful treatment, the therapeutic occlusion can then be regarded as a physiologic one and can, in effect, be judged by the same criteria. In this section the diverse therapeutic methods that can be employed for this purpose will be considered.

In addition to structural occlusal considerations, the masticatory musculoskeletal system may be afflicted with pain or dysfunctional problems. These are commonly brought about by occlusal parafunction, particularly bruxism, as well as by trauma, inflammation, and other organic disorders. Such conditions preclude the existence of a physiologic occlusion, since they affect the normal positioning and function of the mandible; thus, occlusal function may be strongly influenced by these disorders. The subject of Occlusion, therefore, encompasses the management of those painful or dysfunctional conditions that influence, or are influenced by, occlusal form and function. Discussions of treatment modalities directed at relieving such disorders are thus included in this section.

In Part III, special emphasis is given to therapeutic concepts and to treatment modalities that are interdisciplinary in nature, such as interocclusal appliance and occlusal adjustment therapy. Treatment methods that are discipline-related (i.e., prosthodontics, orthodontics, and surgery) are included only to the extent necessary to place them in the context of Occlusion. Thus, detailed discussions of these treatments are not included, because they are better left to specific discipline-based courses and textbooks in these very important subjects.

The chapters included in this section provide an important foundation upon which clinicians can build and develop their clinical judgment and skills relative to the management of occlusal and dysfunctional problems of the masticatory system. Thus, Part III includes these chapters:

Therapeutic Concepts: An Overview
Interocclusal Appliance Therapy
Occlusal Adjustment Therapy
Prosthodontic, Operative, and Orthodontic Therapy
Behavioral Therapy
Physical Therapy
Pharmacological Therapy
Surgical Therapy
Occlusion and Temporomandibular Disorders: A Prologue

Chapter 19

Therapeutic Concepts: An Overview

George A. Zarb and Gunnar E. Carlsson

Clinical experience and epidemiological research indicate that the occlusions of most individuals depart from the criteria used to define a physiologic occlusion, yet appear to be healthy. The concept of adaptation is used to explain this dichotomy (see chapter 13). However, it is believed that a threshold can be exceeded, resulting in a nonphysiologic state, with the sequelae of compromised function and esthetics frequently encountered. These sequelae may be manifested singly or as groups of signs and symptoms, which are associated with faulty structural relationships and/or altered mandibular functional activities, or perceived by the patient as being unesthetic. Likewise, occlusal parafunctional activities may have sequelae that include unfavorable structural changes as well as signs and symptoms of pain and dysfunction. None of these situations is regarded as physiological.

While morphological characteristics and functional activity are frequently considered separately, it must be emphasized that, like the two sides of a coin, they are really inseparable and integral parts of the same therapeutic currency.

Table 19-1 lists some of the clinical signs of a nonphysiologic occlusion and some of the therapeutic initiatives available. It should be emphasized that much controversy exists regarding the selection of a course of one or more treatments. The following reasons account for the controversy:

1. Divergent opinions among clinicians and researchers concerning the importance of dental occlusion for the overall health of the masticatory system
2. Difficulty in diagnostic discrimination of occlusally related problems
3. The fact that different treatment modalities have been reported to be effective for the same or similar clinical conditions
4. The lack of knowledge concerning the natural courses of many conditions

The reader must remember at all times that, because of multiple variables, objective, well-controlled, and accurately documented investigations are difficult to achieve in clinical situations. There is, therefore, a lack of evidence about the long-term efficacy of treatment methods for occlusal problems (Greene, 1976; Griffiths, 1983). Much of the background of the therapy for occlusal and dysfunctional problems has developed on an empirical, rather than on a scientific, basis.

Clinical management of occlusal problems has changed a great deal during the last few decades, and we expect that diagnostic and treatment methods will probably continue to change in the future. New knowledge will emerge from more carefully controlled clinical experiments and studies currently underway in many centers. Hence, the treatment prescriptions listed in Table 19-1 should be regarded as pragmatic and tentative, rather than scientific. They are based on the best clinical knowledge available at this time and represent the currently accepted standards of care.

Table 19-1 Nonphysiologic occlusion

Clinical characteristics	Therapeutic prescription(s)*
• Unacceptable occlusally related esthetic, speech, or masticatory problems • Actively unstable occlusion (extruding, drifting teeth, etc.) • High risk of occlusal instability due to age-related tooth loss • Periodontal conditions related to occlusal functional/parafunctional activity (increasing mobility of fremitus) • Dental condition(s) related to occlusal functional/parafunctional activity (wear, fracture, root resorption, pulpal hyperemia, etc.) • Signs or symptoms of temporomandibular disorders related to mandibular functional/parafunctional activity (pain, muscle tenderness, limited mobility, etc.)	• Interocclusal appliance • Occlusal adjustment • Operative dentistry • Prosthodontics • Interceptive orthodontics • Orthodontics • Behavioral • Physical • Pharmacological • Orthognathic surgery • TMJ surgery

*Treatment sequence is a matter of clinical judgment, which depends on the patient's chief complaint(s), the relative severity of the clinical findings, and other related factors (age, systemic health, etc.).

Objectives of treatment

The primary objective of treatment is to control or eliminate the presenting problems with as simple a method as possible. The twin concepts of risk/benefit and cost/benefit ratios must be applied to all therapeutic decisions. The therapeutic reasoning might be different when confronted with structural, as opposed to functional, problems. Structural problems are often not recognized by the patient, though they are diagnosed by the dentist, perhaps at a routine dental examination. Because of the possible presence of pain and dysfunction, functional problems are frequently recognized by the patient.

Structural occlusal problems

As mentioned earlier, the adaptive capacity of the masticatory system appears to cope with deviations from "ideal" occlusal conditions. It is therefore often advisable, except where a nonphysiologic outcome can be reliably predicted, to wait for some time before taking major therapeutic initiatives. A *supervised* waiting period is especially recommended for patients with structural occlusal problems. Overtreatment is common, even for solving minor deviations from "ideal occlusion" where the normal adaptive capacity would have provided sufficient remedy. For example, followers of gnathology may rebuild the occlusion when it does not conform to preconceived structural standards. However, reliable evidence for such convictions is not available, whereas studies of patients treated with simple or even no occlusal structural methods have shown satisfactory long-term masticatory function (Mejersjö and Carlsson, 1983).

A second popular conviction that needs to be reexamined critically is that tooth loss must always be treated prosthetically. Studies have suggested that the masticatory system adapts well even in the presence of extensive dentition reductions in most individuals (Käyser, 1981; Battistuzzi, 1982).

A third concern regards the treatment of extensive tooth wear. It should be remembered that some degree of wear is natural in all dentitions (even with a modern nonabrasive diet), and that it does not always need treatment. The important factors to consider here are appropriate diagnosis and determination of the *rate* of wear. The latter may require a period of observation and supervision. The dentist can then decide when, if at all, therapeutic intervention is required to restore the lost structure and/or to control the occlusal parafunctional activity that brought it about. The importance of taking steps to lessen the amount of occlusal parafunction, or at least to ameliorate its unfavorable effects, cannot be emphasized too strongly.

The various requirements for a physiologic occlusion have already been described (see chapter 13), and, in a very general sense, a therapeutic occlusion is one that also fulfills these criteria. Many of these criteria can often be readily achieved by occlusal adjustment, although in some patients minor orthodontic or varying degrees of restorative or prosthetic treatment may be required. On occasion, major intervention with orthognathic surgery becomes necessary. The extent to which these objectives have to be fulfilled remain debatable, since they very often depend upon one's concept of cause and effect. For example, some authors claim that signs and symptoms associated with certain types of temporomandibular (TM) disorders have a primary occlusal etiology, and, therefore, advocate continued occlusal adjustment as the primary therapy (Dawson, 1974). Others, however, maintain that occlusal interferences are of little or no importance in the etiologies of these disorders (Greene, 1984). On the other hand, some authors have reported that even minor (albeit incomplete) occlusal adjustment may lead to functional improvement in patients with TM disorders (Magnusson and Carlsson, 1983b).

Several divergent opinions may apply to one patient, owing to the apparent multifactorial etiology of some TM disorders, or to the fact that these conditions often appear to go into remission with or without therapy. However, present knowledge suggests that structural occlusal disharmonies can disturb functions and comfort in the masticatory system. There is some evidence, for example, that osteoarthrosis of the TMJ is initiated by uncompensated loads within the joint and that such loads are increased by tooth loss, particularly the molar teeth (see chapters 6 and 17). The outcome of the occlusion's role ultimately depends on how occlusal contacts are used, and how a person's tissues adapt to them. A patient with missing molars is believed to be at greater risk for osteoarthrosis if bruxism takes place than if it does not occur—an example of the multifactorial nature of these problems.

In the absence of scientific support to justify the routine use of several forms of occlusal therapy to change structural relationships, it is tempting to question its validity as a reliable means to improve occlusal function and comfort. Although noteworthy, clinical success should not be regarded as *proof* of cause and effect. "Proof" must be objectively derived from controlled clinical investigations. Nevertheless, patients do have problems and they do seek help, and the clinician must try to render care within the present state of our knowledge and skills. This often means reliance on objective assessment of empirical clinical observations.

In this context, the role of centric relation as a therapeutic position of the mandible should be briefly discussed. This is an extensively discussed issue in the dental—particularly prosthodontic—literature (Helkimo, 1978; Winstanley, 1985). Again it must be stated that research on this question has not been conclusive. It is well known that in more than 90% of all natural dentitions centric relation (retruded contact position) and centric occlusion (intercuspal position) do not coincide. This suggests that the normal relationship includes a difference. Strangely enough, many educators believe that the reverse is true, and that 90% of patients should be "equilibrated" to be like the other 10%. It is, therefore, not logical to consider retruded contact position as the principal therapeutic position. However, many dentists find it practical and convenient to use retruded contact position as a reference and recording position, and a number use the "long centric" concept as a therapeutic objective (Ramfjord and Ash, 1983; Helkimo, 1978). Certainly, if a viable centric occlusion does not exist in a given patient because of tooth loss or mutilation, another position, such as centric relation, is warranted as an initial position during therapy, to be followed by adjustments to assist the patient during the adaptation process.

Temporomandibular disorders

Temporomandibular disorders encompass a wide range of clinical conditions, often overlapping, that may involve the TMJ or the neuromuscular system associated with mandibular function. It is generally agreed that the most common signs and symptoms associated with TM disorders are

1. Pain and tenderness in the region of the muscles of mastication and/or the TMJs
2. Sounds in the TMJs during mandibular movements
3. Limitations of mandibular movements

Many other symptoms have been recorded in various series of patients (Rugh and Solberg, 1985; Carlsson et al., 1982). Such findings emphasize the heterogeneity of these patients (Greene et al., 1969) and the likely multifactorial etiologies of some types of TM disorders, e.g., myofascial pain-dysfunction and osteoarthrosis (Zarb and Carlsson, 1979).

A discussion of specific treatment methods presupposes an understanding of the nature and causes of the condition to be treated. With this heterogeneity of symptoms and etiologic background, it is easy to understand the wide disparity of opinions about what constitutes reasonable and effective management of these problems. Ideally, treatment should be based on the following general principles: *(1)* correct diagnosis, *(2)* identification of etiologic factors responsible for the condition, and *(3)* elimination or correction of the etiologic factors.

Often none of these treatment principles can be easily fulfilled in patients with masticatory, headache, or other pain. In these cases, etiology may not be readily apparent except to those who have a preconceived idea of cause and effect. Despite these constraints, there are a number of treatment modalities that are reasonably effective in managing TM disorders, both in the short-term and long-term perspectives (Zarb and Speck, 1979; Carlsson, 1985; Mejersjö and Carlsson, 1983).

The major treatment objectives for TM disorders are

1. Control of pain and discomfort, usually by symptomatic reversible treatment
2. Improvement of impaired function by controlling precipitating or supporting factors
3. Treating the residual pathological sequelae

Most clinicians and authors agree that these goals require the lowering of psychological stress and/or modification of oral habits. It should be noted, therefore, that treatment modalities may include behavioral, physical, and pharmacological therapy in an effort to control pain, reduce psychological stress, and enhance function. Thus, in a very loose sense, these modalities may be considered types of occlusal therapy. Depending upon the particular disorder and its possible etiology, some clinicians also add the need for structural occlusal therapy in order to redistribute occlusal forces, correct an occlusal "disharmony," or "improve condylar position."

The characteristics of the occlusion and how it is used may precipitate, or certainly aggravate, some types of TM disorders. There is little doubt that TM disorders, in turn, can modify occlusal functions. Thus, one is compelled to adopt a prudent approach to the treatment of the occlusion as it relates to TM disorders. Although it is a somewhat simplistic notion that a nonphysiologic occlusion is an inevitable candidate for a TM disorder, clinical experience suggests that a lack of awareness on the clinician's part of the possible implications of a nonphysiologic occlusion is too shortsighted. The 1982 American Dental Association's President's Conference on Temporomandibular Disorders stated:

> Although the scientific literature has not shown that occlusal problems cause temporomandibular disorders, clinical data do confirm the two conditions frequently co-exist, but the na-

ture of the relationship between them is unclear at this time (Griffiths, 1983).

In this context, one particular facet of preliminary treatment, particularly for myofascial pain-dysfunction, must be emphasized. Such therapy should, initially at least, comprise only reversible modalities. Because mandibular position and movement may be altered by the pain and dysfunction, a definitive examination of the occlusion in the presence of signs and symptoms is, almost by definition, inaccurate. The determination of whether identifiable occlusal "disharmonies" are a part of the cause of the problem, or whether they are a result of the disorder, simply cannot be made.

After symptom resolution—and in many patients signs and symptoms improve without further treatment being necessary—a more reliable and critical assessment can be made of whether occlusal disharmonies really exist. *If* it can be determined that such disharmonies may have contributed to the cause of the problem, then, *and only then,* should irreversible occlusal therapy be instituted. This determination, however, may be impossible to achieve. An exception is when a patient presents with muscle, and even TMJ, pain symptoms that have developed immediately after inadvertently created iatrogenic occlusal changes or prematurities. It would then be reasonable to relieve such interferences immediately with an occlusal adjustment. These concepts are compatible with the American Dental Association's recommendation that "occlusal adjustment therapy should be considered an irreversible therapy. . . . It should not be used routinely and especially not during the acute stages of most TM disorders" (Griffiths, 1983).

Before treatment is discussed in subsequent chapters, some comment must be made about the placebo implications and symptom fluctuation of some of the occlusally related problems with which patients can present. The morphological features of a nonphysiologic occlusion are visible, tangible, and more or less indisputable. Their correction is frequently challenging, and their resolution lends itself to reasonably reliable assessment. On the other hand, pain or dysfunctional symptoms that may accompany a nonphysiologic occlusion are difficult to assess and even to monitor. One reason relates to the very subjective manner in which a patient views his or her pain or dysfunction. Another reason is the observed symptom fluctuations of most musculoskeletal disorders. These factors must be added to the issues of cause and effect and the role of occlusal parafunction, which also do not lend themselves very well to specific, objective, and reliable clinical assessment at the present time.

In addition, while the contributory, or even the precipitating, occlusal problem may be resolved by therapeutic methods, the symptoms may persist and profoundly influence the patient's perception of the disorder. On the other hand, successful outcomes are reported by many clinicians, often after the use of diverse occlusal and nonocclusal structural and nonstructural treatment methods. These factors further confound our ability to assess the etiological interrelationships involved in these disorders.

In all disorders where pain is a presenting symptom, many patients respond favorably to placebo treatment. It was shown long ago (Beecher, 1955) that, on average, 35% of more than 1,000 patients in 15 clinical studies reported a satisfactory effect of placebo for a variety of different disorders. Many other studies have since verified that all treatments can have a placebo effect. This also holds true for the treatment of some types of TM disorders, particularly those that involve primary muscle hyperactivity (myofascial pain-dysfunction) (Rugh and Solberg, 1979; Epstein, 1984).

The placebo effect has usually been explained by psychological mechanisms of which the doctor-patient relationship is an important part. Recent research (Levine et al., 1978; Bonica, 1980) has identified biochemical changes that are dependent on psychological factors and which may account for the placebo analgesia (increase of pain-reducing endorphins in the central nervous system). The powerful placebo effect operating in ordinary clinical situations should be taken advantage of in all therapy, for example, by developing good rapport with the patient and by starting treatment with simple and reversible procedures whenever possible.

Another often overlooked factor is the considerable spontaneous fluctuation of symptoms in patients with pain-dysfunction problems (Kopp, 1977b). This emphasizes the fact that the condition can often have a natural remission, which makes the clinical evaluation of occlusal treatment extremely difficult. Objective clinical studies of therapeutic efficacy require the use of matched control groups to which the treatment groups may be compared. Furthermore, as with any therapy, the psychological aspects of the therapeutic setting may be critical.

It is extremely important to create a relationship of mutual respect and confidence between the patient and the dentist from the very beginning. Enough time must be given to the patient to talk about his or her problems. The doctor should listen with nonjudgmental interest and patience and provide the necessary questions to supplement the patient's report. After a careful clinical examination, and when the preliminary diagnosis is established, an explanation about the condition, and advice regarding its management, should be given to the patient. It has been shown in several studies that patients who received such an explanation reported reduction of symptoms, but not necessarily of clinical signs of dysfunction (Franks, 1965; Kopp, 1977b). *The importance of this approach cannot be overemphasized.*

Treatment sequence

The sequence in which treatment is applied cannot be a definitive and identical one for each patient. The majority of occlusal problems are not accompanied by pain or overt functional problems. Therefore, standard dental initiatives—for example, operative or prosthodontic procedures, limited occlusal adjustment, and minor orthodontic movement—are the treatments most frequently employed. The accompaniment of, or the superimposition of, pain or dysfunctional problems demand different or wider initiatives, and in these cases the use of interocclusal appliance therapy, rest, counselling, and medication are prescribed. As previously discussed, these are usually employed before any definitive structural occlusal therapy is initiated. In subsequent chapters the diverse treatment methods employed will be discussed at length.

Summary

While the morphologic characteristics of an occlusion may suggest that it qualifies as a nonphysiologic one, clinical experience suggests that it is the way a patient adapts to and perceives such an occlusion that determines the outcome of function and comfort. A therapeutic overview must reconcile the patient's demonstrated ability to adapt to an occlusion with an understanding of whether the apparently nonphysiologic occlusion needs to be treated to a therapeutic one.

Chapter 20

Interocclusal Appliance Therapy

Glenn T. Clark

Theories of interocclusal appliance therapy

An interocclusal appliance is generally considered to be a removable device made of hard acrylic resin, which fits between the maxillary and mandibular teeth (Fig. 20-1). Its purpose is to perform one or more of the following: *(1)* stabilize and improve the function of the temporomandibular joints (TMJ), *(2)* improve the function of the masticatory motor system and reduce abnormal muscle activity, and *(3)* protect teeth from attrition and adverse traumatic loading.

With the growing recognition of the relationship among occlusal stability, mandibular function, and musculoskeletal health, the use of the interocclusal appliance (orthotic appliance*) in diagnosis and therapy has greatly increased. As a diagnostic tool, the interocclusal appliance, or splint, as it is commonly called, can help establish a comfortable, relaxed maxillomandibular relationship. The splint is also used diagnostically as a reversible method to test the muscular and articular responses to changes in the vertical or horizontal positioning of the mandible prior to permanent stabilization of the occlusion with occlusal adjustment, prosthodontics, or orthodontics.

Therapeutically, in cases of traumatic occlusion, the splint can provide a stable, bilateral occlusal contact pattern. Interocclusal appliances have been shown to reduce the activity of the masticatory muscles both at night and during the day; and in cases of significant bruxism, these appliances can protect the teeth from attrition and serve as a reminder against this parafunctional activity.

At present, there are several appliance designs and several distinct therapeutic approaches. Although the major emphasis of this chapter will be the interocclusal stabilization appliance, several appliance designs and five distinct theories with regard to how the various interocclusal appliances work will be discussed.

Occlusal disengagement theory

The occlusal disengagement theory is based on the concept that providing the patient with an interocclusal appliance that has an "interference free, ideal occlusal scheme" will reduce or eliminate all abnormal muscle activity caused by occlusal interferences (Posselt, 1968; Ramfjord and Ash, 1983). The occlusal scheme of the splint is usually designed to have simultaneous, bilateral, multiple posterior tooth contact, with excursive guidance on the canine and/or anterior teeth (Fig. 20-2).

Vertical dimension theory

The vertical dimension theory is based on the concept that by providing the patient with an interocclusal splint designed to restore the previously lost occlusal vertical dimension, abnormal

*An orthopedic device used to support, align, prevent, or correct deformities, or improve the function of movable parts of the body.

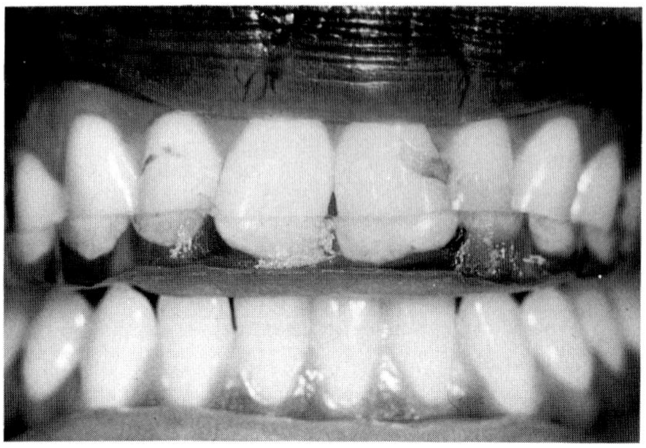

Fig. 20-1 A maxillary full-arch stabilization appliance.

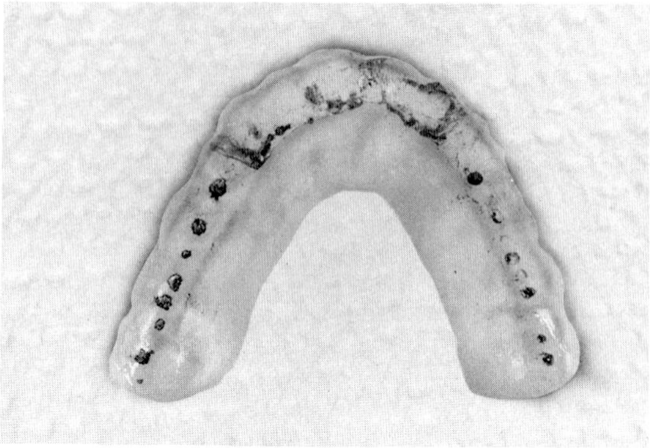

Fig. 20-2 A maxillary full-arch appliance. The contact points in full closure and in all excursive movements are indicated by the black marks.

muscle activity due to the abnormal vertical dimension will be eliminated or reduced (Block, 1947; Christensen, 1970). According to this theory, care is given to selecting an interocclusal opening that reestablishes the "original" occlusal vertical dimension.

Maxillomandibular realignment theory

The maxillomandibular realignment theory states that, for various reasons, the mandible in the position of maximum intercuspation has an abnormal, nonadaptive position relative to the maxilla. It is theorized that only by changing this relationship to a more anatomically and physiologically correct jaw position with an interocclusal appliance will the various dysfunctional musculoskeletal symptoms improve or disappear.

Three approaches can be taken to determine the need for mandibular realignment. First is the traditional use of what in the past was called a "ligamentous determined jaw position" and is often described as a centric relation jaw position (Dawson, 1974). To achieve this position and evaluate its relationship in space to a position of maximum intercuspation, the operator performs a jaw manipulation technique of a hinge-type movement, while attempting to seat the condyles with an upward pressure into the temporomandibular fossa.

The second approach to mandibular realignment is to use various dental, gingival, palatal, and alveolar landmarks drawn on the maxillary and mandibular casts to reorient the casts and construct a realignment splint (Lieb, 1977). The shortcomings of this theory are that subsequent permanent changes in skeletal asymmetries and dental irregularities are expensive and not easily accomplished, and by utilizing the criteria proposed for this theory, a very significant portion of the population would need realignment. Furthermore, no objective clinical efficacy studies have demonstrated that the application of this theory is any more effective than more conservative methods.

A third approach is a muscle-determined positioning of the mandible. A transcutaneous electrical stimulation of low frequency is applied over the preauricular area to stimulate, theoretically at least, the motor division of the trigeminal nerve (Jankelson, 1979). It is postulated that the trigeminal motor nerve excitation produces a jaw-closing trajectory resulting in a neuromuscularly harmonious jaw position. This position is recorded, and a splint is constructed to create this relationship, which is usually well anterior to intercuspal position. Thus, subsequent permanent alteration of the occlusal relationships would be necessary if this theory were applied. Objective clinical efficacy studies are lacking here as well.

Temporomandibular joint repositioning theory

The TMJ repositioning theory is based on the concept that by improving the position of the condyle in the fossa, the function of the TMJ, and presumably the neuromuscular system, will improve (Weinberg, 1979, 1980a, 1980b). There are at least two different theories regarding TMJ repositioning, both of which utilize radiographs of the joint to evaluate the position of the condyle in the fossa. One theory attempts to place the condyle in a specific therapeutic position in the fossa (usually concentric) (Gausch and Kulmer, 1977). This approach is very similar to the other mandibular realignment approaches, in that a high percentage of the normal asymptomatic population would also require repositioning if they were to be evaluated with this criteria. An overriding complication to the application of this condylar repositioning approach is that the most common method of radiographically evaluating the TMJ is with the flat plate transcranial projection. This projection has significant errors associated with it regarding joint position measurements (Palla, 1977). It has also been demonstrated that a large amount of variation in condylar positions exists in the normal asymptomatic population (Blaschke and Blaschke, 1981; Pullinger et al., 1985).

The second application of the TMJ repositioning theory is recommended for the treatment of a specific intracapsular derangement (the reciprocally clicking joint) (Farrar, 1972). This method is typically applied to induce a change in the disk-condyle relationship, which implies putting the mandible into a new position (usually more anterior) for a period of time. If successful, the patient's TMJ function will improve and the disk-condyle complex may continue to function in a click-free manner. One basic premise of the condyle-disk repositioning theory is that a disk repositioning actually occurs. After a period of "healing or adaptation" occurs, the mandible, now functioning in a click-free manner, can be returned to a normal anatomic position by multiple adjustments of the splint. This "successive approximation" approach of TMJ repositioning requires serial adjustments of the appliance, along with periodic radiographic analysis of the condyle position. As this reapproximation of a normal condyle position occurs, it is hoped that the clicking will not begin again. If it does, a more permanent anterior repositioning may be required by irreversible alterations of the occlusion following reuse of the splint.

One of the dangers in following this procedure or any of the other repositioning or realignment procedures is that *the resolution of one problem may produce other more serious occlusal problems.* A significant permanent alteration of the condylar position may stop the clicking in the joint for a period of time but induce long-term dysfunctional remodeling changes in them (McNamara and Carlson, 1979; Mongini, 1980). Further, the stabilization of the occlusion in a position much different from the original maximum intercuspation is both difficult and expensive. These factors must all be considered and explained to the patient before attempting such an approach.

Cognitive awareness theory

Although the previous four theories are the most prevalent ones advanced regarding how different appliances appear to work in clinical practice, a fifth theory, cognitive awareness, can be applied to any and all of the appliances utilized. The cognitive awareness theory is based on the concept that having an interocclusal appliance in the mouth constantly reminds the patient to alter his or her normal behavior so that the opportunity for harmful or abnormal muscle activity with every closure of the teeth is decreased. The increased cognitive awareness of the patient regarding the positioning and use of the jaw, the change in oral tactile stimuli, and the decrease in oral volume can all influence the patient to learn what positions or activities are harmful (Rugh and Robbins, 1982). Learning to alter, reduce, or

Figs. 20-3a to d Various occlusal appliances.

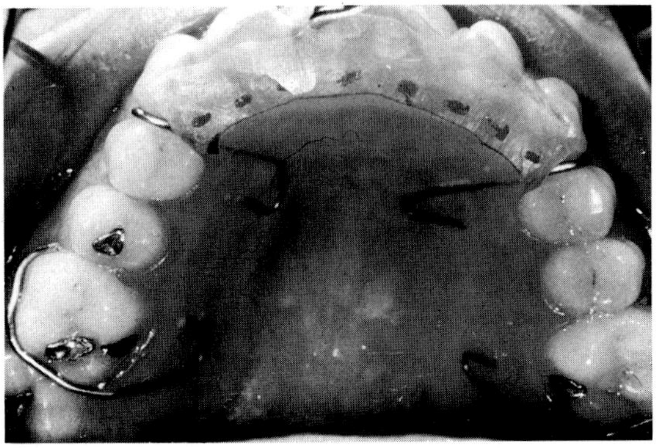

Fig. 20-3a The anterior maxillary biteplane appliance has an acrylic resin platform in the anterior portion only.

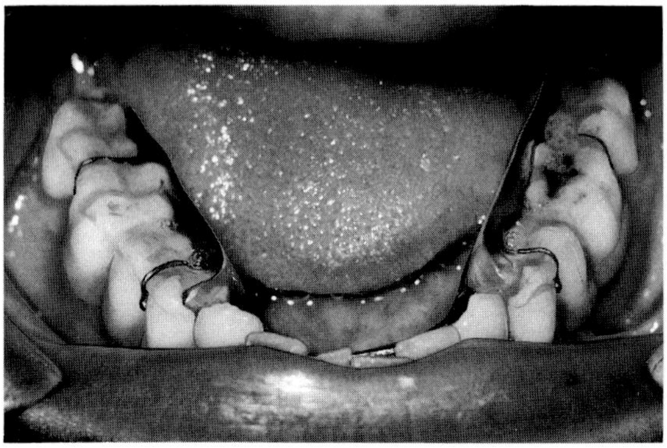

Fig. 20-3b The mandibular posterior occlusal coverage appliance has two acrylic resin platforms in the posterior portion with a connecting metal bar.

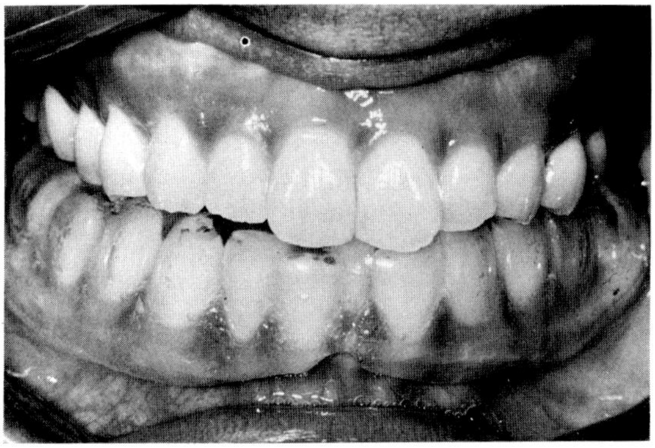

Fig. 20-3c The soft mandibular appliance is made of a flexible polyvinyl material.

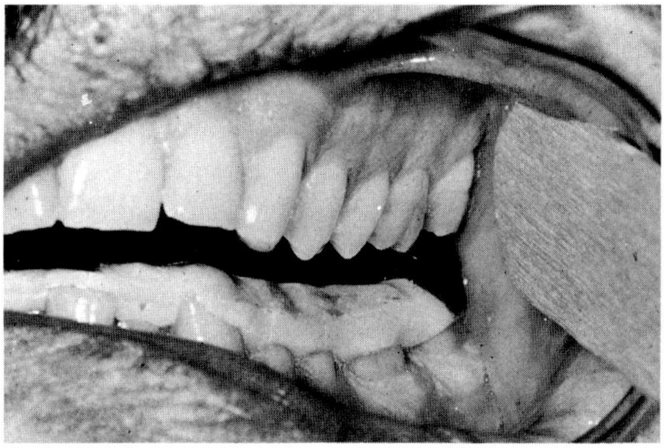

Fig. 20-3d The mandibular pivot appliance has an acrylic resin "pivot" in the second molar region.

change a harmful behavior is generally helpful to most successful therapeutic interventions (Rugh and Solberg, 1976).

Splint designs

Stabilization splints are full-coverage hard acrylic resin appliances that can be constructed to fit on either the maxillary or mandibular arch. They offer a distinct advantage over other appliances because they control and maintain tooth position. A stabilization splint is adjusted to have stable simultaneous occlusal contacts on all opposing teeth. The maxillary appliance provides better stabilization than the mandibular appliance, because all of the mandibular teeth can contact against a flat occlusal surface. A mandibular splint has no vertical stops for the maxillary anterior teeth.

The construction of anterior and lateral canine guidance is usually easier with a maxillary stabilization splint, especially in cases with severe overjet. The full-arch mandibular stabilization splint, however, offers advantages to the patient such as easier speech adaptation and less visibility of the appliance. These splints are typically constructed to occlude in a position of comfortable mandibular closure. This position is usually slightly anterior to an unstrained centric relation jaw position. If the patient has significant muscle splinting, then some initial centric relation guidance may be necessary to approach this position.

Repositioning splints have been used for several years. Their designs may differ, depending on the theory being advocated. The overall design of a repositioning splint usually consists of a hard acrylic resin appliance with indentations or guiding ramps that are used to produce a new mandibular position other than the habitual path-of-closure position (Farrar, 1972; Gausch and Kulmer, 1977; Weinberg, 1979). As previously mentioned, most of the repositioning theories call for further adjustments and alterations of the appliance during treatment to refine this position. Most of these theories suggest wearing the appliance full time, including while eating. When a successful resolution of the disorder occurs, the teeth are moved into this newly acquired position via various prosthetic, orthodontic, or orthognathic surgical procedures.

Many other splint designs are presented in the literature, in addition to the two mentioned above (Figs. 20-3a to d). Soft *resilient interocclusal appliances* have been suggested as a simple technique for use in bruxing patients and in patients with symptoms of joint pain (Krogh-Poulsen and Olsson, 1968; Block et al., 1978). Several other reports address the use of resilient appliances but note they are less durable and not easily adjusted (Ingersoll and Kerens, 1952; Posselt, 1968). These appliances are usually constructed out of a resilient polyvinyl material and are also worn as protective mouthguards during athletics (Bodenham, 1970).

The anterior biteplane is a hard acrylic resin, partial-coverage appliance commonly used for occlusal disengagement, muscle relaxation, and establishing a new vertical dimension (Posselt, 1963, 1968; Krogh-Poulsen and Olsson, 1968). Another common partial-coverage appliance design is the *mandibular posterior appliance,* which usually has two acrylic resin pads covering the posterior teeth (premolars and molars), connected by a thick lingual wire or metal bar (Lieb, 1977).

Appliances that cover only a portion of the dentition have been reported to cause uncontrolled tooth movement (Kanter, 1959; Ramfjord and Ash, 1983). Furthermore, complications exist for *all* interocclusal appliances, regardless of design, that are overutilized by patients. Such complications usually consist of changes in the occlusal scheme due to intrusion or eruption of teeth, caries under the splint, gingival inflammation, or even psychological dependence on the appliance (Brayer and Erlich, 1976).

Overall clinical effectiveness of interocclusal appliances

A majority of the clinical studies that have evaluated splint treatment have studied the full-arch maxillary stabilization appliance. These studies generally use the stabilization splint in combination with one or more other modes of treatment, usually occlusal adjustments and prosthetics (Franks, 1965; Zarb and Thompson, 1970, 1975; Agerberg and Carlsson, 1974; Magnusson and Carlsson, 1980b). The result of this combined therapeutic approach is that between 70% to 90% of the patients studied achieved clinical success (Fig. 20-4). Two studies appear in the literature where full-arch maxillary stabilization splints were the only form of treatment, and their success rates appear similar (Greene and Laskin, 1972; Carraro and Caffesse, 1978). The effect of the interocclusal appliance may be due to dental stabilization and force redistribution or to any number of other factors that have been discussed under the cognitive awareness theory section.

The overall clinical effectiveness of the stabilization appliance is not in question, but there is much debate as to why it is successful and what this implies regarding the need for follow-up therapy. According to the occlusal disengagement theory, if the appliance is successful at

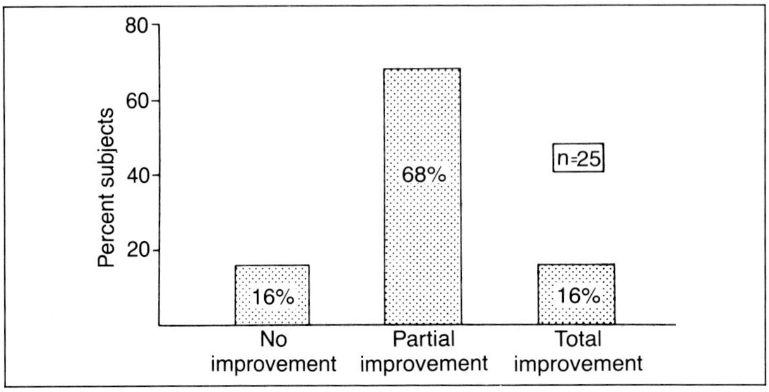

Fig. 20-4 The outcome results from 25 patients who underwent treatment with a stabilization appliance.

reducing the symptoms, then this is proof that a malocclusion exists and that a follow-up occlusal adjustment is required. However, several research articles have questioned the need for follow-up occlusal adjustment therapy (Greene and Laskin, 1972, 1974; Goodman et al., 1976; Cohen, 1978). One clinical report evaluated the effectiveness of maxillary occlusal appliances on two groups of pain-dysfunction patients and found equal effectiveness (80% success for both groups) whether or not the subjects had occlusal interferences (Moffett, 1980). Although still controversial, the results of these studies confirm the need to reconsider this aspect of the occlusal disengagement theory. Certainly, additional research is necessary to compare the long-term results of follow-up occlusal adjustments versus no occlusal adjustments. At present, it must be determined on a case-by-case basis.

As with the occlusal disengagement theory, the success of an occlusal appliance in resolving the patient's symptoms does not prove that the patient's original vertical dimension was overclosed. As mentioned previously, there are several possible explanations for the decrease in symptoms other than that a proper occlusal vertical dimension has been reestablished (Greene and Laskin, 1972, 1974). The most appropriate application of this treatment approach is for a patient suspected of overclosure secondary to a significant loss of posterior occlusal support. In these cases, the concept of "restoring" muscle length seems empirically correct if the mechanical factors, such as periodontal bone support and crown/root ratio, do not contraindicate this change (Storey, 1962). However, a diagnosis of a loss of occlusal vertical dimension is a very difficult determination to make without reliable quantitative methods.

Although there are some cases where few clinicians would argue about whether there is a loss of occlusal vertical dimension, the widespread application of this theory in a great many cases is highly debatable (Rugh and Drago, 1981). The assumption that an abnormal vertical dimension—either too much closure or not enough closure—is the cause of the problem is somewhat incongruous with animal research that has compared muscle adaptation to experimentally induced changes in muscle length (Goldspink, 1976; Ramfjord and Blankenship, 1981). Furthermore, human research on clinical postural rest position with different thicknesses of dentures demonstrates that muscle adaptation to a new vertical dimension is quite good in the masticatory system (Tallgren, 1957). One research study even evaluated the assumption that an interocclusal appliance that exceeds the clinical resting muscle length is harmful (Drago et al., 1979). The results of this study showed a decrease in nocturnal muscle activity with splints made of different thicknesses. No consistent result was evident, and, in fact, in several subjects the thicker splints had the greatest decrease in muscle activity even though they exceeded the interocclusal distance. This is contrary to the belief that occlusal vertical dimension is the key factor in producing dysfunctional symptoms of the masticatory system. Certainly the vertical dimension of occlusion is an important clinical concept to consider when evaluating a patient with a partial or complete denture. Yet, considering the weak experimental evidence, the potential hazards, and the costliness of permanently altering occlusal vertical dimension in the fully or near fully dentate subject, this approach should be deemphasized as a primary concern.

One way to determine if a maxillomandibular realignment is necessary to the success of the treatment is to take the repositioning appliance away after a period of time (Greene and Laskin, 1972). If the symptoms return, then the realignment may in fact be a necessary part of treatment. One must be cautious with this assumption because other explanations may exist. The return of the symptoms doesn't prove that the realignment was necessary, only that an appliance was necessary. A better, but obviously less practical, test would be to construct a nonrealignment appliance and test its effect. Considering the amount of work and expense necessary to realign the teeth to a new position, permanent realignment should be a last resort.

Regarding the TMJ repositioning theory, there is still a need to carefully and objectively demonstrate that a new joint position is a necessary part of the success of the treatment. The danger of this approach, as with all the realignment and repositioning appliances, is concluding that the reason the symptoms disappear is the new position. These methods of treatment must be continually reevaluated for alternative explanations and long-term adverse side effects.

It is safe to say that no one theory can explain the clinical results of interocclusal appliance treatment. The general lack of a single proven theoretical basis for this treatment and an unclear conceptualization behind the splint treatment models being applied make the evaluation of the effectiveness of treatment extremely difficult. This difficulty is even greater because reports and research on splints are rarely done in a controlled environment. Few of the research reports reviewed were designed to test the validity of any of the underlying assumptions. The typical clinical report on the effectiveness of interocclusal appliances involves the introduction of the appliance as well as an entire complex of therapies that usually includes diet modification, counseling about chewing and clenching behavior, and simultaneous or follow-up occlusal adjustments.

Many uncontrolled, nonspecific factors also cloud the research environment in which splints have been studied. Some typical nonspecific factors that can influence treatment results are the placebo effects of treatment, the patient's expectations for success, and the clinician's unstated confidence or predetermined bias in the correctness of the treatment. These variables make it very difficult to evaluate the overall effectiveness of the splint.

Symptom-specific effectiveness

Further evaluation of the literature on the effectiveness of an interocclusal appliance for individual symptoms of TM pain-dysfunction reveals the following information. Research shows that the clicking TMJ is sometimes helped, but not cured, by the traditional stabilization interocclusal appliance, and that TMJ clicking is the least responsive of all symptoms to treatment (Greene and Laskin, 1972; Agerberg and Carlsson, 1974; Goharian and Neff, 1980). Questions have been raised in the literature regarding the need to specifically treat the clicking, but painless, joint (Greene et al., 1982). At present there is no prospective longitudinal evidence to support the common clinical observation that certain clicking joints become progressively dysfunctional (Ireland, 1963; Toller, 1976). Although it is generally agreed that the clicking joint is resistant to treatment, the cost-effectiveness of the time-consuming approach of repositioning splint therapy, the subsequent dental stabilization, and the unknown long-term effects of a potentially altered condylar position must be considered and

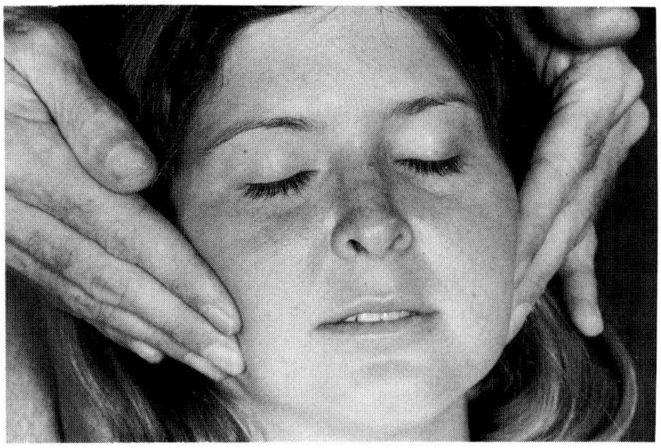

Fig. 20-5a Patients with myalgia usually complain of pain in the masseter-temporalis muscle region, which can be verified by palpation.

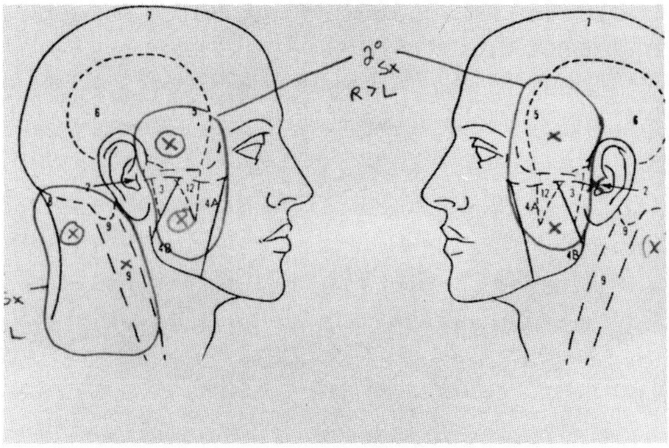

Fig. 20-5b Pain diagram of palpation findings from a patient with myalgia secondary to a chronic tooth-clenching habit.

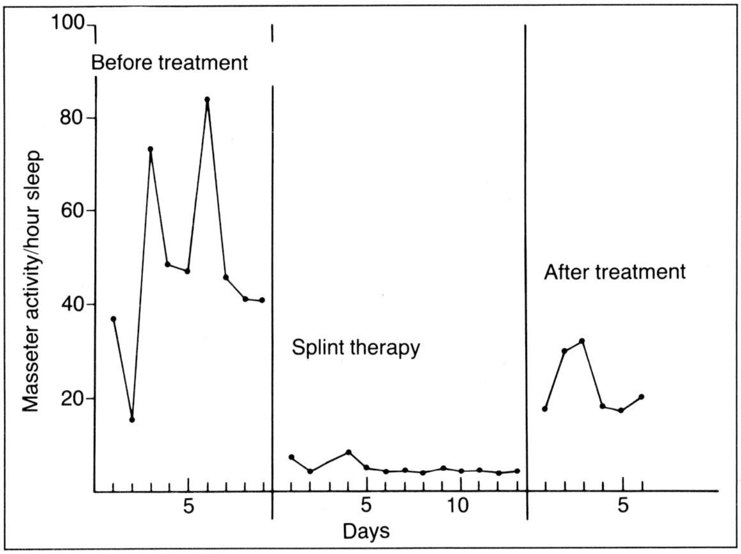

Fig. 20-6 Nocturnal masseter muscle electromyographic levels recorded from a patient with bruxism before, during, and after 2 weeks' use of a maxillary stabilization appliance.

will remain open to question until more research addresses the issue. Currently, several reports have appeared in the literature indicating a long-term success rate of between 35% and 55% for significantly reducing joint sounds and painful symptoms (Clark, 1984, 1986; Moloney and Howard, 1986).

Painful TMJs have been shown to respond to occlusal appliance therapy regardless of design, but questions still exist regarding the effectiveness of these appliances as a sole or primary treatment (Agerberg and Carlsson, 1974; Carraro and Caffesse, 1978; Magnusson and Carlsson, 1980b; Goharian and Neff, 1980). A good comparative study needs to be performed to evaluate the relative effectiveness of the nonsteroidal, anti-inflammatory medications versus occlusal splint therapy for treating joint pain. Obviously, if the pharmacologic approach is not sufficient, then the second-line approach would probably be an interocclusal appliance. As for degenerative joint disease (osteoarthrotic

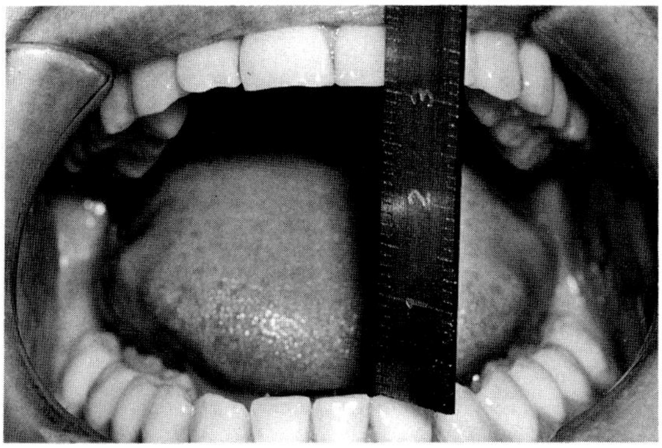

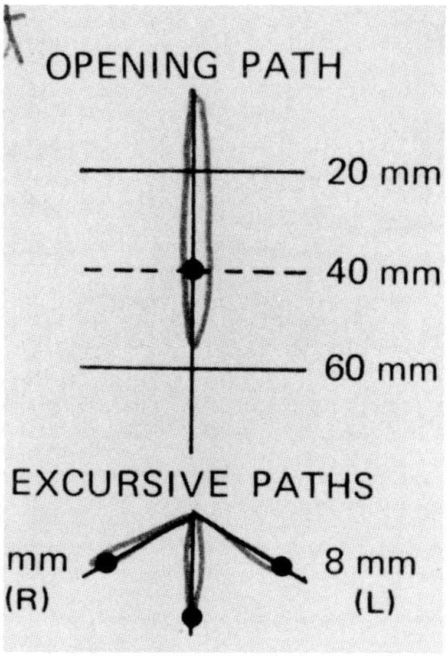

Fig. 20-7a *(above)* Maximum active interincisal opening ability (30 mm) of a patient with trismus.

Fig. 20-7b *(right)* Interincisal opening diagram in the same patient after maxillary stabilization appliance use for 2 weeks.

changes), very little good evidence is yet available regarding the ability of interocclusal appliances to effectively slow down or reverse degenerative TMJ changes evident on radiographs (Kopp, 1977a; Öberg, 1980; Mongini, 1980). Because arthrosis is regarded as an unfavorable response to joint loading, one can make a case that the appliance has a potential beneficial effect by reducing muscular hyperactivity and thus diminishing the loading.

Masticatory muscle pain (myalgia) is by far the symptom with the best experimental evidence to support occlusal splints as a highly effective method of treatment (Figs. 20-5a and b). Myalgia is generally considered to be a function of various local tissue inflammation and vascular alterations in the muscle, as well as referred pain from other sources. A strong association has been demonstrated between muscle hyperactivity and the symptoms of masticatory muscle pain (Clark et al., 1981) (Fig. 20-6). The actual pathophysiological changes in the muscle tissue are not yet agreed upon, but occlusal splints have been used effectively to treat this condition.

The relationship among nocturnal muscle hyperactivity, myogenous pain symptoms, and occlusal splints has been evaluated in two studies (Clark et al., 1979, 1981). The larger study, on 25 myofascial pain dysfunction subjects, demonstrated that 52% of these patients had significantly reduced nocturnal muscle activity levels when full-arch stabilization splints were used. Another related study evaluated eight bruxism subjects and demonstrated a significant reduction in muscle activity with appliance therapy in all of the subjects (Solberg et al., 1975). Several others have also demonstrated a good correlation between occlusal splint therapy and relief of masticatory muscle pain (Greene and Laskin, 1972; Agerberg and Carlsson, 1974). These changes are probably mediated via an alteration in the patient's muscle activity patterns (Fuchs, 1975; Beemsterboer et al., 1976a, 1976b; Carlsson et al., 1979; Kawazoe et al., 1980; Hamada et al., 1982; Rugh, 1982). Those patients with more severe symptoms are less likely to be helped with splints as the sole treatment modality (Clark et al., 1979).

The effect of occlusal appliances on muscle trismus (limited opening) has been discussed in the literature, but not effectively evaluated (Figs. 20-7a and b). On the other hand, occlusal splints have been shown to have a significant influence on improving mandibular muscle coordination (Ransjö and Thilander, 1963; McCall et al., 1976; Beard and Clayton, 1980). The relation-

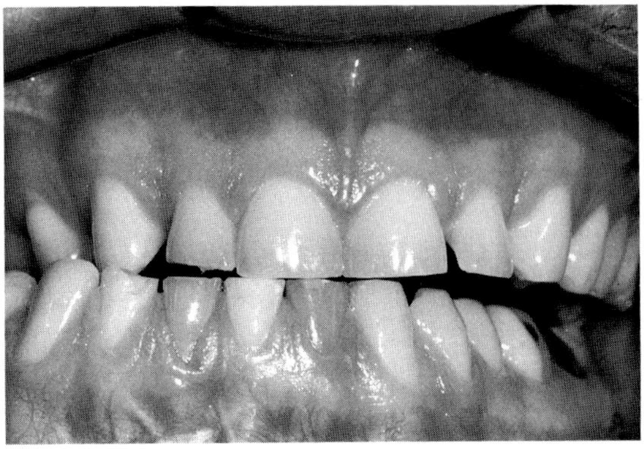

Fig. 20-8 Attrition in a 32-year-old patient with a chronic nocturnal grinding behavior.

ship among mandibular coordination, tremor and weakness, and other such symptoms is not well understood at this time. Finally, interocclusal appliances are commonly used to control attrition and adverse tooth loading, and little question has been raised in the literature regarding this therapeutic application (Ingersoll, 1952) (Fig. 20-8).

The stabilization splint

Design

An interocclusal appliance must be unobtrusive in its appearance yet have adequate strength and rigidity to prevent breakage and maintain stability of the teeth. It should cover all of the incisal and occlusal surfaces of the teeth. The vertical dimension (thickness) of the appliance should be established using the posterior teeth (approximately 2 mm in the molar region). If exceptionally thin, holes may be produced on the occlusal surface of the splint while adjusting it—so, for the maxillary appliance, it may be necessary to extend the acrylic resin into the palatal area about 10 to 15 mm to maintain rigidity and strength (Fig. 20-9), and for the mandibular appliance, any necessary extension on the lingual area should cover at least the attached gingival tissues but not go to the full depth of the vestibule (Fig. 20-10). These extensions onto the lingual and palate are optional and are necessary only to add strength to the appliance. A line drawn on the study casts should mark the extension of the appliance. The facial surface extension should be between 0.5 to 1.0 mm, and, posteriorly, the splint usually extends to the most distal aspect of the last tooth.

For retention, the occlusal stabilization splint may place ball clasps between the canine and the first premolar and between the first and second first molars. The occlusal surface of the maxillary appliance should be flat, with only slight mandibular buccal cusp tip and incisal edge indentations. For the mandibular appliance, slight maxillary molar and premolar lingual cusp indentations are acceptable. As the mandible moves in a laterotrusive direction, all posterior teeth should be separated by a canine-discluding ramp or incline. The shape of this incline should be wide enough to provide stability during most lateral movements and should be gradual and slightly concave. For most normal occlusal schemes, the canines and incisors should be the only teeth in contact during a protrusive jaw movement, and the angle of disclusion should again be gradual and smooth. A recommended technique for processing the wax-up into acrylic resin is to use essentially the same technique as in complete or partial denture fabrication, except that cold-cure acrylic resin can be substituted for heat-cure resin and the flasks are placed under pressure for only 10 minutes to process them (Figs. 20-11a and b).

Insertion

The main requirements for inserting a stabilization splint are that it be well fitting and stable. It should seat fully with no tipping or rocking motion produced as the opposing teeth contact it (Fig. 20-12). If the appliance does tip or rock and this motion cannot be stopped by adjusting the internal surface, then a very light wash with clear

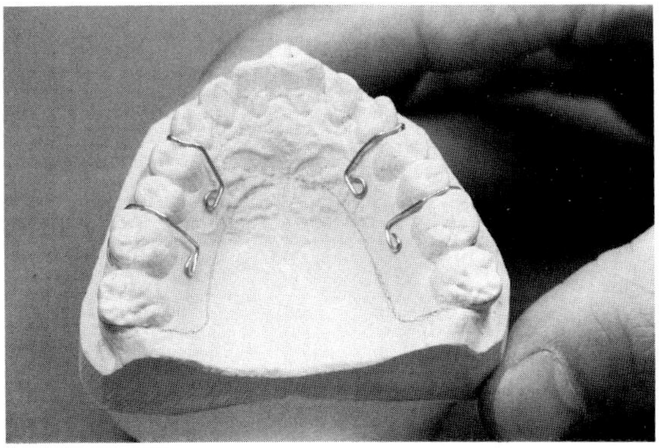

Fig. 20-9 Palatal extension outline and ball clasps prepared for maxillary stabilization appliance.

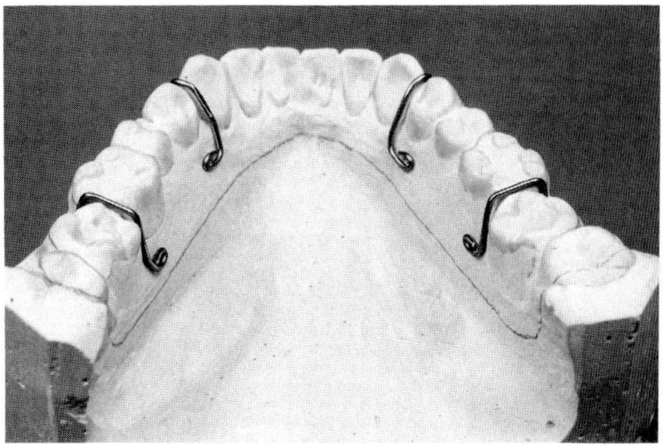

Fig. 20-10 Lingual extension outline and ball clasps prepared for mandibular stabilization appliance.

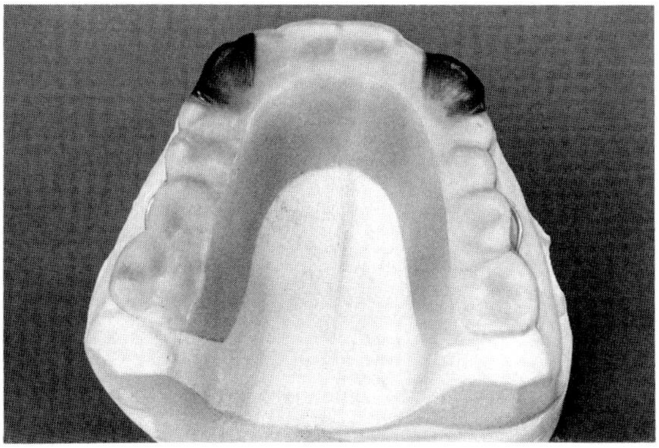

Fig. 20-11a Finished wax-up of a maxillary stabilization appliance. Note anterior guidance ramps.

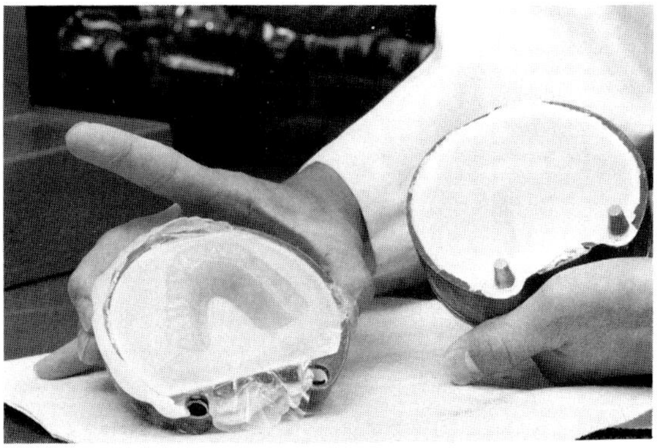

Fig. 20-11b Acrylic resin packing of a flasked maxillary stabilization appliance.

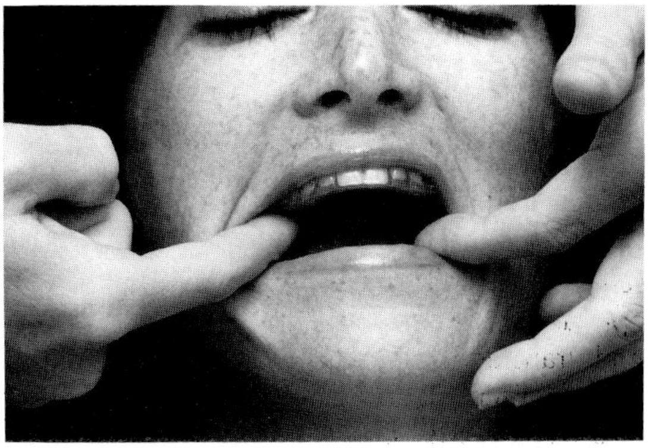

Fig. 20-12 Check the fit of the interocclusal appliance by applying pressure in different quadrants.

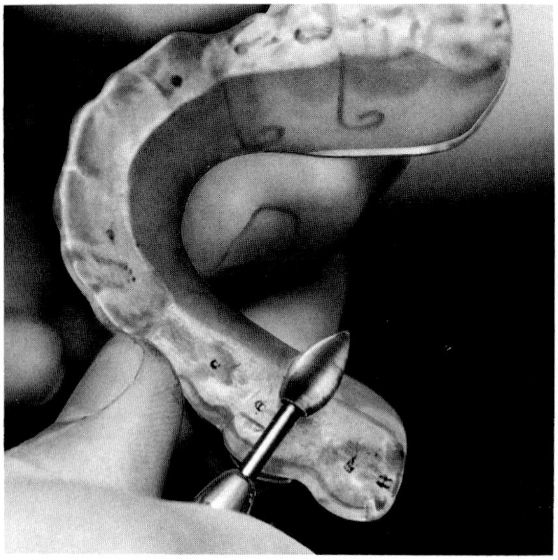

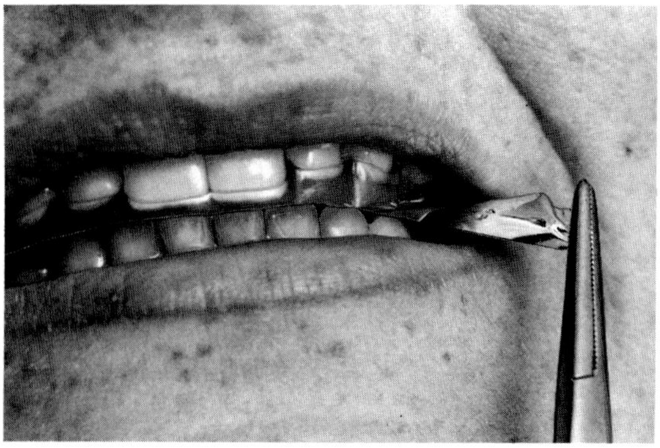

Fig. 20-13 *(left)* Adjustment of a stabilization appliance is usually performed with an acrylic resin bur.

Fig. 20-14 *(above)* Adjust the appliance until all the contact points firmly hold the mylar paper.

self-curing acrylic resin directly in the mouth will produce a very stable splint. Adjust any clasp arms as needed to achieve retention of the appliance in the mouth. Retention should be such that the appliance should snap in and out easily and smoothly. If the splint cannot be dislodged with the tongue, retention is satisfactory.

At the initial insertion appointment, a common problem is too much retention. This occurs when the acrylic resin extends too far onto the facial surface of the anterior and posterior teeth. Reduction of the facial extension of the acrylic resin to a maximum of 1 mm over the incisal edges and 1 to 2 mm over the buccal cusps of the posterior teeth will make the splint more comfortable and more easily inserted and removed. If tightness is still a problem, then reline the entire inner surface of the appliance after relieving all undercuts significantly with an acrylic resin bur.

Patients who require stabilization splint therapy very often have had no experience with removable appliances. The sheer bulk of the appliance, the speech impairment that results, and transient increases in salivary flow frequently discourage the patient from compliance. It is desirable to forewarn the patient of these initial inconveniences before the splint is inserted, but do not overemphasize these aspects.

Adjustment

Observe for gross discrepancies in the position of habitual closure (unguided muscular closure or muscular contact position). Begin by adjusting the appliance into a stable centric relation jaw position. After achieving this, continue the adjustment of the appliance without manipulating the mandible. Place the patient in an upright position and adjust the appliance by using muscular contact position of the mandible (habitual closure).

Continue adjusting until a good distribution of posterior and anterior occlusal stops is obtained (Fig. 20-13). For most patients, the contact area between centric relation and muscular contact position is usually less than 0.5 mm and should be level and smooth. If the patient has poor muscular coordination and is unable to close into a repeatable position, then the habitual closure adjustment should be performed at a subsequent visit.

Mark all excursive movements (lateral and

protrusive) with marking paper. Always mark the muscular contact position in a different color ribbon immediately after marking the excursive contacts. Preserve these contacts and eliminate all excursive contacts in the posterior segments. In the canine and anterior segments, the discluding surfaces should be smooth from the muscular contact positions to the extreme positions. The primary requirement is that the discluding movement over the canine and anterior teeth be *smooth and unobstructed.* Any rocking of the splint when the patient goes to right or left lateral movement indicates the angle of canine disclusion may be too steep and should be flattened with a rubber wheel.

Finally, check muscular contact positions with mylar strips (Fig. 20-14). The mylar strips should just slip through in the anterior segments. For maximum tongue space, remove as much of the anterior lingual acrylic resin as possible. For the maxillary appliance, there must be a 1-mm shelf remaining lingual to the contact points produced by the mandibular incisors. The mandibular appliance will not have vertical stops on the anterior teeth. Reduce the buccolingual width of the posterior acrylic resin surface to approximately 10 mm. Be careful not to alter or destroy the contact areas of muscular contact position during the polishing procedures.

Postinsertion instructions

Make certain the patient has instructions on the care and maintenance of the appliance. Review oral hygiene, cleaning, and care of the appliance. Initially the patient may be asked to wear the appliance as much as possible with the idea that later the use of the appliance will be only on a part-time basis. Make it clear that, should the patient want or need to remove the appliance for any length of time during this phase of treatment, the dentist should be informed. Set up the recall appointment for the patient in 1 to 2 weeks.

At the follow-up adjustment appointment, interview the patient to record the progress of the symptoms under treatment. Often it is best to first determine if the patient could wear the splint, even before asking about the progress with his or her symptoms. If a patient shows poor adaptation to the splint, this may be diagnostic in itself. Review all signs and symptoms and note progress. Remove the splint and examine all its occluding surfaces for shiny facets indicating active bruxing activity. Check the evenness of the muscular contact position contacts and adjust until they are even. Relaxation of the patient's muscles and possible repositioning of the mandible necessitates readjusting the occlusal surface of the appliance to maintain optimal stability. Several additional splint adjustment visits may be necessary at a 2-week interval. When the patient has achieved a reduction in symptoms, determine if they will benefit by long-term part-time appliance use.

The typical patient stays on part-time use of the appliance because of a still-active forceful jaw-closing habit. However, before proceeding to part-time appliance use, ensure that a significant relief of the pain or dysfunctional symptoms has resulted. As mentioned previously, in many cases splint therapy alone is sufficient. If no obvious occlusal instability is present, then it is not necessary to adjust the teeth. If the patient is aware of, or the dentist observes, occlusal instability, an uneven bite, or a tooth with obvious premature contact, then an occlusal adjustment is in order. The details of this aspect of therapy are discussed in the next chapter.

Judgment and improvement of symptoms determine how long the stabilization splint should be worn. For most myogenous conditions, the period of full-time use usually involves at least a 6-week treatment period and two adjustment appointments. After this time, reduce the use of the splint to a part-time basis. At each follow-up visit, reevaluate the original diagnosis and repeat and compare muscle palpation patterns and the subjective patient response to symptoms. After a reasonable period of initial treatment, the splint therapy could be phased out gradually by limiting its use to only that period of time when clenching is most prevalent. If a persistent nocturnal bruxism habit exists, the splint could continue to be used at night.

Summary

Interocclusal appliance therapy is a commonly used modality for many occlusal problems, parafunctional habits, and temporomandibular disorders. When designed and used properly in the appropriate situation, such appliances are usually reversible and generally effective.

This chapter has critically reviewed the most common theories that underlie the use of these appliances. Of the several types discussed, the full-arch maxillary stabilization splint has the most evidence for its efficacy. Thus, the design and use of this type of appliance has been discussed in some detail.

Chapter 21

Occlusal Adjustment Therapy

Glenn T. Clark, Norman D. Mohl, and Richard R. Riggs

Occlusal adjustment therapy, or *coronoplasty,* is a procedure of selective coronal tooth modification (Schuyler, 1935, 1947). This reshaping of one or more teeth is usually performed by selectively removing enamel, which rarely produces dentinal sensitivity. The purposes of occlusal adjustment are to achieve *(1)* a stable, nontraumatic occlusal contact relationship between the maxillary and mandibular teeth in maximum intercuspation and in all functional excursive contact positions; and *(2)* stability of the temporomandibular joints (TMJs) in maximum intercuspation.

For many years the dental profession has believed that there is a correlation between occlusal relationships, mandibular function, muscular activity, and TMJ health (Stuart and Stallard, 1959; Mann and Pankey, 1963; Shore, 1976; Ramfjord and Ash, 1983). Dentists have claimed that occlusal adjustment procedures can both improve masticatory function and reduce individual tooth trauma (Ramfjord, 1961a; Glickman and Zander, 1971; Dawson, 1974; McNamara, 1976). In some cases, occlusal adjustment therapy has been performed to protect the TMJs from excessive wear (Kopp and Wennenberg, 1981; Mongini, 1982). In this last regard, dentists have claimed that remodeling changes produced by adverse TMJ loading can be prevented by stabilizing and improving an unstable or incorrect mandibular position. In addition, several claims have been made that an occlusal adjustment can reduce noxious or harmful dental input and, therefore, improve neuromuscular function (i.e., reduce muscle hyperactivity and bruxism) (Dawson, 1974; Ramfjord, 1961b). The evidence for these claims will be discussed in this chapter.

At present there are several distinct theories explaining the effects of occlusal adjustments on the occlusion: *(1)* traumatic tooth contact theory, *(2)* avoidance of tooth contact theory, *(3)* abnormal mandibular position theory, and *(4)* behavioral effect of occlusal adjustment theory.

This chapter will discuss each of these theories and give specific, practical information on how to recognize and remove traumatic tooth contacts and achieve a stable functional position with maximum intercuspation that is compatible with an acceptable position of the condyles. Finally, it must be remembered that *occlusal adjustment therapy may not be the correct approach for severe maxillomandibular disharmonies.* Combined prosthodontic, surgical, and orthodontic procedures are often required in such cases to achieve a stable long-lasting maxillomandibular occlusal relationship.

Theories of occlusal adjustment

Traumatic occlusal contact theory

The traumatic occlusal contact theory has two goals: *(1)* to remove forceful contacts from individual teeth, and *(2)* to distribute the tooth contact forces in a consistent interference-free occlusal scheme. According to this theory, occlusal adjustment is designed to reduce or eliminate the harmful local effects of traumatic occlusion.

The criterion for a tooth in a traumatic contact relationship is clinical evidence of dental and/or periodontal injury (Orban and Weinman, 1933; Coolidge, 1938; Anderson and Picton, 1958; Glickman, 1972; Picton, 1976; Ramfjord and Ash, 1981). At a local dental level traumatic forces can produce cracked or fractured teeth, root resorption, pulpal hyperemia, pulpitis, pulpal degenerative changes, tooth mobility, fremitus, or alveolar-periodontal pain. Pain can often be elicited with a simple percussion test of tapping on the tooth. Examples and a further definition of traumatic occlusal contacts can be found later in this chapter, under "Traumatic tooth contact recognition."

The local dental and periodontal-osseous effects of traumatic tooth contacts are generally well accepted as indications for occlusal adjustment therapy. The major exception used to be the no-longer-supportable contention that traumatic tooth contact relationships enhance or accelerate apical migration of the periodontal attachment. This issue has been discussed in chapter 16.

Avoidance of tooth contact theory

The avoidance of tooth contact theory is based on the concept that when occlusal contact relationships are perceived as noxious by the trigeminal neurosensory system, the neuromuscular system that controls jaw movements will adapt and develop patterns of mandibular movement to avoid these contacts (Graf and Zander, 1963; Schärer and Stallard, 1966; Schärer, 1974; Storey, 1975). This differs from the traumatic occlusal contact theory in that the primary effect of the "adverse or noxious" tooth contact is at a neurosensory level, involving reflex and accommodative muscular behaviors. The two theories are similar in that the physical description of noxious or adverse tooth contacts is the same.

According to the avoidance of tooth contact theory, the clinical criterion for a tooth contact relationship that is producing avoidance behavior in the mandibular motor system is mandibular incoordination. Mandibular incoordination is the inability to make specific directed mandibular movements in a smooth fashion. Examples of mandibular incoordination are *(1)* inability or difficulty in moving the jaw laterally from intercuspal position with the teeth in light contact, and *(2)* inability or difficulty in closing firmly, rapidly, and accurately into a repeatable intercuspal position, particularly with the head upright (Watt and Wakabayashi, 1978). This mandibular movement disability is thought to be related to avoidance of a noxious or painful tooth contact. However, it must be remembered that mandibular incoordination can, and probably does, occur for many other reasons as well (Edmiston and Laskin, 1978).

Another, more controversial variation of this theory is that a noxious tooth contact will result in an unconscious attempt to grind away this "offending" contact. According to this idea, tooth grinding behavior, or bruxism, is triggered by the interference and can be controlled by an occlusal adjustment (Ramfjord, 1961a). That occlusal interferences produce bruxism has not been satisfactorily demonstrated; current research suggests that bruxism is more often a result of central nervous system disturbance or conditions (Kardachi et al., 1978; Bailey and Rugh, 1980).

Abnormal mandibular occlusal position theory

This theory is based on the premise that, for various reasons, the intercuspal position (ICP) is in an abnormal or nonadaptive position (Beyron, 1954a; Weinberg, 1976; Mongini, 1982, 1983). Although this "abnormal" position is thought to occur whenever a significant malocclusion exists, it is the "deflective occlusal contact" (often iatrogenic) that maintains this "abnormal mandibular position." Deflective occlusal contacts are believed to prevent or deflect the mandible from closing into a "physiologic" intercuspal position. This theory implies that the patient has a "neuromuscular imbalance" and is unsuccessfully attempting to adapt to an abnormal occlusal position. The definition of neuromuscular imbalance and how it produces the pathological muscular effects have never been specified clearly by proponents of this theory. Such specification would allow the abnormal mandibular position theory to be tested.

The occlusal signs most often used as evidence for abnormal mandibular positions are a large vertical or horizontal difference between the voluntary postural or muscular contact position of the mandible and ICP, and/or a large or asymmetrical difference between the manipulated retruded contact position of the mandible (RCP) and ICP. The radiographic sign most frequently used is a bilaterally asymmetrical or nonconcentric positioning of the condyles in the fossa with the teeth in ICP. If these findings are present, there are often some corroborating dental findings that indicate occlusal imperfections (dental midline shift, missing posterior teeth, drifting [unstable] teeth, deep overbite, etc.). Advocates of this theory place great emphasis on a nonconcentric condylar position, even if the occlusion appears normal.

It has been suggested that an abnormal jaw position may produce peripheral muscular effects—muscle hyperactivity, pain, and incoordination. Furthermore, if an abnormal condyle position is present, it may predispose the disk-condyle complex to a functional disturbance (Clark, 1984). The articulating surfaces are then thought to undergo pathologic or nonadaptive remodeling changes in response to the altered joint.

It is theorized that only by changing the existing occlusal contact scheme from a nonadaptive mandibular position into a more correct intercuspal position will the "neuromuscular imbalance" be corrected and the various pathologic effects of the abnormal TMJ relationship disappear. The significance of varying jaw or condyle positions in the absence of overt symptoms is not known. However, research has shown that asymptomatic subjects can have widely variable condyle and jaw positions (Blaschke and Blaschke, 1981).

Thus, the use of nonconcentric condylar positions or asymmetrical dental landmarks (which also occur very frequently in asymptomatic subjects) as sole criteria for occlusal adjustment or other types of occlusal therapy is probably not warranted at the present time. On the other hand, the lack of a cause-and-effect relationship between mandibular position and TM disorders does not mean that occlusal relationships are unimportant. It means that it is simply not possible, based on existing evidence, to use these factors reliably and predictably in the prevention of TM disorders.

Behavioral effects of occlusal adjustment theory

Although the previous three theories are most prevalent, the behavioral effects of occlusal adjustment theory must also be considered (Goodman et al., 1976; Marbach, 1978; Kopp, 1979; Laskin and Greene, 1972). In addition to nonspecific treatment factors (e.g., placebo effects), the positive response seen after occlusal adjustment could also be due to the fact that the adjustment changes the dental contact relationships. Because most adjustments improve the mechanical force distribution of tooth contact, occlusal adjustment therapy will serve, transiently at least, to make the patient more aware that his or her bite is more comfortable. The patient often becomes more occlusally aware due to the changes in oral-occlusal tactile stimulation, which may serve to alter abnormal harmful behavior and help reduce muscular activity. This increased awareness of the patient regarding the position, use, and comfort of the jaws may also help reduce pain or dysfunction symptoms.

Traumatic tooth contact recognition

Evaluation of intercuspal position

Since the patient will function in ICP most of the time, it is important that this position be consis-

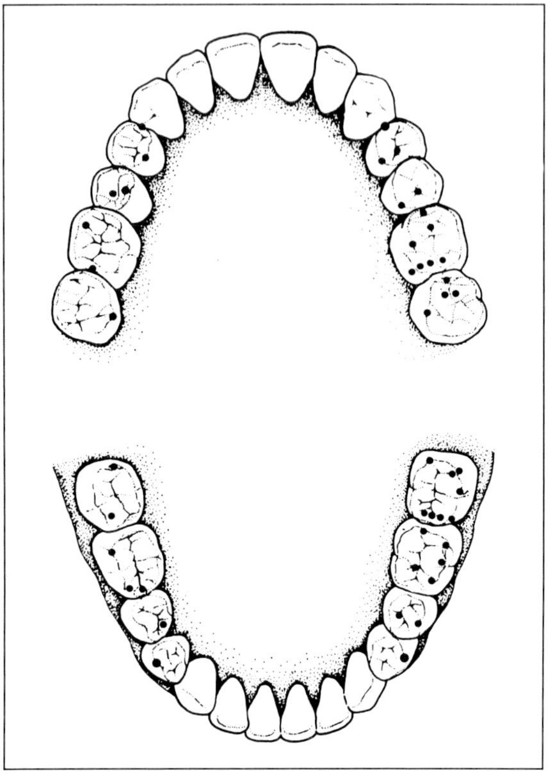

Fig. 21-1 Two types of typical, naturally occurring contact patterns. The right side is a cusp tip–fossa pattern, whereas the left side has a tripod contact relationship in the molar region, with a cusp tip–fossa pattern in the premolar region.

tent and stable. The consistency of closure into ICP may be evaluated in several ways. First, the teeth are examined for broken restorations, large wear facets, flaring of anterior teeth, sore teeth, missing teeth, or loose teeth as indicators of a potential unstable or traumatic occlusion. Second, the patient is asked to tap his or her teeth together slowly and forcefully while in an upright posture. The sound of the resulting tooth contacts should be sharp, reproducible, and solid, suggesting good ICP consistency. If the tooth contacts sound dull or soft, or result in multiple sliding noises, such abnormal sounds may be a result of poor contact relationships, or of poor muscle function and coordination and not of the occlusion. The use of sound to assess occlusal contact in this manner is referred to as *gnathosonics*. Applying a stethoscope to a bony prominence can be a useful tool to hear the sounds (Watt and Wakabayashi, 1978). A visual display of the sound via a microphone is called an *occlusogram* and is an excellent device to measure the consistency of closure into ICP.

Finally, the patient is positioned upright with the Frankfort plane horizontal to the floor and the head unsupported. The teeth are dried, and the patient closes on bilaterally placed articulating ribbon, squeezing the teeth together. The colors of the ribbon are then changed, and the patient is asked to rapidly tap the teeth together. In a consistent closure, these marks should be coincident. They should show appropriate cusp-fossa contacts, and/or cusp-marginal ridge contacts, with the forces being directed down the long axes of the contacting teeth. Further, these contacts should be multiple, and bilaterally distributed on all posterior teeth (Fig. 21-1).

An inconsistent ICP may occur when the contact scheme on some teeth does not direct the forces axially, but laterally instead. This can occur due to the absence of tooth contact in a posterior segment, or to excessive contact on a single tooth. It is often related to a new restoration; all new restorations should be checked both at the time of placement and after 1 week of function, for evidence of heavy wear facets. Extractions or restorations placed completely out of occlusal contact can produce an excessive load on the remaining teeth in contact.

Congenitally missing teeth or developmental malocclusions (e.g., open bites) can also result in traumatic ICP contacts. Occasionally, traumatic ICP tooth contacts can also result from *(1)* a poorly finished or relapsing orthodontic treatment, *(2)* a severe episode of erosive TMJ disease, *(3)* an improperly healed maxillary or mandibular fracture, or *(4)* an orthognathic surgical procedure. Inconsistent closure into ICP can be the result of an appliance-induced change in the occlusion or the jaw position. Two final examples of traumatic tooth contacts are *(1)* local dental or periodontal trauma (primary occlusal trauma) as a result of excessive force generated by the musculature, and *(2)* local trauma with normally well-tolerated functional forces (secondary occlusal trauma) secondary to a loss of periodontal osseous support reducing the load tolerated by a tooth.

Evaluation of lateral guidance

When the mandible moves into or out of ICP, two types of tooth contacts may occur: *(1)* normal guiding tooth contacts, and *(2)* guidance-disturbing tooth contacts. Guiding tooth contacts do just as the name implies—they guide the mandible into and out of maximum intercuspation. Normal tooth guidance during a lateral movement involves contact that can occur in one of several patterns. Most common, at least in younger individuals, is the canine-guided occlusion, where, on a lateral movement, the working side canines are the sole guiding teeth.

Alternative forms of lateral guidance are the canine segment guidance, or the progressive, unilateral, or bilateral group (cross-arch balanced) guidances. Further evaluation of which inclines are actually contacting on the working side guiding teeth is done during lateral jaw movement with particular attention to any fremitus of these teeth. Three guidance patterns are possible: *(1)* distal inclines of mandibular teeth functioning against mesial inclines of maxillary teeth, *(2)* the mandibular cusp tip traveling over the inner aspects of the maxillary teeth, or *(3)* the mesial inclines of mandibular teeth functioning against the distal inclines of the maxillary teeth. Clinical observation suggests that this latter type of excursive guidance has a greater potential for distalization of the mandible on the working side during periods of nocturnal parafunctional activity. It may be the least desirable of all three kinds of guidance.

If a cusp incline does not allow function of the normal working side contacts, it is considered a guidance-disturbing (premature) contact. These abnormal contacts occur for various reasons, usually developmental or iatrogenic. If present, they may exist on the ipsilateral working side or on the contralateral nonworking side of the arch (Figs. 21-2a and b). A guidance-disturbing contact should be evaluated to determine if it is associated with either avoidance behavior (incoordination) or traumatic dental-periodontal effects. If it is, then the dentition should be evaluated to determine if and how an acceptable guidance pattern can be produced. It must be noted that an occlusal adjustment is not always the procedure of choice. For example, in some Class II malocclusion patients who lack ICP contact with the maxillary canines, working side and nonworking side deflective guidance contacts can often be demonstrated. The addition of a restorative material on the lingual surfaces of the maxillary canines to restore contact is a therapeutic option and may be all that is required to establish an acceptable guidance (Fig. 21-3).

Evaluation of protrusive guidance

Protrusive incisal guiding contacts should ideally involve symmetrical contact on at least two or more incisor teeth and their antagonists, while producing separation of the posterior teeth. When present, protrusive guidance-disturbing contacts typically occur on posterior teeth. If appropriate disclusion of the posterior teeth occurs during protrusive guidance, but incisal contact takes place only on one side of the midline, then mobility and fremitus should be evaluated. Separation of the normal protrusive guiding teeth or any deviation from a straight protrusive movement should also be observed. This deviation could be an indication of a guidance-disturbing contact (Figs. 21-4a to c). If evidence of occlusal trauma is present, the clinician should consider an adjustment to remove this contact, and reestablish normal guidance, if possible.

A common example of excursive guidance interferences (either lateral or protrusive) is a mesially tipped mandibular molar resulting from a first molar or second premolar that has been extracted but not replaced (Fig. 21-5). Another example is an extruded maxillary or mandibular tooth opposing an edentulous space. This extruded tooth can result in a disturbing excursive

Figs. 21-2a and b Two possible types of posterior disturbing interferences.

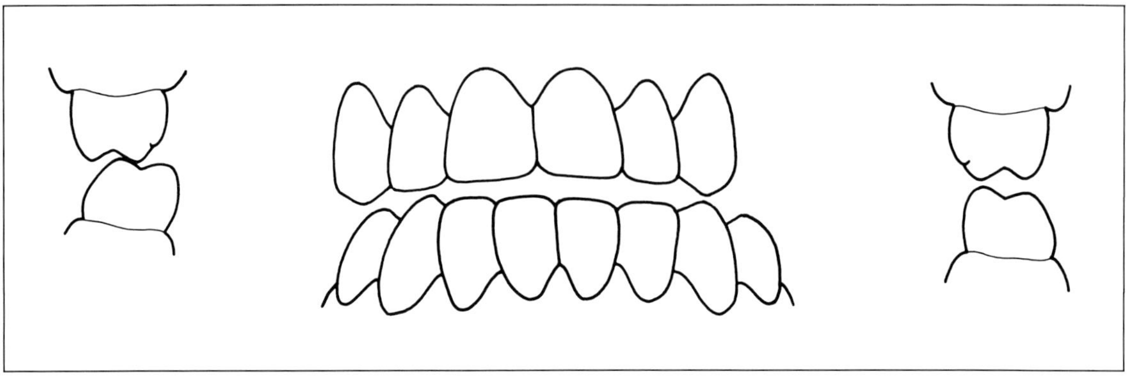

Fig. 21-2a A true nonworking side interference, which prevents contact anteriorly and on the working side.

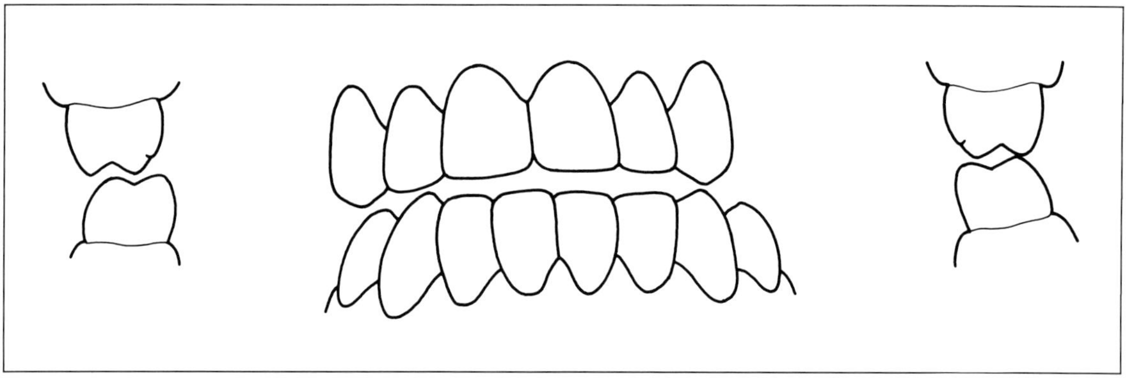

Fig. 21-2b A working side interference, which prevents anterior (including canine) guidance.

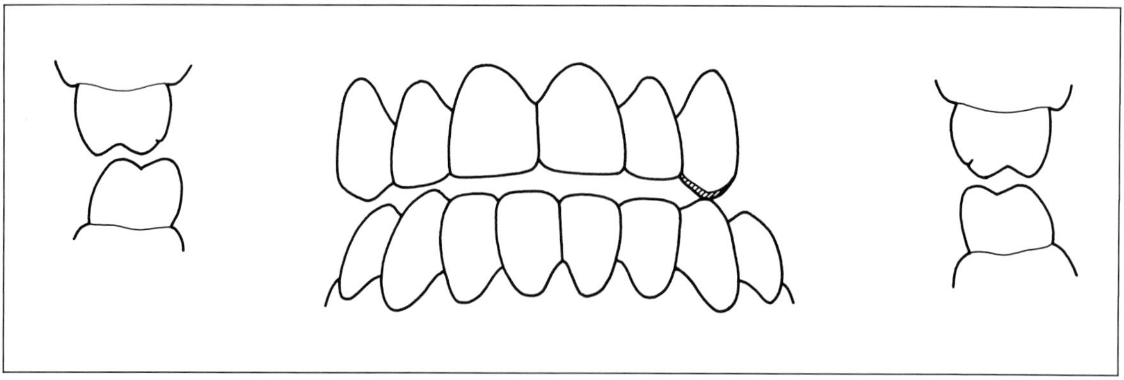

Fig. 21-3 Note the change in guidance that can be produced by addition of restorative material to the lingual aspect of a canine.

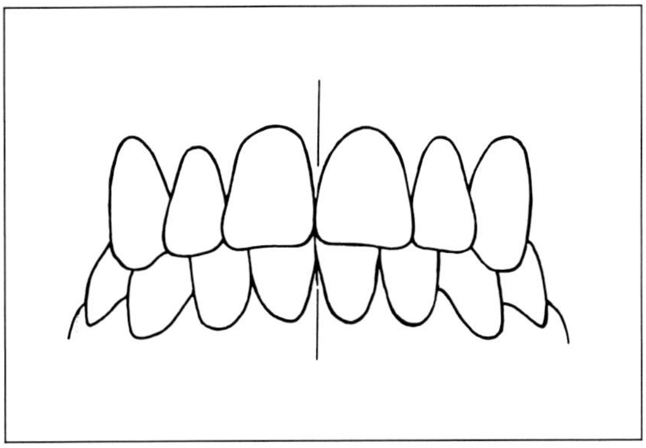

Fig. 21-4a With the teeth in the closed position, the maxillary and mandibular midline are correctly aligned.

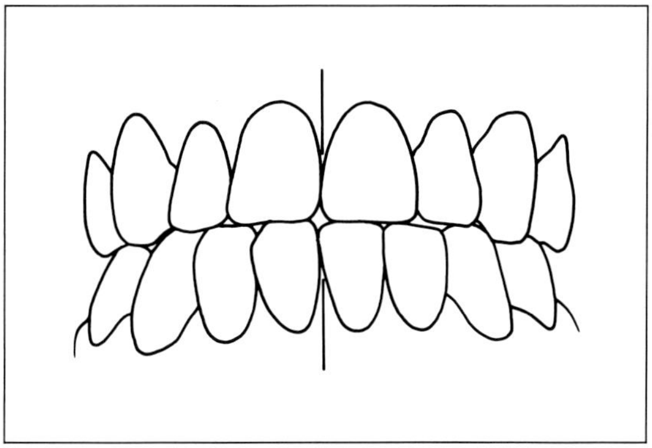

Fig. 21-4b As the mandible moves anteriorly, the midline starts to deviate to the right.

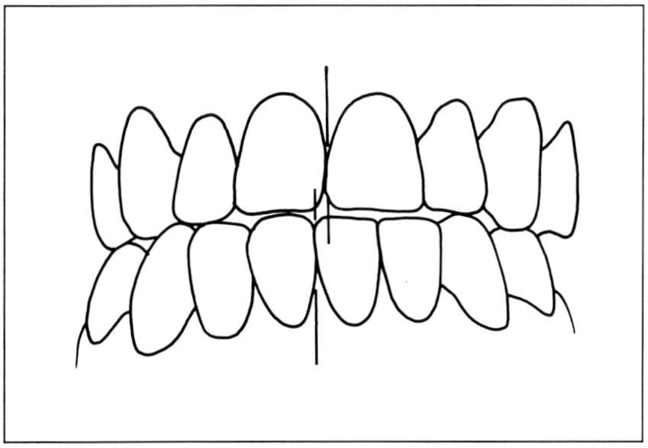

Fig. 21-4c With the teeth in a full end-to-end protrusive position, the mandibular midline is definitely off to the right, indicating a possible deflecting posterior occlusal interference.

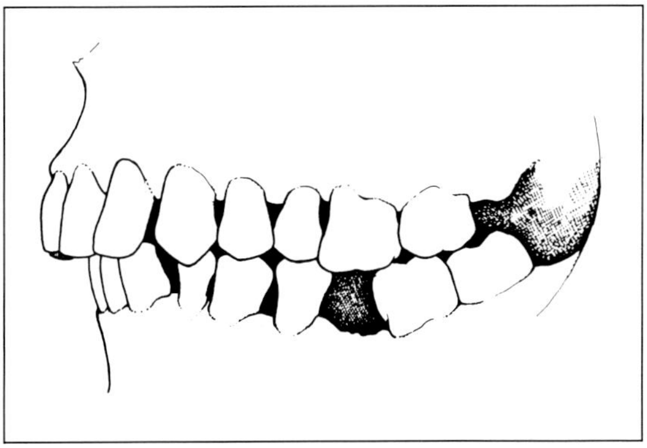

Fig. 21-5 Note the typical posterior tooth collapse that occurs when a mandibular molar is removed and not replaced.

contact. It must be remembered when discussing guidance that even though some guidance contacts are mechanically abnormal, they are not always harmful. The harmful effects usually occur only when enough force is applied to produce a noxious effect. In the absence of reasonable evidence of a noxious effect, occlusal adjustment therapy is inappropriate as a purely preventive or prophylactic treatment. A frequent exception is that when pretreatment decisions regarding moderate to extensive restorative and prosthodontic dentistry are being considered, mechanical considerations regarding guidance become more important.

Evaluation of retrusive guidance

The evaluation of RCP to ICP slide (centric slide) is performed by guiding the mandible posteriorly so that a manipulated hinge arc of closure is possible. The mandible is closed to the point of first contact, or RCP. The patient is then asked to slide the teeth together to achieve full closure into ICP. During this slide, the amount and direction of the movement is evaluated. This retruded jaw movement evaluation looks at an important aspect of the occlusion (i.e., the relationship between condylar position and the teeth).

If the TMJ is healthy and functioning normally, then the manipulated arc of closure can be used to determine if ICP is in a usual position relative to RCP. A healthy TMJ assumes *(1)* normal, smooth (noise-free) translation of the condyles, *(2)* bilaterally similar positioning of the condyles in the fossae, and *(3)* reasonable concentricity of the condyles in the fossae. On a manipulated hinge arc of closure, the distance from the first point of contact to RCP to ICP is normally less than 2 mm in a symmetrical anterior and slightly superior direction. This means that in a retrusive movement (assuming a normal ICP), the initial guiding teeth occur as bilaterally symmetrical contacts on the anterior inclines of the maxillary posterior teeth, and the posterior inclines of the mandibular teeth. If the movement between ICP and RCP is asymmetric or excessively long (>2 mm), one should first look for evidence that ICP has resulted from an iatrogenic change that has been introduced into the occlusion. If an iatrogenic change is present and evidence of occlusal trauma exists, a retruded contact occlusal adjustment to either lessen the amount of the slide or change its direction should be considered. The purpose of this adjustment is to develop an ICP that is more symmetrically positioned in relation to RCP, and to remove any adverse loading on the individual retrusive guiding teeth.

If the TMJ is functioning abnormally, or if there is evidence of muscle pathology, then occlusal adjustment procedures using a retruded jaw position as an anatomic reference position are contraindicated. In these cases, prior reversible treatment, such as with an interocclusal appliance, is usually indicated to reestablish a normal functioning joint and reduce any muscle problems. After resolution of the problem, the need for an occlusal adjustment may be assessed.

When considering the need for a retrusive guidance adjustment or any other occlusal adjustment, one must remember that most of the population will exhibit some irregularity in their occlusion. In biological systems, reasonable function and comfort are the ultimate criteria, not average anatomical values representing ideal form. If a patient is able to adapt to a "less-than-ideal occlusion," the occlusal scheme is considered physiologic. Thus, therapy of the occlusion should not be based on arbitrary anatomical classifications, such as Classes I, II, or III, nor on the amount and direction of slide between RCP and ICP. It should be based on adaptability of the system to be maintained in a state of health and comfort. Remembering this will help prevent needless and unwarranted therapy. Thus, *occlusal adjustment to preconceived idealized standards should not be done on a prophylactic basis.* Such procedures are indicated only when specific criteria exist, or the dentition will be, or has been, altered for other reasons (see chapter 13).

Indications and objectives for occlusal adjustment of the natural dentition

Indications:

1. Nonphysiologic occlusion, in some cases
2. Occlusal trauma (particularly primary occlusal trauma)
3. Occlusal instability
4. After orthodontic treatment, in some cases
5. Before moderate or major prosthetic or restorative procedures, in some cases
6. After prosthetic or restorative procedures, when needed
7. Unacceptable amount of discrepancy between RCP and ICP
8. Unacceptable working side, nonworking side, or protrusive interferences (guidance-disturbing contacts)

Objectives:

1. Improve structural and functional relations of the dentition
2. Bring occlusal forces within limits tolerable to the periodontium
3. Achieve and maintain occlusal stability

4. Permit condyle-disk complex to move and function normally, or within tolerable limits
5. Permit neuromuscular system to function within the adaptive potential of the patient
6. Reduce effects of parafunctional activities of the mandible
7. Improve esthetic needs of patient, if required

Occlusal adjustment procedures

The remainder of this chapter is devoted to practical techniques designed to help the student of Occlusion apply the basic principles of occlusal adjustment to the actual clinical situation. Because of the wide variability among dentitions, no discussion of procedures can describe the specific needs of any given patient. Basic principles, however, can be elucidated and can be applied to most, if not all, clinical cases.

Armamentarium

A slow- or high-speed handpiece (right angle) with a variety of green stones is sufficient to perform any adjustment procedure. An inverted cone or a small round green stone is commonly used. White stones and rubber wheels are required to polish the teeth after the adjustment is completed. The thinnest articulating film or ribbon available is used to mark centric stops and all functional contacts. Paper-holding forceps aid in handling articulating film, paper, or ribbon intraorally. Dry teeth will allow an accurate transfer of marking pigment from the articulating paper. The average patient's saliva flow can be controlled through the use of cotton rolls and other mechanical aids. On occasion, some patients will need the additional support of anticholinergic medication. Fifty milligrams (up to 100 mg) of methantheline bromide or 15 mg (up to 30 mg) of propantheline bromide, 45 minutes to 1 hour before an adjustment, will usually reduce salivary flow. Both drugs are contraindicated in patients with glaucoma and should be used cautiously in patients with cardiovascular disease. Other than these precautions, adverse reactions are rarely seen in single-dose therapy as used in dentistry, and the infrequent side effects are transitory.

Patient management

It is a wise clinician who practices the old adage: "Inform before you perform." The purpose of the adjustment, and what to expect during and after it, should always be explained to the patient. If a patient is prepared for side effects, he or she is much less likely to overreact. Before an adjustment, the patient should understand the proper relationships of the TMJs, teeth, muscles, and how they should function as a unit. An explanation of the probable etiology of any malfunctioning is usually given (e.g., unreplaced missing teeth, periodontal disease). Patients will understand their treatment and appreciate the importance of their treatment if the clinician speaks in terms that they understand. For example: "By improving the way your teeth fit together, your muscles will not have to work as hard to position your jaw as they have been in the past." Assurance that the adjustment will not initiate the decay process is also imperative.

The adjustment will usually result in an occlusion that feels more exact, comfortable, and stable. The patient should be informed that at the first appointment his or her teeth will be adjusted to an initial position, and that a reevaluation appointment will be scheduled in about 2 weeks. During the interim, loose teeth may tighten, muscles may relax, and the occlusion may change slightly and not feel exactly the way it did immediately after the adjustment. It should be impressed upon the patient that this is a normal course, and that the purpose of the reevaluation appointment is to refine and correct for these changes. The refinement or reevaluation appointment gives the patient a sense of security in that it is a time at which any problems will be alleviated.

At the initial adjustment appointment, a few minutes should be taken to demonstrate the type of movements needed to mark the teeth properly. During the procedure, the patient should be encouraged to ask questions. Also, patient feedback can be helpful in locating contacts that may need adjustment. Ask which side hits first and when the opposite side starts to contact. When the occlusion is being "fine tuned," most patients can tell exactly which tooth is in premature function. Involving the patient in the adjustment procedure not only hastens the process, but the interaction and cooperation is psychologically beneficial and reinforces the doctor-patient relationship. This does not imply that the clinician should lose control of the situation by having the patient dominate all of the adjustment decisions. Patients can develop an "abnormal positive occlusal consciousness" following such procedures by constantly checking their bite to find additional interfering areas of contact.

Diagnostic cast adjustment procedures

When extensive coronoplasty procedures are being considered, it is often necessary to do these adjustments on diagnostic casts first. Diagnostic casts help the clinician to determine the amount, location, and sequence of selective grinding, and to visualize the outcome and possible need for restorative procedures following the actual occlusal adjustment on the patient's dentition.

The casts should be accurately mounted on an articulator, usually with a face-bow transfer, in the relationship in which the coronoplasty is going to be performed. As will be discussed later, this may require that the casts be mounted in ICP, in a retruded jaw relationship, or in an appliance-dictated jaw position. Once the mounting procedure is complete, the casts must be treated with extreme care to avoid inadvertent chipping or other damage to the occlusal surfaces. The articulator incisal pin should be set firmly to the incisal table when tapping the teeth together. Marking the casts for adjustment is best performed with a very thin, colored articulating ribbon or paper. Thick marking paper often results in extraneous or false contact marks. Finally, adjustment of the casts is accomplished along the same guidelines and principles as for the actual dentition, detailed later in this section.

General principles of adjustment

The first general principle that must be adhered to is that *occlusal stability must be maintained or created.* By *occlusal stability* we mean the absence of teeth migrating within a dentition other than as compensatory physiological movements secondary to tooth wear. Centric holding (supporting) cusps of a tooth, for example, should not be taken out of ICP contact because this will lead to extrusion or migration of the tooth. To avoid future instability and new interferences, additions to the height of an opposing fossa or ridge with a restoration may be indicated in order to maintain occlusal stability whenever a centric holding cusp is to be reduced. Alternate methods of stabilizing the ICP can be considered in specific situations. Alloy restorations can be used to build up tooth surfaces that are not in contact. If the tooth is not in need of a restorative procedure, the acid-etch microfil resins can be utilized on a limited basis for this purpose.

Whether adjustments are being performed on casts or on natural teeth, an orderly sequence of the procedure will maximize time efficiency and ensure that all aspects of the occlusion are evaluated. Assuming that there are positive indicators to warrant occlusal adjustment therapy, these principles should be followed in the adjustment process:

1. Evaluation is needed to determine if an occlusal adjustment is the best method by which to achieve a consistent ICP. The clinician should visually evaluate the extent of adjustment needed to establish stable contacts. If removal of excessive amounts of tooth structure are required to achieve this, another mode of treatment may be in order (Fig. 21-6).
2. A harmonious intercuspal position must be established and maintained. Whether one is creating a new ICP or stabilizing the existing ICP, the procedure always seeks to establish a consistent contact pattern in this position.

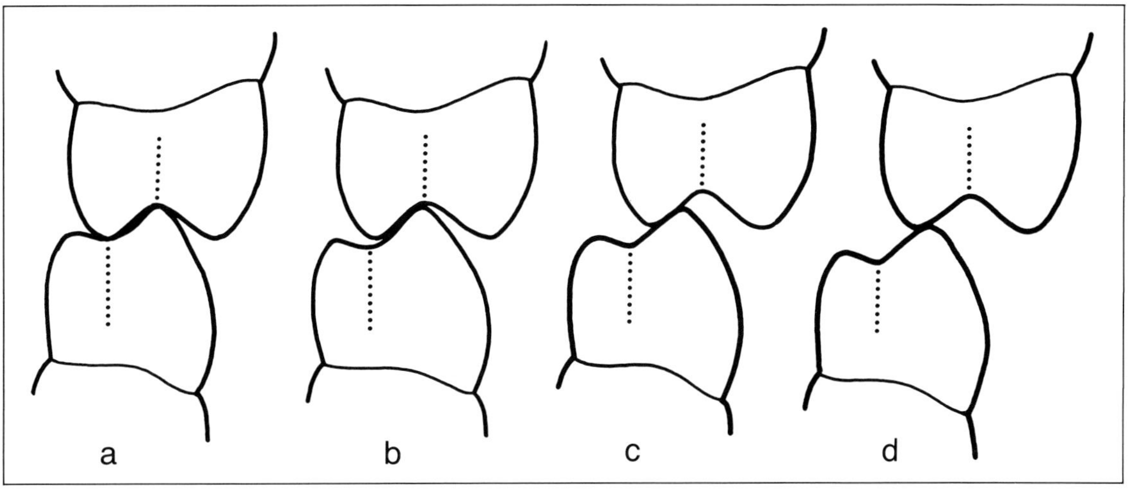

Fig. 21-6 Ideal cusp-to-fossa contact pattern *(a)*; only minor occlusal adjustments are necessary to achieve an ideal contact pattern (that is, one that is not unstable because of the influence of midline planes in ICP) *(b)*; major adjustment would be necessary to stabilize the occlusal relationships *(c)*; occlusal stability is not possible with occlusal adjustment *(d)*.

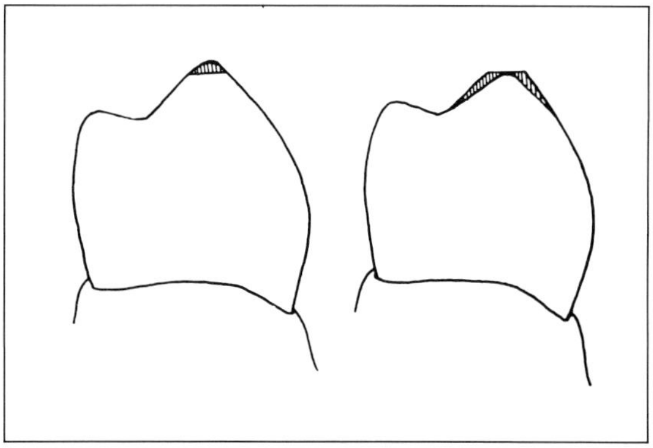

Fig. 21-7 Recontouring of a cusp tip is necessary after reduction of the height.

3. Care should be taken not to widen the occlusal table as the adjustments are being made. The original buccolingual width should be maintained or reduced. Likewise, cusps, ridges, and fossae should not be left flat. If an adjustment must be made on a cusp tip, that cusp should not be flattened, but instead, the original contour should be maintained (Fig. 21-7). When an adjustment is made on a convex surface, such as a triangular or marginal ridge, the original convex contour should be restored by widening the grooves and then rounding the ridges accordingly. Thus, original contour should be restored if possible on all adjusted teeth so that they look similar to the preadjusted natural dentition.

4. *Modification of centric holding cusps should always be approached with caution so as not to remove those cusps from occlusal contact in ICP.*

5. *Once reasonable contact pattern in maximum intercuspation has been established, contacts should not be removed during excursive contact adjustment.*

6. The goal of the excursive contact adjustment phase is to ensure that interference-free excursions can be performed without trauma to individual teeth. In all eccentric positions, the potential exists for removing the contacts providing optimal stability in maximum intercuspation. To prevent this error when recording ICP, the patient should perform the desired eccentric movement using a ribbon color different from that used for ICP. The ICP marks are preserved by removing only the color recorded by the eccentric movement. If a patient presents with maxillary first premolar lateral guidance, and the tooth is mobile, the excursive contacts are adjusted to involve more teeth in sharing the load, if possible. However, if excessive adjustment is required, alternative procedures may be needed to involve other teeth in the excursive guidance pattern.

7. When the adjustment process begins, there may only be several points of contact. As the adjustment proceeds, more points of contact will usually appear. It is necessary to evaluate previously adjusted marks as the adjustment continues. The clinician must measure and monitor the vertical dimension of occlusion in ICP by marking the amount of incisor overlap on the mandibular teeth before, during, and after the adjustment. This is done to prevent closing the vertical dimension during the adjustment.

Recontouring adjustments

Recontouring adjustments are most often necessary when replacing teeth that have been missing for a long period. Typically, the opposing teeth are not in a good occlusal relationship to enable a stable, interference-free occlusal scheme to be developed. Objectives include *(1)* correction of supereruption of opposing teeth into edentulous spaces; *(2)* improvement of marginal ridge relationships, or rotated, malpositioned, or tilted teeth; *(3)* reduction of plunger cusps; and *(4)* esthetic reshaping of malpositioned or chipped anterior teeth.

When recontouring teeth for either esthetic or functional purposes, the use of diagnostic casts is often very helpful in order to note how much reduction of the tooth is needed to accomplish the goal. If too much reduction is required, then a restoration may instead be indicated. During the reduction, the maintenance of normal contour and occlusal table width is important. After final shaping, the tooth must be polished in order to leave smooth functional surfaces. Again, an unstable occlusion should not result from recontouring adjustments—recontouring adjustments may be performed in conjunction with adjustments of ICP.

Intercuspal position adjustment

When an ICP adjustment is to be performed, the existing intercuspal contacts are first marked. Based on these marks, the clinician decides how best to achieve stable and evenly distributed intercuspal contacts on as many of the posterior teeth as possible. Constant examination of the individual contact patterns of each tooth during the adjustment is important in order to attempt to achieve the resulting axial force.

The ICP adjustment is typically performed with the patient in a semireclined position, for operator convenience, even though an upright position is a more functional position. It is not the purpose of this adjustment to change the position of maximum intercuspation but merely to improve it. The patient usually helps determine where adjustments should be made by tapping in an unstrained habitual arc of closure with the head erect. If this arc of closure is different from ICP, or if it is not reproducible, then an interocclusal appliance is first used to establish a reproducible jaw position.

Appliance-determined adjustment

When a patient has been treated with an interocclusal appliance for a period of time, it is sometimes necessary to adjust the occlusion to this appliance-determined position. As discussed in chapter 20, the *stabilization appliance* is not designed to deliberately alter mandibular position; only minimal postappliance adjustments are performed, if any, in these cases. The *repositioning appliance,* on the other hand, often produces significant changes in jaw position in an attempt to find a more therapeutic jaw position.

Depending on the amount of positional change, occlusal stabilization may or may not be achieved with an adjustment. Regardless of the appliance, appliance-determined adjustment is usually performed over several short appointments. This multiple appointment approach is necessary so that a consistent appliance-determined closing pattern can be maintained during the adjustment process. If the appliance is removed and the patient closes too many times, the proprioceptive system will begin to shift the jaw closure back to the former ICP, which is dictated by the old former occlusal contact pattern.

Appliance-determined adjustment is indicated when

1. The patient has prolonged relief from symptoms due to the appliance.
2. The patient repeatedly demonstrates a traumatic occlusal contact, unilateral occlusal contact, or a deflective occlusal contact pattern on initial closure when the appliance is not in place.
3. A reasonable therapeutic trial of part-time appliance use without an occlusal adjustment demonstrates that failure to correct this instability will cause the symptoms to return.

Appliance-determined adjustment is performed by having the patient remove the appliance, then close in the same arc of closure he or she uses when wearing the appliance. Obviously this requires a healthy, proprioceptively accurate mandibular motor system. The adjustments are continued until a consistent repeatable closure can be performed with consistent multiple contacts and no deflection or occlusal trauma is evident on closure.

Retruded contact position adjustment

Sometimes it is necessary to remove retrusive interferences and provide more freedom in the ICP. In these cases, a retruded jaw relation is used as an anatomical reference position for performing the adjustment. As pointed out previously, an RCP adjustment would be considered in cases where there is a significant asymmetrical slide from the RCP to that of maximum intercuspation, and then only in cases where there is a healthy TMJ. One indication for an RCP adjustment may be prior to and after a restorative procedure that could potentially render the existing ICP unstable. This is more likely when multiple restorations are involved.

The actual adjustment is performed by reducing any contact that produces a lateral slide. The goal of this adjustment is to produce even, stable, bilateral contacts on the posterior teeth. Continued adjustment of these RCP contacts is done until only a small symmetrical slide remains between RCP and ICP. After eliminating the lateral component and reducing the magnitude of the slide between RCP and ICP, the patient should be returned to the upright position and asked to tap his or her teeth together several times. While this is being done, the dentist should gently feel the labial surfaces of the maxillary anterior teeth for fremitus. The occlusion is again checked for an asymmetrical slide. In general, this type of adjustment is performed in situations where there has been a significant collapse of the occlusal support system. This type of adjustment should *not* be performed when there is an active TM disorder without prior reversible treatment and resolution of the signs and symptoms.

Mandibular manipulation

In order to observe the RCP and ICP slides, the mandible must be manipulated to place the condyles in centric relation position. A patient with a healthy musculature and joints will allow this procedure to be performed easily. However, much resistance will be encountered with patients exhibiting muscle pain, hyperactivity, or incoordination. If this situation occurs, the best approach is to initiate interocclusal appliance

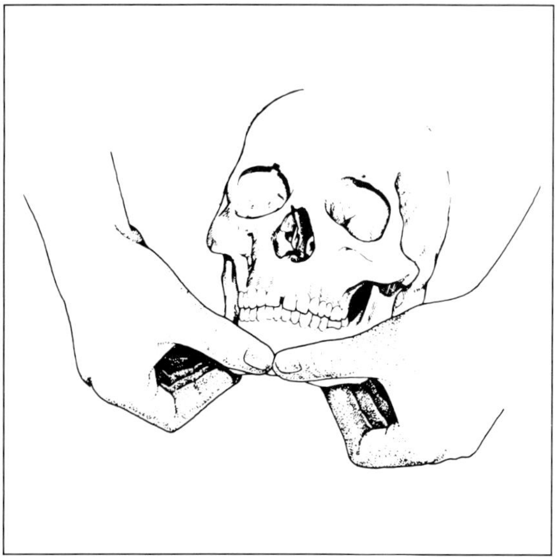

Fig. 21-8a Note placement of the thumbs and fingers of the dentist's hands when guiding the patient in an arc of closure.

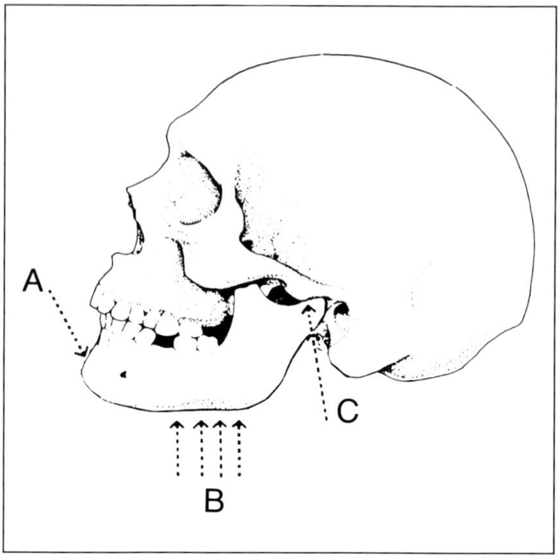

Fig. 21-8b Light force applied by the thumbs *(A)* and by the other fingers *(B)* results in a mostly superior force at the condyles *(C)*.

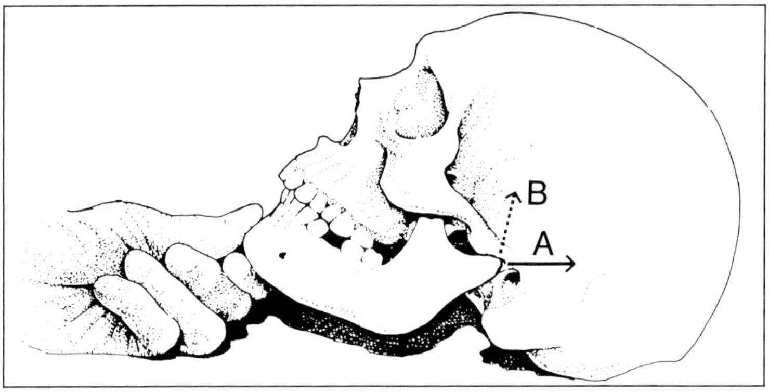

Fig. 21-9 Using the thumb and forefinger of one hand on the anterior part of the mandible will produce a force that is mostly posterior *(A)* and somewhat superior *(B)*. This method of guiding the patient's mandible into a retruded arc of closure is also acceptable, provided that gentle forces are used.

therapy (usually with a stabilization splint) to try to relax the musculature.

Two manipulation techniques are available to place the mandible in centric relation. For the two-hand method, the patient is reclined at a 45° angle and the dentist sits behind the patient. The dentist's thumbs are placed on top of the chin, and the fingers of each hand are placed along the inferior border of the mandible (Figs. 21-8a and b). Light force is now applied upward on the angles of the mandible and downward on the chin. This will result in a force on the condyles in a more superior, rather than a posterior, direction. While maintaining this pressure, the wrists and fingers are kept in a semifixed position and arcing of the mandible is done by moving the forearms. An assistant will be required to hold articulating paper and to dry the teeth.

For the one-hand approach, the patient is again placed in a reclined position, but the dentist sits beside the patient. The dentist should place the thumb on the patient's chin, or on the

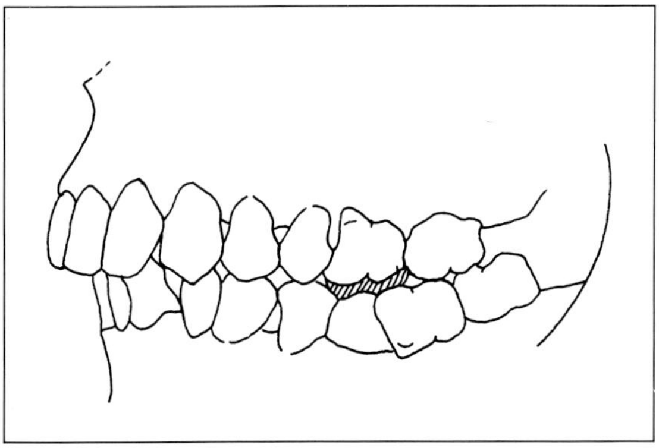

Fig. 21-10a Shortening and recontouring of extruded maxillary first molar prior to construction of a mandibular fixed prosthesis.

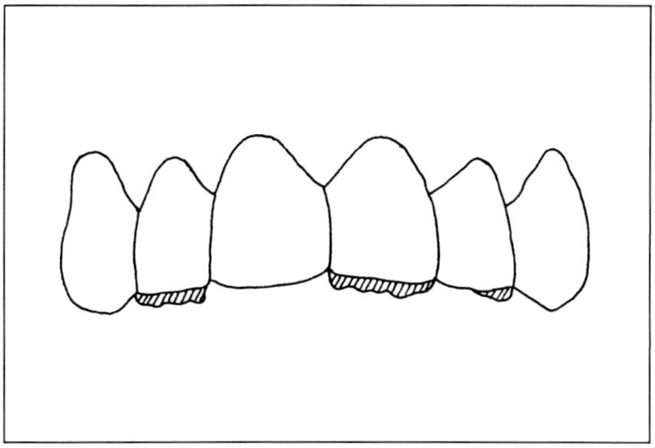

Fig. 21-10b Recontouring of incisal edges of maxillary incisors to improve esthetics.

gingiva below the mandibular central incisors, and with the forefinger under the chin, apply a light force in a direction that will bisect the condyles (Fig. 21-9). This places a force on the condyles in a posterior-superior position. The mandible is slowly arced by flexing the elbow. This technique will allow one free hand to hold the articulating paper. Dramatic differences in jaw positioning have not been demonstrated between the two techniques, even though they apparently apply force to the jaw in different directions. The two-hand technique best simulates the ideal force direction naturally occurring in the TMJ, but both techniques are acceptable methods. Whichever technique is used, the key is *not to apply extreme force*.

Excursive adjustments

These adjustment procedures are performed after a consistent and stable ICP contact is achieved. In many cases the existing ICP is adequate; therefore, it is not necessary to do anything other than the excursive adjustment. The posterior teeth are marked with one color of articulating ribbon in ICP, and another color ribbon is used to evaluate the teeth for guidance-disturbing interferences by having the patient go through lateral and protrusive excursive movements. This type of evaluation should certainly be performed in cases where major restorative treatment is needed and whenever anterior guiding restorations are to be placed.

Whenever excursive adjustments are to be performed, the type of guidance can be predetermined by studying articulated diagnostic casts. Posterior tooth excursive interferences may then be adjusted accordingly, *preserving the ICP contacts*. An excursive interference should be reduced enough to provide 0.5 to 1.0 mm clearance so that no contacts are made under functional loading (chewing or bruxism).

Nonworking side interferences are usually corrected first. Most often these will involve the inner aspects of maxillary lingual cusps and the inner aspects of mandibular buccal cusps, in the region of the last molars. Since both of these are centric holding cusps, particular caution should be exercised during any selective grinding so as not to destabilize the occlusion. Inclines, not cusp tips, should be adjusted, if possible. If cusp tips must be involved, the maxillary lingual cusp *or* the mandibular buccal cusp should be shortened—*but not both*. Reducing both will take those teeth out of occlusion in ICP and lead to their subsequent extrusion and the return of interferences.

Next, working side interferences are evaluated. If adjustment of this side is required, selec-

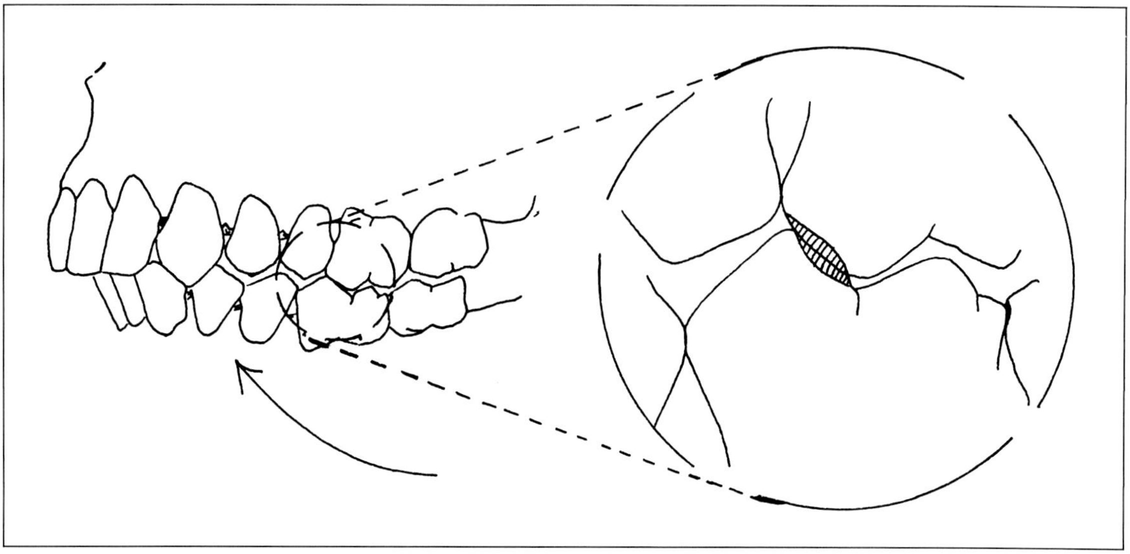

Fig. 21-11 The anterior component *(arrow)* of a slide from RCP and ICP involves forward facing inclines on maxillary teeth and backward facing inclines on mandibular teeth. Adjustment of one or both of these inclines should, whenever possible, avoid reduction of cusp tips, particularly those of supporting cusps.

tive grinding should avoid the centric holding cusps. This implies that adjustment is usually done on the maxillary buccal and/or mandibular lingual cusps (buccal of upper, lingual of lower: B.U.L.L. rule). In the natural dentition, it is not an intention of occlusal adjustment therapy to seek to obtain heavy lingual-to-lingual cusp contact or cross-tooth balance on the working side during lateral excursion. Buccal-to-buccal cusp contact is more than adequate. The canines are most often in contact, either alone (canine guidance) or along with one or more pair of adjacent posterior teeth, depending on individual circumstances.

Sequence of occlusal adjustment procedures

1. Recontouring adjustment and ICP adjustment without changing maxillomandibular relationships (Figs. 21-10a and b). Occlusal stability must be considered in any of these procedures:
   a. Shorten extruded teeth.
   b. Improve esthetics.
   c. Reduce plunger cusps.
   d. Correct marginal ridge relationships.
   e. Correct rotated, malpositioned, or tilted teeth.
   f. Correct facets and abraded teeth.
   g. Round sharp edges when indicated.
   h. Narrow buccolingual diameters when indicated.
   i. Create the ability to voluntarily tap into a consistent ICP with head erect (muscular contact position coincident with ICP).
2. Elimination of asymmetric slide between RCP and ICP:
   a. Identify anterior component to the slide (forward facing inclines on maxillary teeth and backward facing inclines on mandibular teeth) (Fig. 21-11).
   b. Identify right and left component to the slide (left facing inclines on maxillary teeth responsible for slide to left, etc.) (Fig. 21-12).
   c. As a general rule, *widen fossae or embrasure areas to accommodate the occluding*

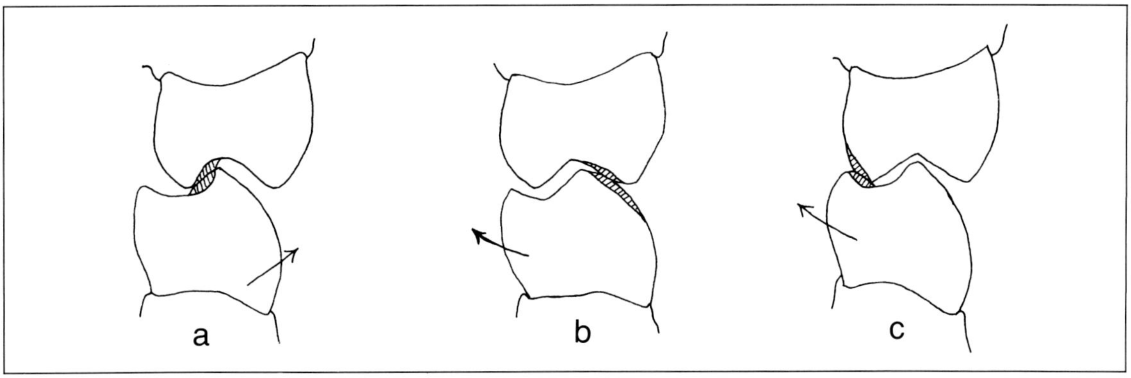

Fig. 21-12 The lateral component *(arrows)* of a slide from RCP to ICP may involve the inner aspects of maxillary lingual cusps and mandibular buccal cusps *(a)*, the inner aspect of maxillary buccal cusps and outer aspect of mandibular buccal cusps *(b)*, or the outer aspect of maxillary lingual cusps and inner aspect of mandibular lingual cusps *(c)*. Note the inclines that may be adjusted in each situation. In all cases reduction of centric holding areas should be avoided.

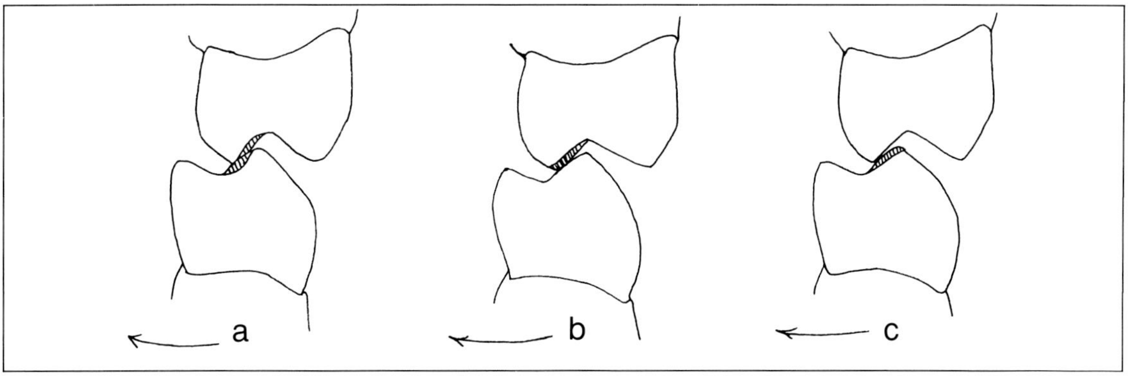

Fig. 21-13 An interference on the nonworking side most often involves the inner aspects of maxillary lingual and mandibular buccal cusps, both of which are centric holding cusps. One or both of these interfering inclines may be adjusted without shortening either cusp tip *(a)*. If a cusp tip must be adjusted, the maxillary lingual cusp *(b)* or the mandibular buccal cusp *(c)* may be shortened, *but not both*.

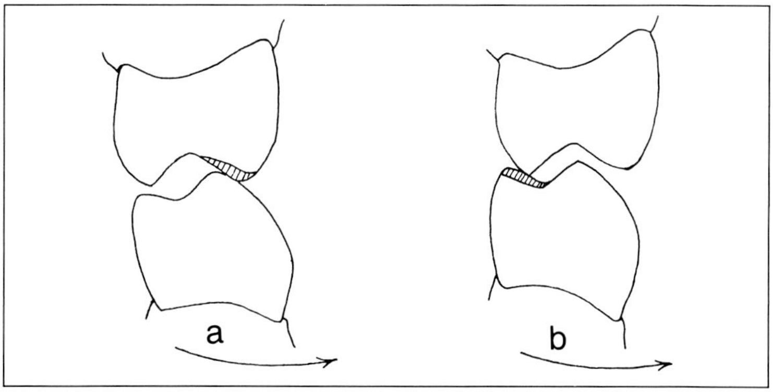

Fig. 21-14 An interference on the working side most often involves the opposing buccal cusps *(a)* and/or the opposing lingual cusps *(b)*. In order to avoid destabilizing the occlusion, adjustment would involve the inner aspect of the maxillary buccal cusps and/or the inner aspect of the mandibular lingual cusp.

cusps (do not grind depth of fossa or tips of cusps if this is avoidable).

3. Elimination of nonworking side interferences: This will typically involve the buccal aspect of maxillary lingual cusps and lingual aspect of mandibular buccal cusps. Since two supporting or centric holding cusps are ordinarily involved in this type of interference, cusp tips should not be touched. If a cusp tip must be ground, adjust either maxillary or mandibular but *not both* in order to maintain occlusal stability in ICP (Fig. 21-13).

4. Elimination of working side interferences:
   a. Avoid adjustment on centric holding cusps, especially cusp tips.
   b. Adjust buccal cusps of maxillary teeth, and/or lingual cusps of mandibular teeth (B.U.L.L. rule) (Fig. 21-14).
   c. Do not try to achieve cross-tooth balance.
   d. Achieving a canine-guided occlusion, complete group function, or a combination of both depends upon individual circumstances of the case.
   e. Recheck for nonworking side interferences.

5. Elimination of protrusive interferences:
   a. Do not remove centric holding areas of posterior teeth.
   b. Seek to achieve bilateral incisive contact, if possible (at least one incisor tooth on each side of midline during protrusion).
   c. Alter incisal guidance only when definite indications exist.
   d. Do not reduce centric holding areas of anterior teeth.

6. Examination for fremitus while patient voluntarily taps teeth into ICP in the *upright position*

7. Polishing of all areas that have been ground

8. When is adjustment complete?
   a. If indicated, asymmetric shift is eliminated.
   b. Nonworking side interferences are eliminated.
   c. Lateral and protrusive movements are smooth.
   d. Incisive contact is bilateral.
   e. Patient can voluntarily tap into ICP with head upright, and without producing fremitus.

9. Cautions:
   a. Adjustment should be done for a definite reason—not prophylactically.
   b. Adjustment should be done cautiously—tooth structure is irreplaceable.
   c. Adjustment should not be done in the presence of TMJ and/or muscle problems—*alleviate problem first by reversible procedures.*
   d. Adjustment should not be completed at one sitting, particularly if major adjustment is needed—give patient a chance to adapt.
   e. Adjustment should not create unfavorable positive occlusal consciousness on the part of the patient, leading him or her to think about and test his or her occlusal contacts frequently.
   f. Occlusal adjustment therapy alone may not be the only mode of occlusal therapy needed—it may need to be used in conjunction with orthodontic, prosthetic, operative, or other modes of therapy.

Summary

This chapter has presented several criteria for determining the need for an occlusal adjustment. If enough of these criteria exist, several methods of adjustment are possible. It should be remembered that in certain clinical situations occlusal adjustment therapy is a highly successful treatment, but in other situations it must be avoided as a primary therapy.

The patient who has a painful or dysfunctional TMJ will usually need prior treatment, such as with an interocclusal appliance (splint), in an attempt to reduce the symptoms and find an optimal mandibular position. This situation may require that an appliance-determined occlusal adjustment be utilized at a later time.

The patient with significant muscular pain problems, incoordination, or other TM disorders that are not directly related to a recent occlusal change will also need to be successfully treated prior to evaluating the occlusion for the need to perform an adjustment.

Occlusal adjustment is a logical treatment when there are local dental and periodontal effects due to adverse loading on individual teeth. Occlusal adjustment therapy can redistribute logically the force or load on teeth, but it would be illogical as a treatment approach to stop a nocturnal bruxism behavior.

Muscle and even joint pain symptoms that have developed immediately after iatrogenic interferences reasonably can be expected to be relieved with occlusal adjustment.

When the occlusal support system changes over a long period of time it is necessary to consider the possibility that subsequent mandibular and condylar positional changes can be harmful. This is especially so when the dysfunctional symptoms are related to a derangement of TMJ function. In these cases, alteration of the jaw position with appliances and subsequent occlusal stabilization appear logical, although they are still considered experimental.

Finally, because research demonstrating the necessity of routinely changing maxillomandibular relations is not available, occlusal adjustment for purely prophylactic reasons should be avoided.

Chapter 22

Prosthodontic, Operative, and Orthodontic Therapy

George A. Zarb and Aaron H. Fenton

This chapter deals with those forms of traditional occlusal therapy most frequently practiced by the dentist. As noted in the introduction to Part III, this discussion will not cover clinical procedures and techniques that are readily available in discipline-based textbooks (i.e., on operative dentistry, orthodontics, fixed and removable prosthodontics). The objective is to deal only with those issues that specifically relate to occlusal form and function and that are of common denominator interest for all dentists.

Over the years several authors have sought to articulate criteria for an optimized therapeutic occlusion. In chapter 13, such an occlusion was described as one that has been modified by therapeutic modalities so that it falls within the parameters of a physiologic occlusion. This description is helped by a set of therapeutic objectives proposed by Beyron (1954a, 1969, 1973) and since modified by others. These objectives consist of

1. Acceptable interocclusal distance
2. Stable jaw relationship with bilateral contact in retruded closure
3. Stable quadrant relationships providing axially directed forces
4. Freedom in retrusive range of contact
5. Multidirectional freedom of contact movement

For many cases where structural occlusal therapy is indicated in order to change a nonphysiologic situation to a physiologic one, Beyron's prescription represents a logical and practical approach. It has been applied in countless clinical situations and, in a sense, has stood the test of time. Because of this it is adhered to by many dental practitioners and educators. Each of Beyron's objectives will be considered in this chapter, particularly in its application to prosthodontic therapy. It must be emphasized, however, that the relevance of these objectives, or any others, cuts across disciplines and techniques, because occlusal therapy outcome objectives all underscore the fundamental goal of achieving *jaw and tooth structural relationships that enhance optimal function and self-perpetrating occlusal harmony.*

All phases of dentistry evaluate the mandibular function of a patient and plan therapy to maximize the functional result. Thus, a therapeutic occlusion is very often achieved as a result of interdependent strategies. In this chapter, three of these important strategies are considered: *(1)* prosthodontic therapy, *(2)* operative therapy, and *(3)* orthodontic therapy. The overlap between these and other therapeutic strategies is the rule rather than the exception. Despite this unified approach, these therapies retain their own inherent characteristics in terms of knowledge, skills, techniques, patient evaluation, and treatment potential.

Prosthodontic therapy

Partial or complete tooth loss is almost invariably the result of disease of the tooth tissues (caries) or

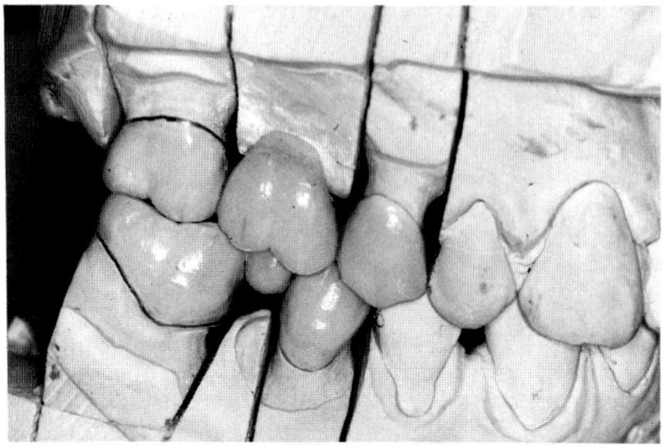

Fig. 22-1a An example of a short-span fixed prosthesis replacing one posterior tooth in each arch.

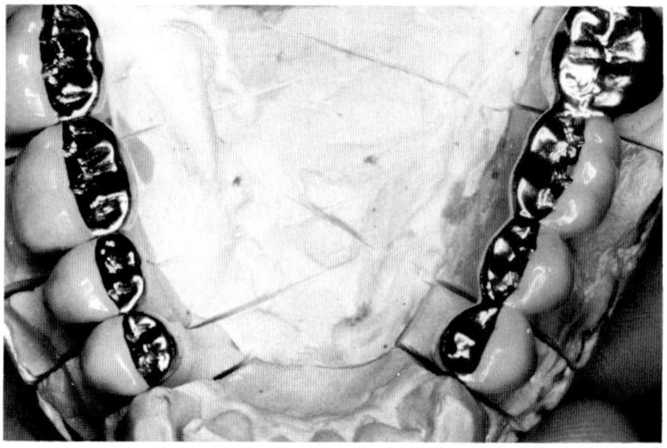

Fig. 22-1b A longer-span fixed prosthesis replacing the second premolars and first molars in both mandibular quadrants.

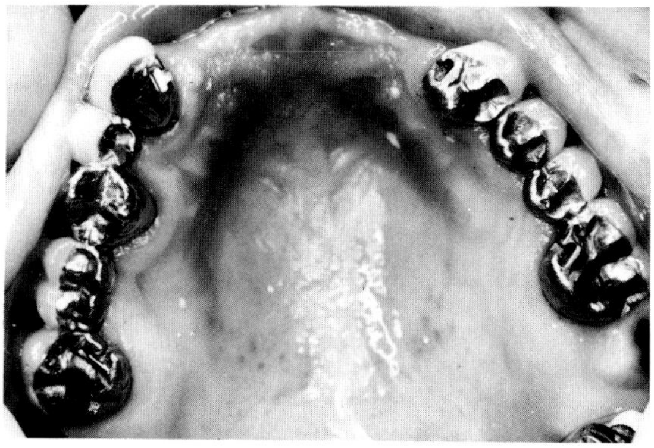

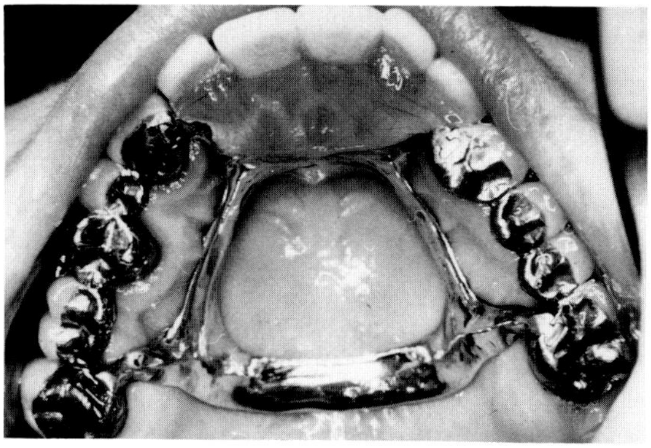

Figs. 22-1c and d Posterior maxillary fixed prostheses replace missing premolars on the left and the first premolar and first molar on the right. The four anterior teeth could not be replaced with a fixed prosthesis because a mechanism for compensating for resorption of the residual edentulous segment was required. A precision retained removable partial denture was used for this purpose.

disease of the supporting tissues (periodontal disease). Occasionally, tooth loss may also result from traumatic incidents or from severe attrition. Both diseases have a long history and their effects have been extensively studied. The incidence of complete edentulism (total loss of the natural dentition) in Western countries is well documented and attests to the profession's ongoing need to treat an increasing number of aging edentulous subjects. We can only speculate on the incidence of partial edentulism, although published evidence does suggest that partial destruction of the dentition and supporting tissues is prevalent.

Over the years, dentists have demonstrated considerable skill at replacing depleted dentitions and in compensating for the resultant deficit in periodontal ligament support. Tooth loss can be mutilating, because it can undermine function and esthetics. It also leads to a reduction of alveolar bone, which forms an integral part of the facial skeleton. This loss is irrevocable. Prosthetic care has, therefore, evolved into an applied clinical skill of variations on a theme of ingenious salvage. This is routinely demonstrated in clinical prescriptions that range from simple to complex multiunit fixed prostheses or complete dentures, to dental rehabilitation of

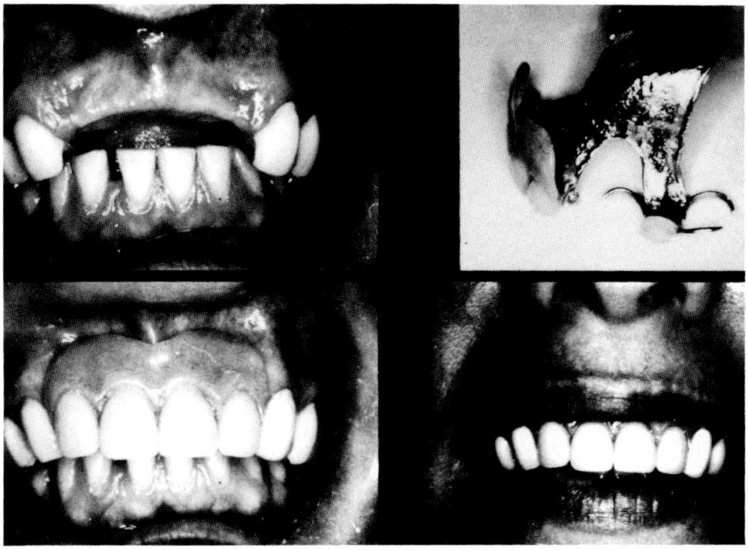

Fig. 22-2 The segment of tooth and alveolar bone loss in the anterior part of the maxilla is restored with a removable partial denture.

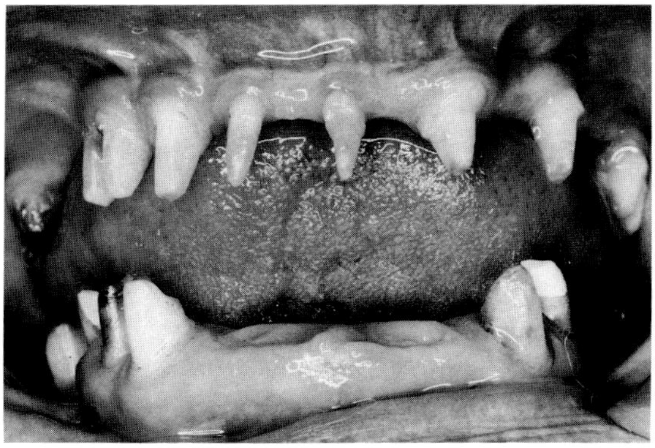

Fig. 22-3a The remaining dentition in an example of full-mouth fixed rehabilitation.

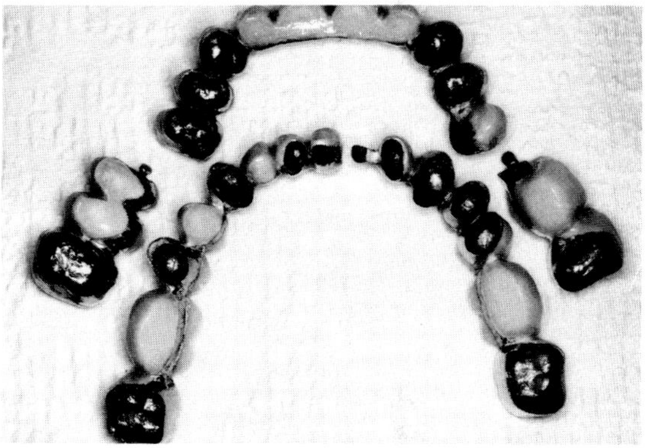

Fig. 22-3b Multiple interlocking castings.

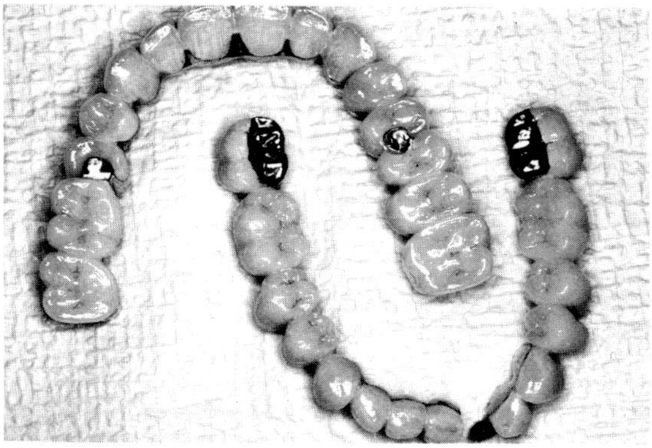

Fig. 22-3c Porcelain occlusal fixed partial dentures.

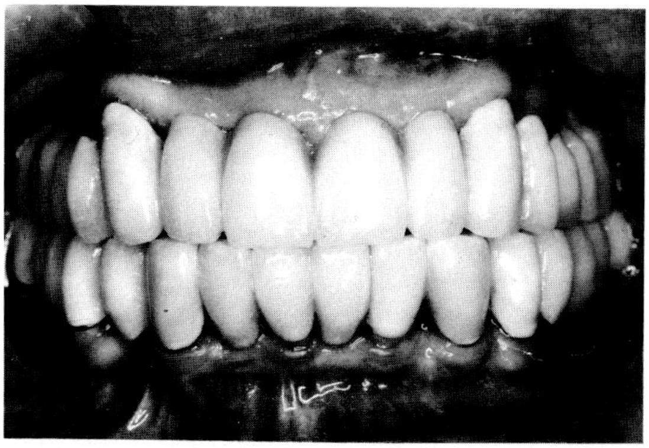

Fig. 22-3d The prostheses in situ.

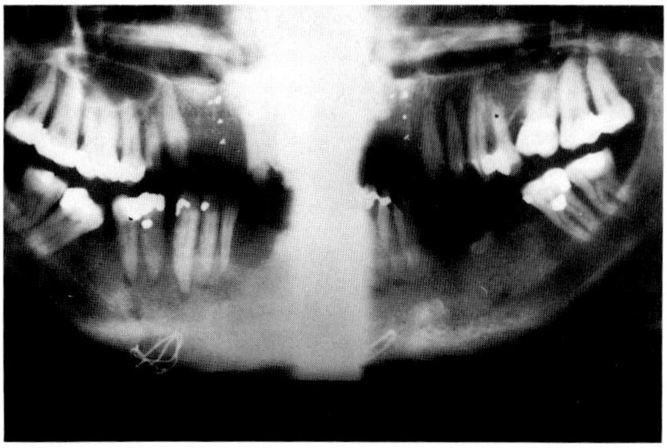

Fig. 22-4a A severe traumatic incident has necessitated the removal of several teeth as evidenced by this postaccident radiograph.

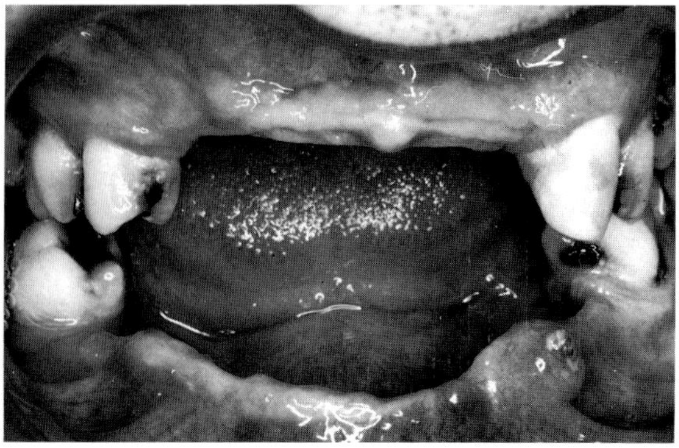

Fig. 22-4b Intraoral view.

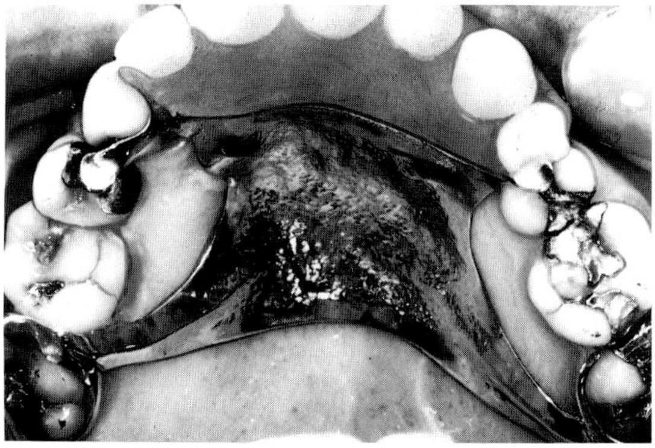

Fig. 22-4c Maxillary view following treatment with removable partial dentures.

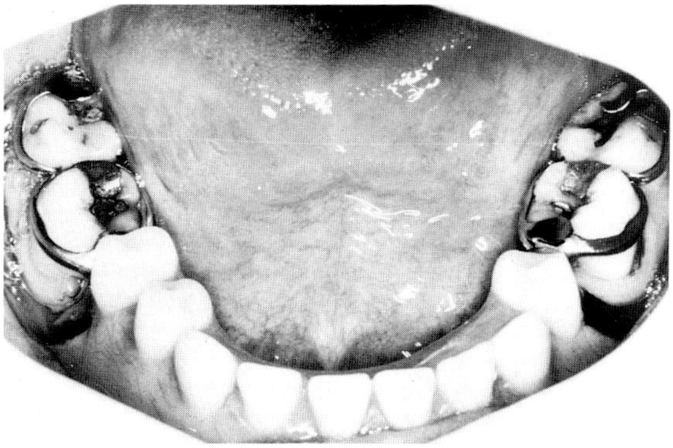

Fig. 22-4d Mandibular view of prosthesis.

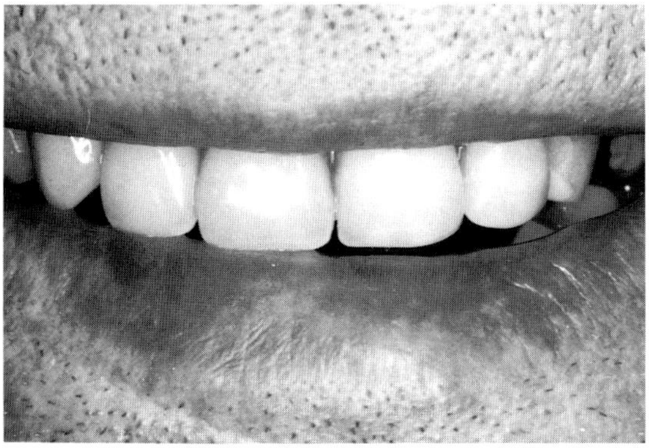

Fig. 22-4e The treatment for this patient ensures both functional and esthetic restoration.

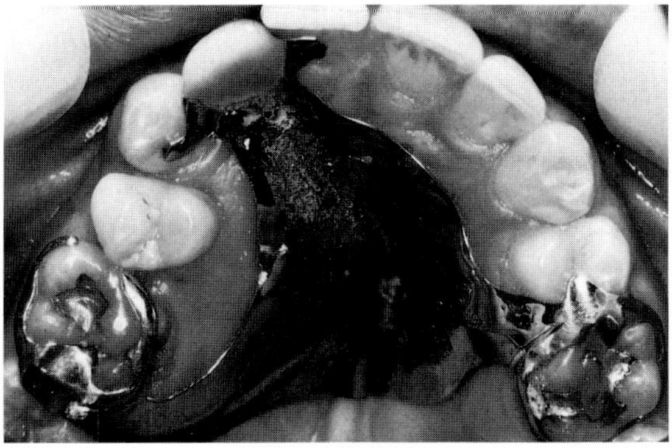

Fig. 22-5a An example of prosthodontic therapy for a cleft lip and palate. Palatal view of the cast removable partial denture covering the congenital defect.

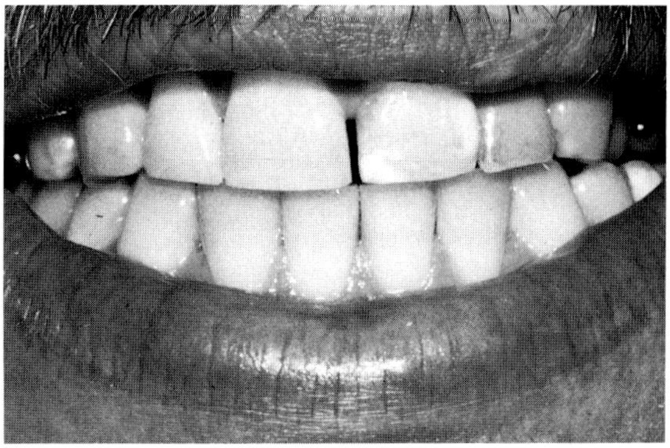

Fig. 22-5b The patient's smile has been restored.

patients suffering from congenital defects, traumatic incidents, or oncologic surgical interventions (Figs. 22-1 to 22-5).

In prosthodontic treatment, considerable skills may be required to reconcile patient expectations with clinical diagnoses and treatment planning as well as with tooth and supporting tissue preparation, biomaterials selection, and their technical applications. However, a common denominator prescription applies in every clinical situation, irrespective of the extent of the required occlusal restoration(s) (Figs. 22-6a to d). This prescription comprises a series of biomechanical objectives for occlusal therapy. As stated in this chapter's introduction, clinical experience endorses these objectives. A brief discussion of the relevance of each is required.

Acceptable interocclusal distance

The interocclusal distance (also popularly referred to as freeway space) is the space or existing gap between the maxillary and mandibular teeth when the mandible is in postural rest position during normal respiration and the patient is upright and alert. It amounts to 2 to 4 mm in a vertical direction if observed at the position of the first premolars (Figs. 22-7a to c). It appears to vary, for most subjects, within a limited range and depends upon a variety of factors. These include craniofacial morphology, head and body posture, alertness, the relative amount of tonic activity of the masticatory musculature, the presence of prostheses, and nasopharyngeal patency. A patient's interocclusal distance may be partially encroached upon as a result of extrusion of unopposed segment(s) of the dentition (Fig. 22-8), as a result of incorrectly designed (too high) restorations, and/or as a result of the dentist's effort to "raise the bite," that is, increase the occlusal vertical dimension. All of the above encroachments on the interocclusal distance, particularly when sudden, can be potentially hazardous. In some patients, they appear to precipitate myofascial pain dysfunction. A correct interocclusal distance is also absolutely essential for complete-denture patients. An excessive interocclusal distance can cause "clicking" of the teeth, loosening of dentures, soreness of denture-bearing tissues, and rapid destruction of the denture-supporting residual alveolar ridges.

An inadequate interocclusal distance may compromise the patient's esthetics, speech articulation, jaw relationship, and mastication. However, the range of individual tolerance is such that an inadequate interocclusal distance is more commonly accepted by a patient. To a large extent, most clinicians and dental educators suggest that a functionally comfortable and esthetically acceptable interocclusal distance should be maintained unless there are specific indications for change.

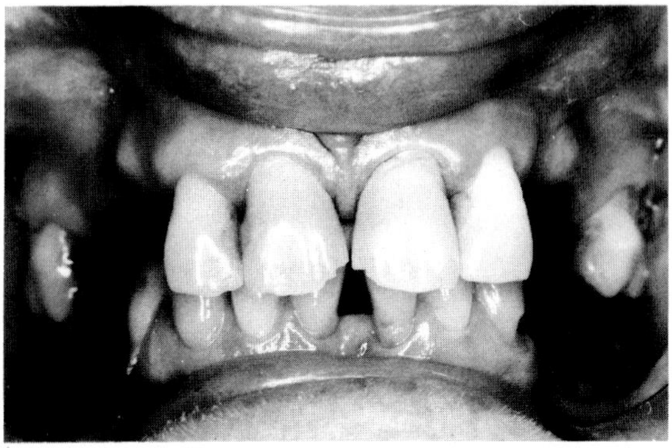

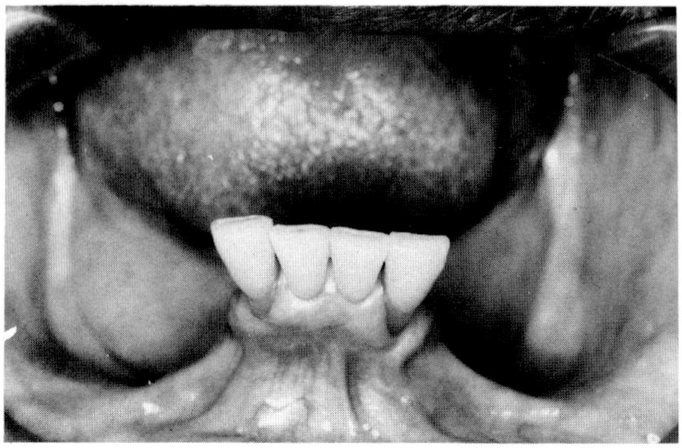

Figs. 22-6a and b Beyron's objectives for occlusal therapy apply to a variety of morphologically different clinical situations, such as these partially edentulous situations.

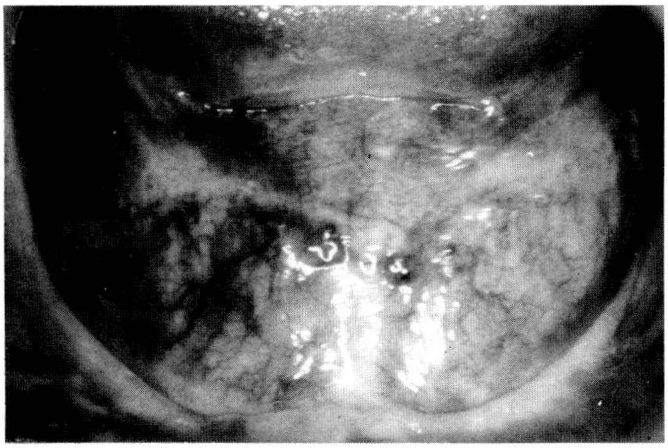

Fig. 22-6c An edentulous situation.

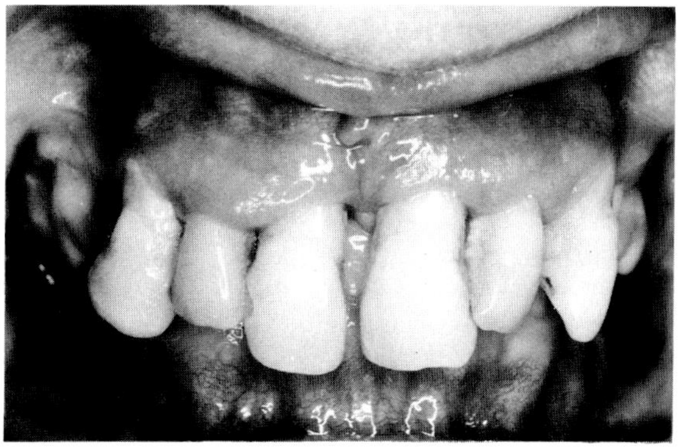

Fig. 22-6d A dentulous situation. The advanced periodontal disease necessitated extraction of the entire dentition with immediate denture replacement.

Certain clinical situations are encountered where a decrease or an increase in the interocclusal distance can be tolerated or actually requested by some patients. Small increments in the occlusal vertical dimension may make a smile more visible or improve the soft tissue profile to a patient's satisfaction. Technically, a small increment may allow for an adequate thickness of a prosthetic occlusion without extra reduction of healthy enamel and dentin. The success of these modifications is contingent upon the amount of interocclusal distance required by the individual patient. For example, a patient with a "natural" interocclusal distance of 4 mm can usually tolerate an occlusal addition, that is, an interocclusal distance encroachment of 1 to 2 mm. The ability of the individual patient to accommodate to the resultant increased occlusal vertical dimension should first be clinically tested with reversible dental procedures prior to the institution of definitive therapy.

Clinical situations are also encountered where an interocclusal distance may appear to be excessive, well beyond the typically observed 2- to 4-mm range. This usually occurs *(1)* as a result of a developmental anomaly (e.g., inadequate

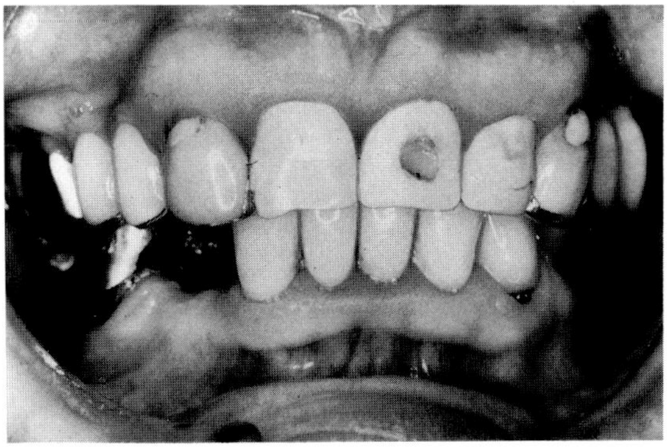

Fig. 22-7a The variable interocclusal distance tends to fall within a 2- to 4-mm range for most patients. In this pretreatment view the patient is sitting upright in a relaxed position with his mandible at rest and the teeth *not* contacting.

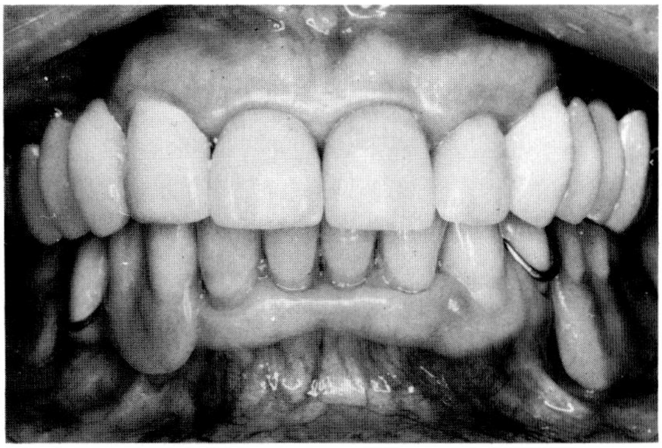

Fig. 22-7b Posttreatment view. The 2-mm interocclusal distance was retained.

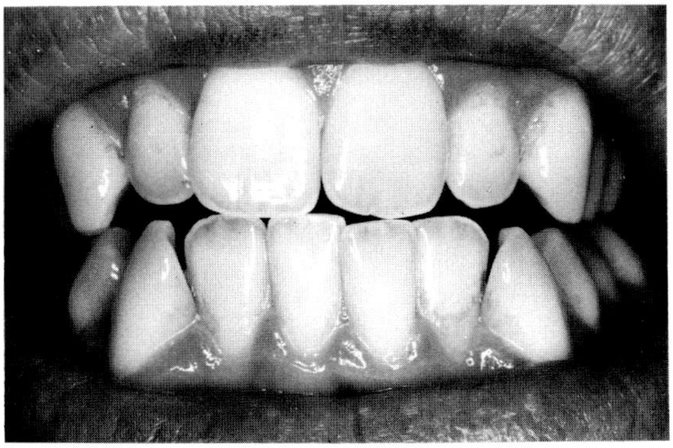

Fig. 22-7c The interocclusal distance in a dentate patient.

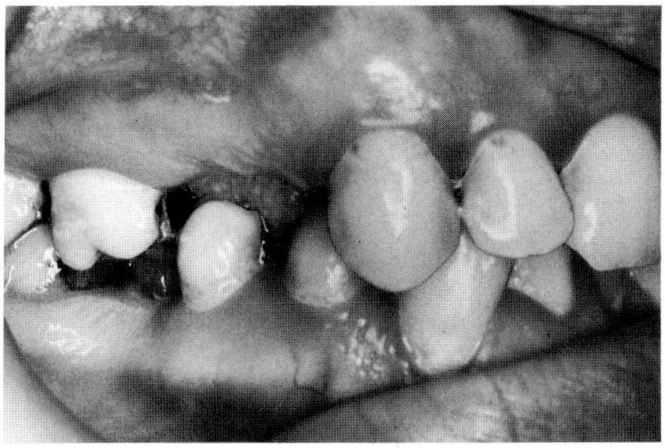

Fig. 22-8 Premature loss of posterior support for the dentition resulted in extrusion of teeth, which has encroached upon the interocclusal space.

midfacial growth associated with a cleft palate; Figs. 22-9a to d), *(2)* from loss of bilateral posterior tooth quadrant support (Figs. 22-10a to c), or *(3)* because of rapid advanced tooth wear or attrition (Fig. 22-11). These situations, especially *1* and *3*, are usually asymptomatic.

When treatment becomes necessary it is done by *recovery* of lost occlusal vertical dimension via the establishment of a clinically determined optimal interocclusal distance. In other words, the patient's occlusal vertical dimension at the initial examination is restored to a physiologically "normal" range. This is not an arbitrary prescription but one that is based upon traditional and clinically reliable methods of evaluating and establishing optimal vertical dimension positions (Hickey et al., 1985). This endeavor is frequently prognosticated by the fabrication of an acrylic resin interocclusal appliance that is worn by the patient to determine the feasibility of the planned reduction in the interocclusal distance (Figs. 22-12a to h).

When the loss in the occlusal vertical dimension results from loss of posterior tooth support, a patient is more likely to be at risk to develop a temporomandibular (TM) disorder, particularly

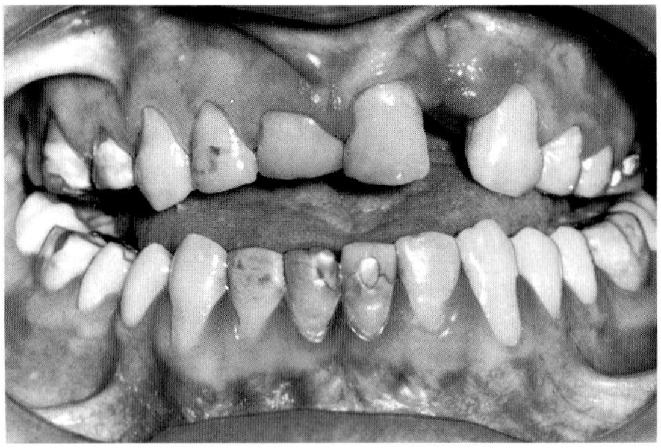

Fig. 22-9a Deficient midfacial growth. Facial view.

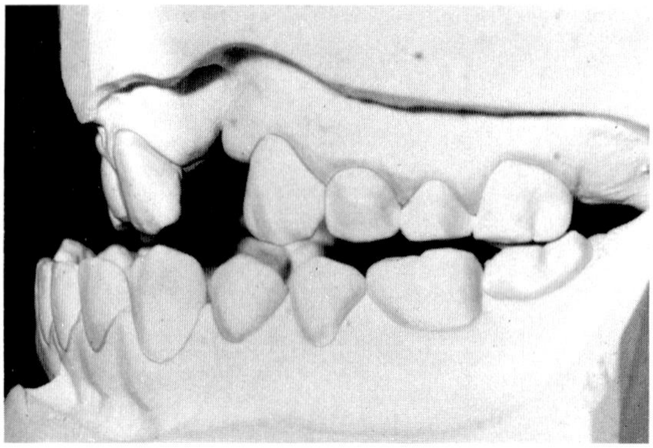

Fig. 22-9b Anterior dental arch defect.

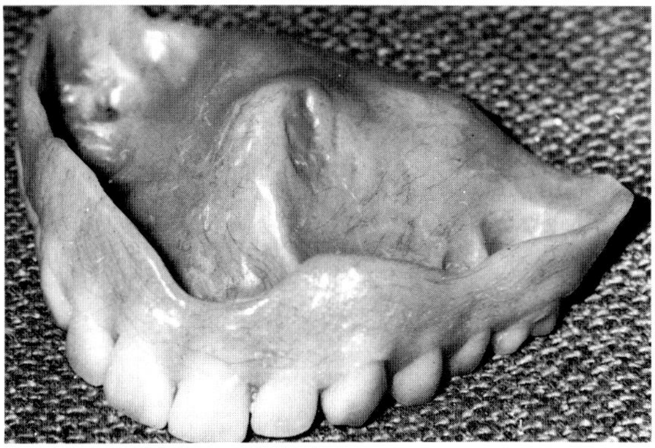

Fig. 22-9c Maxillary overdenture to restore missing facial growth.

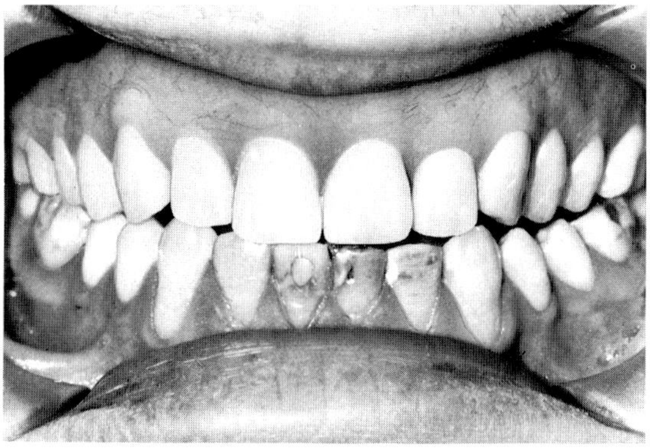

Fig. 22-9d Intraoral view of facial restoration.

osteoarthrosis. The relationship between a "collapsed" occlusal vertical dimension and TM disorders has often been regarded as a clear-cut cause-and-effect situation by the profession. However, scientific evidence for such a conclusion is far from compelling, and clinical experience suggests that each individual situation has to be diagnosed as such—not as part of a routine and dogmatic formula solution to justify "opening the bite" or otherwise increasing occlusal vertical dimension.

Stable jaw relationship with bilateral contact in retruded closure

An acceptable occlusal vertical dimension along the path of the terminal hinge movement of the mandible may be regarded as the position of centric relation (see chapters 6 and 9). This position can be located irrespective of whether the teeth are present. Clinical research indicates that the majority of tooth contacts occur in and around the position of maximal intercuspation (centric occlusion) and that in the vast majority of individuals with natural dentitions, tooth contacts in centric relation do *not* coincide with those in centric occlusion. The Posselt envelope of motion is a useful teaching diagram (Fig. 22-13) to outline the sagittal and the horizontal extreme envelopes of mandibular movement. These movements are only influenced by the presence of the dentition at a specific occlusal contact level, which may be the naturally occurring one or the one determined by the dentist.

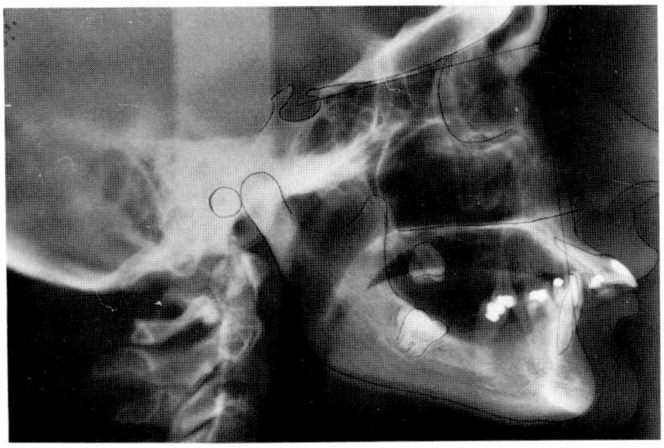

Fig. 22-10a A patient with a dual bite and bilateral loss of posterior tooth quadrant support.

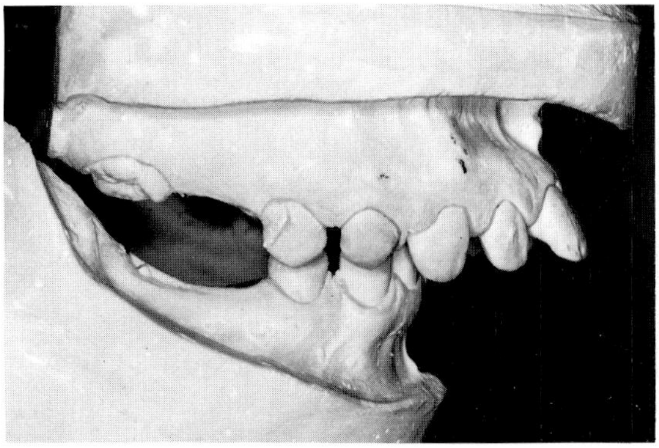

Fig. 22-10b The morphologic Class II, division 1 appearance is dramatically emphasized.

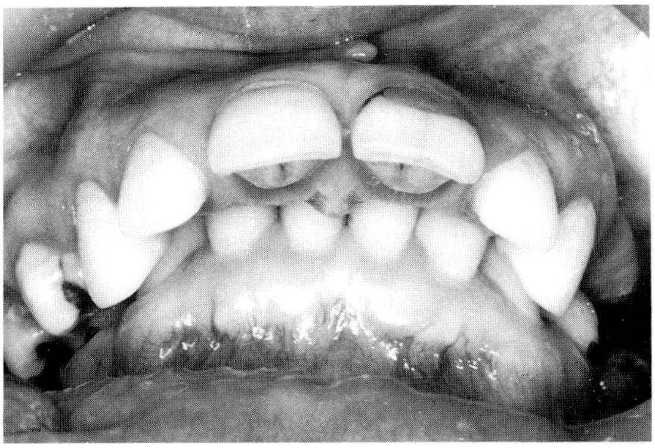

Fig. 22-10c The risk of palatal gingival trauma is an untoward consequence.

In the case of single tooth or single quadrant restorations, the choice is to utilize and not change the patient's preexisting intercuspal position. The only caution here is that the restoration(s) not increase the extent or direction of the original "slide in centric." In other words, maxillomandibular relationships should not be changed by the prosthodontic therapy.

Over the years, considerable controversy has raged about the significance of the centric relation position (see chapter 12) and its clinical use. Current clinical wisdom still regards a *passive* patient-dentist guided retruded closure of the mandible as the optimal position to be used in many therapeutic situations. This certainly applies when there are an insufficient number of residual natural teeth and the position of centric occlusion (intercuspal position) can no longer be confidently determined.

Quite logically, the temporomandibular joints (TMJs) and musculature should be healthy before prosthetic treatment is undertaken. Unhealthy TMJs complicate the registration of jaw position records and may even preclude them. Structural and functional harmony of osseous structures, intraarticular tissues, and ligaments must exist if centric relation is to be useful as a therapeutic position. If these specifications cannot be fulfilled, a recordable centric relation record is not feasible. Hence, the importance of routine evaluation of a patient's TMJ function (see chapter 14) is an integral part of prosthodontic therapy. If signs or symptoms of a TM disorder are present, they should be treated, as outlined in other chapters of Part III of this textbook.

Centric relation is also often used as a therapeutic position in the presence of an existing and recordable intercuspal position when an extensive number of occlusal surfaces are to be restored. For example, when planning multiple restorations (i.e., of one or both arches) where a naturally occurring difference exists between centric occlusion and centric relation, they are often made to more nearly coincide via occlusal adjustment therapy before prosthodontic treatment is started. In this situation, the dentist has three choices of where to design morphologic maximum intercuspation: *(1)* at centric relation alone, *(2)* at the preexisting centric occlusion alone, or *(3)* to a broader flattened area of occlu-

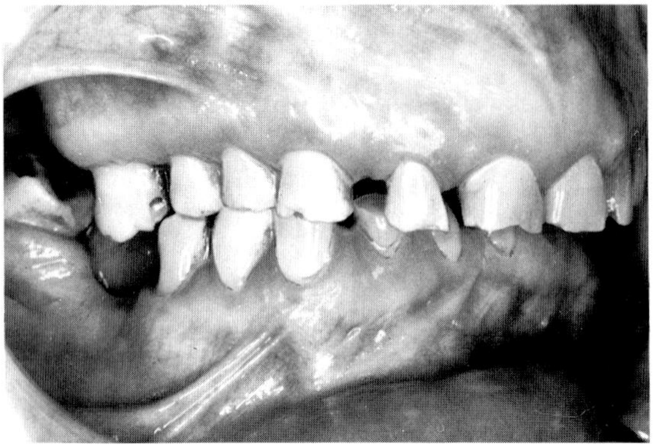

Fig. 22-11 Although advanced tooth wear is frequently insidious and appears to be compensated for by alveolar bone growth, its clinical appearance tends to suggest an increase in interocclusal distance. A patient's morphologic facial height can remain unchanged in spite of the dramatic reduction in enamel, as seen in this patient. Other patients are not so lucky and can end up with loss of both tooth tissue and morphologic facial height (i.e., the interocclusal distance is increased).

sal contact that can accommodate the mandible at centric relation *and* at a position slightly anterior to centric relation ("long centric" or "freedom in centric" concept, see chapter 12). Decisions on which choice to employ will depend upon the number of occlusal surfaces to be restored or replaced as well as upon the area, location(s), and resultant contact and slide direction associated with the centric relation/centric occlusion noncoincidence. Whatever the choice, three principles should be adhered to, namely *(1)* that the final restored intercuspal position be positive in order to maintain a stable occlusion, *(2)* that during guided retruded closure simultaneous bilateral occlusal contact occurs, and *(3)* that voluntary closure, when the head is erect, will accurately and consistently end in the intercuspal position.

Stable quadrant relationships providing axially directed forces

It is axiomatic that teeth can withstand more load without unfavorable vectors when forces are applied in an axial direction and within the root housing. One of the most fundamental examples of this form-and-function phenomenon is the position of the centric holding or supporting cusps of posterior teeth vis-à-vis the other cusps. The fact that the mesiolingual cusp of a maxillary first molar, which can sustain maximum load during occlusal function, is located very near to the center of the occlusal surface, is tangible evidence of this basic principle.

Thus, in the fabrication of a therapeutic occlusion by prosthodontic therapy, or by any occlusal therapy for that matter, every effort should be made to adhere to this objective. Such adherence will greatly assist the dentition to withstand and adapt to occlusal forces produced by functional as well as parafunctional activities. Several strategies are available in order to advance this objective.

A definite bilateral intercuspation on multiple posterior occlusal surfaces during centric occlusion closure helps to enhance optimally distributed and axially directed forces on the dentition as well as on individual posterior teeth. These characteristics also increase the probability of maintaining a stable occlusion. These objectives are fundamental ones although clinicians may differ on the best ways to achieve them.

For example, a great number of dentists believe that occlusal stability and optimally directed occlusal forces are best achieved when closure to centric occlusion takes place at, or within 1 mm anterior to, centric relation. Such views are based upon numerous empirical clinical observations. An alternative to this, also advanced by many clinicians, is that therapeutic modification of an occlusion to a "long centric" concept will, because of the resultant occlusal loading by cusp tips on multiple flattened surfaces, ensure even greater likelihood that such loads are optimally distributed and applied along

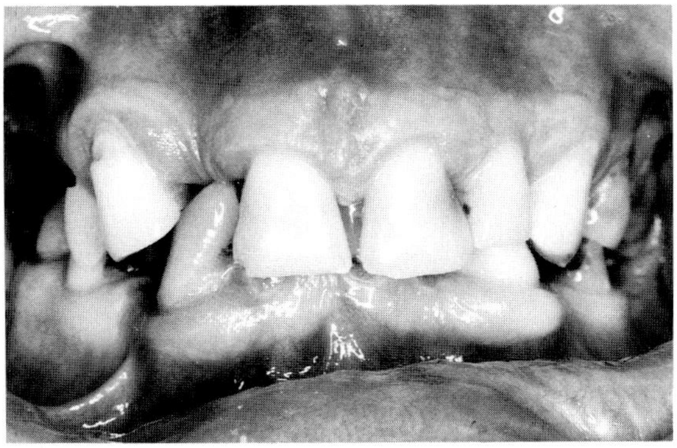

Fig. 22-12a Vertical restoration of occlusion. Intraoral view of posterior collapse.

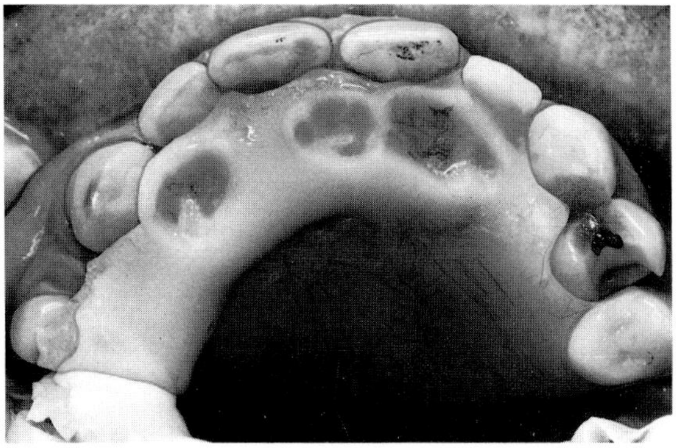

Fig. 22-12b Autocure acrylic resin is used intraorally to generate a prosthesis.

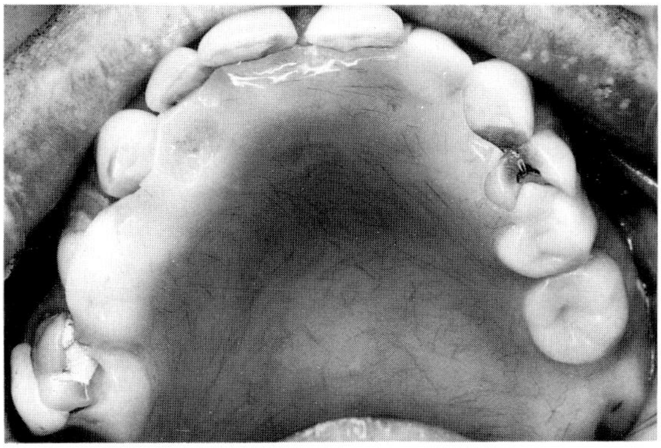

Fig. 22-12c The prosthesis is adjusted and worn by the patient for 3 months to assess tolerance.

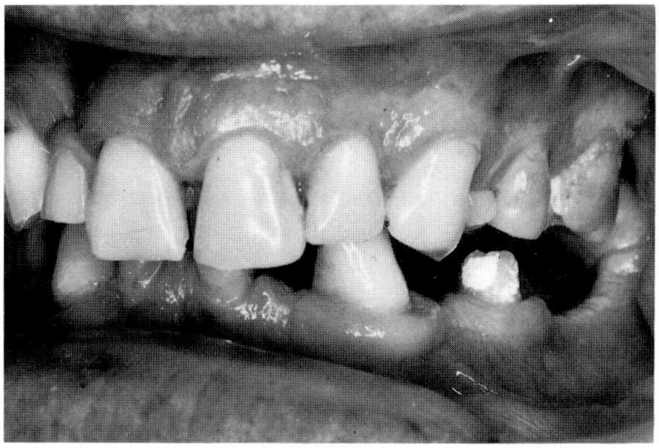

Fig. 22-12d Vertical dimension available at the mandibular left second premolar for a crown.

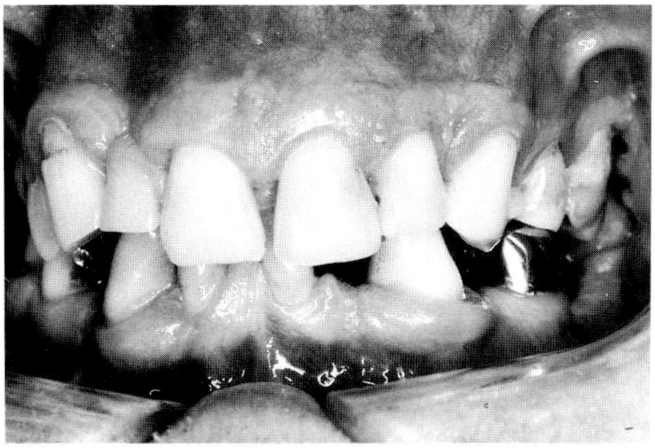

Fig. 22-12e The cast crown for the second premolar made to the vertical dimension as determined by the acrylic resin partial denture.

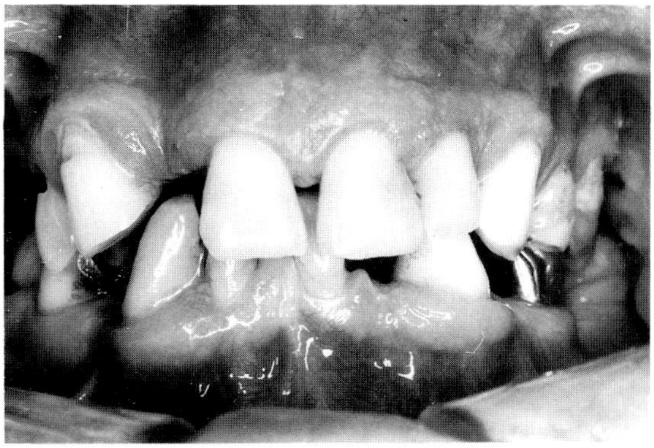

Fig. 22-12f Compare this position to that shown in Fig. 22-12a.

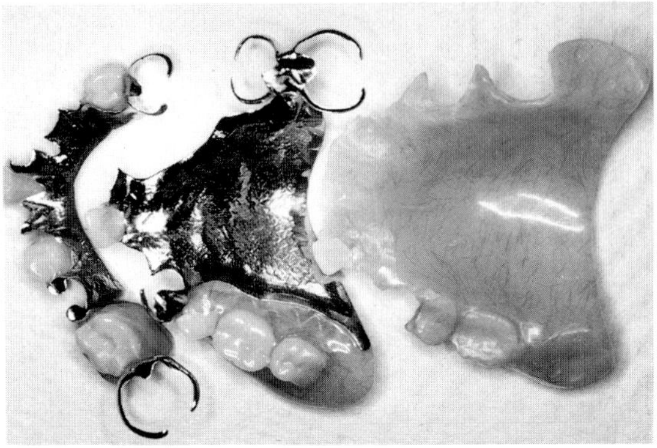

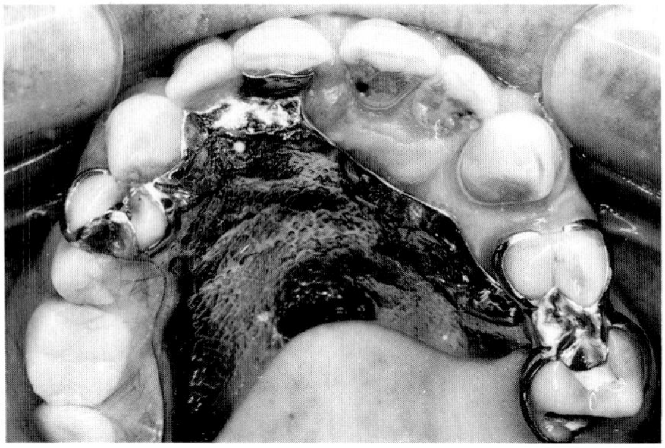

Figs. 22-12g and h Cast removable partial dentures to maintain vertical features and designed to restore occlusal contacts and retain stable tooth positions.

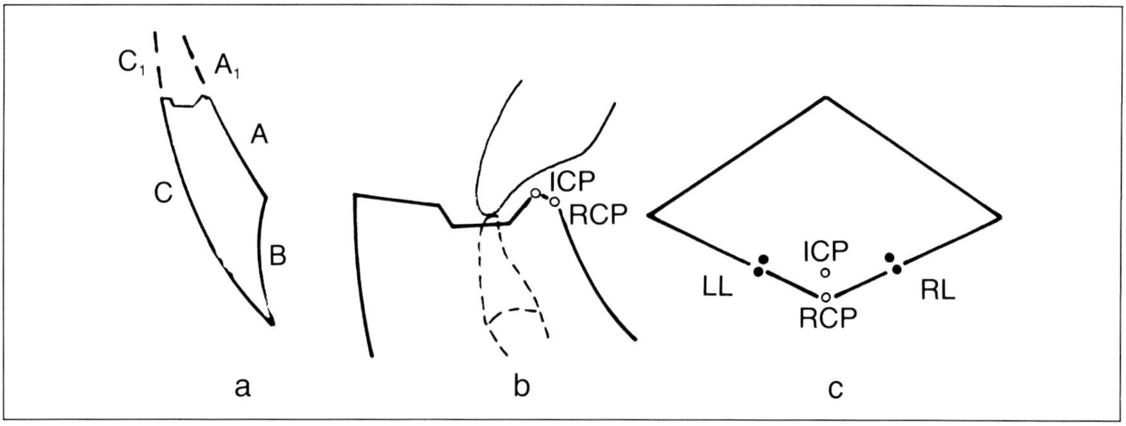

Fig. 22-13 The hypothetical extension of the arc of opening and closing (A_1 in retrusion and C_1 in protrusion) if the tooth-stops (the "impediment" to overclosure) were to be removed, as would occur if the Posselt envelope were to be recorded on an edentulous, nondenture wearing patient—diagrammatic sagittal view *(a)*. *(A)* arc of opening and *(B)* closing; *(C)* arc of protrusive opening or closing. The arcs of opening and closing after the condyle begins to translate as well as rotate; *(RCP)* retruded contact position/centric relation; *(ICP)* interocclusal contact position/centric occlusion *(b)*. Extension of the protrusive arc of opening and closing—diagrammatic occlusal view *(c)*; *(RL)* right lateral and *(LL)* left lateral excursive movements.

the long axes of the posterior teeth (Dawson, 1974; Ramfjord and Ash, 1983). Others take the view that the objectives are best achieved by having a more definitive position of maximum intercuspation. Proponents of this concept often advance the idea of "tripodization" of the contact of cusps in their opposing fossae. This implies that, in intercuspal position, each cusp-to-fossa relationship should be characterized by three areas of equal contact around, but not at, the tips of the cusps. Such an approach appears to be very logical when seen in diagrammatic representations (Fig. 22-14). Technically, however, it is very difficult to accomplish (Burch, 1980) and, if not correctly achieved, may have the opposite effects than those intended.

In addition, such a rigid approach may limit the dentist's options in the design and composition of some prostheses. For example, tripodization will invariably necessitate the use of cast metal occlusal surfaces since the wedging effect of such contacts could promote fracture of porcelain surfaces. In this case, a dome-shaped cusp fitting into a "socket" reduces the development of high tensile stresses and is less likely to lead to fractures of porcelain occlusal restorations (McLean, 1984).

Other strategies are often employed to enhance the agreed upon objectives. One is to alter cusp-to-marginal edge relationships (typically found in most natural dentitions) to cusp-to-fossa relationships in prosthetic restorations. Such therapeutic structural modifications seek to inhibit the potential wedging effect of cusps that contact adjacent pairs of marginal ridges by placing such contacts into opposing fossae in order to direct the occlusal loads along the long axes and within the root housing of the teeth. Teeth that exhibit mobility or fremitus due to occlusal trauma are the most likely candidates for such modifications when restorations are required.

It is also very important to keep in mind that the correct position of the occlusal table and of the supporting cusps vis-à-vis the root housing is central to the issue of optimal and axially directed occlusal forces. As already noted, it is not an accident of nature that the mesiolingual cusp of a maxillary first molar, for example, is located much closer to the center of the occlusal surface than are its other cusps. Such form and function principles must be kept in mind when prosthetic restorations are fabricated.

In some cases, the sought after objectives are easily achieved. In others, however, the clinician's basic understanding and creativity are severely tested. For example, many dentitions are so mutilated that irregular and anomalous tooth-to-tooth and/or arch-to-arch relationships develop (Figs. 22-15a to d). The restoration of such dentitions frequently results in nontextbook morphologic location of cusps and fossae (e.g., crossbite relationships, canted cusps, cusp-to-cusp contacts, etc.). The latter situation is similar to one frequently encountered in an occlusion designed for complete dentures. Thus, clinical experience suggests that the selection of an occlusal design *must* be modified according to the structural and functional requirements of each individual situation. The tendency to rigidly adhere to a standardized occlusal pattern for all treated patients is neither logical nor correct. The essential goal is for the mandible to close in a manner that ensures that the occlusal contact promotes occlusal stability and produces occlusal forces that are directed favorably to the supporting tissues.

Freedom in retrusive range of contact

This objective attempts to reconcile the following clinical observations:

1. Maximal intercuspation occurs most frequently in centric occlusion and not in centric relation.
2. Preliminary tooth contact in centric relation, the retruded contact position, leads to a mandibular slide into maximal intercuspation. This "slide in centric" usually occurs in a straight anterior and superior direction but may include a large lateral component. Slides straight in front of the retruded contact position that are less than 1 mm and tolerated by the patient are generally regarded as innocuous.
3. The contacts responsible for the slide may be unilateral or bilateral and may include variable numbers of teeth. These tooth contacts (or prematurities) in centric relation are frequently referred to as *occlusal discrepancies,* implying that they should be routinely eliminated. *There is no compelling evidence to support such an approach, and, thus, occlusal adjustment for this purpose is not recommended as a strictly prophylactic procedure* (see chapters 13 and 21).
4. The registration of jaw records in centric relation is a practical, convenient, and reliable starting point for planning the simplest to the most complex fixed or removable prosthetic restorations.
5. Simple restorations (e.g., a crown, one quadrant with a fixed prosthesis) are usually

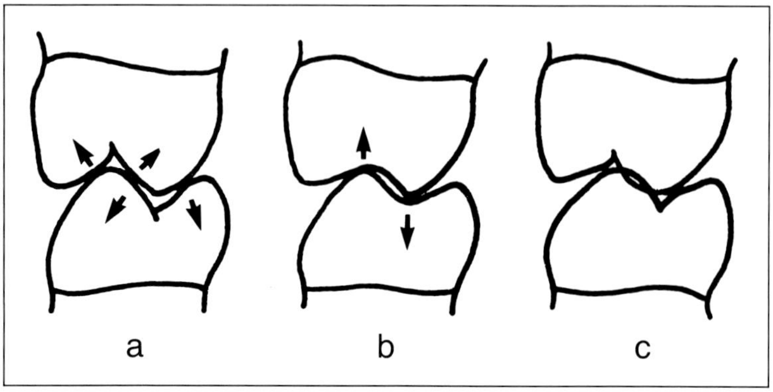

Fig. 22-14 Diagram of frontal plane view of cusp-fossa relationship. Three-point contact to ensure that axial loading occurs *(a)*. A flat fossa allows for cusp tip to also load the tooth axially and at the same time precludes the risk of a wedging effect on the material used for the restoration *(b)*. This alternative restorative technique, usually used when a natural tooth is to be opposed by a crown, places the contacting point near the cusp tip *(c)*. In both *b* and *c* freedom in the RCP/ICP contact range can be designed (i.e., supporting cusps are free to move slightly in the central fossa at about the same level).

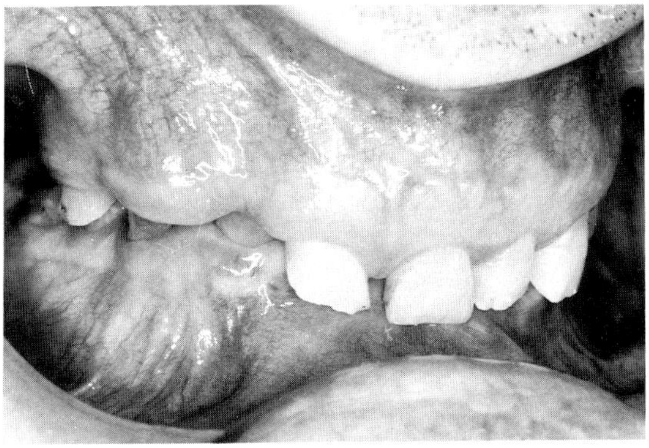

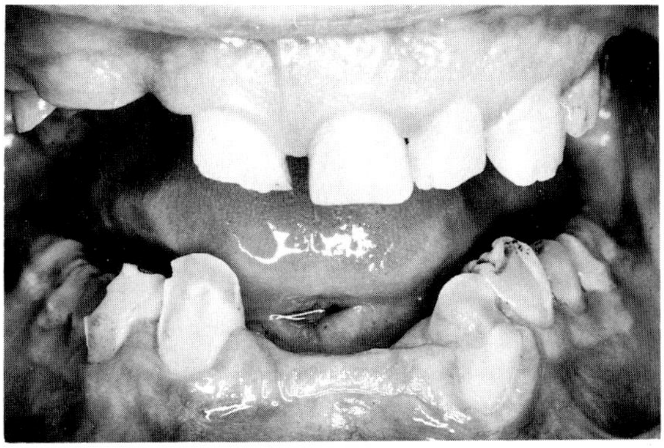

Figs. 22-15a and b A mutilated dentition showing excessive wear with occlusion on dentin and gingiva.

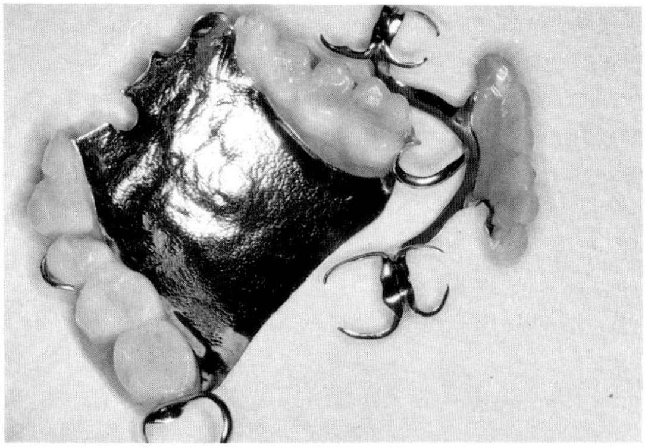

Fig. 22-15c Overlay partial prostheses modified for occlusion: large rests, palatal extensions, and widened acrylic resin teeth.

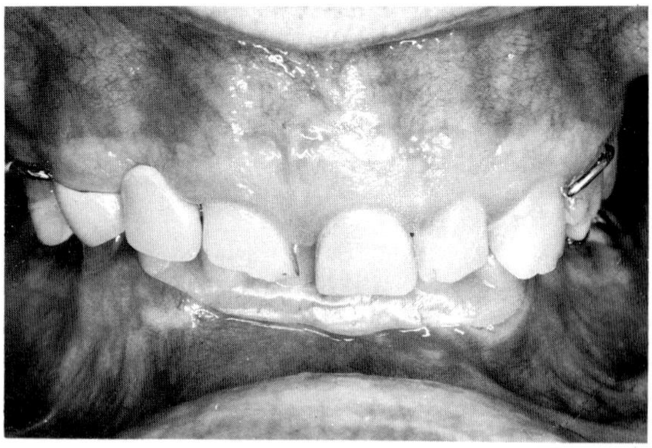

Fig. 22-15d Overlay of appropriate maxillary teeth to regain occlusal vertical position. Compare this with Fig. 22-15a.

contoured to conform to the prevailing natural teeth as existing maximum intercuspation dictates.

6. Complex prosthetic restorations (multiple occlusal surfaces involving one or both dental arches) more often require an occlusal morphologic design that ensures maximal occlusal contact at centric relation. This is a traditional prosthodontic viewpoint and is certainly justified where the original centric occlusion no longer exists (e.g., an edentulous arch). It is most probably justified where the residual natural dentition has been mutilated and the existing centric occlusion is no longer deemed to be a reliable position to which prosthetic reconstruction should be fabricated. This concept, however, has been overinterpreted to mean that occlusal adjustments to make centric occlusion and centric relation coincident or near coincident should be routinely and prophylactically prescribed for the natural dentition so as to avoid the risk of the prematurities catalyzing parafunctional habits and eventual TM disorders. Past publications (during the last 25 years) have perpetuated this overinterpretation with consequent unnecessary selective grinding of occlusal surfaces in a futile attempt to prevent or to stop bruxism or other occlusal parafunctional habits.

7. Most dental clinicians and educators elect to use centric relation as a *starting point* for prosthodontic therapy, particularly when it is extensive. Maximal intercuspation is initially established in this position and occlusal morphology is then altered so that a very small area of accommodation is created (anteriorly and sometimes laterally) which allows for maximal intercuspation anterior to the centric relation position. This is the notion behind the practical concept of a "long centric" or a "broad or wide centric." This freedom in the retrusive range, with maximum intercuspation slightly (0.5 to 1.0 mm) anterior to and directly in front of centric relation, appears to be physiologically viable. It reduces the rigidity imposed upon a patient's occlusal function when centric relation and centric occlusion are made coincident in therapeutic situations. It is also technically feasible and allows for realistic and relatively uncomplicated clinical and laboratory procedures (see chapter 12).

Application of the long centric concept, the concept of centric relation/centric occlusion coincidence, or any other concept that modifies existing maxillomandibular relationships should not be based upon perfunctory clinical decisions. Such decisions should be based on a definite rationale. In prosthodontic therapy, they are ordinarily not applied unless an entire dental arch is involved or parts of both arches are to be restored. Clinical judgment must be used to determine when and under what conditions any of these concepts are to be utilized under the unique circumstances presented by a specific patient.

Multidirectional freedom of contact movement

This objective seeks to enhance the ability of the mandible, when it is in occlusal contact, to move in all desired directions without structural occlusal impediments to such movements. Multidirectional freedom implies that mastication should be able to be carried out on either side of the arch, and, very importantly, that occlusal parafunctional activity (specifically tooth grinding) can occur without excess loading of teeth with premature contacts or occlusal interferences. Such contacts can lead to cusp fracture, tooth fremitus or mobility, fracture of restorations, etc., due to the large forces that may be generated during bruxism. The multidirectional tooth contacts that may occur during bruxism (e.g., protrusive and/or lateral tooth grinding) can be simulated by moving articulated maxillary and mandibular dental casts over one another.

Every prosthetic restoration (from a single crown to a complete denture) should be created with this very clear-cut objective in mind: that the restored or replaced teeth should *not* be an impediment to free gliding movements of the mandible. The contact relationships of residual natural teeth, assuming that they are satisfactory, are usually used as guides for the occlusal morphology of opposing teeth that are to be replaced or restored (Zarb et al., 1978). When such tangible tooth guides are not present, for example, one arch or both arches are to be totally restored or are in need of multiple restorations, articulators of increasing levels of sophistication are employed. The guidance features of the articulator (canine guidance, incisal guidance, condylar inclination, condylar angulation, intercondylar distance, etc.; see chapter 9) are used to record and/or replace those guidance factors no longer available from residual natural teeth.

The dentist has options with regard to the choice of the level of articulator sophistication to be employed. As a rule, the selection of more articulator complexity will be *directly* related to the complexity of the case and *indirectly* related to the number of sound residual natural teeth that are not involved in the restorations.

Articulator systems exist that permit detailed recording of a patient's mandibular border movements and accurate transfers of such recordings to the articulator. Many very good clinicians believe that subsequent prosthetic occlusions designed on such an articulator must follow these movement trajectories faithfully when cusp, fossa, and groove morphology and position are fabricated. Other dentists, of equal ability, feel that this approach is too rigid and tend to use arbitrary, anatomically averaged, or several overlapping settings on whatever articulator system they employ.

Whatever articulator system or concept is followed, one thing remains clear. The incisal and canine guidances have a more immediate and profound effect on posterior occlusal morphology and on multidirectional contact movements than do the condylar guidance factors. The reason is simple. The anterior teeth are closer to the posterior teeth than are the condyles. In major prosthodontics, decisions are first made regarding acceptance or nonacceptance of any existing anterior guidance. Such decisions will be based on an evaluation of many factors associated with the anterior teeth, such as esthetics, speech articulation, root/crown ratios, fremitus or mobility, wear facets, etc. After the existing, altered, or newly created incisal and canine guidances are established, the appropriate articulator guidance settings are placed on the articulator. These, along with the condylar guidance settings, will serve to assist in the creation of occlusal surfaces that permit smooth, unimpeded protrusive and lateral excursive movements of the mandible.

During these lateral excursions, what appears to be essential is not the number of teeth in contact but the even gliding character of the jaw movement. In the natural dentition, lateral working side contacts can involve the canines, one or both premolars, and even one or more molars. Such contact movements most often disclude the teeth on the contralateral or nonworking side. It must be remembered that the contacting area(s) on the teeth changes as lateral movement progresses. Furthermore, the number of contacting teeth decreases as the excursion continues. Contact movement beyond a range of 1 to 2 mm is usually accompanied by a "canine rise" or contact on the canines alone. Sometimes the incisors may also be involved. In protrusive movements, contacts occur on a wide range of incisor, and sometimes canine, teeth depending upon arch sizes and interarch relationships.

Figure 22-16 is a schematic drawing of possible working side contact movement areas on canines and premolars and of the occlusal surfaces of maxillary and mandibular arches. Although specific tooth contacts can be identified (see chapters 4 and 21), for reasons of convenience it must be emphasized that these contacts vary, because occlusion is not something fixed and solid, like a gearbox. Reported diurnal and nocturnal variations in occlusal contacts (Berry, 1986) preclude the making of dogmatic statements such as the need for tripodization of all posterior tooth contacts.

The presence of a naturally occurring or restored, well-defined canine guidance facilitates occlusal design in virtually every facet of prosthodontic care. The exception to this statement is the complete denture, where cross-arch stabilization requires a balanced occlusion.

Generally speaking, prosthodontic therapy involving the natural teeth aims at early canine guidance in lateral contact movements, provided that the canines have adequate bony sup-

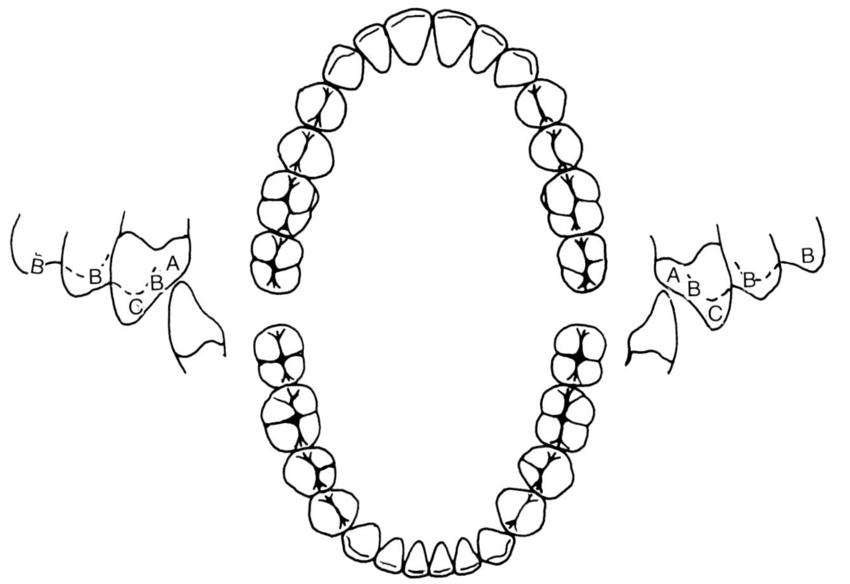

Fig. 22-16 A schematic drawing of possible working side contact movement areas on canines and premolars, and the occlusal surfaces of maxillary and mandibular teeth. The side diagrams reflect the recommendation for a functional range of 1 to 2 mm between the intercuspal position *(A)* and the lateral horizontal position *(B)*, where group contact is established. Beyond this range, a canine rise takes over *(C)* and the posterior teeth are discluded.

port and normal mobility. If not, this guidance may be shared by posterior (and in some cases anterior) teeth depending upon root/crown ratios and arch and tooth relationships (Burch, 1980).

It is clear that prosthodontic therapy aims at optimizing occlusal stress distribution during functional and parafunctional jaw movements. Such therapy can, and in fact should, be modified to meet individual requirements (Table 22-1).

However, the notion of harmonious function as an outgrowth of neuromuscular and biomechanical harmony demands an equation that can be applied predictably and pragmatically. Beyron's therapeutic objectives can be considered integral and essential components of such an equation. Their application allows for the establishment of harmonious occlusal relationships with relatively simple and practical therapeutic modalities.

Operative therapy

Most operative dentistry procedures are performed within the context of an already existing physiologic occlusion. The treatment of dental caries and the restoration of lost tooth structure typically involves individual teeth or multiple teeth treated sequentially. In the presence of a physiologic occlusion (as defined in chapter 13) no consideration need be given to changing maxillomandibular or occlusal relationships. However, it is imperative that all operative therapy be performed carefully and exactly so as not to destabilize the occlusion or alter the occlusal relationships in a way that will upset the adaptive equilibrium already exhibited by the masticatory system. In chapter 14, several morphologic features were identified that affect one tooth or a few teeth and which, in turn, may stretch the limits of adaptation of a physiologic occlusion.

Table 22-1 Jaw relation records and occlusal morphology in prosthodontics

Restoration/ prosthesis	Position ICP/RCP	Records	Articulator	Occlusal morphology
Single crown	ICP	Hand articulate maxillary and mandibular casts	Simple hinge	Conform to morphology of opposing teeth
Fixed partial (one quadrant)	ICP	Hand articulate casts + anterior guidance	Semiadjustable with 20° condylar inclination	Conform to morphology of opposing natural teeth that have been recontoured if extruded or otherwise malaligned or malformed
Removable partial (not free-end saddle)	ICP	Hand articulate casts + anterior guidance	Semiadjustable with 20° condylar inclination	Select preformed denture tooth anatomy, adjust to conform to opposing natural teeth that have been recontoured if malaligned or malformed
Removable complete maxillary & mandibular	RCP + postinsertion long centric	Face-bow transfer + centric relation record + occlusal vertical dimension + anterior guidance based upon esthetics and speech articulation	Semiadjustable with 10°–30° condylar inclination	Select 0°–20° denture teeth, achieve cross-arch balance and cross-tooth balance in lateral excursion
Removable complete maxillary opposing natural mandibular	RCP + postinsertion long centric	Face-bow transfer + centric relation record + occlusal vertical dimension + anterior guidance based upon esthetics and speech articulation	Semiadjustable with 10°–30° condylar inclination	Select anatomic preformed denture teeth, adjust to conform to well-aligned and formed natural teeth, achieve cross-arch balance during lateral excursion
Fixed partial multiple units or several quadrants	RCP + assessment for possible long centric	Face-bow transfer + centric relation record + anterior guidance + condylar inclination and angulation by positional or pantographic records	Semi- or fully adjustable with anterior and posterior guidance mechanisms	Concept of mutually protected occlusion, often with cusp-to-fossa posterior occlusal relationships

When these limits are exceeded, the "spillover" into a nonphysiologic occlusal state may occur. Operative dentistry procedures should not require further stretching of the limits of adaptation. Thus, the prevention of iatrogenically produced problems is inherent in good operative therapy.

Tooth loss and, just as frequently, faulty dental procedures and restorations can elicit adverse changes in both mandibular function and dental arch integrity. Current research underscores the fact that few, if any, of the associated morphologic changes have a significant direct effect upon the etiology of periodontal disease, although effects on tooth mobility and fremitus are quite clear. It is therefore tempting to conclude that a program of plaque control is all that is needed for patients with these morphologic variables. However, comfort, functional considerations, and both patients' and dentists' esthetic perceptions frequently dictate the need for operative intervention. A maximum number of well-aligned teeth that are pleasing to their possessor appears to be a strong incentive for treatment on the part of both the public and the profession. This is not a frivolous issue, and any patient's perception of the esthetic needs of his or her dentition deserves serious consideration by the clinician.

From a functional standpoint, the restoration of occlusal contact morphology and consistency are considered routine clinical treatment objectives. Such treatment frequently requires adjunctive occlusal adjustment therapy, which ensures redistribution of occlusal forces or load on the teeth. Although occlusal adjustment per se is probably contraindicated as a treatment for bruxism, it has a role in diminishing the unfavorable effect of bruxism on the dentition. Thus, occlusal interferences in maximum intercuspation and/or excursive contact movements are considered unfavorable if these contacts constantly occur in an adversely forceful manner, such as during bruxism. Thus, iatrogenic interferences (those produced by the dentist), which disrupt maximum intercuspation contact or smooth excursive movements, may produce dental or periodontal pain because of adverse loading. Many dentists believe that such interferences can also cause muscle or TMJ pain, particularly when they are large and introduced suddenly. However, direct evidence of these relationships is not presently available. Although restorations that only disrupt an excursive contact movement appear to be less likely to elicit overt clinical symptoms (Clark and Adler, 1985), signs of fremitus or mobility may certainly result from such interferences.

Much has been made of occlusal interferences produced by "high" restorations. Often neglected is concern for "low" restorations, that is, ones in which properly located occlusal contact is not achieved. Such a restoration will, initially, be quite comfortable to the patient and the dentist will feel secure because it is not high. Unfortunately, however, this may have caused an unstable situation because the restored tooth, or its opponent, can now extrude, tip, or otherwise change position. These changes can now lead to interferences that did not previously exist. This same scenario can also be applied to faulty interproximal contacts, faulty cusp-to-marginal ridge relationships, or to any situation that can lead to an unstable occlusion or to other signs or symptoms of a nonphysiologic occlusion. It is thus extremely important that all operative procedures, *including those for individual teeth,* be performed to established criteria for such restorations in order to avoid any possible unfavorable sequelae.

Operative therapy may also be part of the dentist's armamentarium for treating an already existing nonphysiologic occlusion. This may or may not be associated with changes in maxillomandibular relationships. As explained in the section on prosthodontic therapy, a decision to change such relationships should be deliberate and, if indicated, be performed prior to finalizing the operative therapy. Thus, subsequent operative dentistry procedures can be accomplished within the newly changed occlusal relationships. Acute operative needs, of course, must be taken care of without delay.

When operative dentistry is used as one of several treatment modalities to change a nonphysiologic occlusion to one that is physiologic,

Beyron's therapeutic objectives should be kept in mind. Such procedures are directed at fulfilling the needs of the entire masticatory system as well as the very important needs of an individual tooth.

As previously noted, the specific techniques and procedures used in operative therapy are not considered here. The reader is encouraged to review current textbooks in operative dentistry that deal with this subject.

Orthodontic therapy

It has been reported that approximately 70% to 80% of a studied North American population exhibits morphologic malocclusion by the time they are young adults (Popovich and Grainger, 1959). This observation does not imply an epidemic of occlusal problems. It simply describes the fact that a large number of individuals in their late teens demonstrate morphologic departures from a conceptualized ideal occlusion. The majority of these individuals possess a physiologic occlusion that, with good patient care and regular dentist maintenance, should last a lifetime. Most of these individuals would not need orthodontic treatment unless it is necessary to improve dental esthetics and restore normal facial contours and skeletal malrelations.

However, some of these patients may have an occlusion that is close to crossing the threshold into one that is nonphysiologic or that is already nonphysiologic. These individuals benefit from orthodontic treatment on both esthetic and functional grounds. In fact, when a patient with a malocclusion loses one tooth or several teeth, orthodontic intervention can become an essential part of treatment (Jenkins, 1978).

In adults, most forms of orthodontic treatment have the following objectives: *(1)* dentofacial esthetic improvement, *(2)* optimal stress distribution over residual dentition, and *(3)* less frequently, to align abutment teeth so as to facilitate subsequent operative or prosthodontic therapy. To date, there is no compelling evidence to indict morphologic malocclusion (as determined by the Angle classification, hence most frequently a nonideal but a physiologic occlusion) as causing periodontal disease (Ramfjord and Ash, 1981) or TM disorders (Griffiths, 1983).

In recent years, however, dentists have recognized that many patients' overall periodontic and prosthodontic treatment plans benefit from adjunctive minor tooth movement as an integral part of the objective of improving tooth stability and function, as well as esthetics. Two common indications are the realignment of inadequate pontic spaces (Figs. 22-17a to e) and uprighting of mandibular molar abutments (Figs. 22-18a and b).

Some specific aspects of developmental or postdevelopmental morphologic malocclusions are listed in Table 22-2. Their treatment by orthodontics may in fact be essential for optimal periodontic and/or prosthodontic results. Orthodontic therapy is invariably preceded by elimination of plaque and the establishment of a hygienic phase of home care. However, it precedes periodontal surgery or prosthodontic procedures. Two specific rules apply in orthodontic treatment: *(1)* teeth are never moved away from basal bone because a favorable tooth-to-bone relationship is mandatory, and *(2)* the induced controlled tooth movement should not be countered by the forces generated from the occlusion so as to preclude instability and relapse.

Occlusal adjustment is often required during or after orthodontic treatment. The removal of interfering inclines can facilitate tooth movement. The goal of occlusal stability is sought for retention of the orthodontic result. This can often be enhanced by occlusal adjustment therapy. Interocclusal appliances are also frequently employed because they can be designed to eliminate unfavorable occlusal contacts (e.g., when correcting a crossbite or uprighting a tilted molar). Extensive fixed orthodontic appliances are necessary if comprehensive skeletal and dental arch improvements are planned. Extreme changes are best managed by a combined surgical-orthodontic team (see chapter 26).

As in most forms of dental therapy, a biologic price may be exacted as a result of the mechanical movement of teeth. This price includes

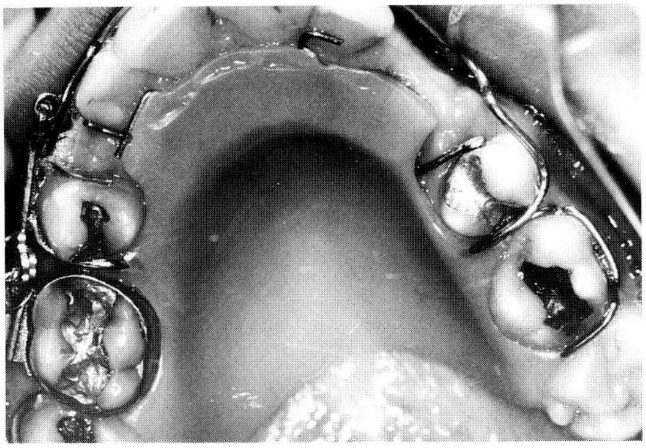

Fig. 22-17a Preprosthetic orthodontic treatment for a patient whose early loss of maxillary canines and first premolars reduced pontic space for an optimal prosthesis. Reflected view of the fixed and removable orthodontic appliances in the mouth.

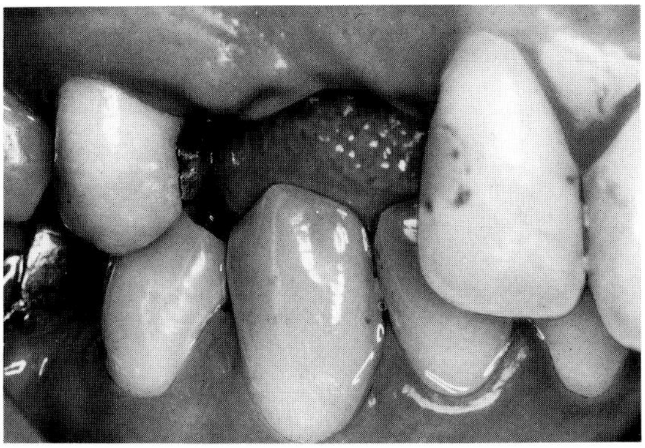

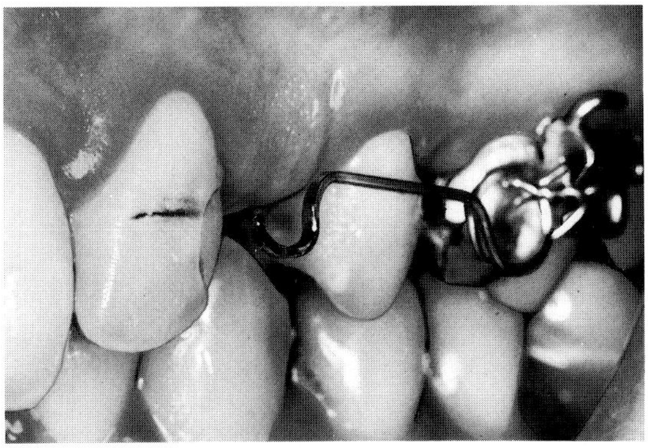

Figs. 22-17b and c Right and left buccal views of the recovered pontic spaces, which are filled with right canine, first premolar, and left canine teeth.

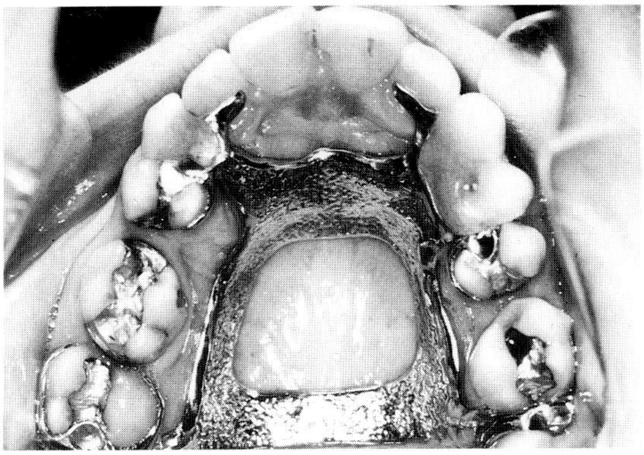

Fig. 22-17d The decision was made to end up with small interproximal spaces distal to the maxillary second premolar; however, there is no esthetic compromise.

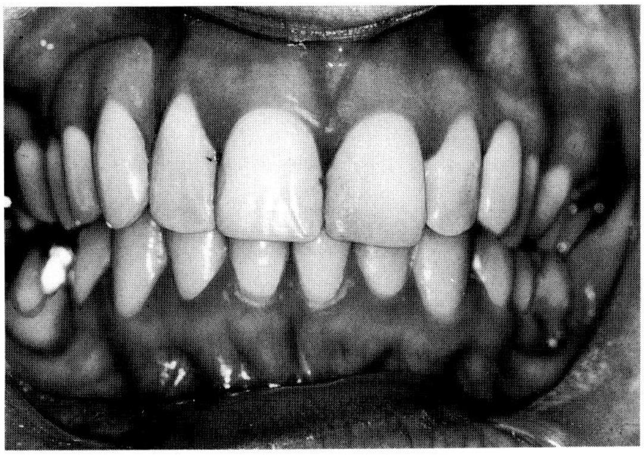

Fig. 22-17e The final restoration in place.

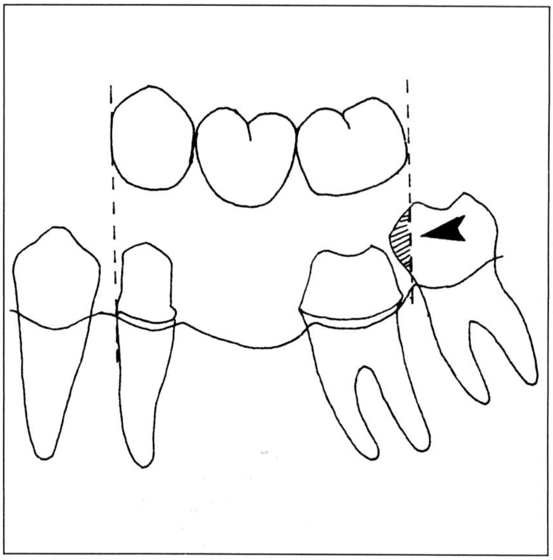

Fig. 22-18a A diagrammatic representation of the consequences of a tilted molar that is to be used for abutment service for a fixed prosthesis. The tooth distal to the prosthesis *(arrow)* will interfere with the line of insertion.

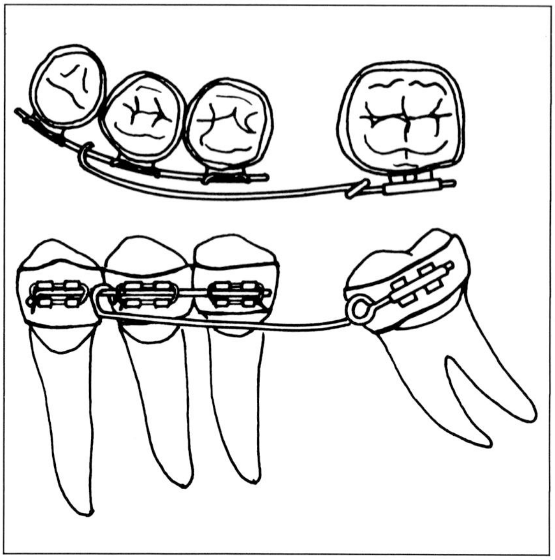

Fig. 22-18b The molar is uprighted orthodontically with the more anteriorly placed teeth splinted together for anchorage service.

Table 22-2 Some sequelae of occlusal changes that benefit from orthodontic therapy

Occlusal changes	Prosthodontic difficulties	Gingival/ periodontal	Functional impairment	Esthetic problems
Malaligned teeth	X		X	X
Protrusion of maxillary anterior teeth with resultant diastemata	X	X	X	X
Impinging deep overbite		X	X	
Anterior open bite and/or lack of lip seal		X	X	
Decreased posterior occlusal support	X		X	X

1. *Excessive resorption.* The very nature of orthodontic force involves a balance between bone resorption and deposition. The close structural relationship between bone and cementum in this force application context may be disturbed and undesirable resorptive sequelae can result. Some teeth (e.g., permanent incisors) appear to be more vulnerable than others. Furthermore, some types of tooth movement (e.g., rapid tipping, intrusion, and root torque) can result in excessive force concentration on small areas with an increased risk of crestal bone loss or cementum resorption.

2. *Tooth devitalization, with or without pulpal*

calcification. Excessive orthodontic forces can lead to high levels of pressure in the periodontal ligament. If this occurs in the apical region, the pulpal vascular supply may be endangered. Pulpal hyperemia may lead to degeneration of pulpal tissue and devitalization, tooth discoloration, and even deposition of calcium.

3. *Dehiscence and fenestration.* When teeth are moved too far (e.g., buccally) they may actually pass through the cortical plate of bone and partially lose their periodontal support. This is more likely to take place in the anterior region, but is an unlikely occurrence.

4. *Enamel decalcification.* Plaque and caries control combined with good dietary instruction and maintenance will preclude this risk.

5. *Surgical treatment.* This involves the additional risk of damaged tooth roots in the surgical field and occasional dramatic and tragic osteonecrosis with loss of sections of the alveolus.

Angle's classification of malocclusion, which remains an extremely valuable concept, deals only with static maxillomandibular relationships in the intercuspal position. Thus, considerations of intercuspal position/retruded contact position slides, nonworking side disclusions, etc., seemingly so important to prosthodontists, have not been considered on a routine basis by most orthodontists. Despite this, the outcome of major orthodontic therapy appears in most cases to produce occlusal relationships that function well and that naturally exhibit characteristics of the mutually protected occlusion (see chapter 12).

Should the orthodontist, like the prosthodontist, be concerned with Beyron's therapeutic objectives listed in the introduction to this chapter? The answer is a qualified yes. A minority of orthodontists believe so strongly in traditional prosthodontic standards that they seek to use gnathological principles as a basis for the final positioning of the teeth. At the present time, however, there is no evidence that mandibular lateral movement patterns of postorthodontic patients are more efficient or comfortable if they follow gnathologically determined border pathways. Thus, most orthodontists have not adopted the gnathological concept that accurate recordings of condylar position and movement trajectories are essential parameters to which occlusal relationships in orthodontic therapy should be directed.

On the other hand, ignoring such objectives as a stable jaw relationship with bilateral contact in retruded closure and multidirectional freedom of contact movement may be shortsighted, because in the presence of bruxism these could become significant. Because of concern over the potentially unfavorable sequelae that can occur as a result of clenching or grinding parafunctional habits, it appears appropriate that orthodontically derived occlusions should have characteristics that will best be able to withstand these extra loading forces. Therefore, it is recommended that each orthodontic case, prior to discharge, be examined with the mutually protected concept of occlusion and Beyron's objectives in mind.

The following are criteria for a mutually protected concept of occlusion, as discussed in chapter 12:

1. In the intercuspal position, primary occlusal loading, axially directed, should be absorbed by contact supporting areas on posterior teeth only. Anterior teeth should contact very lightly and should not bear these potentially heavy forces.
2. In protrusion, the overbite-overjet relations of the incisors should produce an incisal guidance that is steep enough to cause disclusion of all posterior teeth.
3. In lateral excursion, the overbite-overjet relationship of the contacting teeth on the working side should be sufficiently steep to cause disclusion of all nonworking side teeth.

Summary

The traditional forms of occlusal therapy (namely, prosthodontic, operative, and orthodontic therapy) have been reviewed. Emphasis has been given to those aspects of treatment that most influence occlusal and mandibular position and function. The occlusal outcome criteria were discussed within the context of Beyron's therapeutic objectives. These include

1. Acceptable interocclusal distance
2. Stable jaw relationships with bilateral contact in retruded closure
3. Stable quadrant relationships providing axially directed forces
4. Freedom of retrusive range of contact
5. Multidirectional freedom of contact movement

The overriding goal of these therapies and objectives is to create a therapeutic occlusion that has all of the characteristics of a physiologic occlusion, if not the theoretically ideal.

Chapter 23

Behavioral Therapy

John D. Rugh

Occlusal therapy is commonly directed at strengthening the structural integrity of the dentition and its supporting structures. Through appropriate operative, prosthodontic, orthodontic, and surgical procedures, a therapeutic occlusion can usually be achieved. Unfortunately, however, a therapeutic occlusion does not necessarily result in a pain-free, appreciative patient. Many orofacial pain conditions, as well as many occlusal problems, appear to be related to oral motor activities of central nervous system origin. These must also be managed.

The integrity of the dentition and of structural improvements made by the dentist often depend more on the patient's oral behavior than upon the characteristics of the occlusion or upon the technical quality of structural occlusal therapy. Even the most ideal dental restorations can be destroyed, sometimes within a few months, by an aggressive bruxer. Thus, both short-term pain management and the long-term success of structural occlusal therapy often depend on the identification and management of self-destructive, insidious, oral parafunctional activities. Because occlusal parafunction is intimately related to the health and comfort of the masticatory system, control of parafunctional behaviors is often required. Chapter 18 discussed methods to identify occlusal parafunction in patients. This chapter describes behavioral procedures to control occlusal parafunctions.

Foundations for successful therapy

Several principles underlie the successful administration of dental and behavioral therapies. *Patient education* is particularly critical in dealing with orofacial pain and occlusal conditions because of the significant behavioral and emotional aspects of these conditions. It is not uncommon for patients with such pain to display great fear and intense anxiety over their pain conditions. Fear and anxiety are particularly strong when the cause of the pain is unknown or not understood (Fig. 23-1). It is thus important to address the patient's fears and anxiety early in the therapeutic procedure. This may be accomplished through education and may involve discussing the pathophysiology of the condition with the patient in terms and analogies he or she will understand. The patient should be assured that he or she is not suffering from some unknown or life-threatening disease. It is helpful to review radiographs and other diagnostic information with the patient. This demonstrates to the patient that the clinician has carefully studied the results of diagnostic tests.

The patient should be asked if there are questions about the radiographs or diagnostic tests. This provides additional opportunity for the patient to describe particular fears or concerns about the pain condition. In this regard, it is always important to simply ask the patient what

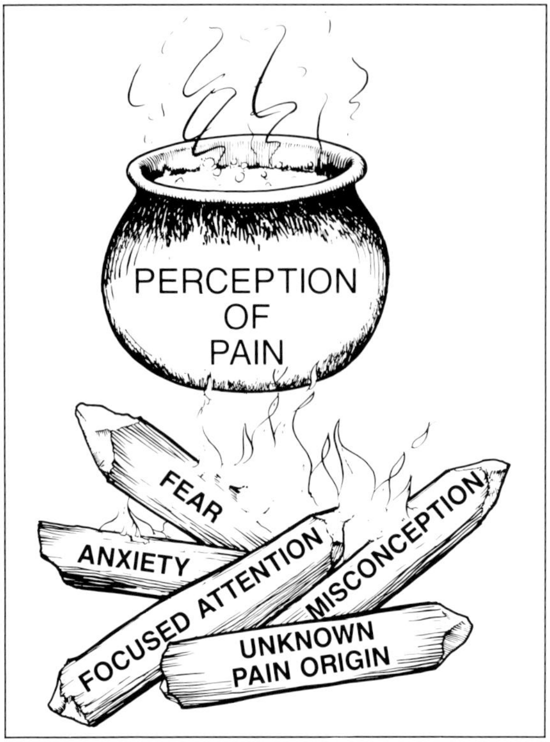

Fig. 23-1 The patient's perception and response to tissue damage is modified by several cognitive factors that must be dealt with directly through discussions with the patient.

he or she feels is the problem and what caused it. This important question allows the dentist to identify patients with delusions or bizarre beliefs such as "bone worms" causing their pain.

Patients with an intense fear of cancer or other serious diseases must be identified early so that the clinician can address the patient's concern through a discussion of appropriate diagnostic results. It is not unusual for a patient's attention to be so focused upon a fearful disease that little headway can be made in diagnosis or treatment. Also, it is important to remember that fear and anxiety influence whether a given stimulus is perceived as painful by the patient (Beecher, 1969). When the patient's fears and anxiety about the condition are reduced, a dramatic improvement in the patient's perception of the condition and response to treatment is often observed.

Another key factor in all treatments that involve changing human behavior is *patient motivation*. The long-term management of many oral habits and occlusal conditions requires substantial commitment and personal effort on the part of the patient. The dentist must provide information, enthusiasm, personal support, and appropriate reinforcement contingencies to help motivate the patient.

There are several methods to help motivate patients. Patient education regarding the long-range outcome of his or her behavior is useful. Pictures and case studies help illustrate the long-term consequences of neglecting to attend to the problem. Written instructions and patient behavioral contracts are useful. In the "patient contract," the dentist agrees to provide certain restorative services and treatments while the patient agrees to accomplish certain specific behavioral changes. These might include, for example, daily brushing and flossing, wearing a splint, or completing a stress control program. These contracts are not meant to be legally binding and are not presented in a formal manner. Rather, they are intended to inform the patient of the importance of change and to establish the patient as an active participant in the success of a treatment.

Motivation and compliance can also be improved by phoning the patient early in therapy. These phone calls let the patient know that you are concerned and that the behavioral change is important.

The manner in which the dentist presents the treatment program is often critical to patient motivation and compliance. Contrast the following two statements:

> "Oh, yes, . . . you'll need to control the bruxism, because it may compromise the restorative work."
>
> versus
>
> "Ms. Smith, it is essential that you stop bruxing. If you continue bruxing, it will destroy the new crowns we have made."

Notice the difference in the strength of these two statements. The choice of strong exacting words and direct simple statements convey the importance of change to the patient. Also, use of the patient's name directs the patient's attention and helps establish rapport.

In addition to presenting directions forcefully, instructions for behavioral change should be presented in a positive, confident manner. Compare, for example, the following two statements:

"Let's see if this habit can be changed."

versus

"Ms. Smith, I am confident that you can change this habit."

Again, notice the use of the patient's name. In addition, notice that in the stronger second statement, it is clear that the patient is responsible for the change; the first statement does not indicate who is responsible for the change. This helps establish the concept of self-control and self-responsibility. With most behavioral change programs, the patient is ultimately responsible for behavioral change. It is important to reinforce this concept with the patient.

Modification of specific behaviors

Several methods are available to assist patients in modifying specific oral habits and behaviors. There are also several dental appliances and biomedical instruments that are effective. These procedures and devices are discussed in this section. However, before attempting to design a program to help patients modify an oral habit, it is important to review the fundamental principles upon which most human behavior is established and maintained.

Reinforcement theory

Most daily human behaviors appear to be controlled by what psychologists refer to as "reinforcement contingencies," that is, the positive or negative consequences of the behavior for the individual. The behavior of stopping at red traffic lights, for example, may be controlled by the desire to avoid an accident or traffic ticket (negative reinforcers). The behavior of studying for a pathology exam may be maintained by the desire for an *A* on the test (positive reinforcer). Both healthy and unhealthy behaviors are subject to such contingencies. It follows that one way to change a behavior is to change the reinforcement contingencies related to the behavior. This is the principle underlying behavior modification techniques, which, when systematically applied, have proved powerful methods to eliminate undesirable behaviors and establish desirable healthy behaviors (Bandura, 1969; Chesney, 1984). A simple example of behavior modification principles is a parent making use of the family car contingent upon improved grades. Another example is good oral hygiene maintained by the positive reinforcement of fresh breath or the negative reinforcement of fear of periodontal disease. It must be noted that different people will have a unique inventory of reinforcers. What reinforces some may not reinforce others. Note also that reinforcement contingencies may be internal (fear of periodontal disease) or external (control of car).

The reinforcement contingencies that appear to control many oral behaviors are internal. Chewing ice, for example, may be reinforced by some oral gratification (internal contingency) that cannot easily be controlled by the dentist. This makes changing the behavior difficult for the dentist to accomplish. The responsibility ultimately must lie with the patient.

Changing human behavior is further complicated when the reinforcement contingency that established a behavior is different from the contingency that maintains the behavior. For example, a patient may begin chewing on the right side of the mouth because of the loss of a first molar on the left side. Unilateral chewing may continue after a fixed partial denture is placed because the muscles on the unused side have become atrophied and fatigue quickly with use. In a similar fashion, an anterior open bite may be established through thumb-sucking but maintained by a tongue-thrust swallow. Considerable thought must be given to the identification of the reinforcement contingencies that maintain behaviors.

Another important consideration in changing behavior is the strength of the positive or negative reinforcement. *To change a behavior, the therapist and/or patient must establish reinforcement contingencies that are stronger than those currently maintaining the behavior.* If the positive value of changing the oral behavior is not sufficiently strong, it is unlikely that a change in the behavior will be accomplished. This basic principle of human behavior accounts for one of the greatest frustrations faced by health care professionals. Clinicians recognize early in practice that patients often do not act in their own long-term best self-interest in health matters. Immediate gratification from an unhealthy behavior is often stronger than the long-term reinforcement of good health.

Several positive and negative reinforcers can motivate oral behavioral change. The patient may wish to alleviate a current pain condition, to prevent tooth wear, or to prevent joint damage. Improved esthetics or increased masticatory efficiency may be important for other patients. In many cases, however, these contingencies are not sufficiently rewarding to motivate the patient to expend the effort required to change behavior. The dentist quickly realizes that each patient is influenced differently by different contingencies and priorities in life. The chances for a successful behavioral change can be improved if attention is given to ensure that reinforcement contingencies are appropriately strong and recognized by the patient. Also remember that praise from the clinician is often an extremely powerful, positive reinforcement for behavioral change. In some cases patients are more apt to change habits for the doctor than for themselves.

When dealing with oral habits, one of the most difficult problems is that patients are often unaware of the habits. The habits often occur when attention is directed elsewhere or when the patient is asleep. Most behavioral change techniques require that the patient be aware of the behavior. Many of the specific therapeutic techniques described below are designed to help increase patient awareness of the behavior.

Behavioral extinction

In addition to establishing powerful new positive or negative reinforcers, behavioral change may also be accomplished by removing current positive reinforcement contingencies that maintain the undesirable behavior. This process, called *behavioral extinction,* is exemplified by the young man who stops opening pop bottles with his teeth when the peer group that reinforced the behavior in high school changes as he goes to college. The college peer group may not socially reinforce the behavior, and it will thus be extinguished.

Substitute behaviors

Another important method of behavioral change that is useful with oral habits is the establishment of an incompatible or substitute behavioral pattern. For example, a patient's daytime isometric clenching can be reduced in lateral excursive position by simply asking the patient to chew gum. Lateral isometric clenching is a behavior incompatible with gum chewing, and its frequency will thus be reduced. Simply advising the patient to "keep the teeth apart" while not chewing or swallowing is sometimes sufficient to reduce clenching. Keeping the teeth apart is a behavior incompatible with clenching, and clenching is thus reduced.

Another example of substitute behavior treatment is the reduction of thumb-sucking by the use of a pacifier (Popovich and Thompson, 1973). When using substitute or incompatible behaviors, care must be taken to make sure that the incompatible behavior is not more damaging to the teeth or joints than the original behavior. A wide variety of incompatible or competing behaviors can be used to help reduce the occurrence of undesirable oral behaviors.

Self-monitoring

One of the most powerful and cost-effective methods of behavioral change is self-monitoring

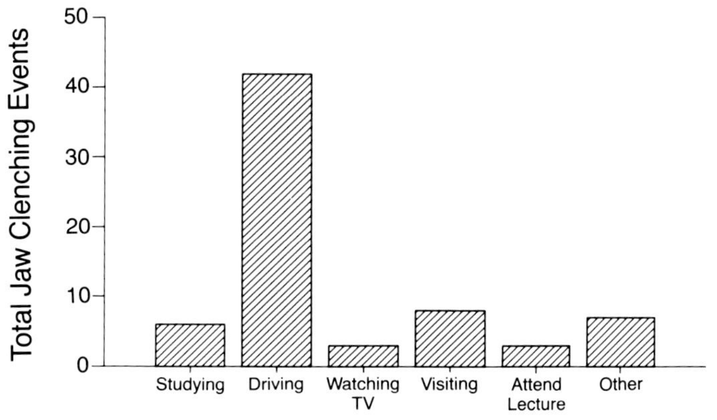

Fig. 23-2 Tally of total jaw clenching events with different daily activities during a 3-day period. This student's self-monitoring log was a valuable tool to increase awareness of the clenching and the conditions under which it most frequently occurred.

(Adesso et al., 1979; Rosen, 1981; Bornstein et al., 1986). With this therapy, the patient is asked to keep a log or diary of the undesirable behavior. The log may be hourly, daily, or weekly, depending on the behavior. The objectives are to *(1)* identify how frequently the behavior occurs, *(2)* identify the conditions or situations under which it occurs, *(3)* identify the reinforcing stimuli maintaining the behavior, and *(4)* help control the behavior. An example of a behavioral log is shown in chapter 18 (see Fig. 18-7). Data from the log can be plotted over time or as a function of activity, as shown in Fig. 23-2. Cyclic variations in frequency sometimes help pinpoint reinforcement contingencies that may be maintaining the behavior.

The behavioral log has several important functions. By requiring patients to keep track of the occurrences of the behavior, they become more aware of it. They are better able to recognize the conditions that elicit the behavior and thus better able to control it. In addition, the graphs plotted from the patient's log document changes in the frequency of behavior, serve as feedback to the patient, and allow the dentist to assess the patient's progress. Logs also serve to document specific oral habits for the dental records.

Massed practice

Patient awareness of an undesirable habit may also be increased by having the patient practice the behavior in front of a mirror (Ayer and Levin, 1975). While practicing, the patient concentrates on the sensations from the muscles and teeth that occur with the undesirable behavior so that the behavior can be more readily detected during the day. For many adult oral habit problems, a simple awareness of the problem activity and knowledge of its long-term consequences are all that is required for change.

Portable biofeedback devices

Biofeedback instruments have been used in many clinics to help patients modify oral habits and oral pain conditions (Gale, 1986). Small portable electromyographic (EMG) feedback devices such as that shown in Fig. 23-3 may be used in the patient's natural environment to alert the patient to clenching or grinding (Solberg and Rugh, 1972). This device detects the EMG activity associated with muscular contraction. If the EMG level exceeds a preset threshold, a tone

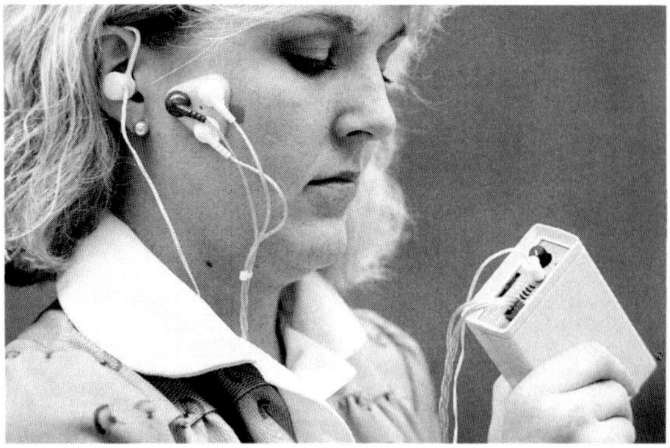

Fig. 23-3 Patient awareness of destructive oral habits may be increased through a portable EMG feedback device. An earphone signals the patient when muscle tension exceeds a preset threshold.

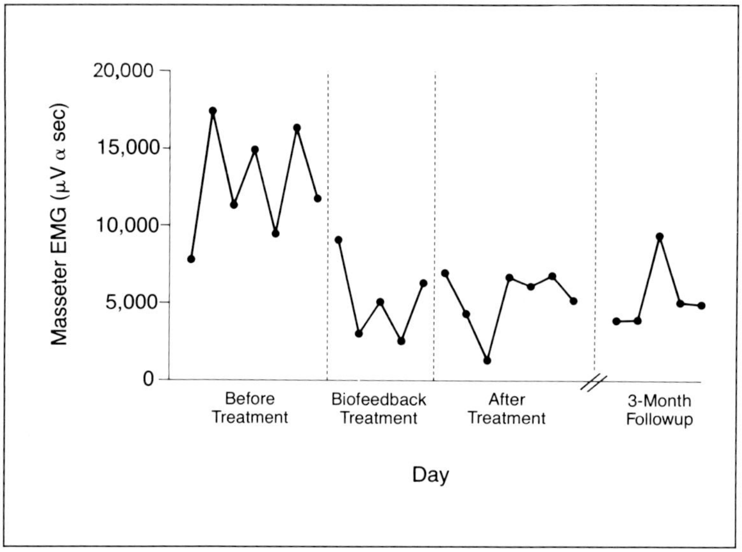

Fig. 23-4 Daily (2-hour) EMG recordings of the masseter muscle of a male 24-year-old tooth clencher before, during, and after treatment are plotted. A 5-day treatment consisted of using a portable EMG biofeedback unit, which signaled clenching events. The reduction in clenching was maintained at a 3-month followup.

sounds through a speaker or an earphone, alerting the patient to the undesirable behavior. The device can be used with oral behaviors that are primarily produced by increased masseter or temporalis muscle activity. This includes teeth clenching or grinding, biting on foreign objects, and some lip-, cheek-, and tongue-biting behavior (Fig. 23-4). The small changes in muscle activity associated with unusual posturing of the mandible are not easily distinguished from muscle activity associated with smiling, swallowing, or speaking. For this reason, these small portable devices are not well suited to modify low-level muscular tension (tonic activity), or unusual posturing habits such as protrusive thrusting or lateral positioning of the mandible.

The portable EMG biofeedback device may be particularly helpful, in combination with a self-monitoring diary, to help control habits of which the patient is unaware. The major limitation of these instruments is that some patients feel uncomfortable about wearing the device in public.

Portable EMG feedback devices have been found useful in suppressing nocturnal bruxism (Clarke and Kardachi, 1977; Rugh and Johnson, 1981; Moss et al., 1982). However, bruxism usually returns when the feedback device is not used (Rugh and Solberg, 1975; Funch and Gale,

1980). For this reason, it is recommended that the devices be used in combination with other, more long-term management techniques, such as stress control or interocclusal appliances. The exception would be when the patient's history suggests that the bruxism behavior is transitory. In these cases, the portable EMG biofeedback units would provide a cost-effective management approach. These instruments may also help document the existence of nocturnal bruxism for the patient.

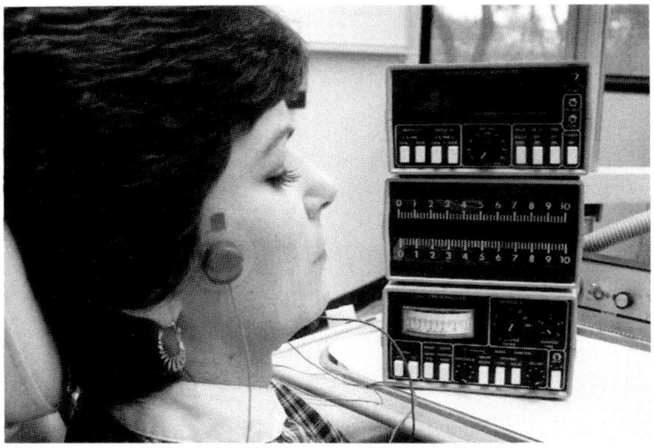

Fig. 23-5 Relaxation of jaw and facial muscles in the dental office using EMG biofeedback usually results in a relaxed jaw opening of 4 to 8 mm.

Clinical biofeedback devices

Deep muscle relaxation training can be accomplished in the clinic using larger, more elaborate, and more sensitive EMG biofeedback devices. In contrast to the portable EMG devices, which may be used for several hours each day or night to modify clenching or grinding activity, the clinical EMG instruments are usually used for several 20- to 30-minute training periods in the office. These sensitive instruments are used to teach patients deep relaxation of the jaw and facial muscles.

Several procedures for clinical EMG biofeedback have been described by clinical investigators (Carlsson et al., 1975; Gessel, 1975; Berry and Wilmot, 1977; Dahlström and Carlsson, 1984; Rugh and Lemke, 1984). The procedures usually involve a setup similar to that depicted in Fig. 23-5. The EMG activity picked up by surface electrodes placed over the jaw and/or facial muscles is amplified and converted to an auditory tone and is displayed visually on a meter. The frequency of the tone and the number on the meter rises and falls, depending upon the level of EMG activity in the muscles being monitored. The patient is thus provided with detailed information about the level of muscular tension and is given instructions to reduce this level of tension. The goals of the training are *(1)* to learn to relax the jaw muscles to a very low EMG level, *(2)* to do this in a short time period, and *(3)* to increase awareness of tension in jaw and facial muscles. Instructions are given to help patients practice and generalize this relaxation training to their home and work settings. The success of this type of therapy seems to depend on how well patients can apply the relaxation technique learned in the clinic to their everyday environment.

Reviews of the literature conclude that EMG biofeedback relaxation methods are relatively effective with many TM disorder patients, particularly those with myofascial pain-dysfunction (Rugh and Lemke, 1984; Gale, 1986). Biofeedback has been shown to be as effective as occlusal appliance therapy for both short-term (1 month) and long-term (1 year) followups. It has been found useful in patients who have been refractory to other forms of therapy (Carlsson et al., 1975) and as an adjunct to more traditional occlusal therapy (Berry and Wilmot, 1977). In addition, one study demonstrated that occlusal contact patterns were improved following a muscle relaxation program involving EMG biofeedback (Berry and Singh, 1984). Clinical EMG biofeedback without a general relaxation program does not appear to be effective for TM disorders related to nocturnal bruxism (Dahlström and Carlsson, 1984). The American Dental Association's Council on Dental Care Programs (1982) has listed biofeedback and other behavior modification techniques as recommended initial treatments for symptoms of masticatory pain and dysfunction. As with dental therapy, biofeedback and other behavioral therapies are not useful by themselves with patients who are clinically depressed. These patients very often require antidepressant medication and should be referred to a psychiatrist (Gessel and Alderman, 1971).

Table 23-1 Characteristics of chronic pain patients

Homebound	Explores fringe therapies
Physical inactivity	Drug dependency
Social inactivity	Depression
Multiple doctors	
Secondary gain	

Procedures for general relaxation therapy

In many patients, a specific oral habit and/or its reinforcement contingency cannot be identified. The patient complains of diffuse muscular tension in the jaw muscles. Generalized muscular tension is believed to be a result of general arousal and anxiety (Yemm, 1985). The focus of therapy, thus, is not directed at modifying a specific habit; rather, the focus is on providing a general relaxation and stress control program for the patient.

General relaxation programs often involve several components. These include Jacobson's relaxation exercises, self-hypnosis, assertiveness training, biofeedback, learning of coping skills, and sometimes general counseling. Patients whose life-styles are particularly demanding or stressful are also asked to make major changes in their commitments and schedules. A careful history often reveals that some patients are simply attempting to accomplish too much. It is not uncommon to find a patient working two jobs, raising three children without a partner, and yet attempting to maintain a 3.7 grade point average in college night school courses.

Patients should be encouraged to identify specific aspects of their lives that are stressful or anxiety provoking. Sometimes patients are well aware of specific problems and willing to discuss ways of solving these. The dentist may provide encouragement and offer possible practical solutions. Solutions often involve patients' reevaluating priorities in their lives. The dentist, a successful, respected professional, is in a unique position to advise the patient on many practical "real life" problems that may bother the patient. The dentist's judgment and advice are often readily accepted. In fact, some patients find it easier to discuss certain problems with their dentist than with other health professionals or with religious advisors.

Referral to a psychologist or psychiatrist should be considered for patients with symptoms of depression and/or chronic pain. Depression may be evaluated by asking the patient about his or her general mood, changes in sleeping and eating patterns, energy level, and general capacity for pleasure (Blasberg et al., 1983). Patients with a long history of unsuccessfully treated pain are particularly susceptible to depression and chronic pain behavior. Characteristics of chronic pain patients are listed in Table 23-1. Considerable progress has been made in managing these patients (Keefe and Gil, 1985).

General relaxation programs usually involve weekly 1-hour visits to the office or clinic, supplemented with daily home self-practice sessions. Audio tape relaxation exercises are often used during the home practice sessions. Programs are usually individualized, but they often require from 6 to 10 weeks. Some programs recommend that patients return for brief training periods at 3- and 6-month intervals, to ensure that the patient has not slipped back into old habits. Reviews of the clinical research studies using general relaxation programs suggest that these methods are effective with several TM disorders, especially myofacial pain-dysfunction (Scott and Gregg, 1980; Moss et al., 1983; Gale, 1986). However, these behavioral therapies are not usually effective, nor intended to relieve severe pain, locking, inflammatory conditions, or other TM disorders that are unquestionably structurally caused. Physical medicine and pharmacological management must be employed to

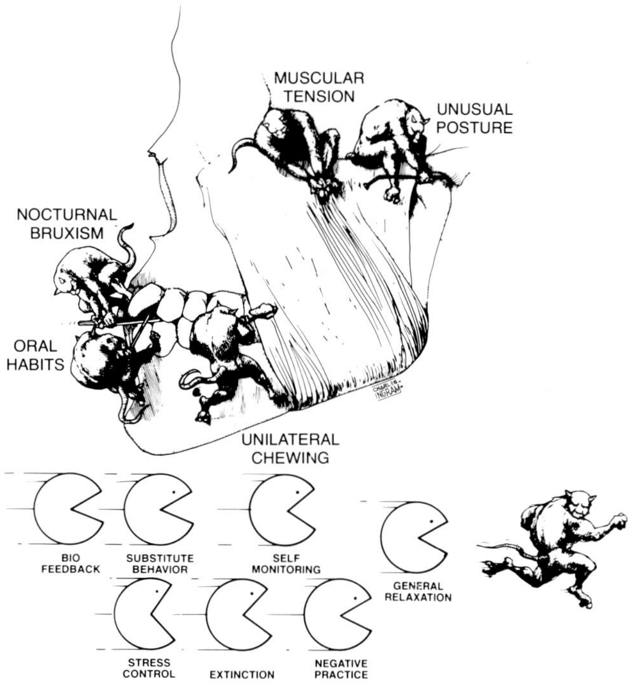

Fig. 23-6 Challenges to the structural integrity of the teeth and supporting structures may be managed through several behavioral strategies, as portrayed by this 20th century adolescent's perspective.

control acute pain conditions and inflammation. Relaxation and stress control programs are, however, useful after acute conditions have been controlled, providing a method of long-term patient management. These therapies are also ideally suited to be used in conjunction with traditional dental or occlusal therapies. Brooke et al. (1977) have provided evidence to indicate that the success of such therapies could be improved by the addition of relaxation training.

Stress control and relaxation programs are believed to be particularly useful for the stress-related nocturnal bruxist patient. Clinical observations of these patients suggest that bruxism is often related to stressful life periods or events. While bruxism can be temporarily suppressed with antianxiety medication, nocturnal EMG feedback, or an interocclusal appliance, long-term management often requires that the patient make significant changes in his or her life-style.

Biofeedback and relaxation training have been recommended primarily for stress-related muscle hyperactivity or myofascial pain-dysfunction conditions. These procedures may also be useful in the management of patients who have internal joint derangements. There are no well-controlled studies documenting this; however, when successful, EMG biofeedback and relaxation programs result in relaxed muscles and reduced trauma to the joint.

Patient selection for behavioral programs

It is not easy for patients to make major changes in their life-styles. Financial, child-rearing, and social obligations are often exceedingly difficult to alter. For this reason, patient selection and patient motivation are extremely important when considering a behavioral change or stress control program. Patients who generally do well in stress control programs appear to be those whose history indicates evidence of self-control (i.e., they have successfully quit smoking, lost weight, stopped nail biting, or demonstrated other self-regulating behaviors). As mentioned earlier, patients with significant depression are not well suited for these programs unless the depression is also treated.

Selection of an appropriate treatment program is very individualized. Groups of patients with occlusal problems and/or facial pain are not homogenous, but, rather, often represent extremes in terms of life-style, motivation, stage of illness, reaction to symptoms, oral habits, past treatments, hostility, and occlusal conditions. These and many other factors must be considered when determining a therapeutic program. Dealing with these conditions often is very challenging. Because of the complexities of these conditions, the success of treatment programs must be frequently evaluated and often adjusted. Unfortunately, assessment of treatment effects for conditions such as bruxism or TM disorders is difficult because of their cyclic natures. Signs and symptoms often go into remission with or without treatment, making it very difficult to determine if improvement is due to the therapy or to the cyclic or self-limiting nature of the problem.

Summary

In this chapter, general principles and specific treatment procedures have been described to help manage occlusal and facial pain conditions. Many of these conditions and treatments are portrayed in Fig. 23-6. For some therapies there are long-term studies demonstrating efficacy. For most, however, there is a lack of well-controlled, long-term, clinical trials. Justification for use of many of these treatments comes only from clinical opinion, a few case studies, or from the success of the therapy in management of other similar medical or behavioral disorders. The clinician must routinely review literature to update treatment methods and philosophies.

Chapter 24

Physical Therapy

Kenneth Abramovitch, Robert P. Langlais, and G. Robert Bradley

As discussed in Part III, the musculoskeletal components of the masticatory system may be afflicted with pain or dysfunctional problems that can strongly affect occlusal position and limit jaw function. Many factors may bring about or contribute to masticatory musculoskeletal pain problems, and the dentist is frequently called upon to diagnose and treat these problems. One mode of therapy is the use of physical agents and methods—physical therapy—to relieve pain and assist in the restoration of normal function after illness or injury. Although well-controlled clinical trials have not been completed, physical therapy is recognized as an effective, conservative method of treatment for many painful and dysfunctional problems of the masticatory system (Danzig and Van Dyke, 1983; Hargreaves and Wardle, 1983; Hall, 1984; Selby, 1985; Solberg, 1986). The conservative and reversible nature of this type of treatment has also been a compelling reason for its use in dentistry.

This chapter describes physical therapeutic methods that have been found to be most useful in the clinical situation and briefly summarizes the hypotheses underlying their assumed effectiveness. Thus, it will serve as an introductory reference source to the role of physical therapy in the field of Occlusion. The various forms of physical agents and methods are outlined in Table 24-1.

Table 24-1 Physical agents and methods for TM disorders

Exercise	Heat
Anesthetic adjuncts	Manipulation
Analgesia	Acupuncture

The role of physical therapy in temporomandibular disorders

Pain is usually the major symptom for which a patient will seek treatment. With regard to the temporomandibular joint (TMJ) and other regions of the masticatory system, pain is often associated with hyperactive muscles and limitation of jaw movement. Chronic, long-term muscle spasm often leads to muscle contracture, a condition whereby the muscle shortens, becoming mechanically much less flexible and, therefore, less capable of normal function. Trauma and long-term intermaxillary fixation may also lead to contracture (Solberg, 1986). Physical therapy is often directed specifically at relieving these muscular conditions.

Signs and symptoms often associated with masticatory muscle and joint disorders are also trismus, decreased chewing force, and referred pain to regions of the head and neck. Historically, it has been believed that the interaction of this pain and muscle hyperactivity or spasm can lead to a self-perpetuating pain-spasm-pain cycle (Schwartz, 1955). Also, injury to a joint often leads to protective functional compensation by adjacent joint musculature in an attempt to stabilize or maintain regular joint function. This compensation has been referred to as muscle guarding or joint splinting. Physical therapy as a treatment regimen may also be directed at breaking these feedback cycles (Selby, 1985).

When using physical therapy, one must recognize the nature and extent of both the treatment regimen and the disease entity itself. Those modes of treatment that successfully provide analgesic effects that are sufficient for a large number of conditions do not always treat the initial cause of the problem. Consequently, they do not necessarily provide a cure. Painful symptoms of TMJ osteoarthrosis, for example, may be relieved with some of the analgesic modes of therapy, but they never address the organic etiology. Joint clicks from muscular incoordination, however, can often be successfully treated by exercises that retrain physiological mandibular movement. Physical therapeutic methods such as massage and heat application directly treat the primary problem in traumatically associated disorders. Some physical therapy modalities may also be employed to help relax tense, hyperactive muscles in order to assist the dentist in positioning the mandible for occlusal therapy.

From the preceding discussion, it is clear that physical therapy can increase the therapeutic armamentarium of the dentist in certain painful and dysfunctional disorders of the masticatory system. In many cases, it is used as an adjunct to other treatments.

Exercise therapy

Exercise, the repetitive, therapeutic movement of body parts, has many applications in the treatment of muscular conditions. Exercise therapy is frequently used to treat the major muscle groups of the body (Gardiner, 1973), including the muscles of mastication (Schwartz, 1959). Regardless of the exercise prescribed, it must have a specific purpose. For the masticatory system, three types are recommended: *(1)* exercises to retrain coordinated rhythmic muscle function; *(2)* exercises to increase range of motion—*isotonic exercises;* and *(3)* exercises to increase muscular strength—*isometric exercises.*

The exercises for the masticatory muscles outlined here are easy to perform. However, it is important for the patient to be consistent in performing an *exercise set*—the prescribed number of repetitions for the prescribed number of cycles in an exercise session. The biggest drawback to the therapeutic use of exercise is the failure to properly motivate a patient, which can lead to problems in patient compliance.

Relearning rotation exercise

When there are signs or symptoms related to trauma or myofascial pain dysfunction, some authors feel that the principal problem is due to asynchronous isometric contractions of the musculature during function (Chayes and Schwartz, 1968; Yavelow et al., 1973). This, of course, would preclude the presence of any organic disease process in the TMJ itself. It is hypothesized that these uncoordinated mandibular movements are evidenced by either deviation and/or joint popping. This type of joint popping must be differentiated from other causes of joint sounds such as those created by arthritic changes, internal derangements, or chronic subluxation/dislocation. These other types of joint noises require different kinds of treatment. Conscious mandibular relearning exercises were suggested by Yavelow et al. (1973) for the deviation and popping caused by condylar rotation and translation occurring at different times in either joint. According to them, if the patient can learn to synchronize the rotating movement on initial mandibular opening, then a coordinated translational movement void of any clicking or deviations will follow.

To perform the relearning exercise, the patient first assumes a relaxed closed position sitting or standing in front of a mirror. The fingertips of

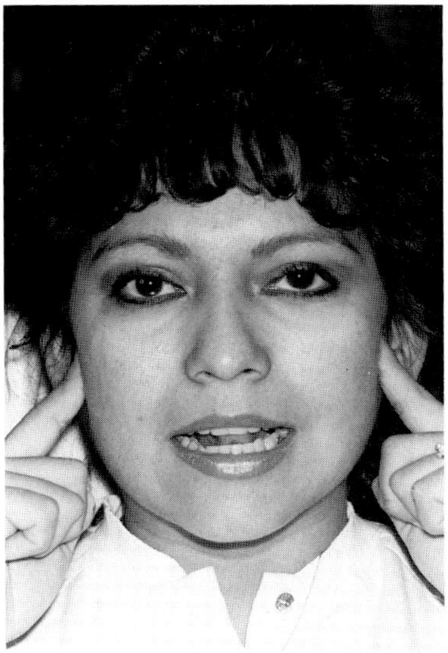

Fig. 24-1 To perform the mandibular relearning exercise, the patient places fingertips over the condyles to detect deviation or translation, and the tip of the tongue is placed at its most posterior extent on the palate.

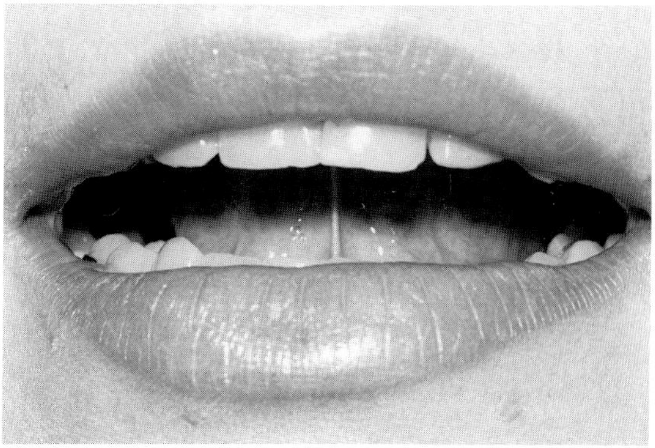

Fig. 24-2 Maximum opening distances in the mandibular relearning exercise are often limited to only a few millimeters. Note again the position of the tongue on the palate, which helps keep the condyles from translating during the exercise.

either hand are placed adjacent to the ipsilateral condyles and the tip of the tongue is placed as far back as possible on the palate. In this position the fingertips can palpate the nonworking condyle if deviations occur. The tongue position helps to keep the condyles from translating during rotation (Fig. 24-1). From this starting position, the patient slowly opens to a comfortable opening limited primarily to the rotation of the condyles. Any lateral deviation or translation of the condyles will be detected by the fingertips or by observation in the mirror. During the first attempts at this exercise, the maximum opening distance where the condyles do not translate or deviate may be limited to only a few millimeters (Fig. 24-2). From this opened position, the patient then rhythmically closes to a point just before tooth contact. This opening/closing movement is repeated in a rhythmic manner for 1 minute. A longer exercise interval may increase the fatigue of some muscles, which would jeopardize the proper exercise technique of rhythmic and synchronous mandibular movement. However, the exercise can be repeated every 10 to 15 minutes as often as desired (Chayes and Schwartz, 1968).

Placement of toothpicks in the interproximal midlines of the dental arches is often helpful for the patient to align the jaws and avoid deviations. However, this procedure can be very confusing to patients whose interproximal midlines are off; therefore, toothpick placement is optional.

During this opening exercise, when relearning mandibular rotation, it is important that the patient refrain as much as possible from translational and lateral movements of the condyles during routine functional mandibular movements such as eating and speaking. It may also be necessary for the patient to restrict the diet to soft foods. With the proper use and application of this technique, the pain will often diminish; and if the range of painless rotational movement were restricted, then it should begin to increase. Joint popping may also diminish and eventually disappear.

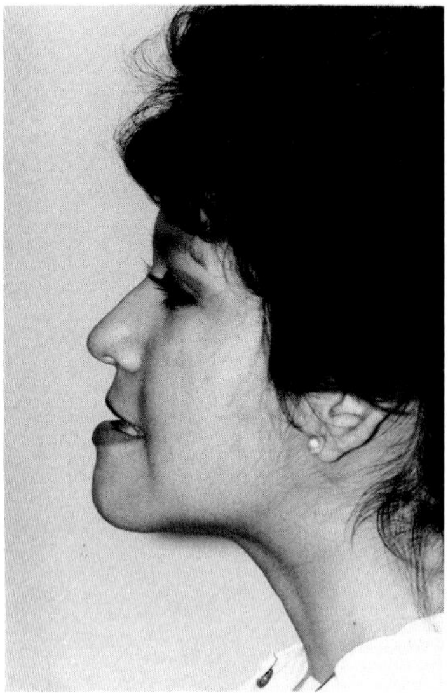

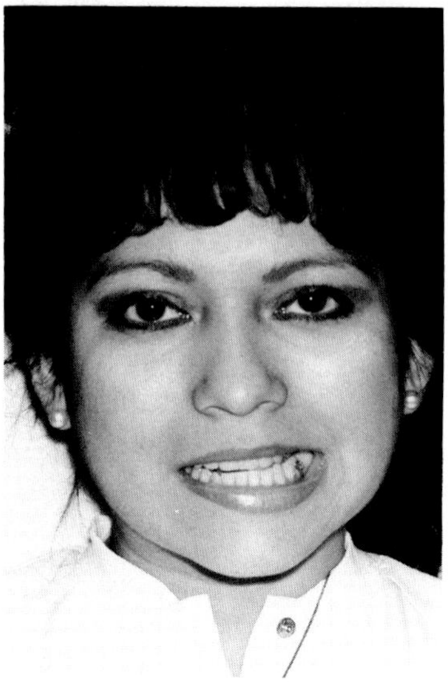

Fig. 24-3a *(left)* Maximum protrusion of the mandible is held for 3 seconds.

Fig. 24-3b *(right)* Maximum painless lateral excursion is repeated for both sides, if indicated.

Stretching exercises

These exercises are designed to increase the range of motion of the mandible in the lateral and protrusive directions (Schwartz, 1959). The range of motion may be increased by the dual phenomena of greater condylar translation and reduction of muscle hyperactivity.

As in the previous type of exercise, a straight relaxed posture either sitting or standing is preferred. When performing protrusive stretching exercises, it is important to protrude the mandible in a smooth, rhythmic manner. The mandible should be moved to the maximum protrusive position without eliciting pain and then held in this position for 3 seconds before retruding back to the original position (Fig. 24-3a). This movement is repeated ten times to complete one set. Five sets of ten repetitions, four times per day, is the suggested regimen; however, the number of sets per exercise period can be modified slightly for each patient.

During this stretching exercise, it is the 3-second holding of the stretch without eliciting pain that gradually increases the excursive range of motion. The patient will usually notice an improvement in the mandibular range of motion. This improvement can, of course, be measured clinically, giving further confidence to the patient.

It is important that the patient be consistent in performing the exercises. Long, complicated instructions that are difficult to remember, although perhaps more biologically sound, merely compromise the success of the exercise therapy. It is therefore suggested that the patient perform these exercises a minimum of four times per day, with five sets of ten repetitions each exercise period. This type of regimen is easily accommodated into one's daily schedule, at the three mealtimes and bedtime.

Stretching exercises for lateral excursions are performed in a similar manner. The mandible is held in the maximum painless lateral excursive position for 3 seconds, then rhythmically returned to the postural rest position. This exercise should be done for both sides, if indicated (Fig. 24-3b).

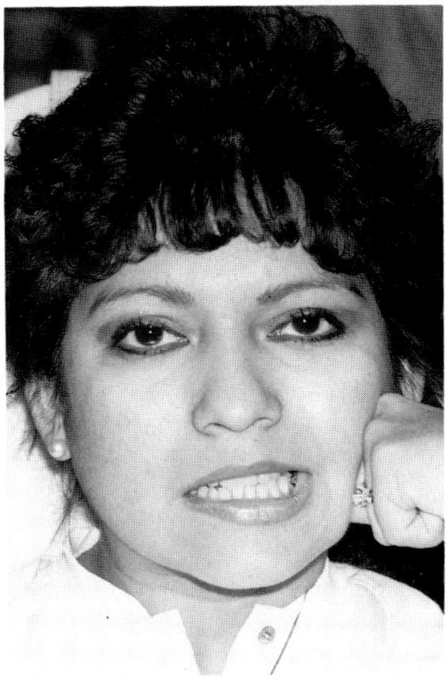

Fig. 24-4a A clenched fist provides resistance for muscle strengthening.

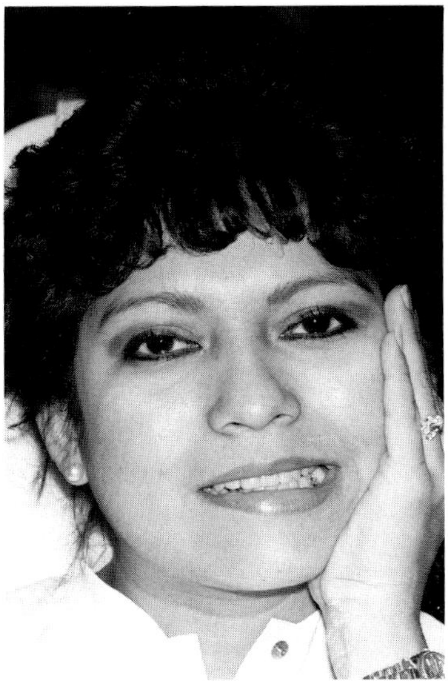

Fig. 24-4b The open palm as an alternate method of resistance.

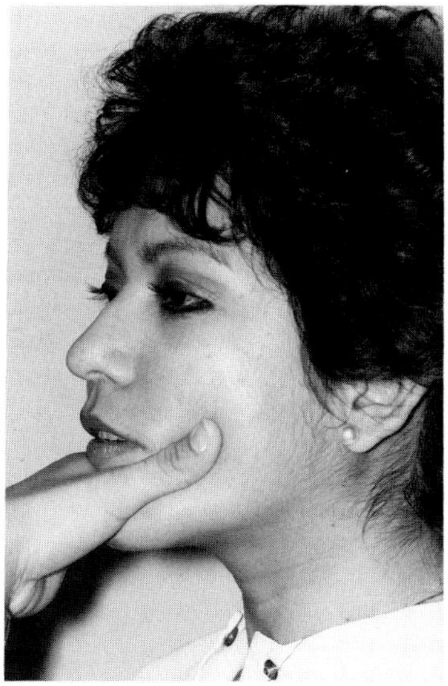

Fig. 24-4c Resistance to protrusion may be provided by the V formed by the index finger and the thumb.

Muscle strengthening exercises

Once stretching exercises can be performed comfortably using smooth, rhythmic movements, they can be performed against voluntary resistance to increase muscle strength. The degree of resistance applied must not inhibit painless synchronous movement. Excess force is not necessary. Resistance may be achieved by using either a clenched fist or an open palm against the chin and resisting 180° to the movement of the mandible. These positions are shown in Figs. 24-4a and b.

The patient must concentrate on not applying too much resistance. Excess resistance will strain the muscles the exercise is designed to help. Because muscle strengthening exercises should not be done before the patient has learned the stretching exercises, it is possible to concentrate on not applying too much resistance while also performing the exercise correctly.

Resistance against protrusion may be provided by placing the base of the V formed by the thumb and index finger into the mentolabial sulcus (Fig. 24-4c). During retrusive movement, anterior resistance may be applied by finger pressure to the labial aspects of the mandibular incisors. Stable resistance against closing movements may be provided by a tongue blade or any other similarly shaped object placed across the incisal/occlusal edges of the anterior/premolar mandibular dentition and held with adequate finger support.

Neck exercises

It is common for patients with TM disorders to report pain and tenderness of the muscles of the neck (Kaye et al., 1979). The reasons for this are not clear, although it is probably related to the cervical spine of the vertebral column being functionally and anatomically related to the mandible. One of the functional relationships is between head position and mandibular range of movement. Maximum range of mandibular movement is increased when the neck is extended slightly posteriorly. As a consequence, most people slightly extend the head during extreme mandibular movements. Theories of TM disorder etiology based upon neck and head postural problems have been proposed (Rocabado, 1984). However, these theories have not been tested through the usual scientific methods. Nonetheless, many patients with TM disorders have neck complaints that are improved or resolved through physical therapy exercises.

There are two basic types of neck stretching exercises that can be performed. One is flexion and hyperextension in the sagittal plane, and the other is lateral rotation in the coronal plane. To laterally rotate the head, it is important to straighten the back and slightly bend the neck forward (i.e., flex). The head is then rotated to one side toward the shoulder, to the farthest stretched position without eliciting pain. It is held here for 3 seconds and then returned to the center. This should be repeated ten times. After a very brief rest to assure total concentration and maximum performance, the same exercise is done toward the opposite shoulder.

For the flexion-hyperextension exercises, the back must again be straightened and the chin tilted along the midline toward the chest to the maximum flexed position without eliciting pain, and held for 3 seconds. Then the neck is hyperextended by tilting the head posteriorly to its most posterior painless limit for 3 seconds.

Anesthetic adjuncts to exercise therapy

It has been hypothesized that long-term muscle hypertonicity and spasm may lead to localized tender areas in the muscle, called *trigger points*. Referred pain from these points can involve adjacent facial or neck muscles (Bonica, 1957; Travell and Simons, 1983). One of the problems of using stretching exercises for symptomatic muscles has been the inability to perform them because of associated discomfort. Adjunctive anesthetic agents are available for use in these cases to increase range of motion in painful muscles.

Vapocoolant sprays

Vapocoolant sprays are useful for controlling trigger points and other sources of pain (Travell and Simons, 1983). Sprays such as Fluori-Methane* are very easy and relatively safe to apply if proper precautions are taken. The theoretical principle behind vapocoolants is that they act as counterirritants to the noxious stimuli of the trigger points. The application of a vapocoolant bombards the cutaneous receptors over the trigger point with both cold shock and topical anesthesia (Kraus, 1941). Although the pain elimination is only temporary, it is at this point that appropriate stretch exercises increasing the range of motion in muscles with the trigger points can be accomplished. Vapocoolant sprays are seen as an effective adjunct to exercise therapy (Travell, 1960; Travell and Simons, 1983).

Before application of a vapocoolant, the patient's conjunctival, nasal, and oral mucosa must be protected, so as not to have contact with spray vapors. The spray is applied to the masseter and/or anterior temporalis muscle from a working distance of about 12 to 18 in., in a sweeping motion from the trigger point toward the areas of referred pain (Fig. 24-5a). After the initial spraying, the patient will perform an exercise in the direction mandibular movement is painful. Often it is necessary to help guide the motion of the exercise (Fig. 24-5b). As the range of movement is increased, other painful areas may be uncovered. In that case, spray must be reapplied to these areas in order to extend the movement. This procedure is continued until movement can be performed with the normal range of motion. It is usually common to have to spray the masseter and sometimes temporalis area two to three times before obtaining a significant increase in the range of motion. At the end of the exercises, the sprayed areas should be warmed with lukewarm heat packs to avoid frosting the skin or chilling the muscle. The spray-and-stretch procedure can be performed

*Gebauer Chemical Co., Cleveland, Ohio.

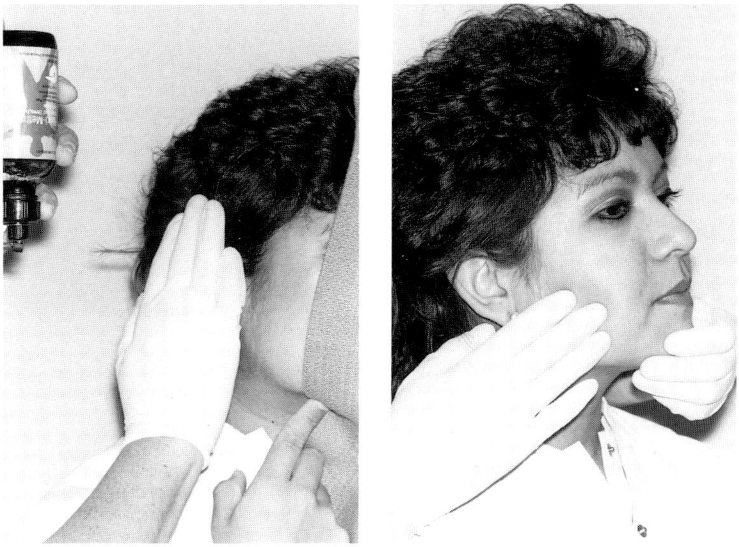

Fig. 24-5a *(left)* Application of vapocoolant spray with proper protection of nasal, conjunctival, and oral mucosa.

Fig. 24-5b *(right)* Guidance of mandibular motion after vapocoolant spray application.

on a daily basis in conjunction with properly prescribed exercises, until the acute pain emanating from myofascial trigger points has been controlled.

Trigger point injections

The injection of local anesthetic agents without vasoconstrictors into myotrigger points is another mode of treatment available for painful muscles not readily amenable to exercise therapy. Typical local anesthetic agents that are used for dental anesthesia are the agents of choice, such as 1% lidocaine or 0.5% mepivacaine hydrochloride. The infiltration of these agents into muscle tissue has an immediate analgesic effect. These agents are also vasodilators and as such have muscle relaxing properties. In conjunction with local anesthetic infiltration, the technique of dry needling also appears to be of some therapeutic benefit (Kraus, 1970). It is believed that needle piercing of a muscle in spasm will alter membrane potential significantly enough to temporarily block motor nerve conduction.

Before injection, the trigger point must be clearly isolated by palpation. Usually trigger points feel nodular upon palpation. In most cases, trigger points are tender and painful enough that they are easy to accurately locate. Once isolated, some type of sterile marker should be placed over the skin or mucosa in that area.

A 23- to 25-gauge needle is slowly injected into the trigger point. There is usually an initial sharp pain when the trigger point is contacted. The patient should be warned to expect this sharp pain, as it is a useful diagnostic sign in properly locating the trigger point before infiltration. Repeated dry needling is gingerly performed with alternating aspiration and injection of the required amount of solution as it is deposited in the trigger point tissues. For smaller muscle areas, 1 to 2 ml of solution is usually sufficient. However, up to 10 ml have been used for trigger points in larger muscle groups. Pain relief is almost immediate. Once the trigger points have been anesthesized, the patient should be able to painlessly carry out a regimen of prescribed exercises (Travell and Simons, 1983).

Stretch following trigger point injections is an integral part of the treatment. The muscle is passively stretched to its full length and sprayed with vapocoolant to relax remaining tense fibers.

Hot packs are then applied to reduce postinjection soreness. After a few minutes, the patient actively moves the muscle through its full range of motion several times to reaccustom the muscle to its normal length.

Frequent, repeated use of this technique is not recommended because a more persistent muscle spasm may result. However, it is indicated for the short-term relief of trigger point discomfort. When trigger point injections are used, further benefits should also be derived from the resulting anesthesia. Consequently, muscle stretching exercises should be carried out as in the case with vapocoolant sprays.

Recent research suggests less post-injection soreness from "jet" injection of the local anesthetic when compared to conventional trigger point injections (Ready et al., 1983). "Jet" injection systems force the fluid into the tissues at high velocity and have been used in other areas of the body. This method possesses equal efficacy in pain reduction of trigger points when compared to conventional means and may prove to be valuable in future management of trigger point pain.

Physical agents for analgesia

Three physical agents are available for analgesia in the treatment of orofacial pain commonly associated with TM disorders. They are transcutaneous electrical nerve stimulation, ultrasound, and iontophoresis. These techniques have been found reasonably successful when used in other parts of the body and, consequently, may also be applied to the masticatory system (Kahn, 1980; Travell and Simons, 1983; Selby, 1985).

Transcutaneous electrical nerve stimulation (TENS)

Transcutaneous electrical nerve stimulation is often referred to by its acronym, TENS. It has been used for analgesia in different types of orofacial pain, such as trigeminal neuralgia, atypical facial neuralgia, and herpetic neuralgia (O'Neil, 1981; Black, 1986). TENS also appears to be effective as a local analgesic for the pain related to TM disorders (Wessberg et al., 1981; Gold et al., 1983). Activation of the opioid antagonist system, enkephalins and endorphins, was once regarded as a possible mechanism of action of TENS; however, it has been shown using naloxone hydrochloride, an opioid antagonist, that this pathway is most likely not involved (Hansson et al., 1986).

A major difference between TENS and other forms of electrical stimulation is that TENS is designed primarily for sensory stimulation, rather than motor stimulation. Some motor stimulation may occur, but it is of a small enough magnitude to be noncontributory. If significant motor stimulation does occur concurrently with the transcutaneous stimulation, this may impair the analgesic effect and even exacerbate the pain.

The exact stimulation frequencies are often empirically determined among patients and conditions. In the orofacial region, though, frequencies range between 10 and 100 Hz. The duration of the pulse also varies. The treatment can be applied for anywhere from 15 to 40 minutes. An analgesic effect of several hours is often reported by chronic pain sufferers (Loeser et al., 1975). In experimental studies, analgesia has lasted up to 72 hours (Block and Laskin, 1980; Gold et al., 1983). However, the possible placebo effects of this therapy must not be ignored. Hansson and Ekblom (1983) showed temporary alleviation of orofacial pain in 40% of subjects in the placebo, or control, group of their study. This highlights the point that this type of physical therapy is purely analgesic in nature and primarily useful for symptomatic treatment.

The technique of TENS, with its low biocompatible electrocurrent, has virtually no side effects. The major problem that can arise is skin irritation from the adhesives or conducting agents that are placed between the skin and the surface electrodes. Although relatively safe, TENS is contraindicated for patients with cardiac pacemakers or who are pregnant. TENS therapy has also been reported to produce adverse ef-

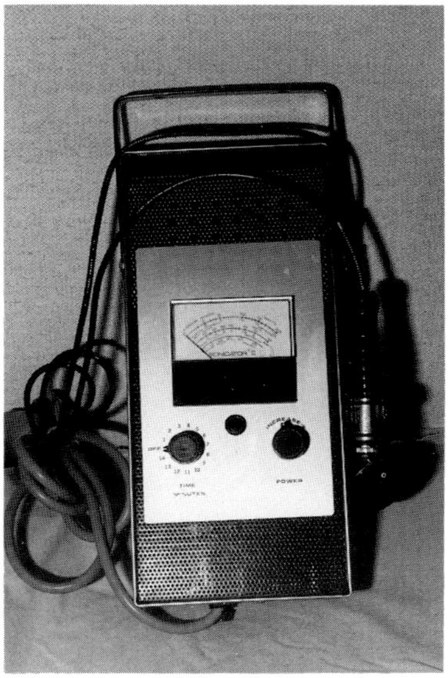

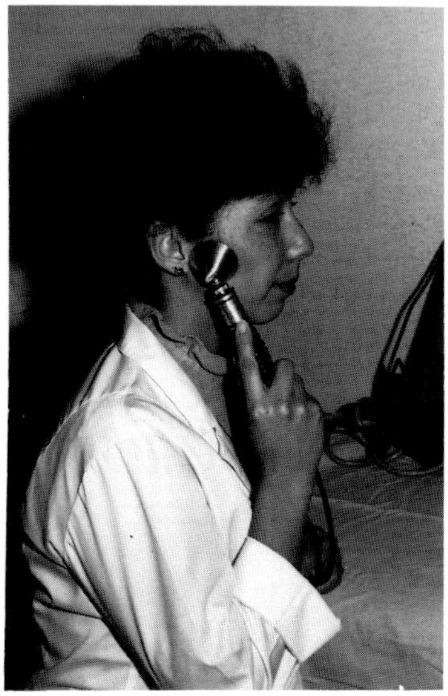

Fig. 24-6a *(left)* Ultrasound unit.

Fig. 24-6b *(right)* Patient applying ultrasound to herself.

fects in patients with rheumatoid arthritis (Griffin and McClure, 1981). In addition, caution is necessary to avoid placing TENS electrodes over the carotid sinus. Manufacturers' directions should always be followed.

Ultrasound

Sound waves at inaudible frequencies are referred to as *ultrasound*. The rationale of ultrasound therapy involves the conversion of mechanical energy in the tissues. A high-frequency electrical current driven through a transducer composed of piezoelectric crystals creates mechanical oscillations. These oscillations can be transferred through connective tissue, whereupon tissue resistance creates a localized rise in temperature. This heat production, when within physiological tolerance, is believed to be therapeutic. Ultrasound also is believed to have analgesic effects for masticatory pain. When used at low outputs, ultrasound seems to provide marked relief for pain in and around the TMJ (Erickson, 1964). A 3- to 5-minute application of ultrasound at 0.2 W/cm^2 provides hours of analgesia (Esposito et al., 1984).

A common ultrasound unit is shown in Fig. 24-6a. When applying a transducer head to the surface of the skin, oil is used as a coupling medium to decrease interface impedance. During application, the transducer head is used in a stroking motion to prevent excessive heat buildup in any one area of the tissue. In accessible areas, patients can apply the transducer head themselves (Fig. 24-6b).

Ionizing radiation generated from ultrasonic transducers has been a problem in the past with older machines. Biological damage to various tissues, including bone, has been documented (Stewart and Stratmeyer, 1982). However, properly calibrated machines operating at peak intensities of less than 2 W/cm^2 minimize the probability of these damaging effects. For the therapeutic use intended here, the harmful effects of ionizing radiation are not a problem.

Iontophoresis

Iontophoresis is the electrical introduction of various ions from the skin into the connective tissues. Many drugs once in their ionized form are amenable to iontophoresis. The technique

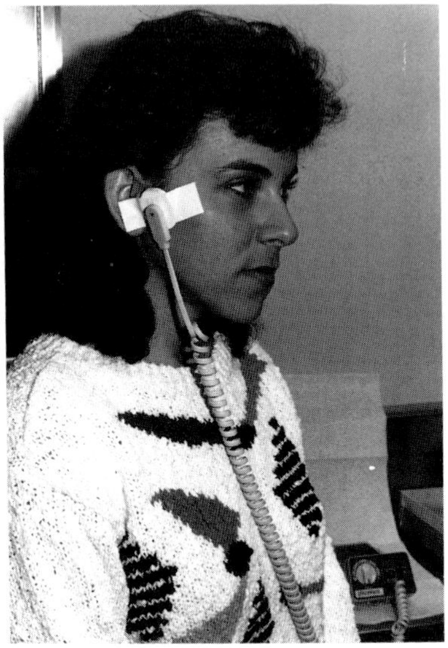

Fig. 24-7 Iontophoresis unit attached to area overlying TMJ.

involves passing a direct current through an electrolytic solution. The current causes ions to migrate according to their electrical charges.

Many topical drug agents such as local anesthetics, corticosteroids, antibiotics, and vasoconstrictors are ideal for iontophoresis because they possess a positive charge that will then migrate into an electrical field (Gangorosa, 1983). Once in the electrical field, they can be made to migrate in the direction of the negative electrode, which takes them to the tissue areas requiring their therapeutic effect.

Recently, the improved localized injection techniques for the introduction of local anesthetics (trigger point injections) and corticosteroids (inflammation) have made the use of injections more popular. However, the use of iontophoresis still appears to be a beneficial technique. Iontophoresis can produce a local therapeutic drug concentration very safely with virtually no systemic toxicity (Gangorosa, 1983). In addition, it is useful for needlephobic patients. Iontophoresis has been used successfully with lidocaine hydrochloride for trigeminal neuralgia and also for the introduction of hydrocortisone to inflamed TMJs (Fields et al., 1972; Kahn, 1980). Figure 24-7 shows a typical iontophoresis unit and the placement of the electrodes for the introduction of therapeutic ions around a TMJ. A typical session lasts approximately 30 minutes.

Heat

Externally applied heat is a useful form of energy with beneficial physiological effects (Travell and Simons, 1983). It should be used frequently in association with the host of other physical therapeutic techniques for painful muscles and joints. Mild heat has a sedative effect on the irritative conditions of both sensory and motor nerves. The sedative effect on motor nerves is felt to be useful for myospasm and muscle soreness.

The localized effects of heating are usually beneficial prior to performing exercise, and should probably be used routinely for this purpose. Because of the analgesic and relaxant properties, heat application can be applied at almost any time of the day, whenever a patient feels it is necessary. Hot water bottles, electric heating pads, and hydrocollator packs (canvas-enclosed packs of silica gel) are all useful for this purpose. However, these methods transmit heat by conduction, and consequently are only useful for superficial heat application. When it becomes necessary to heat deeper structures, such as the lateral and medial pterygoid muscles, heat from the conversion of electromagnetic radiation is more effective than heat from conduction. Diathermy and ultrasound are two electrotherapeutic forms of heat.

In ultrasound, the high-frequency oscillations of the transducer head get converted to heat when transmitted through the tissue. This can effectively heat any biological tissues to a depth of 5 cm. To do this, an intensity of 1.0 to 1.5 W/cm^2 must be used, which is higher than the wattage used for analgesia. Heat application in this manner may decrease the convalescence period associated with painful joint disorders (Hargreaves and Wardle, 1983; Esposito et al., 1984). Ultrasonic heat is useful for its spasmolytic effect in decreasing muscle hypertonicity. It should be applied to a particular site for 5 minutes a day. If symptoms persist after 1 to 2 weeks of ultrasound applications, then it is doubtful that further use of ultrasound will be helpful.

Like ultrasound, diathermy is a form of electrotherapy that provides therapeutic heat application to deeper symptomatic tissues. Ultrasound uses a high-frequency mechanical energy that is converted into heat. In diathermy, heat is produced by the tissue resistance to a high-frequency electrical current passing through the symptomatic tissues. In general, diathermy has not been used much for the smaller anatomical areas of the masticatory system.

Manipulation

Contracture was discussed earlier as a loss of muscle flexibility. It can arise in the masticatory muscles from long-term joint immobilization after trauma and/or intermaxillary fixation. Contracture can also result from long-term chronic muscle spasm and alterations in body posture. Regardless of the cause, a muscle with contracture has lost its mechanical ability to stretch.

Once a muscle has reached this state, it will not respond favorably to the same type of treatments applicable for trigger points and myospasm. Heat and vasodilatation are of little consequence. Voluntary stretching exercises are also of little value, because the muscle has temporarily lost its voluntary range of motion. Mobilization techniques then become necessary, requiring actual manipulation by a therapist to literally stretch the resting muscle. Repeated manipulation will eventually restore a more physiological length that permits a more normal range of motion.

In instances where many treatment periods may be required to adequately increase range of motion, a team approach between the dentist and the physical therapist is the approach of choice. There are a number of different techniques for mandibular manipulation useful to physical therapists. These techniques involve skillful fingertip manipulation and pressure application to different parts of the mandible. For a more detailed discussion of these techniques, the reader should refer to Maitland (1977).

Acupuncture

The multifactorial etiology of most TM disorders has prompted recent research comparing acupuncture with conventional methods of treatment. As with TENS, the therapeutic effects of acupuncture on pain and dysfunction are usually explained by neural and humoral pathways. Implications have been made involving the gate control theory of pain and release of neurohumoral factors, such as endogenous morphinelike compounds, as mechanisms. Mediation of pain impulses by the autonomic nervous system has also been reported to be involved in acupuncture (Kao and Kao, 1979).

The efficacy of acupuncture treatment for TMJ pain caused by osteoarthrosis and rheumatoid arthritis has been reported to be reasonably good (Corcos and Brandwein, 1976). However, the criterion for assessment of efficacy was a subjective rating scale completed by each patient. In a randomized study, acupuncture was compared with conventional treatment modalities in the management of TM disorders (Raustia et al., 1985). The results indicated that patients favored conventional therapy; however, there was no statistical difference in pain relief or improvement in function. At this time, with no sound clinical research reported, it may be concluded that acupuncture may be of limited value in the management of TM disorders and other associated problems. However, the few studies available suggest that acupuncture is worthy of future research in the management of these disorders.

Conclusions

The use of physical therapy for TM disorders is

an important component of therapy. With adequate preparation, physical therapeutic techniques can be applied by most dental practitioners. Careful treatment selection is, however, indicated—secondary only to the proper diagnosis of the particular disorder. The dental profession must continue to study the clinical effects and underlying physiological mechanisms of physical therapeutic techniques in order to enhance the management of patients with pain and dysfunction of the masticatory musculoskeletal system. In cases where familiarity with the different techniques is lacking, close cooperation with professional physical therapists is necessary.

Chapter 25

Pharmacological Therapy

John M. Gregg and John D. Rugh

Pharmacological therapy is a major component of the comprehensive management of many masticatory system musculoskeletal problems. Pharmacological agents are used to assist in diagnosis, to manage acute pain and anxiety, to control local and systemic disease, and as part of some rehabilitation programs. They can be powerful tools for the clinician; however, they must be used with a sound understanding of their action and as part of a planned comprehensive therapy program. This chapter reviews the principles of pharmacological management for myofascial and several other temporomandibular (TM) conditions. Indications and contraindications for the major classes of drugs are reviewed.

Bases for pharmacological management

Step 1: Identification of causative factors

This step often requires considerable thought. Etiological factors may be complex and diverse. They may include trauma, responses to psychosocial stressors, and certain "constitutional" physiological factors, such as underlying systemic disease and genetic predisposition. The appropriate drug must be selected based on the specific etiology. For example, if domestic conflict, anxiety, or depression are central factors, then a drug regime that includes psychopharmacological agents will be more effective. If extreme trismus and capsular edema are identified with nocturnal bruxism, then an anti-inflammatory agent coupled with an antianxiety drug at bedtime may be useful. If host defenses are reduced from a systemic (constitutional) disease, such as poorly controlled diabetes mellitus, then the associated TM disorder may respond only when the systemic disease is better controlled. Clearly, no single drug known at present can compensate for the full range of causative factors in masticatory musculoskeletal pain. The clinician must carefully evaluate each case. The patient's history is the most valuable diagnostic aid.

Step 2: Identification of primary sources of pain

Effective drug management recognizes the tissue distribution of pain. Although pain is often presumed to arise primarily in intramuscular or tendinous receptors, pain also may emanate from the TMJ capsule, dental periodontium and periosteum, and perivascular receptors. Although biogenic amine release occurs at all tissue-receptor interfaces, drug management should differ depending on whether the pain is capsular, vascular, or muscular. In the first case, emphasis may be on anti-inflammatory agents; in the second, on antiserotonergic agents; and in the third, on anxiolytic agents.

Pain may also be very localized in one or a few trigger points, or it may be disseminated and multifocal. Focal pain may respond well to local anesthetic block injections, whereas systemic and centrally acting agents are more appropriate for multifocal forms.

Step 3: Identification of the stage of the disease

Acute and chronic pain represent markedly differing psychophysiological conditions and require equally divergent drug management strategies (Sternbach, 1974). For example, patients with acute pain of a few days' duration tend to demonstrate inflammation, edema, trismus, anxiety, and a generalized sympathomimetic response. Drugs are best prescribed in a "titration" fashion, much like postoperative pain medication, and are directed toward minimizing further injury, reducing edema, mobilizing parts, reducing anxiety, and blunting catecholamine release. Anxiolytics, anti-inflammatories, local anesthetics, and even narcotics may be used with acute pain conditions.

Chronic pain, by contrast, is associated with muscle atrophy and fibrosis, physical and social immobility, depression, and a generalized parasympathetic dominance (Black, 1975; Fordyce, 1976). With chronic pain, drug therapy must enhance attempts to mobilize the patient. Sedative analgesics must not be given pro re nata (p.r.n.), if at all, with chronic pain conditions. Antidepressant agents given on a rigid schedule are believed to be more appropriate. Thus, the stage of the illness is clearly an important factor in determining appropriate management. Again, the patient's history is most often the key to understanding the stage of the illness.

Pharmacological agents

Five drug classes appear to have the greatest efficacy for managing the pain and dysfunction associated with TM disorder:

1. Local anesthetics
2. Analgesics
3. Anti-inflammatories
4. Anxiolytics
5. Antidepressants

An overview of each drug used in TM disorders, and a tabular summary of each agent's primary action are provided in the following sections.

Local anesthetics

Local anesthetics have a long history of use in pain management (Bonica, 1959). Their specific indications in therapy are the presence of acute myospasm as indicated by recent restriction of jaw motion, palpable painful trigger points, or muscular dysfunction related to condyle dislocation. Local anesthetics can serve a number of useful purposes: pain control, diagnosis, prognosis, and therapy (Black and Bonica, 1973).

Palliative blocks should be given mainly for acute or recurrent episodes of pain, and not only may afford immediate pain relief to the patient, but also may secure the time needed to institute additional therapies. Palliative blocks can be repeated at intervals of 2 to 4 days, but more frequent applications run the risk of local muscular tissue toxicity or fibrosis. The blocks also may be helpful in diagnosis by defining the locus and degree of importance of a given muscle in generating pain. The prognosis in a given case may be derived in part from the effects of the block. The longer and more profound the pain relief, the more likely it would appear that repeated blocks or physical therapy interventions would also help.

Blocks may also be therapeutic in cases of musculoskeletal pain conditions (Ghia et al., 1979). Injections are typically given at weekly or biweekly intervals for a period of 2 to 8 weeks. Agents most commonly used are lidocaine 2% and, with increasing popularity, the longer-acting bupivacaine hydrochloride 0.5% and etidocaine hydrochloride 0.5% (Lund et al., 1973; Laskin et al., 1977). Some protocols have included corticosteroids, such as methylprednisolone acetate, along with the anesthetic, although there is no clearly documented advantage over using the anesthetic alone. Indeed, there are data to support the notion that therapeutic effects of block injections in painful muscles are not due at all to the drug, but to a muscular or placebo response to the needling trauma instead (Ghia et al., 1976; Leavit, 1979).

A key injection site for diagnosis and therapy is the lateral pterygoid muscle block. The injection is given just posterolateral to the pterygoid hamulus. The penetration should be approximately 1.5 in. into a paracondylar position. Also useful is the occipital block for triggers in the superior attachments of sternocleidomastoid, trapezius, and posterior cervicalis muscle groups. Masseteric attachment and lateral TMJ capsular blocks also have application. The intraarticular block, although helpful in defining the role of the auriculotemporal nerve in pain transmission, has little effect on muscle function.

Analgesics

Although the analgesics may be a source of abuse and misuse, they nevertheless play a major role. In terms of pain management, it is useful to divide analgesics into subclasses of strongly addictive, moderately addictive, and nonaddictive (Halpern, 1977).

Strongly addictive agents, including morphine, methadone hydrochloride, meperidine hydrochloride, and fentanyl citrate, are contraindicated for most cases of focal or isolated myofascial pain. They should be avoided where depression is a factor and where there is concurrent addiction or dependence on other centrally acting agents, such as alcohol. They should also be avoided in long-term use with chronic patients.

The major narcotics *should* be used where there has been an exacerbation of musculoskeletal pain associated with proven neoplastic, traumatic, or infectious conditions.

Moderately addictive analgesics are widely prescribed, but rarely indicated, for routine myofascial pain management. They should be used for a specific time, usually less than 3 weeks, and should be prescribed as frequent low doses on a rigid, fixed time schedule. They are indicated for posttraumatic or postsurgical conditions where pain is expected to be short-lived and diminishing in intensity as healing occurs. Every attempt should be made to replace this drug class with nonaddictive, anti-inflammatory analgesics, local anesthetic blocks, and nonpharmacologic therapies.

Nonaddictive analgesics available for "baseline" analgesia have increased dramatically in the past decade (Cooper, 1978; Houde, 1980). A common denominator for these agents is their apparent similarity of action as suppressors of prostaglandin action on the peripheral nociceptors. There is also evidence that they may exert some central nervous system effect on nonopiate receptor pain modulating systems. As such, these agents combine mild anti-inflammatory and analgesic actions that reportedly equal that of codeine in analgesia. This class of agents, particularly the nonsalicylates, is not widely used for myofascial and other TM disorders, perhaps because patients and clinicians alike view them all as "just aspirin." In addition, the slow resorption time minimizes the effect on myospastic pain if taken p.r.n. when pain becomes intolerable. However, experience with chronic arthritic pain suggests that, when taken prophylactically to build a constant blood level of 1,200 to 2,000 mg daily, these agents can be an effective means of "baseline" pain suppression (Cooper, 1978). They would, of course, be especially useful if chronic inflammation were present or suspected. Slow-release and long-acting preparations, such as piroxicam, taken twice a day, are particularly useful.

Anti-inflammatories

Glucocorticoids, given as a single intraarticular injection of the TMJ, have a long and successful use in the treatment of inflammatory-phase osteoarthrosis (Henny, 1954; Keagy and Keim, 1967). However, a review of the literature fails to produce a definitive study of glucocorticoids' effect on myofascial pain conditions. Numerous uncontrolled reports suggest that injection of painful and swollen muscle trigger points with single boluses of approximately 20 to 40 mg methylprednisolone is rapidly effective (Black and Bonica, 1973; Kraus, 1973).

Corticosteroids have also been advocated by some for use as topical creams in inflammatory TMJ pain. Agents such as 0.05% fluocinonide and 0.025% triamcinolone are recommended for iontophoresis. However, no controlled studies of effects on muscle pain are available.

Nonsteroidal oral anti-inflammatory agents, as reviewed under "Analgesics," are clearly indicated for TM disorders, particularly where acute capsulitis or abrupt increases in painful and swollen muscle trigger areas exist. Agents such as ibuprofen, naproxen, and indomethacin should be prescribed over a minimum of 2 weeks on a low-dose, rigid schedule of two to four times daily.

Anxiolytics

Antianxiety agents are probably the most prescribed drugs for myofascial pains. Four types are most prominent: antihistamines (infrequently used), propanediols (older and moderately used), benzodiazepines (overwhelmingly the most prescribed), and alcohol (heavily patient selected). There is no question that the benzodiazepines can and should be used to manage acute exacerbations of TM disorders when crises in job, family, or general health have precipitated anxiety and psychophysiological upheaval. An effective protocol is diazepam, 2.5- to 10-mg tablets, two to six times daily—titrated to anxiety rather than pain, and such that speech is coherent and mental functions intact.

In a study of 90 myofascial pain-dysfunction patients, Greene and Laskin (1971) reported that meprobamate, an anxiolytic and muscle relaxant, can effectively relieve symptoms in a significant number of patients. It is important that the patient understand the supportive psychological basis on which these drugs are being used, and that this therapy last no more than 7 to 10 days' duration. Beyond this arbitrary point, there is an increasing drug tolerance and dependency, and the initial pain relief and relaxation of muscles often undergo a "rebound" return of myospastic pain (Gregg, 1978). Benzodiazepines, when used with chronic patients, and particularly in patients with depression, may result in a dangerous deepening of mood, physical complaints, concomitant central nervous system drug use, and sleep disorder. Stress-related nocturnal bruxism may be controlled for a few weeks with benzodiazepines; however, alterations of slow-wave sleep patterns with chronic benzodiazepine use may compound destructive nocturnal dyskinesias (Satoh and Harada, 1973; Moldofsky et al., 1975).

Antidepressants

Depression may generate or perpetuate chronic myofascial pain (Moldofsky et al., 1975; Gregg, 1978). Antidepressant drugs have a more than 20-year history of excellent effectiveness and safety in both acute and chronic pain cases, and are a cornerstone of chronic pain therapy in multidisciplinary pain clinics (Lascelles, 1966). Antidepressants can be expected to reduce anxiety, reverse both mood and vegetative signs and symptoms of depression, alter sleep dysfunction, potentiate the effects of analgesics, and replace abused central nervous system drugs (Halpern, 1974; Gessel, 1975). On the negative side, peripheral fluid retention and allergic responses are frequent side effects.

Three antidepressant types have been used: tricyclics, monoamine oxidase inhibitors, and lithium salts. The tricyclics are most widely used and are highly effective for patients with "typical" depression where mood, vegetative, and sleep dysfunctions are seen (Gessel, 1975). A useful schedule is a bedtime-only prescription of amitriptyline hydrochloride or doxepin hydrochloride, titrated to a level of tolerance from 50 to 150 mg. Improvement may be observed within 1 week, but may take up to 30 days. Therapy should be sustained for 3 to 4 months, followed by tapering to a low-dose maintenance or a placebo. The tricyclics are often combined with phenothiazine psychotropic agents to enhance their analgesic and tranquilizing effects.

Monoamine oxidase inhibitor agents, such as phenelzine sulfate, may be effective against the more "atypical" and "masked" depressives, which do not usually respond to tricyclic antidepressants beyond placebo levels.* The monoamine oxydase inhibitors must be used with caution because of their catecholamine-sensitizing side effects.

A newer class of drugs, the triazolopyridines, such as trazodone hydrochloride, are known as "heterocyclics" and have some properties of both anxiolytics and antidepressants. There are no published reports of their use with TM pain, but they nevertheless show promise.

Other pharmacological agents

Antipsychotics

Pain complaints among acutely psychotic patients are very rare. Indeed, these patients have been known to perform gruesome feats of self-mutilization without overt pain suffering. On occasion, however, a borderline psychotic patient will present with bizarre forms of pain, including some resemblance to one of several TMJ or myofascial pain-dysfunction conditions. These patients will usually respond to a supportive program of major psychotropic drugs and behavioral management (Cavenar and Maltebie, 1976; Raft et al., 1979). Primary drugs in this group are the phenothiazines or major tranquilizers, the thioxanthines, and the butyrophenones, such as haloperidol. Ironically, a few patients treated with phenothiazines may show extrapyramidal side effects severe enough to produce tardive dyskinesias and spasticity of masticatory muscles that will intensify myofascial pain.

Antimigraines

Some patients with TM disorders are found to have a vascular component to their condition. In some cases, classic migraine, periodic migrainous neuralgia (clusters), carotidynia, or carotid arterial disease are found concomitant with the TM disorder. They may not necessarily be directly related. Three common agents are used in vascular pain of this type: *(1)* ergotamines, *(2)* serotonin antagonists, such as methysergide, and *(3)* propanolol.

The ergotamine tartrates are still the primary diagnostic and therapeutic controller of classic frontal-temporal migraines. However, dependency and cardiovascular side effects are often seen, as well as a gradual loss of drug effectiveness. Serotonin antagonists such as methysergide are effective against the difficult-to-manage, periodic migrainous, and atypical midfacial syndromes. There is an unfortunate tendency for rare, but severe, connective tissue toxicities with this agent. Propanolol has been found in the past 10 years to be a benign and often effective first-line drug for milder and atypical, stress-induced, vascular facial pain (Diamond and Medina, 1976). At 40 to 120 mg daily, it can be rapidly effective with few side effects. It is contraindicated in the asthmatic patient.

Anticonvulsants

Many patients with facial pain symptoms have been prescribed anticonvulsants, such as phenytoin and carbamazepine. This usually represents a mistake in diagnosis made by the patient's physician, who, upon hearing the patient's description of a "stabbing pain in the ear," presumes the disease to be tic douloureux (trigeminal neuralgia). Other than the expected improvement from sedation or placebo, there is no proven therapeutic effect from the anticonvulsants in TM disorders.

Muscle relaxants

Neuromuscular blocking agents, such as the nondepolarizing agent succinylcholine chloride, can aid in emergency reduction of acute condylar dislocations. However, such agents should only be used in a setting where endotracheal intubation can easily be accomplished.

*D. Raft, The University of North Carolina Multidisciplinary Pain Clinic, Chapel Hill, unpublished data.

Among the centrally acting muscular relaxants, such as methocarbamol or carisoprodol, there lacks convincing evidence that their mild effects on muscular pain are due to a specific action on motor systems (Tseng and Wang, 1971). Rather, their effects are probably due to placebo or nonspecific sedation.

Drug abuse and detoxification

A major barrier to effective pharmacotherapy of TM disorders is, ironically, drug misuse (Halpern, 1974). Although intense physical addiction, with all its secondary social and psychological ramifications, is relatively rare among TM disorder patients, a tenacious form of psychological dependency on certain drugs is common. The most obviously abused agents are the narcotic analgesics, particularly the oral codeine preparations and codeine substitutes, such as oxycodone hydrochloride, dihydrocodeine, and propoxyphene (Ready and Hare, 1979).

An undetermined number of patients with TM disorders seek and receive parenteral narcotics, such as meperidine and pentazocine, in emergency rooms and in isolated private offices.

Anxiolytic "tranquilizing" agents such as the benzodiazepines, the propanediols, and alcohol are probably the most widely abused or misused agents among patients with TM disorders, although accurate statistics are not available. Dental, medical, and pharmaceutical clinicians tend to feel "safer" prescribing these agents, because physiological dependence and central nervous system depression are less overt, and their use by the higher socioeconomic strata of our society, including professionals such as themselves, is more "acceptable." Nevertheless, these agents are known to exacerbate underlying depression, particularly sleep disorders, that may be directly linked to some myofascial pain-dysfunction conditions.

Tranquilizer and alcohol "hangover" may be a factor in reinitiating myospasms at shorter intervals because of vascular release of biogenic amines such as serotonin. Studies have shown that abuse of sedative-analgesic agents emerges as part of the chronic pain syndrome when patients are permitted or encouraged to take drugs as a p.r.n. response when pain becomes intolerable (Black, 1975; Fordyce, 1976). The brief intervals of euphoria or feeling of well-being afforded by the drug become, in this case, the unconscious "reward" for having pain, and appear to ensure that pain cycles become more frequent and drugs less effective.

Detoxification from drug abuse/dependency can be a complex and frustrating task, and there are few specialists or treatment centers available for referral of the average patient. General principles of detoxification developed for patients with chronic pain differ from protocols for "hard-core" addicts (Halpern, 1974, 1977). Many socially functional patients with TM disorders can safely and effectively be withdrawn from the sedative-narcotic agents abruptly. Substitution agents, such as nonnarcotic, anti-inflammatory analgesics, and/or antihistamines, such as hydroxycine or diphenhydramine, have been advocated as a rigid time-contingent "pain cocktail" (Taylor et al., 1980). Other schemes rely on a bedtime-only substitution of low-dose tricyclic antidepressant "cocktails" such as amitriptyline hydrochloride at 50 to 100 mg, or, more recently, doxepin hydrochloride at 50 to 100 mg. All of the detoxification schemes rely heavily on a firm compliance "contract" between doctor and patient (Fordyce, 1976).

Placebos

Placebos are substances that lack active pharmaceutical elements but that often have profound effects on the condition being treated. Beecher, in 1955, demonstrated that 30% to 40% of subjects exposed to placebo treatment in experimental situations exhibited benefits.

Placebo effects are very powerful; they are so powerful, in fact, that some patients have had to stop taking the placebo medication because the "side effects" were too great. The mechanisms underlying the action of placebos are not completely understood. Past theories have focused on cognitive effects; however, placebo analgesia may also be mediated by the release of endorphins. Response to placebos in experimental studies has been found to extend beyond the patient's subjective experience, as laboratory values and other measures of objective physiological change have been found to occur, leading to both therapeutic and adverse effects (Wolf, 1959).

Presently, placebos are thought to work through biochemical changes mediated through the patient's belief system and cognitions. The placebo effect may occur in the absence of any drug therapy, or can be associated in various ways with medications used in the therapy.

Although commonly thought of primarily as pain relievers, virtually all potentially reversible symptoms and diseases investigated using double-blind studies have shown some response to placebos. Although 30% to 40% of patients will respond very dramatically to placebo effects, it is difficult to predict those patients most likely to respond to placebos. This difficulty is due primarily to the unpredictable and inconsistent effects exhibited by these substances, and partly to the fact that the same person may respond or fail to respond to placebos in different circumstances.

Studies in recent years have been directed to examining the effect that the doctor/patient relationship may have on the placebo response. An open, caring relationship, where the patient understands the condition and is given a sense of control over the illness, is more likely to create a positive placebo response, with improved therapeutic results. Furthermore, it has been proposed that the placebo response may be composed of a complex triad of clinician, therapeutic setting, and therapy rendered, with the response being learned through experience.

When used properly and where indicated, placebos may produce extremely powerful therapeutic effects. The appearance of the agent has been shown to affect the patient's reaction to the treatment being rendered. Large, colorful placebos are generally more effective than more ordinary appearing ones. Injections are considered most effective. Clinicians should utilize a patient's cognitions and placebo effect to achieve the most powerful therapeutic effects from pharmaceutical agents. *Placebos play an integral part in any treatment modality.*

Summary

A wide range of pharmacological agents is available to assist in the diagnosis and management of myofascial pain dysfunction or other types of TM disorders. Such disorders may have profound effects on mandibular and occlusal function. Effective use of these agents involves three major steps. The clinician first must identify the predominant etiological factors, second must identify the primary sources of pain, and third must determine the stages of the disease. Of particular importance in the use of medication is the distinction between acute and chronic pain.

The following guidelines are suggested in the management of myofascial and other TM pain conditions:

1. Drugs should be used in the context of a total treatment plan that may include physical therapy, interocclusal appliance therapy, occlusal therapy, surgical treatments, and behavioral management. Medication should not be presented to the patient as isolated, "curative" treatments.
2. The full range of available agents should be applied in a flexible manner. Clinicians should avoid stereotyped "cookbook" reliance on single or favorite agents.
3. The type and balance of drug therapy must be matched with the specific predominant causes, the tissue distribution of pain, and the stage of acuteness-chronicity of the condition.
4. Drug abuse and dependency should be identified, and detoxification undertaken, as a first phase of pharmacological management.
5. The dentist should rely on appropriate consultation and/or referral when pharmacological therapy requires specific knowledge and expertise on the use of these agents.

Chapter 26

Surgical Therapy

Joseph E. Van Sickels and M. Franklin Dolwick

Surgical therapy that corrects "structural abnormalities of the jaws and resulting facial disharmonies" is called *orthognathic surgery* (Jablonski, 1982). Achieving a more ideal occlusion is one of the principal goals of orthognathic surgery. The surgical portion of the procedure, either by itself or in combination with orthodontics, attempts to achieve optimal interdigitation of the teeth for patients with underlying skeletal deformities.

Early orthognathic surgical procedures were limited to the mandible or segmental operations in the maxilla. Today, osteotomies that move the midface, maxilla, and mandible are performed in hospitals throughout the world. As surgical procedures have become more sophisticated and widespread, the need to accurately and systematically describe each case has become paramount (Epker and Wolford, 1975). Components of the face have been divided as follows: upper face and cranium, nasomaxillary complex, maxillary dentition, mandibular dentition, and mandible (Proffitt et al., 1980). Segmentalizing the facial complex allows the surgeon to address where a particular deformity occurs. The entire face can and may be moved in managing craniofacial anomalies, but common dentofacial discrepancies involve the lower four portions.

Esthetically, a patient should be viewed from both a frontal and a profile position. Particular attention should be given to the frontal view, as this is how patients see themselves. A systematic approach notes the degree of right-to-left differences and facial balance (Epker and Wolford, 1975) (Fig. 26-1). Patients should be examined with the lips relaxed and the mandible gently retruded. This is important, because patients with skeletal discrepancies will often alter their posture in order to functionally or esthetically mask an underlying skeletal deformity. Burstone (1967) believes that up to 3.5 mm of interlabial distance is normal when the patient is at rest and the mandible is in centric relation. Subjects with an excessive interlabial gap (lip incompetence) habitually purse their lips to achieve labial closure. Gingival inflammation around the maxillary incisors is sometimes seen in these patients when there is a poor oral seal (Fig. 26-2).

Large occlusal differences between centric relation and centric occlusion may likewise cause a false clinical impression. For example, a subject with a right-sided occlusal prematurity in centric relation may have a 3- to 4-mm left-sided shift of the mandible to full intercuspation. Viewed frontally, in centric occlusion, the patient would appear asymmetrical; however, the facial skeleton is normal.

In profile, the balance between the upper, middle, and lower thirds of the face should be assessed (Fig. 26-3). Detailed articles and textbooks describe facial norms and may be used to evaluate patients more completely than is possible in this brief review; for further information it is suggested that the reader consult one of them (Proffit et al., 1980; Epker and Wolford, 1975). It is important to understand that esthetic norms are based on average population samples. In analyzing an individual patient, several factors must be considered, including the patient's family, racial heritage, and sex.

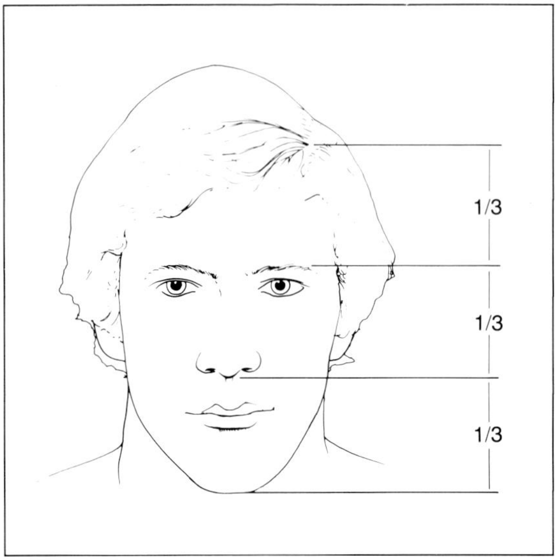

Fig. 26-1 Facial balance, frontal view.

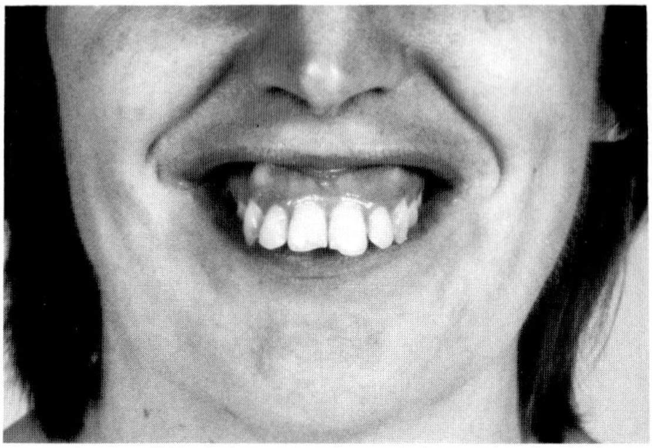

Fig. 26-2 Subject with lip incompetence, accentuated with smile.

Numerous cephalometric analysis systems have been advanced to evaluate patients. Early systems were developed to examine skeletal and dental features, evaluate growth and development, and assess orthodontic treatment. More recent techniques and procedures have been specifically designed to appreciate jaw and facial deformities (Burstone et al., 1978; Delair et al., 1981; McNamara, 1984a). Most of these systems relate the maxilla and mandible to the cranial base, and maxillary and mandibular dentition to each other, to their skeletal bases, and to the cranial base. A premise implied by this method is that there is some stable anatomical base with which to relate these structures. With many facial deformities, this is not so. When the cranial base is abnormal, corrective measures are taken to relate skeletal measurements to a true horizontal reference plane. To do so, patients, both clinically and cephalometrically, are examined in a "natural head position" (Moorrees and Kean, 1958). This reproducible head posture is one assumed by an individual when looking at distant objects or when looking into his or her own eyes in a mirror. A true horizontal reference plane is then drawn using the natural head position.

Although traditional cephalometric systems emphasized hard tissue, soft tissue landmarks are equally important. Once soft tissues are analyzed, formulas and techniques are used to predict what will happen to the soft tissue following bony movements. Recently, computer programs have been used to allow surgeons and orthodontists to trace and predict hard and soft tissue movement. This is an area that will receive much attention in the future.

Clinically, skeletal anomalies should be described by their horizontal or vertical components rather than in simple terms, such as "maxillary prognathism" or "Angle Class II malocclusion." These phrases may be adequate to delineate dental relationships, yet they give little clue as to functional skeletal positions. For example, a patient with an Angle Class II malocclusion may have horizontal maxillary excess, horizontal mandibular deficiency, vertical maxillary excess or deficiency, or various combinations of the above. In fact, several studies have noted that patients possessing characteristics of

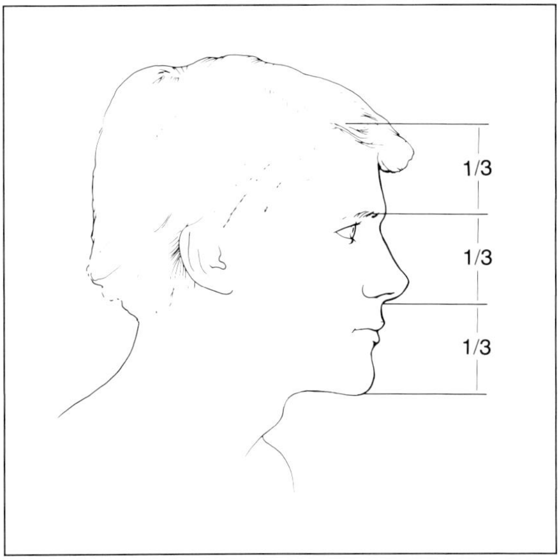

Fig. 26-3 Facial balance, profile view.

an Angle Class II malocclusion are not a homogeneous skeletal sample (Wolford et al., 1978; McNamara, 1981). A study of surgical patients with Class II molar and canine positions noted that the most common skeletal variables found in this group were horizontal maxillary deficiency, vertical maxillary excess, and horizontal mandibular deficiency (Lawrence et al., 1985). Likewise, surgical subjects with a Class III malocclusion have been studied and noted to have combinations of skeletal deformities, the most common of which were horizontal maxillary deficiency, vertical maxillary excess, and horizontal mandibular excess (Ellis and McNamara, 1984). Obviously, a single treatment plan for all individuals with a particular malocclusion would be inadequate.

Timing of orthognathic surgery in growing and nongrowing patients

A child who has had a traumatic injury to the condyles with subsequent lack of growth should be treated as soon as the developmental problem is first noted. Failure to do so will almost certainly result in a severe facial deformity as the rest of the face grows (Fig. 26-4). Likewise, a congenitally missing joint or portion of the mandible should be addressed early in the child's development to allow harmonious facial growth to occur (Fig. 26-5). Gross facial deformities can be corrected at an early age with the realization that secondary procedures may be needed at or near the termination of growth (Fig. 26-6). It is with moderate skeletal deformities that concerns arise as to when and what type of orthodontics should be used, or as to when and if surgery should be performed.

In this regard, it is important to understand the difference between *dental* and *skeletal* corrections of jaw deformities. Orthodontic treatment designed to mask a skeletal deformity by moving teeth is usually contraindicated in a growing child. Flaring maxillary incisions and retracting mandibular incisors in the prepubertal years in a child with a Class III malocclusion will result in a situation in which the teeth interdigitate, but the result may not be esthetically acceptable. The dental relationship would have to be reversed before the skeletal position can be corrected by surgery (Fig. 26-7). Orthodontics in this age group should, in most cases, be designed to keep the teeth structurally aligned to the underlying bone.

When excessive mandibular growth exists, it is usually best to wait until growth has stopped before therapy is begun. However, with deficient growth of the mandible, early intervention may be considered. Functional orthodontic appliances designed to advance the mandible have been shown to stimulate growth of the condyle in growing monkeys (McNamara and Carlson, 1979). Similar appliances have shown a positive influence on *some* growing children (McNamara et al., 1985). Such appliances may help some cases of mandibular deficiency but should be used with caution. Results are not predictable, and, in some patients, their use results only in dentoalveolar changes (Vargervig and Harvold, 1985; Reemer et al., 1985). They also require

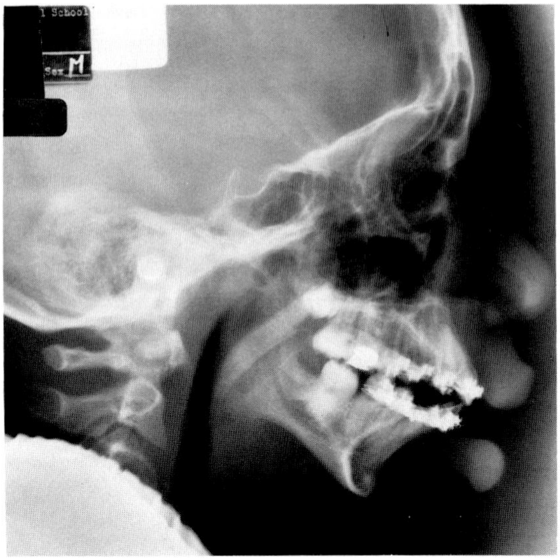

Fig. 26-4 Fourteen-year-old patient who at age 5 had condylar trauma; subsequent growth was restricted.

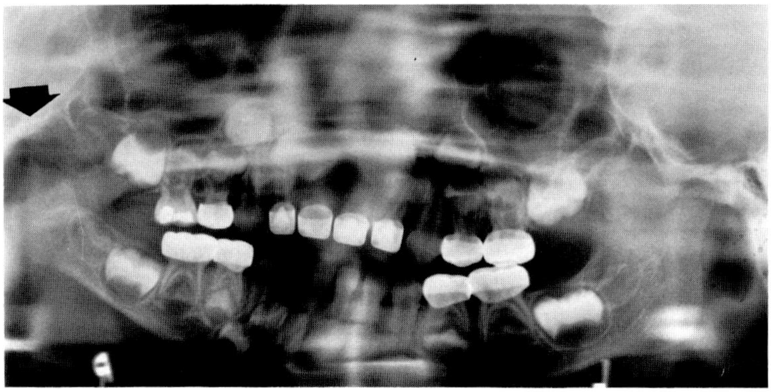

Fig. 26-5 Panorex of 8-year-old child, type 2 hemifacial microsomia. Poorly formed condyle and glenoid fossa *(arrow)*.

good patient cooperation and, to be of any value, must be used at the correct age. Their effectiveness in adults is highly questionable. McNamara (1984b) has shown minimal skeletal and dental adaptations that were insufficient to resolve malocclusions when functional appliances were used in adults.

Traditionally, surgical manipulation of the jaws has been deferred until growth was completed, as it was thought that surgery would have a deleterious effect on the subsequent growth and development of the operated structures. These ideas have been challenged. O'Ryan and Epker (1982) feel that deliberate alteration of the ascending ramus in mandibular deficiency patients with early surgery can positively influence further growth. In contrast, surgical intervention in growing patients with horizontal mandibular excess must be viewed with caution, as late postoperative growth of the mandible will result in unacceptable results (Freihofer, 1977). Advancement of the mandible in growing patients with horizontal mandibular deficiency has yielded harmonious postsurgical skeletal results (O'Ryan and Epker, 1982; Freihofer, 1977; Wolford et al., 1978). Although these results are

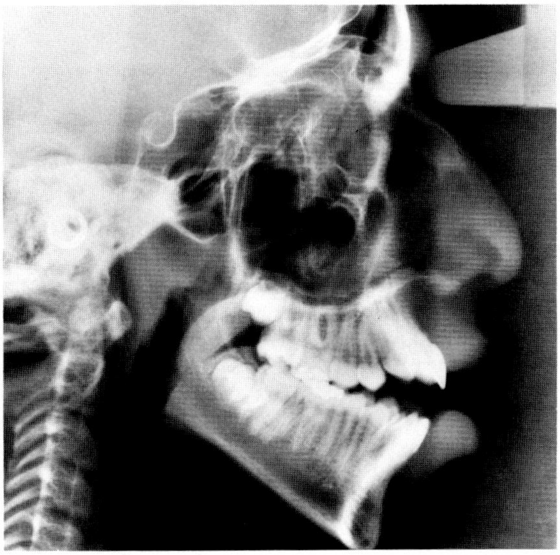

Fig. 26-6 Thirteen-year-old Beckwith-Wiedemann syndrome patient with 10-mm open bite. Patient underwent two surgical jaw corrections with reduction glossectomy.

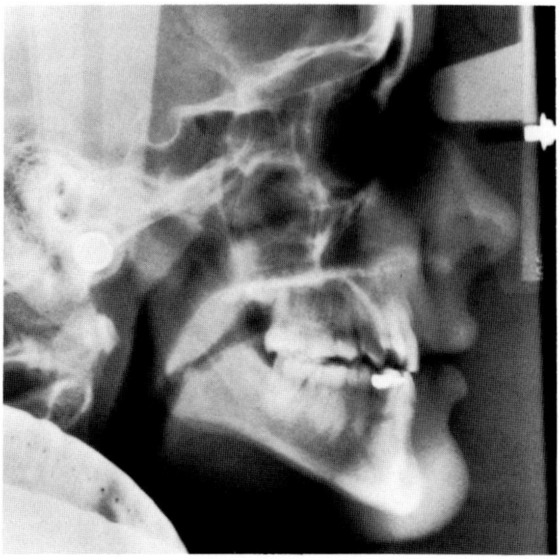

Fig. 26-7 Seventeen-year-old girl who had undergone 5 years of orthodontics starting at age 10 and was unhappy with the final result.

encouraging and certainly discredit the dictum of waiting until growth is completed in the patient with horizontal mandibular deficiency, surgery to the mandible in very young patients should be approached with great caution. It can, however, be a viable option if the child's maturity and social support system are positive factors.

Early surgical intervention in the maxilla is a newer concept. In general, one is limited by dental eruption when operating on growing patients. Epker et al. (1982) reported no significant effect on mandibular growth in sixteen 10- to 16-year-old patients who underwent maxillary impaction for correcting vertical maxillary excess. Nanda et al. (1983) and Nanda and Sugawara (1983) investigated superior anterior surgical repositioning of the maxilla in adolescent monkeys. They found that both the maxillae and mandibles of the experimental monkeys grow harmoniously, although the amount and direction of growth changed when compared with controls.

The timing and sequencing of treatment is less controversial in nongrowing patients. Although patients are frequently treated by an orthodontist and by an oral and maxillofacial surgeon, any number of dental and medical specialists may be involved in therapy. Surgical goals are to create optimal skeletal and esthetic results. The surgeon must work in concert with an orthodontist if orthodontics is involved, or with a prosthodontist/general practitioner if the case involves fixed or removable prostheses.

In most cases, acute operative dentistry and periodontal needs should be managed first. This includes scaling, oral hygiene, and establishing a zone of attached gingiva (Fig. 26-8). Establishing good oral hygiene early in therapy is important in patients undergoing orthodontic and surgical therapy, because the intraoral appliances will make home care more difficult later. Complex restorative or prosthetic dentistry should be deferred until after the surgical and orthodontic management. Temporary restorations are completed to remain in place through the surgical phase. Once these steps have been taken, the sequencing of the orthodontics and surgery is

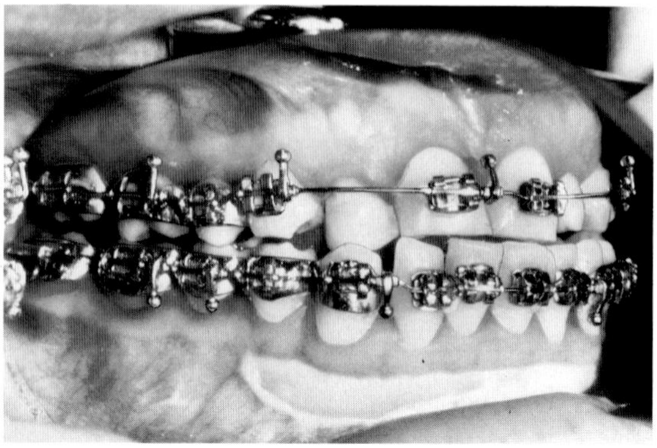

Fig. 26-8 Presurgical patient in whom a gingival graft was placed 1 year prior to this photograph.

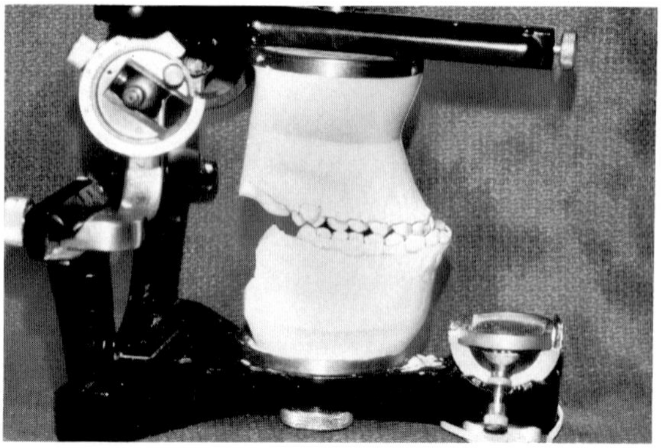

Fig. 26-9 Presurgical casts—trimmed.

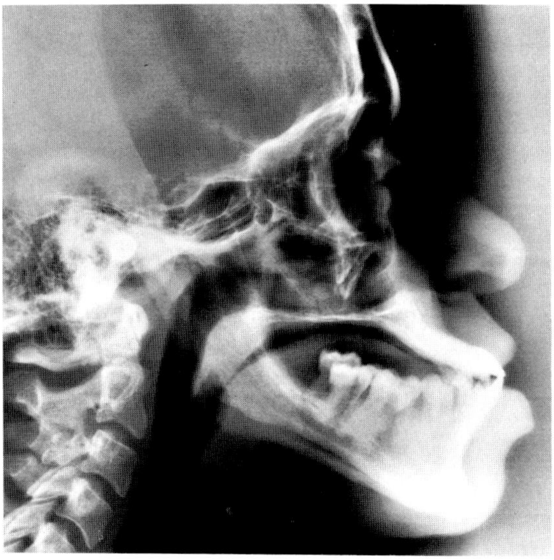

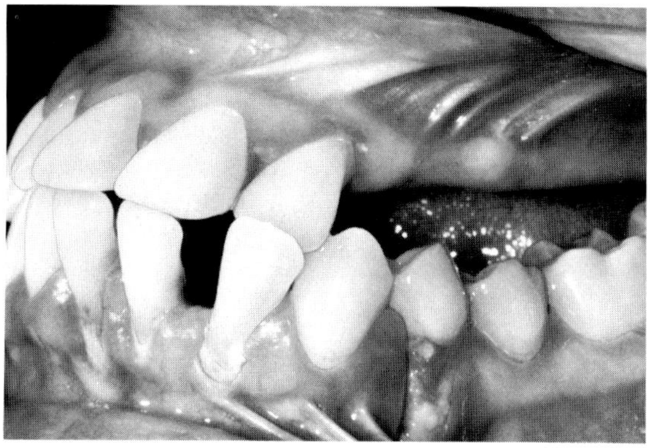

Fig. 26-10a *(left)* Lateral cephalometric radiograph of preprosthetic case.

Fig. 26-10b *(above)* Intraoral photograph. The teeth were maintained until after surgery.

planned. Although each patient is approached on an individual basis, in general presurgical orthodontics is aimed at removing rotations, aligning, and leveling arches. Final detailing of the occlusion is completed after surgery. Orthodontic brackets remain in place during the surgical phase with a variety of attachments that can be used during surgery to interdigitate the teeth as prescribed by the predetermined needs of the case. Sequencing of treatment in this fashion allows improved surgical results by guiding the jaws with orthodontic elastics during the immediate postoperative period. Certain orthodontic procedures may be facilitated postsurgically, when the bony skeleton and surrounding soft tissues are in a more functional relationship.

Approximately 3 weeks after the last arch wire change has been completed, final casts are mounted on a semiadjustable articulator. The casts are anatomically trimmed to simulate the contour of the maxilla (Fig. 26-9). The 3-week time period ensures that no tooth movement will

Figs. 26-11a to d Correction of supererupted maxillary premolars in preparation for orthognathic surgery. (Courtesy of Steven Rhodes, D.D.S.; surgery by Joseph E. Van Sickels, D.D.S.)

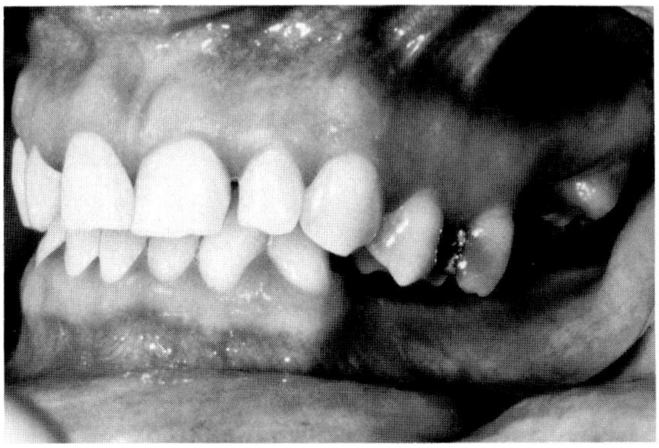

Fig. 26-11a Supererupted maxillary premolars.

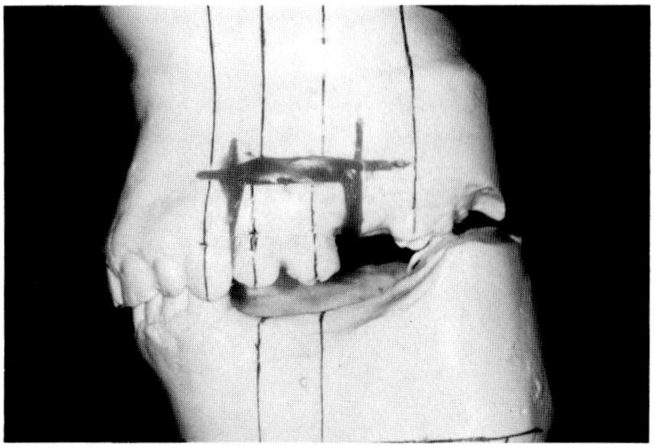

Fig. 26-11b Surgery on mounted casts.

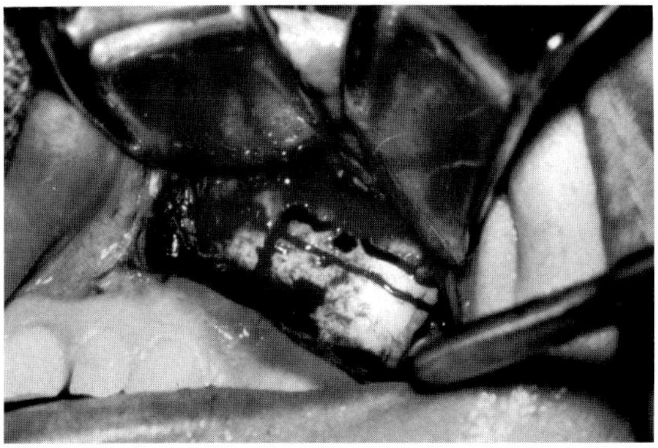

Fig. 26-11c Interoperative photograph.

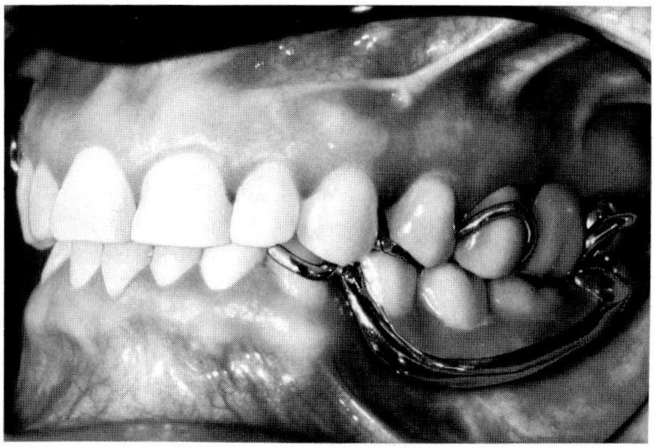

Fig. 26-11d Final prostheses.

occur after the impressions are taken. A final cephalometric radiograph is also obtained in preparation for surgery. Based on the clinical assessment and the radiographic analysis, the surgeon will decide which portion of the skeleton will be moved. The interdigitation of the occlusion should be determined by the orthodontist. If the dental arches do not relate well to one another, or if there are different planes in the occlusion, the maxillary cast can be cut into segments. In preparation for segmental surgery of the maxilla, the orthodontist will have created space between the apices of the teeth. Obviously, the less space there is between teeth, the more likely that injury to the teeth or periodontal structures may occur. When 3 mm or less exists between root apices, there is a greater chance of creating a periodontal defect during an osteotomy.

These same principles and techniques may be applied to preprosthetic cases where skeletal deformities exist. Segments or whole arches may

Figs. 26-12a to d Correction of supererupted mandibular molars in preparation for orthognathic surgery. (Courtesy of Steven Rhodes, D.D.S.; surgery by Joseph E. Van Sickels, D.D.S.)

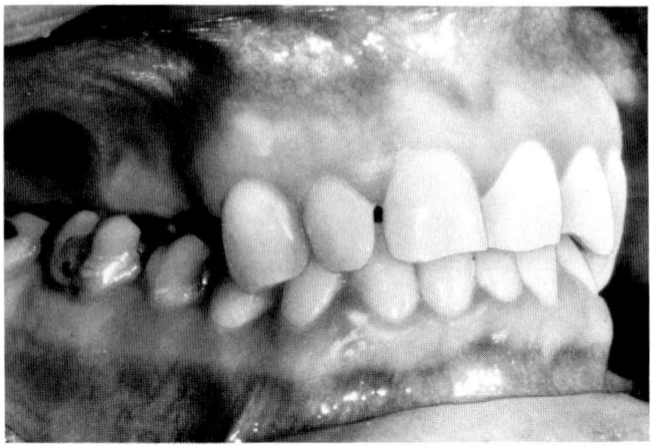

Fig. 26-12a Supererupted mandibular molars.

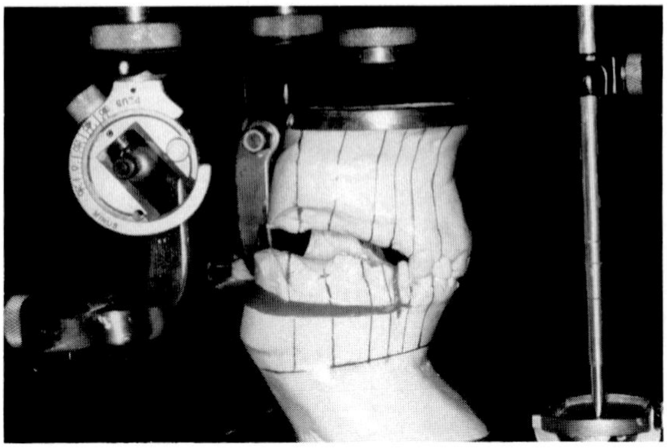

Fig. 26-12b Surgery on mounted casts.

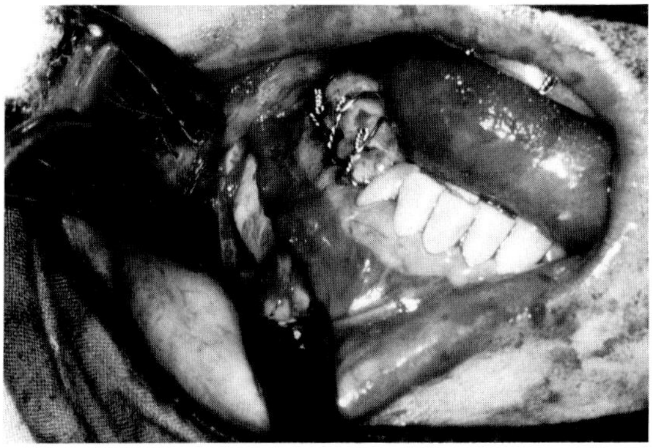

Fig. 26-12c Interoperative photograph.

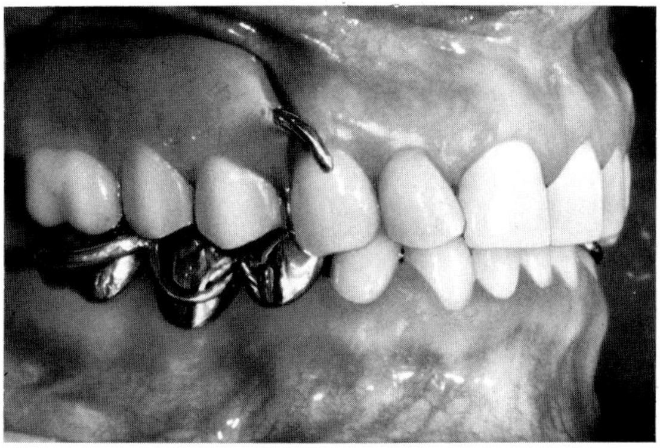

Fig. 26-12d Final prostheses.

be moved in order to improve an occlusal scheme. Here again, preliminary oral hygiene, scaling, and operative dentistry needs should be addressed early in a patient's therapy. Definitive prosthetic or restorative dentistry should be delayed until after the surgical procedure. Following initial therapy, teeth that are candidates for extraction should be noted but not necessarily extracted. Even hopelessly involved teeth are often used during the surgery to stabilize the skeletal movement (Figs. 26-10a and b). In such cases, the arches are set up so that following extraction they will be aligned for prosthetic rehabilitation.

Following unrestored loss of posterior mandibular teeth, the maxillary posteriors may erupt until they are in contact with, or in close proximity to, the mandibular ridge, making construction of a prosthesis impossible. As the erupting teeth generally bring alveolar bone with them, there are several treatment alternatives. Among them are extraction of the teeth with a radical alveoloplasty, or grinding the teeth off to the gingiva with intentional endodontics, followed by the construction of copings for an overdenture. Surgical intrusion of a one- or two-tooth segment, however, preserves the vitality of the teeth and allows more flexibility in the final prosthetic result. The repositioned tooth or teeth may be used for a removable or fixed prosthesis, so the surgeon must discuss the final position of the segment with the prosthodontist or general practitioner. Alignment, both within the maxillary arch and against the opposing mandibular ridge, is an important consideration in the treatment planning for these cases. Occasionally, a space between teeth can be closed, but due to root apices, this is the exception rather than the rule. Most often, one should plan to leave enough space for a pontic as part of a bridge (Figs. 26-11a to d).

A less common situation is eruption of posterior mandibular teeth (Figs. 26-12a to d). Technically, this is a more difficult surgical procedure. The vascular supply is more tenuous, and the inferior alveolar nerve can be injured. Surgical considerations are similar to the previous example, in that alignment must be considered within the mandibular arch as well as against the opposing ridge. Marginal ridges of the teeth next to the osteotomy need to be aligned as much as possible. To establish a good contact, at least one of the teeth next to the osteotomy will usually need a crown.

Although the previous two situations are seen relatively frequently in a typical prosthetic situation, many individual cases may lend themselves to surgical prosthetic procedures. Modern surgical techniques allow many single-tooth or small segmental procedures to be completed as part of an overall prosthodontic treatment plan.

Orthognathic surgical procedures

Many procedures have been designed and continue to be used to reposition the maxilla and mandible. As examined in the preceding sections, although interdigitation of the occlusion is important, achieving an esthetically pleasing result is equally important. Hence, considerable emphasis is placed on the preoperative evaluation in order to move the appropriate jaw(s).

Traditionally, patients underwent surgical procedures coupled with 6 weeks of having their jaws wired together. Bony union was achieved, but oral hygiene was impaired, speech was difficult, weight loss occurred, and mandibles were stiff on opening for a period after the wires were removed.

More recently, several authors have suggested rigid fixation of osteotomized bony segments with a minimal period of having the jaws wired together, in order to increase patient comfort, speech, and bony union, and to decrease relapse (Spiessl, 1976; Jeter et al., 1984). A study comparing rigid and nonrigid fixation of mandibular osteotomies showed that patients having rigid fixation and mild physical therapy showed significantly less reduction in their ability to open than patients undergoing nonrigid fixation with no rehabilitation (Aragon and Van Sickels, 1987).

Several techniques have been developed to move the mandible, either entirely or in segments. Of these, the most popular is the sagittal split osteotomy, which can be used to advance or retrude the mandible. The following cases illustrate its use.

Case 1

A 16-year-old girl was referred from her orthodontist for evaluation of her horizontal mandibular deficiency. The lateral cephalogram showed a deep bite, which was confirmed on clinical examination (Figs. 26-13a and b). An 8-mm advancement was planned for the mandible. Prior to surgery, her orthodontist aligned and leveled her arches. The surgery employed was a bilateral sagittal split osteotomy, with placement of three 2-mm screws on each side. Her jaws were wired shut for 24 hours. At 6 weeks, her orthodontist began changing arch wire to refine the occlusion and finish the case. Two years after surgery, her jaws were stable (Figs. 26-13c and d).

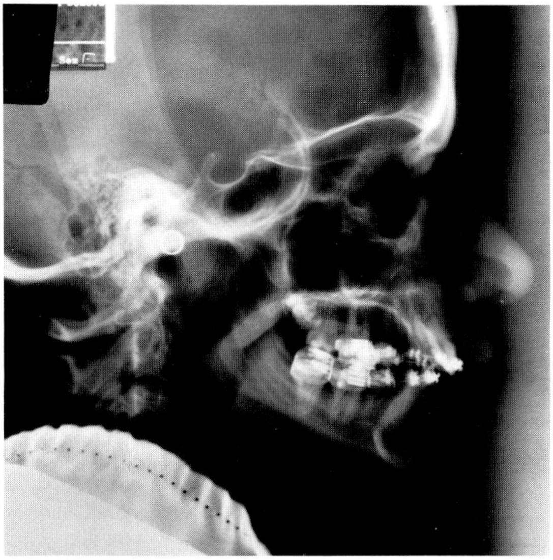

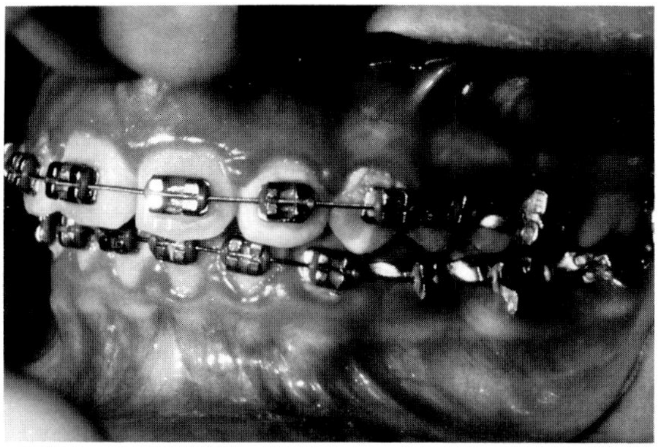

Fig. 26-13a *(left)* Preoperative lateral cephalogram showing horizontal mandibular deficiency in a 16-year-old girl.

Fig. 26-13b *(above)* Preoperative occlusion.

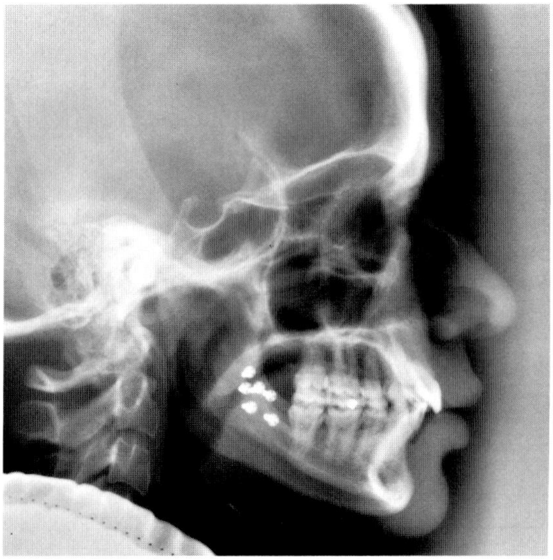

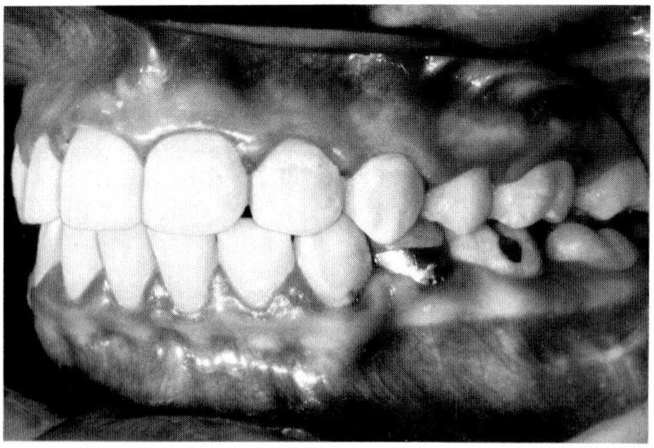

Fig. 26-13c *(left)* Two-year postoperative radiograph.

Fig. 26-13d *(above)* Postoperative occlusion.

Case 2

A 22-year-old graduate student was referred from his orthodontist for evaluation of his horizontal mandibular excess. A component of posterior vertical maxillary excess was noted on his cephalogram and clinical exam; however, due to the minimal maxillary component, a mandibular procedure was judged the treatment of choice. Surgical options included a vertical subcondylar ramus osteotomy, in which the ramus is resected from the sigmoid notch to the inferior portion of the gonial angle, or a sagittal split osteotomy. Bilateral sagittal splits were chosen and the patient was rigidly fixated. His jaws were wired together for 24 hours. He returned to school the following week. Postoperative radiographs show a stable result 1 year after the surgery (Figs. 26-14a and b).

Maxillary deformities may be found in isolation or in combination with other skeletal deformities. The most popular procedure to move the maxilla is the Le Fort I maxillary osteotomy. With it the maxilla can be moved anteriorly, posteriorly, superiorly, or inferiorly, and may be placed in segments. Vascular studies have shown that the periosteal blood supply from the palate will allow the majority of movements needed to achieve an optimal occlusion. Rigid techniques (small plates) have also been used with maxillary osteotomies. Clinically and statistically, maxillary osteotomies have been shown to be more stable when rigidly fixated.

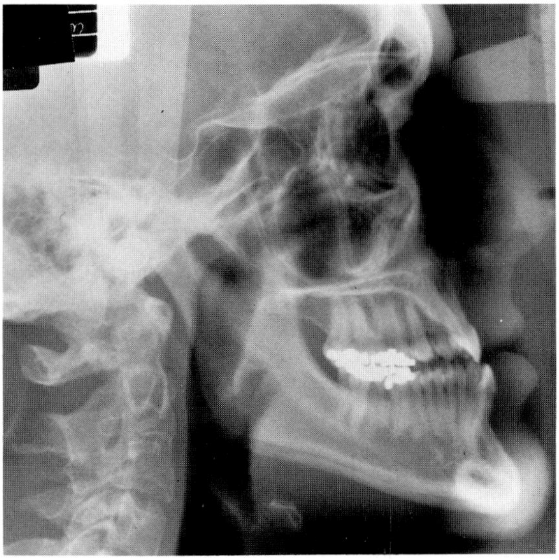

Fig. 26-14a Preoperative radiograph of a 22-year-old man.

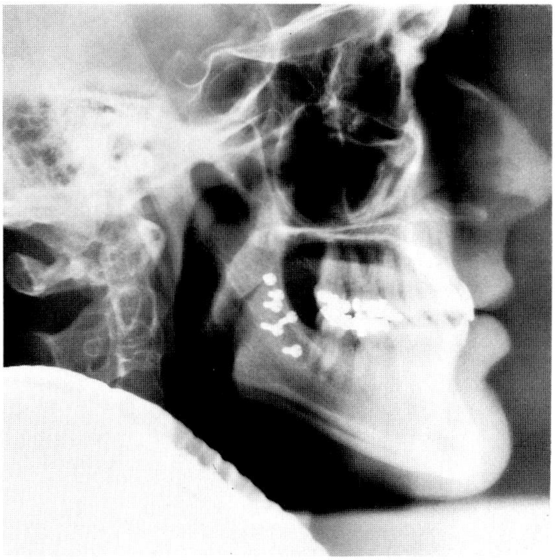

Fig. 26-14b One-year postoperative radiograph.

Case 3

A 16-year-old boy was referred from his orthodontist for evaluation of his maxillary deformity. Clinical and radiographic evaluations revealed horizontal and vertical maxillary excess. Surgery was planned to move his maxilla superiorly 5 mm and posteriorly 5 mm. This was accomplished through a Le Fort I maxillary osteotomy, and his teeth were wired together for 24 hours. Finishing orthodontics was started 4 weeks after his surgery and completed 6 months later (Figs. 26-15a and b).

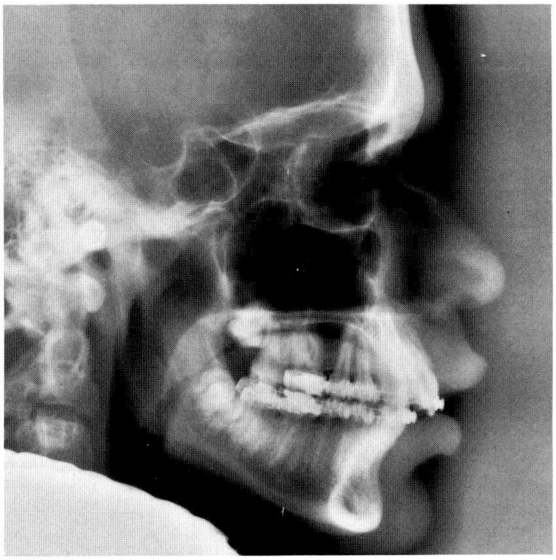

Fig. 26-15a Preoperative radiograph of a 16-year-old boy.

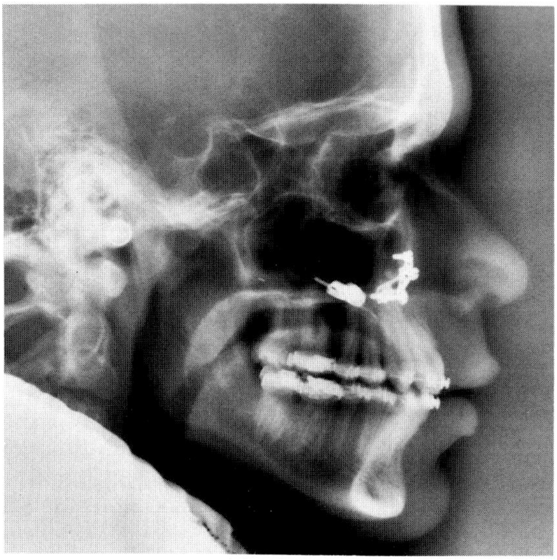

Fig. 26-15b Postoperative radiograph.

Case 4

A 24-year-old woman was referred from her orthodontist for evaluation of her combined skeletal deformity. Clinical and radiographic examinations revealed horizontal and vertical maxillary excess, horizontal mandibular deficiency, and gonial deficiency (Figs. 26-16a to d). Her surgical procedures included a Le Fort I maxillary osteotomy to move her maxilla superiorly and posteriorly, a bilateral sagittal split osteotomy moving her mandible anteriorly, and an augmentation genioplasty further advancing her chin. Total anterior movement of her chin was 14 mm. Two years postoperatively, her results were stable (Figs. 26-16e to h).

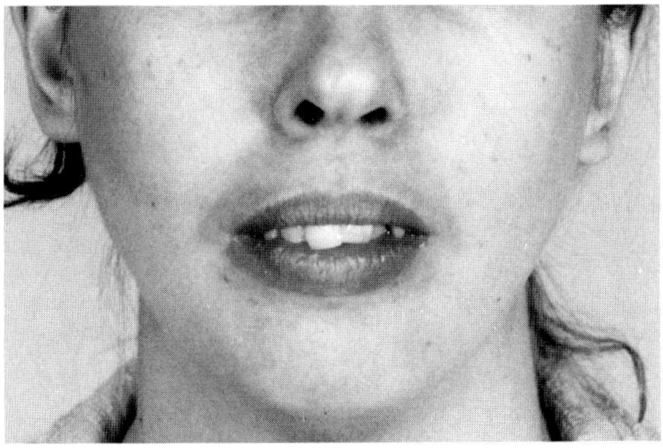

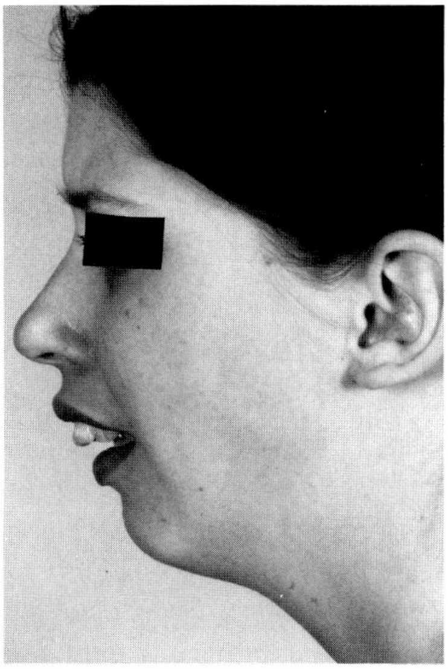

Fig. 26-16a *(above)* Preoperative frontal photograph of a 24-year-old woman.

Fig. 26-16b *(right)* Preoperative profile photograph.

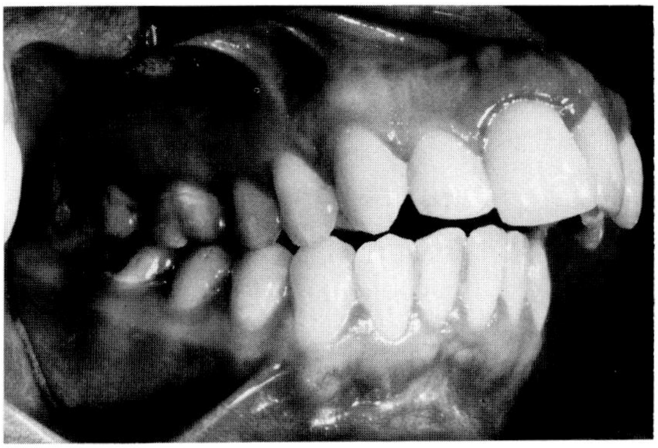

Fig. 26-16c Preoperative occlusion.

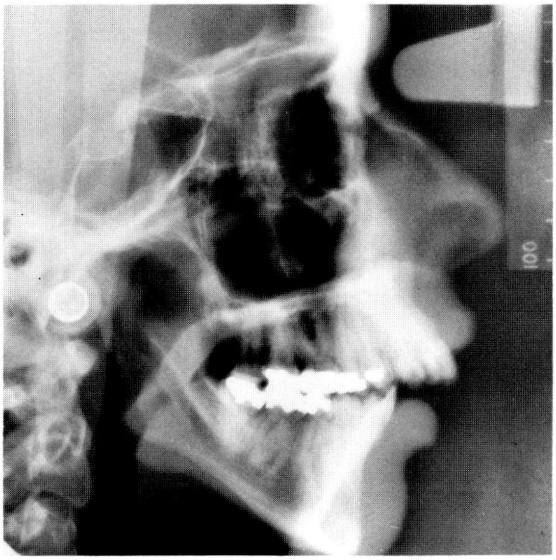

Fig. 26-16d Preoperative lateral cephalogram.

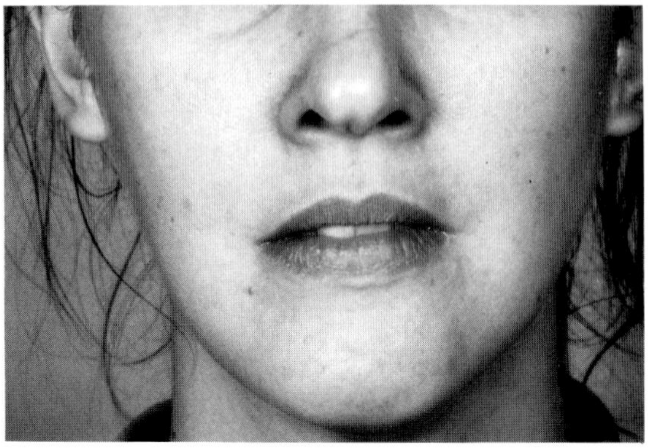

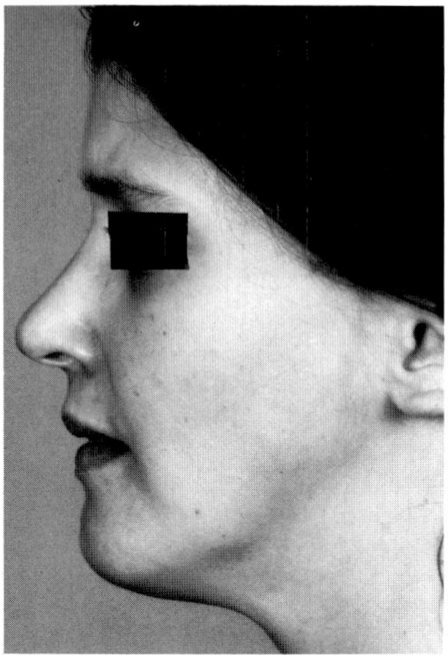

Fig. 26-16e *(above)* One-year postoperative frontal photograph.

Fig. 26-16f *(right)* One-year postoperative lateral photograph.

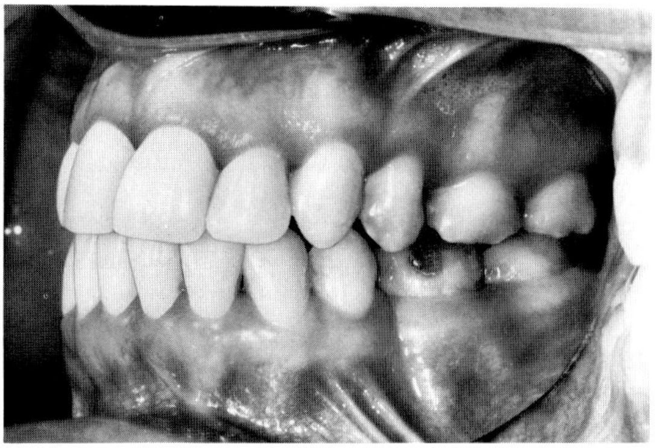

Fig. 26-16g Postoperative occlusion.

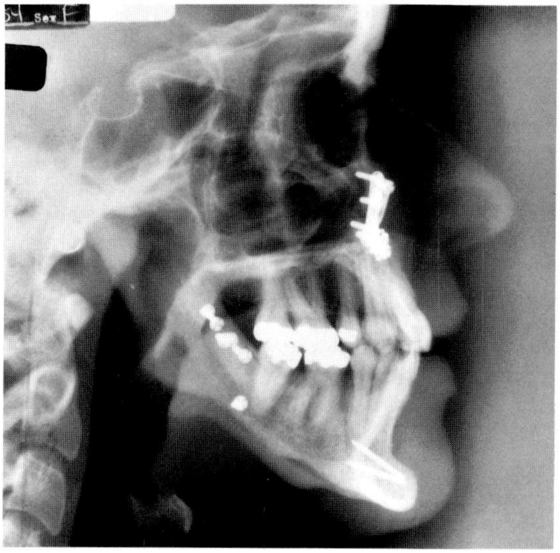

Fig. 26-16h Postoperative lateral cephalogram.

Skeletal disharmonies and temporomandibular disorders

Occlusal disharmony theories suggest a causal relation between malocclusion and temporomandibular joint (TMJ) or masticatory muscle pain and dysfunction. Using this reasoning, one would expect that the worse the malocclusion, the more likely a patient would be to develop a TM disorder. Most studies of patients undergoing orthognathic surgery have not shown an increase in TM disorders over their incidence in general populations; some studies have noted an increase of pretreatment pain and dysfunction symptoms (Laskin et al., 1986). However, centers that treat patients with TM disorders have not noted a malocclusion incidence in their presenting population that exceeds its incidence in the general population (Greene and Marbach, 1982).

These seeming discrepancies may be explained on the basis of the criteria used to categorize a patient with a TM disorder. Much lower percentages of the population are judged to have TM disorders when stringent criteria, rather than every deviation from ideal function, are used for diagnosing clinically significant pain and dysfunction (Gross and Gale, 1983; Greene and Turner, 1983).

This is not to imply that a more ideal occlusion does not help distribute the forces of mastication or occlusal parafunction and secondarily help a patient with a TM disorder. Improvement of TM symptoms in populations undergoing orthognathic surgery have been noted, but for some patients, TM symptoms may worsen or remain unchanged (Timmis et al., 1986). Therefore, surgical therapy for skeletal disharmonies specifically to alleviate the pain or dysfunction associated with TM disorders is not warranted.

Temporomandibular joint problems

Surgical intervention may be indicated or may be the treatment of choice for several types of TM disorders, most especially those of intracapsular origin. These include a wide range of problems, such as neoplasm, developmental anomalies, advanced osteoarthrosis, arthritis, ankylosis, chronic dislocation, and fracture. However, surgery for internal derangements of the articular disk has become the most common procedure involving surgical entry into the TMJ. Issues surrounding the etiology, diagnosis, and management of internal derangements are also intimately related to the subject of Occlusion. Thus, special attention will be given to surgery for internal derangements in this discussion.

Many patients who present with TM disorders have primary muscle problems commonly referred to as myofascial pain-dysfunction. These muscular disorders are generally managed quite well with a variety of reversible *nonsurgical* treatment methods. Other types of TM disorders (e.g., internal derangement of the articular disk) originate primarily *within* the TMJ, and surgery may be indicated.

Successful surgical therapy for this condition requires a coordinated plan between the patient's dentist and the oral and maxillofacial surgeon. The successful treatment of patients with internal derangements initially consists of nonsurgical therapy; experience has shown that most patients benefit from appropriate nonsurgical therapy.

The decision to surgically treat the TMJ is dependent upon documentation of the disk derangement and assurance that it is a major source of the patient's pain and/or dysfunction. The symptoms should be of such magnitude as to constitute a disability to the patient and should have been refractory to appropriate nonsurgical therapy. It should be emphasized that many patients with diagnosed internal derangements may also have a component of myofascial pain-dysfunction, the management of which must be considered in the overall treatment plan.

The criteria for surgical intervention into the TMJ are somewhat subjective, but not so general as to include all patients whose nonsurgical treatment has failed. The primary factor is determining that the pain and/or dysfunction is originating within the joint. This determination is made from the clinical history, physical examination, and, generally, some type of joint imaging. In taking the clinical history, the key factor is that the patient describes the pain as being within or around the joint. The pain usually becomes worse with mandibular function and decreases while at rest. The patient may also report the sensation of catching or locking within the joint.

As for the physical examination, the key factors are joint tenderness to palpation, abnormal joint range of motion, and/or mechanical interferences to smooth movement. Loading the joint as in normal chewing usually produces increased pain. The more specifically the signs and symptoms are localized to the TMJ area, the better the surgical prognosis. Stated in another way, the more diffuse the signs and symptoms, the poorer the surgical prognosis. Various forms of imaging (arthrography, computerized tomography, magnetic resonance imaging) are often used to confirm the presence of joint pathology.

The various surgical techniques include TMJ arthroscopy, disk repositioning with plication, and diskectomy. The specific pathology found within the joint dictates the surgical procedure. The most conservative procedure that will correct the pathology is the preferred method. Final determination of the appropriate procedure is based on inspection of the joint at operation.

The newest and most conservative form of TMJ surgery is arthroscopy. Arthroscopy is the placement of a small telescope (1.7 to 2.7 mm in diameter) into the superior joint space and the observation of the joint structures through this telescope. The procedure is useful as a diagnostic aid, and there is some evidence that it can also be useful as a treatment method. At present, however, the indications for arthroscopy are not clearly defined. The most common arthroscopic procedures are lavage of the superior joint space and lysis of adhesions. Although the results are still unpredictable, early experience is very encouraging.

Open TMJ surgery is most commonly performed through a preauricular incision. The approach to the joint consists of sharp and blunt dissection of the overlying tissues in such a way as to protect important anatomical structures, such as the facial nerve. The most commonly performed TMJ surgery is disk repositioning and plication. In this procedure, the joint proper is entered, the displaced articular disk identified, and the disk repositioned into a more normal position. This is accomplished by removing a wedge of tissue from the posterior attachment of the disk and then suturing the disk back to the posterior attachment tissue. Frequently, the disk is also recontoured. When gross osteoarthrosis is present, the surfaces of the articular eminence and/or condyle are recontoured. The tissues are then closed in layers.

Postsurgically, the patient is instructed to minimize motion of the jaw for the first week or two. After this initial period, the patient is started on an active physical therapy program consisting of vertical, lateral, and protrusive exercises in order to obtain a good range of mandibular movement. The patient is placed on a soft, nonchew diet for approximately 6 weeks. The diet is then gradually broadened, until a normal diet is reached, within 3 to 6 months. Stabilization of the occlusion is important; an interocclusal appliance is indicated if the occlusion does not have even bilateral contacts. The appliance is usually placed 2 to 3 weeks after the surgery and should be adjusted to the patient's existing habitual occlusion. In other words, no mandibular repositioning, either posteriorly or anteriorly, should be attempted. Final correction of the occlusion should not be completed less than 6 months postsurgically.

In general, the results of this procedure have been good, with 85% to 90% of the operated patients having less pain and improved jaw function. Approximately 50% of the operated patients are totally pain-free postsurgically.

Complications following TMJ surgery are uncommon. About 1% to 5% of operated patients will have temporary facial nerve weakness, usually involving the temporal branch. Other branches may also be involved, and occasionally the weakness may be permanent. Most patients will have minor changes in their occlusion postoperatively, but these can be corrected with occlusal adjustment. All patients will have temporary anesthesia of the preauricular skin. This anesthesia disappears in about 6 weeks to 6 months.

Severe complications are rare and occur more often after complete removal of the disk (diskectomy). The most common complication is fibrous ankylosis of the operated joint, resulting in restricted mandibular movement. Major malocclusion may also occasionally occur as a result of condylar resorption.

The clinician who manages patients with TM disorders is obligated to know which conditions and circumstances may or may not benefit from surgery. Any potential benefit must be related to *(1)* the chronicity and severity of the symptoms, or disability that the patient is experiencing; *(2)* the relative effectiveness of past treatment; *(3)* possible surgical risk factors; and *(4)* the risk/benefit and cost/benefit ratios of possible alternate therapies. The reader is encouraged to consult current texts on surgical therapy of the TMJ.

Summary

Surgical procedures in use today can correct virtually any orthognathic deformity a patient may have. A systematic examination and a treatment plan derived from a complete data base are essential to determining the proper treatment for a patient. Coordination of treatment between practitioners is equally important. Optimal occlusal form and function, as well as acceptable esthetics, remain the goals of this surgical therapy.

Patients may present with both skeletal deformities and TM disorders. Although improvement in pain-dysfunction symptoms has been noted in populations undergoing orthognathic surgery, for some patients TM symptoms may worsen or remain unchanged.

Temporomandibular disorders may present in isolation or in combination with other problems. Successful surgical therapy stresses an accurate diagnosis of the problem and a coordinated plan between the patient's dentist, oral and maxillofacial surgeon, and any other health care providers involved in the patient's management.

Chapter 27

Occlusion and Temporomandibular Disorders: A Prologue

George A. Zarb and Norman D. Mohl

In *The Lives of a Cell,* Lewis Thomas (1974) wrote:

> It has been our perpetual habit to try anything, on the slimmest of chances, the thinnest of hopes, empirically and wishfully, and we have proved to ourselves over and over again that the approach doesn't work well. Bleeding, cupping and purging are the classical illustrations, but we have plenty of more recent examples to be embarrassed about. We have been hoaxed along by comparable substitutes for technology right up to the present. There is no question about our good intentions in this matter; we all hanker, collectively, to become applied scientists as soon as we can, overnight if possible.

Dr. Thomas' observations about the planning of science are provocative ones because they deal with principles that apply to all health disciplines. The entire discipline of Dentistry, including Occlusion, has been firmly rooted in empiricism. This was inevitable because the realities of clinical practice demanded that dentists not wait for objective evidence about etiology and efficacy of treatment. Dentists were obliged to respond to the injuries, diseases, or symptoms that afflicted their patients, frequently achieving varying degrees of success. Unfortunately, however gratifying it may be to patient and clinician, clinical success is not necessarily scientific proof of cause and effect. Hence the need for treating our subject both as a developing science as well as an art.

In preceding chapters we sought to articulate our contention that the subject of Occlusion does have a biological basis, and that the scientific method can and should be applied to its study (see Preface). We hope that we have succeeded in this objective and have provided the reader with more enlightened insights into unresolved issues, even if we frequently resorted to justifying our hypotheses, conclusions, or treatment methods with the inevitable "clinical experience suggests. . . ." It must be remembered that Occlusion is a very young science, and its pursuit as such does not preclude the virtues of keen clinical observation and experience. However, by the same token, any health discipline that does not constantly question standards and methods derived from clinical observations alone usurps its claim to scientific advancement.

In chapter 13 we identified a conceptual framework for describing occlusion. It comprised four categories: *(1)* theoretically ideal, *(2)* physiologic, *(3)* nonphysiologic, and *(4)* therapeutic occlusion. A theoretically ideal occlusion is probably infrequently encountered, given the enormous range of definitional or descriptive possibilities resulting from genetic influences. However, we pointed out that in the absence of normative data, a theoretically ideal occlusion is clinically useful in order to identify a yardstick of idealized parameters against which variations may be compared.

A physiologic occlusion, on the other hand, is one that represents a state of harmony or adaptation and does not require therapeutic intervention. It is therefore free of pathological manifestations or dysfunctional problems. It is esthetically satisfactory to the patient. This can even occur in the presence of some missing teeth and/or a malocclusion, but in such situations the patient would have adapted to the particular morphologic variation.

What is particularly challenging about Occlusion as a clinical discipline is the dentist's ability to prognosticate whether asymptomatic structural and/or functional modifications associated with a physiologic occlusion could indeed render the individual's masticatory system more vulnerable in the context of time, or a particular event, such as a macrotraumatic incident (e.g., sudden loss of teeth) or a microtraumatic incident (e.g., episodic bruxing). It is more logical for a dentist to prescribe treatment for a patient whose partial edentulism or malocclusion are accompanied by subtle or overt signs and symptoms of dysfunction. The patient's occlusion in such a situation is readily diagnosed as a nonphysiologic one. Nonadaptation is the dominant feature, and it manifests itself as a spectrum of complaints from problems with speech articulation to masticatory dysfunction, from occlusally related esthetic concerns to pain and discomfort. Various clinical initiatives and prescriptions are available to convert a nonphysiologic occlusion into a therapeutic one. A therapeutic occlusion should now behave as predictably as a physiologic one, but several unanswered questions linger and must be articulated:

1. Is there enough compelling longitudinal information to justify our concept of physiologic occlusion, which includes a broad range of morphologic and functional adaptations?
2. Are the normative data for physiologic occlusions in adults with some missing teeth and/or malocclusion adequate to justify nonintervention?
3. Is it possible that signs and symptoms of a nonphysiologic occlusion are only interim ones that will be adjusted to over time?
4. Is a therapeutic occlusion as trouble-free, in a long-term context, as a physiologic one?
5. If a therapeutic occlusion is achieved (e.g., all missing posterior teeth are replaced), is the efficacy of the dental treatment matched or diminished by the risk of the treatment itself (e.g., the risk of caries or periodontal disease resulting from some prosthetic procedures)?

We consider these concerns to be compelling ones and expect that reasoned debate and research will provide answers in the near future.

Had we considered the subject of Occlusion in a narrow mechanical context, a "how-to" handbook would have replaced this text. We would have started with a premise that 28 to 32 teeth should occupy a specific orientation and relationship and gone on to presume that numerical, positional, or structural departures from this "norm" would lead to adverse consequences. We then would have sought to synthesize technical information and methods mainly from the disciplines of orthodontics, periodontics, operative dentistry, and prosthodontics. With the help of jaw tracking devices, articulators, and modern restorative materials we would have provided blueprints for the maintenance and restoration of depleted dentitions. However, the work of several colleagues in recent years has underscored the significance of the observation that it is not only the structural components of the masticatory system that count, but above all it is the way a patient adapts to his or her occlusion that is important. In other words, it is incorrect to assume that the occlusion is something fixed and solid, like a gearbox.

Behavior (what a patient does to, or with, an occlusion) plays an important role in the overall clinical understanding and treatment of occlusion. This notion must be regarded as a seminal concept in this field's scientific development. Figure 27-1 shows an attempt to reconcile the two faces—functional and structural—of occlusally related disorders. Like two sides of a coin they can be looked at separately, but the reader must remember that they comprise integral parts of the same clinical currency.

In various chapters we have referred to the clinically observed close relationship that may appear to exist between occlusion and TM disor-

A **B**

Structural or morphologic factors ± Functional factors

May lead to the development of a

Nonphysiologic occlusion

⇓

Patients may present with either A or B predominating, or an ill-defined mixture of A and B.

General treatment sequence should include:

1. Symptomatic therapy (reduction of pain/discomfort)
2. Control of contributory factors
3. Treatment of pathologic sequelae
4. Maintenance of restored state of adaptation

This sequence is prescribed irrespective of the precise cause of the problem. Possible causes:

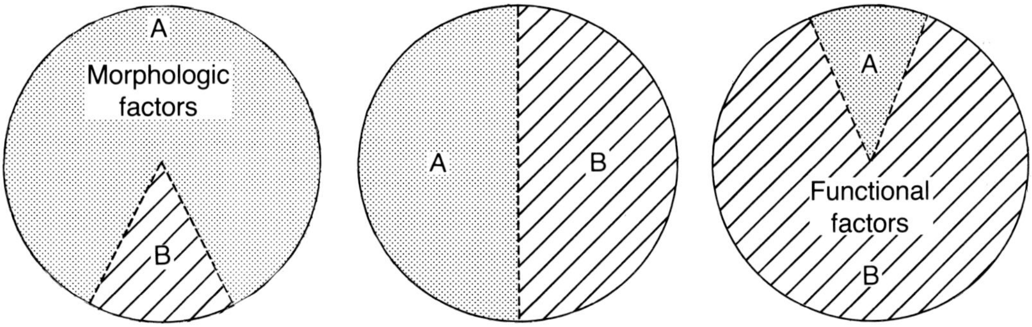

Specific therapy

• Explanation and advice • Range of dental methods	• Explanation and advice • Limited use of irreversible dental methods • Reversible dental methods (e.g., interocclusal appliance therapy)	• Explanation and advice • Nondental methods • Reversible dental methods

Fig. 27-1 Treatment principles based upon relative roles of structural and functional factors.

ders. This relationship is complex and incompletely understood. It has led to polarized views, although the view that occlusion is intimately involved in a cause-and-effect relationship with TM disorders has tended to dominate clinical dental thinking in the past quarter century.

Our interpretation of the current scientific literature precludes belief that structural or positional occlusal factors precipitate parafunctional activity such as bruxism. We do feel, however, that evidence exists to support the notion that bruxism can bring about pains, impaired function, and structural changes in diverse components of the masticatory system. Consequently, we readily concede that a section on TM disorders does not really belong in an Occlusion text. However, we feel that the readers may find a brief and general review of TM disorders to be quite germane. This should enhance the readers' appreciation of the fascinating range of research acitivites that the areas of occlusal and TM disorders offer.

Temporomandibular disorders

The prevalence of TM disorders in humans has not been accurately measured and remains unknown. Although complaints or observations of facial pain, altered patterns of mandibular movement, and joint noise (crepitus or clicking) are cited by several authors as being prevalent, the idea that such disorders are a quasiuniversal disease, perhaps on a par with caries and periodontal disease, is certainly not correct. Temporomandibular disorders include several etiologic features, some of which frequently overlap, but most of the disorders present with similar signs and symptoms. Clearly, some behave differently from others, and some are more significant than others with regard to endangering masticatory function. Published epidemiological studies tend not to be impressive, mainly because diverse forms of TM disorders have been pooled. Consequently these reports are not meaningful in determining the true risk to the masticatory system in a given population.

There is very little agreement as to what causes a TM disorder. False causal relationships are not uncommon and unproven theories abound. A convenient way of looking at proposed etiologies lists them in chronologic order.

Mechanical displacement theory

In 1925, Decker attributed unexplained deafness to lack of occlusal support. Nearly 10 years later, Costen (1934) added pain to the syndrome. He stressed the idea that distal condylar displacement following loss of posterior teeth led to condylar impingement on the auriculotemporal nerve or direct pressure on ear structures and the eustachian tube. Several authors (Sicher, 1948; Zimmerman, 1951; Schwartz, 1959; Steger et al., 1974) have clearly demonstrated that the anatomic basis of Costen's syndrome is not acceptable. Nonetheless, the concept of mandibular overclosure as a factor in causing symptoms of a TM disorder has persisted, and it remains the only dentally related syndrome listed in the *Dictionary of Medical Syndromes* (1981).

Several clinicians have extended the idea of distal mechanical displacement of the condyle to include both frontal and sagittal changes in condylar position (Gerber, 1971; Weinberg, 1973; Kundert and Palla, 1977). The mechanical displacement concept is based on two hypotheses. The first states that a normal condyle-fossa relationship exists in a static habitual occlusal position. This relationship can be altered by loss of molars and premolars, insufficient number of opposing posterior tooth contacts, premature tooth contacts with deviations and/or rotations of the mandible, and nonworking side occlusal interferences. The resulting disharmony between condylar position and the occlusion leads to adverse muscle activity directly on the TMJ.

The second hypothesis is that it is possible to radiographically determine a patient's individual optimal condylar position. This claim has proven to be scientifically elusive in spite of several anecdotal reports. Blaschke and Blaschke (1981) and Pullinger et al. (1985) have demonstrated that, in asymptomatic patients, the condyle-temporal bone spatial relationships show widely varying positions of the condyles within their respective fossae when the teeth are in centric occlusion.

The mechanical displacement theory remains an unproven one. Its development reflected the dominant role enjoyed by gross anatomy as the first basic science to exert a profound influence on clinical dentistry. The advent of neurophysiological dental research from the late 1950s on has tended to eclipse the observations of gross anatomists' extrapolations from their dissections to clinical practice. As a result, newer theories introduced since the 1960s have emphasized the role of the musculature more emphatically.

The neuromuscular theory

The contributory role of mandibular displacement is subtler in this theory's conceptual framework. Hence, any type of occlusal interference can cause parafunctional activity such as grinding or clenching. However, a background of psychic tension, stress, or anxiety is a required adjunctive factor. This theory recognizes the idea that it is not possible to deny the influence of the occlusion on functional remodeling of the TMJs (Carlsson and Öberg, 1974; Bjorn, 1974; Blackwood, 1963; Moffett et al., 1964). It also recognizes the variable influence of occlusion on masticatory muscle behavior (Ramfjord, 1961b; Krogh-Poulsen and Olsson, 1968; Hannam, 1984). Nonetheless, a compelling cause-and-effect relationship has not yet been demonstrated in spite of the immense popularity of this theory among dentists.

Even the claim that muscle spasms result from occlusal abnormalities remains a controversial one. For example, Yemm (1971a, 1971b) could not find electromyographically determined evidence of abnormal muscle activity even though the muscles he examined had been diagnosed by clinicians as being tender and "in spasm." These tender muscles are recognized as "hot spots" (Berry and Yemm, 1974) and may be caused by areas of small hemorrhages or torn fibers. Christensen (1971) identified such areas of muscle tenderness following voluntary tooth clenching in human volunteers as evidence of an increase in intramuscular tissue fluid following hyperactivity. This theory cannot explain why a TM disorder can occur in one patient and not in another, even with more severe presence of occlusal discrepancies and/or bruxism.

Current interpretation of published research in this area has led to a more conservative approach to occlusal therapy. The American Dental Association's "Report of the President's Conference on the Examination, Diagnosis, and Management of Temporomandibular Disorders" (Griffiths, 1983) stresses the importance of limited and reversible forms of therapy and underscores the need for scientific testing of any treatment modality. The report emphasizes that occlusal adjustment and permanent occlusal appliances are treatments for which there is no supporting evidence. Because both these treatment modalities are a proposed, integral part of the neuromuscular theory, the reader should recognize the profound implications of the report on the ongoing significance of this theory.

The muscle theory

The muscle theory claims that the primary etiologic factor lies in the muscles of mastication themselves. Kraus (1963) described a "hypokinetic" disease, which he attributed to the imbalance between a lack of adequate muscle exercise and overstimulation of daily life in this century. He identifies a TM disorder as only one such disease that can involve the jaw, head, and neck. He claims that under stress, the muscles of the jaw never relax; therefore, tension will increase until a painful spasm occurs. These patients manifest general muscle response in addition to specific ones (Schwartz, 1959).

A broader interpretation of this theory holds that such stress-induced muscle hyperactivity may be selective, with the gut as a "target" organ; or else the bronchioles, the skin, or cerebral vessels may be involved with appropriate symptoms following. It then becomes reasonable to assume that actual damage to muscle structure can occur if feeble and untrained muscles are required to sustain contracted episodes.

Bell (1969) expanded the theory further when he claimed that disruption of normal masticatory function could result from spasm associated with yawning, uncoordinated movements, acute illness, somatic and visceral pain, etc.

Travell (1960) proposed that the elicited pain in such muscles in spasm acts as a trigger point and follows a pattern of referral to a variety of other sites. In this theory many of the encountered TM disorders are not even remotely related to dental occlusion problems.

The psychophysiological theory

The psychophysiological theory has been supported by a large body of interesting research and speculation by several authors, notably Franks (1964), Laskin (1969), Greene and Laskin (1972), and Molin et al. (1973). It supports an opposite opinion to the one proposed in the neuromuscular theory; that is, it maintains that emotional disturbances lead to grinding of teeth which in turn may lead to occlusal interferences. These interferences may then act as sustaining factors. It has certainly been demonstrated that hyperactivity can be centrally initiated and provoked by everyday psychological and social difficulties (Yemm, 1979). Furthermore, support for this theory also comes from some experimental and clinical evidence that demonstrates that patients can benefit from reassurance (Franks, 1964), counseling (Greene and Laskin, 1974), and placebo drugs and splints.

Recent research in psychogenic facial pain (Feinmann and Harris, 1984) increases the dentist's awareness that stress or emotional illness can cause pain. Because dentists often have little or no training in, or knowledge of, psychology or psychiatry, they are unlikely to be familiar with the administration of antidepressants that have well-proven value in the control of pain. Although it has been reported that many patients respond favorably to counseling and a placebo, the report of Feinmann and Harris demonstrates that under strictly controlled conditions, significantly more pain patients, including a substantial nonpsychiatric group, respond to an antidepressant without structural occlusal therapy.

Summary

All of these theories have a hypothetical basis and do not necessarily reflect any clinical significance. However, one recurrent component is evident in each of the theories: *our masticatory system and its occlusion may be made to perform excessive or redundant work.* If hyperactivity or parafunction is initiated (irrespective of the source of the catalyst—central, peripheral, or both), the common denominator of expression is muscle overwork. In turn this may lead to muscle fatigue and/or adverse stresses in teeth, TMJ, or other tissues. This may be a temporary or intermittent event that may lead to adaptation or to mild clinical symptom development. It may also be asymptomatic but may "stretch" or weaken the system so that if the parafunctional event recurs, or else a macrotraumatic episode is sustained, adaptation is no longer possible, and overt clinical symptoms develop. The hyperactivity may be a sustained one so that an escalating degree of tissue injury may develop. In this context a prescribed therapeutic occlusion may very well restore structural defects, but ongoing symptoms may not be completely resolved. A state of chronic pain has then been reached by the patient, and treatment strategies will differ profoundly from those routinely prescribed for occlusal or TM disorders.

Zarb and Carlsson (1979) wrote:

> It appears that mandibular dysfunction is a musculoskeletal disorder which involves tissue injury. The cause of the injury may be of a macro- or a micro-nature, or both, and the resulting lesions may be expressed through inflammatory, proliferative and degenerative tissue changes. Furthermore, the effects of the dysfunction often outlive the precipitating cause, with frequent development of chronic pain or discomfort. The dysfunction also in-

volves a psychological response which is distinct but inseparable from the structural response, with an implied need for clinicians and researchers to see mandibular dysfunction in the context of a vicious circle of aetiological factors, with overlapping at both the symptom description and treatment levels.

Treatment strategies have expanded from the dental occlusal reconstructive effort to the use of drugs, electrical stimulation, biofeedback, hypnosis, acupuncture and psychological help. These "modern" alternatives have long histories. Acupuncture is ancient, electric eels have been used for pain control, and psychological help has always been a major tool of witch doctor and faith healer.

The results of these approaches have often conflicted, and although vigorous debate has led to improved management of dysfunction, knowledge of the mechanism and its treatment still leave a lot to be desired. It remains clear that facial pain, TM disorders, and occlusal dysfunction are still areas requiring extensive research endeavors, with the precise role of occlusion in maintaining a healthy masticatory system remaining a fascinating, if incompletely explained, problem.

With the help of our contributors we have arrived at a comprehensive review of intelligently interpreted research in the field of Occlusion. We recognize the inevitable limitations of this endeavor since we share Mapother's aphorism: "Cured by any therapy are those who: never had the disease; still have it; never had the treatment; or would have recovered without it."

References

Abe, K., and Shimakawa, M. Genetic and developmental aspects of sleep-talking and teeth-grinding. Acta Paedopsych. 33:339–344, 1966.

Academy of Denture Prosthetics. Glossary of Prosthodontic Terms. 4th ed. St. Louis: C.V. Mosby Co., 1977.

Adesso, V.J., Vargas, J.M., and Siddall, J.W. The role of awareness in reducing nail-biting behavior. Behavior Therapy 10:148–154, 1979.

Agerberg, G. Maximal mandibular movements in young men and women. Swed. Dent. J. 67:81–100, 1974.

Agerberg, G., and Carlsson, G.E. Functional disorders of the masticatory system. II. Symptoms in relation to impaired mobility of the mandible as judged from investigations by questionnaire. Acta Odontol. Scand. 31:335–347, 1973.

Agerberg, G., and Carlsson, G.E. Late results of treatment of functional disorders of the masticatory system. J. Oral Rehabil. 1:309–316, 1974.

Agerberg, G., and Carlsson, G.E. Symptoms of functional disturbances of the masticatory system. A comparison of frequencies in a population sample and in a group of patients. Acta Odontol. Scand. 33:183–190, 1975.

Agerberg, G., and Carlsson, G.E. Chewing ability in relation to dental and general health. Analyses of data obtained from a questionnaire. Acta Odontol. Scand. 39:147–153, 1981.

Ahlgren, J. Mechanisms of mastication. Acta Odontol. Scand. 24 (Suppl. 44):1–109, 1966.

Ahlgren, J. The silent period in the EMG of the jaw muscles during mastication and its relationship to tooth contact. Acta Odontol. Scand. 27:219–227, 1969.

Ahlgren, J., Omnell, K. A., Sonesson, B., and Toremalm, N.G. Bruxism and muscle hypertrophy of the masseter muscle. Pract. Otorhinolaryngol. 31:22–29, 1969.

Alling, C., and Mahan, P.E. (eds.) Facial Pain. 2nd ed. Philadelphia: Lea & Febiger, 1977.

American Association of Dental Schools. Curricular Guidelines in Occlusion. J. Dent. Ed. 47:561–565, 1983.

American Dental Association Council on Dental Care Programs. Providing benefits for diagnosis and treatment of temporomandibular joint (TMJ) disorders under prepayment programs. Chicago: American Dental Association, May, 1982.

American Dental Association Council on Dental Education. Dental Education in the United States: 1976. Chicago: American Dental Association, 1976.

Anderson, D.J. Periodontal sensory mechanisms. pp. 345–361 *In* A.H. Melcher and W.H. Bowen (eds.) Biology of the Periodontium. New York: Academic Press, 1969.

Anderson, D.J., and Picton, D.C.A. Masticatory stresses in normal and modified occlusion. J. Dent. Res. 37:312–317, 1958.

Angle, E.H. Treatment of Malocclusion of the Teeth and Fractures of the Maxillae: Angle's System. 6th ed. Philadelphia: S.S. White Dental Manufacturing Co., 1900, pp. 37–40.

Angel, J.L. Factors in temporomandibular joint form. Am. J. Anat. 83:223–246, 1948.

Appenteng, K., Lund, J.P., and Séguin, J.J. Behaviour of cutaneous mechanoreceptors recorded in mandibular division of Gasserian ganglion of the rabbit during movements of lower jaw. J. Neurophysiol. 47:151–166, 1982a.

Appenteng, K., Lund, J.P., and Séguin, J.J. Intraoral mechanoreceptor activity during jaw movement in the anesthetized rabbit. J. Neurophysiol. 48:27–37, 1982b.

Aragon, S.B., and Van Sickels, J.E. Mandibular range of motion with rigid/nonrigid fixation. Oral Surg. Oral Med. Oral Pathol. 63:408–411, 1987.

Ashcroft, G.W., Eccleston, D., and Waddell, J.L. Recognition of amphetamine addicts. Br. Med. J. 1:57, 1965.

Atkinson, H.F., and Shepherd, R.W. Masticatory movements and the resulting force. Arch. Oral Biol. 12:195–202, 1967.

Ayer, W.A. Thumb-finger sucking and bruxing habits in children. pp. 7–22 *In* P. Bryant, E. Gale, and J. Rugh (eds.) Oral Motor Behavior: Impact on Oral Conditions and Dental Treatment. NIH Publication no. 79-1845. Washington, D.C.: U.S. Government Printing Office, 1979.

Ayer, W.A., and Levin, M.P. Theoretical basis and application of massed practice exercises for the elimination of tooth grinding habits. J. Periodontol. 46:306–308, 1975.

Bailey, J.O., Jr., and Rugh, J.D. Effect of occlusal adjustment on bruxism as monitored by nocturnal EMG recordings. J. Dent. Res. 59 (Special Issue A):317, 1980.

Bailey, J.O., Jr., McCall, W.D., Jr., and Ash, M.M., Jr. The influence of mechanical input parameters on the duration of the mandibular joint electromyographic silent period in man. Arch. Oral Biol. 22:619–623, 1977.

Bandura, A. Principles of Behavior Modification. New York: Holt, Rinehart, and Winston, 1969.

Barbenel, J.C. Analysis of forces at the temporomandibular joint during function. Dent. Pract. 19:305–310, 1969.

Barghusen, H.R., and Hopson, J.A. The endoskelton: the

comparative anatomy of the skull and the visceral skelton. pp. 265–326 *In* M.H. Wake (ed.) Hyman's Comparative Vertebrate Anatomy. 3rd ed. Chicago: The University of Chicago Press, 1979.

Basmajian, J. Muscles Alive. 3rd ed. Baltimore: Williams & Wilkins Co., 1974.

Bates, J.F., Stafford, G.O., and Harrison, A. Masticatory function—a review of the literature. I. The form of the masticatory cycle. J. Oral Rehabil. 2:281–301, 1975a.

Bates, J.F., Stafford, G.O., and Harrison, A. Masticatory function—a review of the literature. II. Speed of movement of the mandible, rate of chewing and forces developed in chewing. J. Oral Rehabil. 2:349–361, 1975b.

Bates, J.F., Stafford, G.O., and Harrison, A. Masticatory function—a review of the literature. III. Masticatory performance and efficiency. J. Oral Rehabil. 3:57–67, 1976.

Battistuzzi, P. Het gemutileerde gebit. (The mutilated dentition. A descriptive epidemiologic study.) Thesis. The Netherlands: University of Nijmegen, 1982.

Baume, L.J. Physiological tooth migration and its significance for the development of occlusion. I. The biogenetic course of the deciduous dentition. J. Dent. Res. 29:123–132, 1950.

Beard, C.C., and Clayton, J.A. Effects of occlusal splint therapy on TMJ dysfunction. J. Prosthet. Dent. 44:324–335, 1980.

Beecher, H.K. The powerful placebo. J. Am. Med. Assoc. 159:1602–1605, 1955.

Beecher, H.K. Anxiety and pain. J. Am. Med. Assoc. 209:1080, 1969.

Beemsterboer, P.L., McNamara, D.C., Holden, S., and Ash, M.M., Jr. The effect of bite plane splint on the electromyographic silent period duration. J. Oral Rehabil. 3:349–352, 1976a.

Beemsterboer, P.L., Solberg, W.K., and Rugh, J.D. Occlusal splint therapy: nocturnal electromyographic response and symptom improvement. J. Dent. Res. 55:B101, 1976b.

Begg, P.R. Stone age man's dentition. Am. J. Orthod. 40:298–312, 373–383, 462–475, 517–531, 1954.

Bell, W.E. Clinical diagnosis of the pain-dysfunction syndrome. J. Am. Dent. Assoc. 79:154–160, 1969.

Bell, W.E. Orofacial Pains: Differential Diagnosis. 2nd ed. Chicago: Year Book Medical Publishers, Inc., 1979.

Belser, U.C., and Hannam, A.G. The influence of altered working-side occlusal guidance on masticatory muscles and related jaw movement. J. Prosthet. Dent. 53:406–412, 1985.

Bergman, B., Carlsson, G.E., and Hedegard, B. A longitudinal two-year study of a number of full denture cases. Acta Odontol. Scand. 22:3–26, 1964.

Bergman, B., Hugoson, A., and Olsson, C.O. Caries and periodontal status in patients fitted with removable partial dentures. J. Clin. Periodontol. 4:134–146, 1977.

Berkowitz, B.K.B., Holland, G.R., and Moxham, B.J. A Colour Atlas and Textbook of Oral Anatomy. London: Wolfe Medical Publ. Ltd., 1978.

Berlin, R., and Dessner, L. Bruxism and chronic headache. Lancet 11:289–291, 1960.

Berlin, R., Dessner, L., and Aberg, S. Chronic headache and dysfunction of the temporomandibular joint. Acta Med. Scand. 154:167–176, 1956.

Bernstein, P.R., McCall, W.D., Jr., Mohl, N.D., Bishop, B., and Uthman, A.A. The effect of voluntary activity on the masseteric silent period duration. J. Prosthet. Dent. 46:192–195, 1981.

Berry, D.C. Mandibular dysfunction pain and chronic minor illness. Br. Dent. J. 127:170–175, 1969.

Berry, D.C. Occlusion: fact or fallacy. J. Craniomand. Prac. 4:54–64, 1986.

Berry, D.C., and Poole, D.F.G. Attrition: possible mechanisms of compensation. J. Oral Rehabil. 3:201–206, 1976.

Berry, D.C., and Singh, B.P. Effect of electromyographic biofeedback therapy on occlusal contacts. J. Prosthet. Dent. 51:397–403, 1984.

Berry, D.C., and Wilmot, G. The use of a biofeedback technique in the treatment of mandibular dysfunction pain: a preliminary report on the Myotron 220. J. Oral Rehabil. 4:255–260, 1977.

Berry, D.C., and Yemm, R. Changes in facial skin temperature associated with unilateral chewing. J. Oral Rehabil. 1:127–129, 1974.

Bessette, R.W., Bishop, B., and Mohl, N.D. Duration of masseteric silent period in patients with TMJ syndrome. J. Appl. Physiol. 30:864–869, 1971.

Beyron, H.L. Characteristics of functionally optimal occlusion and principles of occlusal rehabilitation. J. Am. Dent. Assoc. 48:648–656, 1954a.

Beyron, H.L. Occlusal changes in adult dentition. J. Am. Dent. Assoc. 48:674–686, 1954b.

Beyron, H.L. Occlusal relations and mastication in Australian aborigines. Acta Odontol. Scand. 22:597–678, 1964.

Beyron, H.L. Optimal occlusion. Dent. Clin. North Am. 13:537–554, 1969.

Beyron, H.L. Occlusion: point of significance in planning restorative procedures. J. Prosthet. Dent. 30:641–652, 1973.

Bishop, B. Basic Neurophysiology. Garden City, N.Y.: Medical Examination Publ. Co., 1982.

Bjork, A. Variability and age changes in overjet and overbite. Am. J. Orthod. 39:779–801, 1953.

Bjork, A. Facial growth in man, studied with the aid of metallic implants. Acta Odontol. Scand. 13:9–34, 1955.

Bjork, A., and Helm, S. Need for orthodontic treatment as reflected in the prevalence of malocclusion in various ethnic groups. Acta Socio-Med. Scand. 1 (Suppl. 1):209–214, 1969.

Bjork, A., Krebs, A., and Solow, B. A method for epidemiologic registration of malocclusion. Acta Odontol. Scand. 22:27–41, 1964.

Bjork, A., and Palling, M. Adolescent age changes in sagittal jaw relation, alveolar prognathy, and incisal inclination. Acta Odontol. Scand. 12:201–232, 1955.

Bjorn, A. Dental health in relation to age and dental care. Odontol. Revy 25 (Suppl. 29):1–17, 1974.

Black, R.G. The chronic pain syndrome. Surg. Clin. North Am. 55:999–1011, 1975.

Black, R.G., and Bonica, J.J. Analgesic blocks. Postgrad. Med. J. 52:105–110, 1973.

Black, R.R. Use of transcutaneous electrical nerve stimulation in dentistry. J. Am. Dent. Assoc. 113:649–652, 1986.

Blackwood, H.J.J. Arthritis of the mandibular joint. Br. Dent. J. 115:317–326, 1963.

Blackwood, H.J.J. Cellular remodeling in articular tissue. J. Dent. Res. 45:480–489, 1966a.

Blackwood, H.J.J. Adaptive changes in the mandibular joints with function. Dent. Clin. North Am. 10:559–566,

1966b.
Blasberg, B., Remick, R.A., and Miles, J.E. The psychiatric referral in dentistry: indications and mechanics. Oral Surg. Oral Med. Oral Pathol. 56:368–371, 1983.
Blaschke, D.D., and Blaschke, T.J. Normal TMJ bone relationships in centric occlusion. J. Dent. Res. 60:98–104, 1981.
Blaschke, D.D., and White, S.C. Radiology. Chapt. 12 *In* B.G. Sarnat and D.M. Laskin (eds.) The Temporomandibular Joint. 3rd ed. Springfield, Ill.: Charles C Thomas Publ., 1979.
Block, L.S. Diagnosis and treatment of disturbances of the temporomandibular joint, especially in relation to vertical dimension. J. Am. Dent. Assoc. 34:253–260, 1947.
Block, S.L. Differential diagnosis of craniofacial-cervical pain. Chapt. 18 *In* B.G. Sarnat and D.M. Laskin (eds.) The Temporomandibular Joint. Springfield, Ill.: Charles C Thomas Publ., 1979.
Block, S.L., Apfel, M., and Laskin, D.M. The use of a resilient rubber bite appliance in the treatment of MPD syndrome. J. Dent. Res. 57:A71, 1978.
Block, S.L., and Laskin, D.M. The effectiveness of transcutaneous nerve stimulation (TNS) in the treatment of unilateral MPD syndrome. J. Dent. Res. 59 (Spec. Issue A; Abstr. No. 999):519, 1980.
Bodenham, R.S. A bite guard for athletic training. A case report. Br. Dent. J. 129:85–86, 1970.
Bohl, C.F., and Knap, F.J. Evaluating occlusal relationships, mandibular dysfunction, and temporomandibular joint pain by palpation. J. Prosthet. Dent. 32:80–86, 1974.
Bonica, J.J. Management of myofascial pain syndromes in general practice. J. Am. Med. Assoc. 164:732–738, 1957.
Bonica, J.J. Clinical applications of diagnostic and therapeutic nerve blocks. Springfield, Ill.: Charles C Thomas Publ., 1959.
Bonica, J.J. (ed.) Pain. New York: Raven Press, 1980.
Bonwill, W.G.A. Geometric and mechanical laws of articulation. Anatomical articulation. Trans. Odont. Soc. Penn., pp. 119–133, 1885.
Bornstein, P.H., Hamilton, S.B., and Bornstein, M.T. Self-monitoring procedures. pp. 176–222 *In* A.R. Ciminero, K.S. Calhoun, and H.E. Adams (eds.) Handbook of Behavioral Assessment. New York: John Wiley & Sons, 1986.
Bosma, J.F. Deglutition: pharyngeal stage. Physiol. Rev. 37:275–300, 1957.
Bosma, J.F. Fourth Symposium on Oral Sensation and Perception: Development in the Fetus and Infant. Washington, D.C.: U.S. Government Printing Office, 1973, p. 419.
Boyer, C.C., Williams, T.W., and Stevens, F.H. Blood supply of the temporomandibular joint. J. Dent. Res. 43:224–228, 1964.
Bramble, D.M., and Wake, D.B. Feeding mechanisms in lower vertebrates. *In* M. Hildebrand, D.M. Bramble, K.L. Liem and D.B. Wake (eds.) Functional Vertebrate Morphology. Cambridge, Mass.: Harvard University Press, 1985.
Brandon, S. Unusual effect of fenfluramine. Br. Med. J. 4:557–558, 1969.
Bratzlavsky, M. Pauses in activity of human jaw-closing muscles. Exp. Neurol. 36:160–165, 1972.
Brayer, L., and Erlich, J. The nite guard: its uses and dangers of abuse. J. Oral Rehabil. 3:181–184, 1976.
Brehnan, K., Boyd, R.L., Laskin, J., Gibbs, C.H., and Mahan, P. Direct measurement of loads at the temporomandibular joint in *Macaca arctoides*. J. Dent. Res. 60:1820–1824, 1981.
Breault, M.R. Eagle's syndrome: review of the literature and implications in craniomandibular disorders. J. Craniomandib. Pract. 4:323–337, 1986.
Brekhus, P.J., Armstrong, W.D., and Simon, W.J. Stimulation of the muscles of mastication. J. Dent. Res. 20:87–92, 1941.
Brill, N., Lammie, G.A., Osborne, J., and Perry, H.T. Mandibular positions and mandibular movements. Br. Dent. J. 106:391–400, 1959.
Brooke, R.I. Postinjection trismus due to formation of fibrous band. Oral Surg. Oral Med. Oral Pathol. 47:424–426, 1979.
Brooke, R.I., Stenn, P.G., and Mothersill, K.J. The diagnosis and conservative treatment of myofascial pain dysfunction syndrome. Oral Surg. Oral Med. Oral Pathol. 44:844–852, 1977.
Bryant, P., Gale, E., and Rugh, J. (eds.) Oral Motor Behavior: Impact on Oral Conditions and Dental Treatment. NIH Publication no. 79-1845. Washington, D.C.: U.S. Government Printing Office, 1979.
Burch, J. Periodontal considerations in operative dentistry. J. Prosthet. Dent. 34:156, 1975.
Burch, J.G. The selection of occlusal patterns in periodontal therapy. Dent. Clin. North Amer. 24:343–356, 1980.
Burch, J.G., and Lundeen, H.C. Mandibular movements in the monkey. J. Prosthet. Dent. 25:183–188, 1971.
Burke, R.E., Levine, D.N., Tsairis, P., and Zajac, F.E., III. Physiological types and histochemical profiles in motor units of the cat gastrocnemius. J. Physiol. 234:723–748, 1973.
Burstone, C.J. Lip posture and its significance in treatment planning. Am. J. Orthod. 53:262–284, 1967.
Burstone, C.J., James, R.B., Legan, H., Murphy, G.A., and Norton, L.A. Cephalometrics for orthognathic surgery. J. Oral Surg. 36:269–277, 1978.
Butler, J.A., and Zander, H.A. Evaluation of two occlusal concepts. Paradontol. Acad. Rev. 2:5–19, 1968.
Cachel, S. A paleoecological model for the origin of higher primates. J. Human Evol. 8:351–359, 1979.
Calder, N. Einstein's Universe. New York: The Viking Press, 1979, p. 141.
Carlsen, D.B., and Meredith, H.V. Biologic variation in selected relationships of opposing posterior teeth. Angle Orthod. 30:162–173, 1960.
Carlsson, G.E. Bite force and chewing efficiency. pp. 265–292 *In* Y. Kawamura (ed.) Frontiers of Oral Physiology. Vol. I. Physiology of Mastication. Basel, Switzerland: S. Karger, 1974.
Carlsson, G.E. Mandibular dysfunction and temporomandibular pathosis. J. Prosthet. Dent. 43:658–663, 1980.
Carlsson, G.E. Masticatory efficiency: the effect of age, the loss of teeth and prosthetic rehabilitation. Int. Dent. J. 34:93–97, 1984.
Carlsson, G.E. Long-term effects of treatment of craniomandibular disorders. J. Craniomand. Pract. 3:337–342, 1985.
Carlsson, G.E., Hedegard, B., and Koivumaa, K.K. Studies in partial denture prosthesis. IV. Final results of a four year longitudinal investigation of dentogingivally supported partial dentures. Acta Odontol. Scand. 23:443–472,

1965.
Carlsson, G.E., and Helkimo, M. Funktionell undersökning av tuggapparaten. *In* J.J. Holst (ed.) Nordisk klinisk odontologi. Copenhagen: A/S Forlaget for faglitteratur, 8 (I):1–21, 1972.
Carlsson, G.E., Ingervall, B., and Kocak, G. Effect of increasing vertical dimension on the masticatory system in subjects with natural teeth. J. Prosthet. Dent. 41:284–289, 1979.
Carlsson, G.E., Kopp, S., and Öberg, T. Arthritis and allied diseases. pp. 269–320 *In* G.A. Zarb and G.E. Carlsson (eds.) Temporomandibular Joint Function and Dysfunction. Copenhagen: Munksgaard, 1979.
Carlsson, G.E., Kopp, S., and Wedel, A. Analysis of background variables in 350 patients with TMJ disorders as reported in self-administered questionnaire. Community Dent. Oral Epidemiol. 10:47–51, 1982.
Carlsson, G.E., and Öberg, T. Remodelling of the temporomandibular joints. Oral Sciences Rev. 4:53–86, 1974.
Carlsson, G.E., and Öberg, T. Remodelling of the temporomandibular joint. Chapt. 5 *In* G.A. Zarb and G.E. Carlsson (eds.) Temporomandibular Joint Function and Dysfunction. Copenhagen: Munksgaard, 1979.
Carlsson, S.G., Gale, E.N., and Öhman, A. Treatment of temporomandibular joint syndrome with biofeedback training. J. Am. Dent. Assoc. 91:602–605, 1975.
Carraro, J.J., and Caffesse, R.G. Effect of occlusal splints on TMJ symptomatology. J. Prosthet. Dent. 40:563–566, 1978.
Cavenar, J.O., and Maltebie, A.A. Another indication for haloperodol. Psychosomatics 27:128–130, 1976.
Charteris, J., Wall, J.C., and Nottrodt, J.W. Pliocene hominid gait: new interpretations based on available footprint data from Laetoli. Am. J. Phys. Anthropol. 58:133–144, 1982.
Chase, M.H., and McGinty, D.J. Somatomotor inhibition and excitation by forebrain stimulation during sleep and wakefulness: orbital cortex. Brain Res. 19:127–136, 1970.
Chase, M.H., Monoson, R., Watanabe, K., and Babb, M.I. Somatic reflex response—reversal of reticular origin. Exp. Neurol. 50:561–567, 1976.
Chayes, C.M., and Schwartz, L.L. Management of mandibular dysfunction: general and specific considerations. pp. 335–355 *In* C.M. Chayes and L.L. Schwartz (eds.) Facial Pain and Mandibular Dysfunction. Philadelphia: W.B. Saunders Co., 1968.
Chesney, M. Behavior modification and health enhancement. Chapt. 22 *In* J.D. Matarazzo, S.M. Weiss, J.A. Herd, N.E. Miller, and S.M. Weiss (eds.) Behavioral Health: A Handbook of Health Enhancement and Disease Prevention. New York: John Wiley & Sons, 1984.
Choukas, N.C., and Sicher, H. The structure of the temporomandibular joint. Oral Surg. Oral Med. Oral Path. 13:1203–1213, 1960.
Christensen, J. Effect of occlusion-raising procedures on the chewing system. Dent. Pract. 20:233–238, 1970.
Christensen, L.V. Facial pain and internal pressure of masseter muscle in experimental bruxism in man. Arch. Oral Biol. 16:1021–1031, 1971.
Christensen, L.V. Jaw muscle fatigue and pains induced by experimental tooth clenching: a review. J. Oral Rehabil. 8:27–36, 1981.
Clark, G.T. Treatment of jaw clicking with temporomandibular repositioning: an analysis of 25 cases. J. Craniomandib. Pract. 2:263–270, 1984.
Clark, G.T. The temporomandibular joint repositioning appliance: a technique for construction, insertion and adjustment. J. Craniomandib. Pract. 4:37–46, 1986.
Clark, G.T., and Adler, R.C. A critical evaluation of occlusal therapy: occlusal adjustment procedures. J. Am. Dent. Assoc. 110:743–750, 1985.
Clark, G.T., Beemsterboer, P.L., and Rugh, J.D. Nocturnal masseter muscle activity and the symptoms of masticatory dysfunction. J. Oral Rehabil. 8:279–286, 1981.
Clark, G.T., Beemsterboer, P.L., Solberg, W.K., and Rugh, J.D. Nocturnal electromyographic evaluation of myofascial pain dysfunction in patients undergoing occlusal splint therapy. J. Am. Dent. Assoc. 99:607–611, 1979.
Clarke, N.G., and Kardachi, B.J. The treatment of myofascial pain-dysfunction syndrome using the biofeedback principle. J. Periodontol. 48:643–645, 1977.
Cohen, S.R. Follow-up evaluation of 105 patients with myofascial pain-dysfunction syndrome. J. Am. Dent. Assoc. 97:825–828, 1978.
Coleman, R.D. Temporomandibular joint: relationships of the retrodiskal zone to Meckel's cartilage and lateral pterygoid muscle. J. Dent. Res. 49:626–630, 1970.
Coolidge, E. Traumatic and functional injuries occurring in the supporting tissues of human teeth. J. Am. Dent. Assoc. 25:354–357, 1938.
Cooper, S.A. Peripheral vs. central analgesics: is anything better than aspirin and codeine? *In* T.E. Nelson and P.C. Bourgault (eds.) Current Concepts of Analgesic Action. 4th Symp. of Pharmacol. Toxicol. Therap. Group, I.A.D.R. 4:41–51, 1978.
Corcos, J., and Brandwein, A. Treatment of temporomandibular joint pain by acupuncture. Am. J. Acupuncture 4:157–160, 1976.
Costen, J.B. A syndrome of ear and sinus symptoms dependent upon disturbed function of the temporomandibular joint. Ann. Otol. (St. Louis) 43:1–15, 1934.
Crompton, A.W., and Parker, P. Evolution of the mammalian masticatory apparatus. Am. Sci. 66:192–201, 1978.
Dahlberg, B. The masticatory effect. Acta. Med. Scand. (Suppl. 139):1–154, 1943.
Dahlström, L., and Carlsson, S.G. Treatment of mandibular dysfunction: the clinical usefulness of biofeedback in relation to splint therapy. J. Oral Rehabil. 11:277–284, 1984.
Dalessio, D.J. Wolff's Headache and Other Head Pain. 3rd ed. New York: Oxford University Press, 1972.
D'Amico, A. The canine teeth—normal functional relation of the natural teeth of man. J. South Calif. Dent. Assoc. 26:6–23, 49–60, 127–142, 175–182, 194–208, 239–241, 1958.
D'Amico, A. Functional occlusion of the natural teeth in man. J. Prosthet. Dent. 11:899–915, 1961.
Danzig, W.N., and Van Dyke, A.R. Physical therapy as an adjunct to temporomandibular joint therapy. J. Prosthet. Dent. 49:96–99, 1983.
Dawson, P.E. Evaluation, diagnosis and treatment of occlusal problems. St. Louis: C.V. Mosby Co., 1974.
DeBoever, J. Experimental occlusal balancing-contact interference and muscle activity. Parodontologie 23:59–69, 1969.
DeBoever, J.A., McCall, W.D., Jr., Holden, S., and Ash,

M.M., Jr. Functional occlusal forces: an investigation by telemetry. J. Prosthet. Dent. 40:326–333, 1978.

Decker, J.D. Traumatic deafness as a result of retrusion of the condyles of the mandible. Ann. Otol. Rhinol. Laryngol. 34:519–527, 1925.

Delair, J., Schendel, S.A., and Tulasne, J.F. An architectural and structural craniofacial analysis: a new lateral cephalometric analysis. Oral Surg. Oral Med. Oral Pathol. 52:226–238, 1981.

Dellow, P.G. Control mechanisms of mastication. Ann. Austr. Coll. Dent. Surg. 2:81–95, 1969.

Dellow, P.G. The general physiological background of chewing and swallowing. pp. 6–21 *In* B.J. Sessle and A.G. Hannam (eds.) Mastication and Swallowing: Biological and Clinical Correlates. Toronto: University of Toronto Press, 1976.

Dellow, P.G., and Lund, J.P. Evidence for central timing of rhythmical mastication. J. Physiol. 215:1–13, 1971.

Delson, E. (ed.) Ancestors: The Hard Evidence. New York: Alan R. Liss, Inc., 1985.

Delson, E. Human phylogeny revised origanism. Nature (London) 322:496–497, 1986.

Dempster, W.T., Adams, W.J., and Duddles, R.A. Arrangement in the jaws of the roots of the teeth. J. Am. Dent. Assoc. 67:779–797, 1963.

Diamond, S., and Medina, J.L. Double blind study of propanolol for migraine prophylaxis. Headache 16:24–29, 1976.

Dictionary of Medical Syndromes. 2nd ed. Sergio Magalini (ed.) Philadelphia: Lippincott, 1981.

Djupesland, G. Contractions of the tympanic muscles in man. Oslo: Universitetsforlaget, 1967.

Domning, D.P., and Hayek, L.-A.C. Horizontal tooth placement in the Amazonian manatee *(Trichechus inungius).* Mammalia 48:105–127, 1984.

Donnarumma, G.C., Burdette, B.H., and McCall, W.D., Jr. Bite force and silent period durations: comparisons in normal subjects and TMD patients. J. Dent. Res. 65 (Spec. Issue):180, 1986.

Dorland's Illustrated Medical Dictionary. 20th ed. Philadelphia: W.B. Saunders Co., 1985.

Downs, W.B. Variations in facial relationships: their significance in treatment and prognosis. Am. J. Orthod. 34:812–849, 1948.

Drago, C.J. The effect of posterior tooth form on the chewing cycle in the frontal plane. Master's Thesis. San Antonio: University of Texas Graduate School of Biomedical Sciences, Dec. 1981.

Drago, C.J., Rugh, J.D., and Barghi, N. Nightguard vertical thickness effects on nocturnal bruxism. J. Dent. Res. 58 (Spec. Issue A):315, 1979.

Droukas, B., Lindee, C., and Carlsson, G.E. Relationship between occlusal factors and signs and symptoms of mandibular dysfunction. A clinical study of 48 dental students. Acta Odontol. Scand. 42:277–283, 1984.

Droukas, B., Lindee, C., and Carlsson, G.E. Occlusion and mandibular dysfunction: a clinical study of patients referred for functional disturbances of the masticatory system. J. Prosthet. Dent. 53:402–496, 1985.

Dubner, R., Sessle, B.J., and Storey, A.T. The Neural Basis of Oral and Facial Function. New York: Plenum Press, 1978.

DuBrul, E.L. Origin and adaptations of the hominid jaw joint. pp. 5–34 *In* B.G. Sarnat and D.M. Laskin (eds.) The Temporomandibular Joint. Springfield: Charles C Thomas Publ., 1979.

DuBrul, E.L. The craniomandibular articulation. Chapt. 4 *In* Sicher's Oral Anatomy. 7th ed. St. Louis: C.V. Mosby Co., 1980.

DuBrul, E.L., and Menekratis, A. The Physiology of Oral Reconstruction. Chicago: Quintessence Publ. Co., 1981.

Duquette, P., and Goebel, W.M. Pulpitis simulating the myofascial pain dysfunction syndrome: report of three cases. J. Am. Dent. Assoc. 87:1231–1239, 1973.

Edmiston, G.F., and Laskin, D. Changes in consistency of occlusal contact in myofacial pain dysfunction syndrome. J. Dent. Res. 57:27–30, 1978.

Edmund, A.G. Sequence and rate of tooth replacement in the Crocodilia. Life Sci. Div. 56. Toronto: The Royal Ontario Museum, 1962.

Egermark-Eriksson, I. Mandibular dysfunction in children and in individuals with dual bite. Swed. Dent. J., Suppl. 10, 1982.

Egermark-Eriksson, I., Carlsson, G.E., and Ingervall, B. Function and dysfunction of the masticatory system in individuals with dual bite. Eur. J. Orthod. 1:107–117, 1979.

Egermark-Eriksson, I., Carlsson, G.E., and Ingervall, B. Prevalence of mandibular dysfunction and orofacial parafunction in 7-, 11- and 15-year-old Swedish children. Eur. J. Orthod. 3:163–172, 1981.

Ellis, E., and McNamara, J.A. Components of adult Class III malocclusion. J. Oral Maxillofac. Surg. 42:295–305, 1984.

Epker, B.N., Schendel, S.A., and Washburn, M. Effects of early surgical superior repositioning of the maxilla on subsequent growth. III. Biomechanical considerations. *In* J.A. McNamara, Jr. (ed.) The Effect of Surgical Intervention on Craniofacial Growth. Monograph 12, Craniofacial Growth Series. Ann Arbor: Center for Human Growth and Development, The University of Michigan, 1982.

Epker, B.N., and Wolford, L.M.: Middle-third facial osteotomies: their use in the correction of acquired and developmental dentofacial and craniofacial deformities. J. Oral Surg. 33:491–514, 1975.

Epstein, J.B. Understanding placebo in dentistry. J. Am. Dent. Assoc. 109:71–74, 1984.

Erickson, R.I. Ultrasound—a useful adjunct in temporomandibular joint therapy. Oral Surg. Oral Med. Oral Pathol. 18:176–179, 1964.

Ericson, S., and Lundberg, M. Structural changes in the finger, wrist, and temporomandibular joints. A comparative radiologic study. Acta Odontol. Scand. 26:111–126, 1968.

Eriksson, P.-O., Eriksson, A., Ringqvist, M., and Thornell, L.-E. Special histochemical muscle-fibre characteristics of the human lateral pterygoid muscle. Arch. Oral Biol. 26:495–507, 1981.

Eriksson, P.-O., Eriksson, A., Ringqvist, M., and Thornell, L.-E. Histochemical fibre composition of the human digastric muscle. Arch. Oral Biol. 27:207–215, 1982.

Eriksson, P.-O., and Thornell, L.-E. Histochemical and morphological muscle-fiber characteristics of the human masseter, the medial pterygoid, and the temporal muscles. Arch. Oral Biol. 28:781–795, 1983.

Esposito, C.J., Farman, A.G., and Veal, S.J. Occlusion in the dental curriculum: 1980–1981. J. Prosthet. Dent. 49:419–426, 1983.

Esposito, C.J., Veal, S.J., and Farman, A.G. Alleviation of

myofascial pain with ultrasonic therapy. J. Prosthet. Dent. 51:106–108, 1984.

Everett, N.B. Functional Neuroanatomy. Philadelphia: Lea & Febiger, 1965.

Farrar, W.B. Differentiation of temporomandibular joint dysfunction to simplify treatment. J. Prosthet. Dent. 28:629–636, 1972.

Farrar, W.B. Craniomandibular practice: the state of the art; definition and diagnosis. J. Craniomandib. Pract. 1:5–12, 1982.

Feinmann, C., and Harris, M. Psychogenic facial pain: presentation and treatment. Br. Med. J. 288:436–438, 1984.

Fields, R.W., Savara, B.S., and Tacke, R. Regional electroanalgesia and its potentialities in control of orofacial pain. Oral Surg. Oral Med. Oral Pathol. 34:694–703, 1972.

Fish, D.R., and Mendel, F.C. Mandibular movement patterns relative to food types in common tree shrews. Am. J. Phys. Anthropol. 58:255–269, 1982.

Fish, S.F. Partial dentures. I. The problem. Br. Dent. J. 128:243–246, 1970.

Fordyce, W.E. Behavior Methods for Chronic Pain and Illness. St. Louis: C.V. Mosby Co., 1976.

Forssberg, H., Grillner, S., and Rossignol, S. Phase dependent reflex reversal during walking in chronic spinal cats. Brain Res. 85:103–107, 1975.

Forssell, H. Mandibular dysfunction and headache. Finn. Dent. Soc. 81 (Suppl. II), 1985.

Frankel, V.H., and Nordin, M. Basic Biomechanics of the Skeletal System. Philadelphia: Lea & Febiger, 1980, p. 70.

Franks, A. The dental health of patients presenting with temporomandibular joint dysfunction. Br. J. Oral Surg. 5:157–166, 1967.

Franks, A.S.T. The social character of temporomandibular joint dysfunction: a comparative study. Dent. Practit. 15:94–100, 1964.

Franks, A.S.T. Conservative treatment of temporomandibular joint dysfunction: a comparative study. Dent. Pract. 15:205–210, 1965.

Freihofer, H.P.M. Results of osteotomies of the facial skeleton in adolescence. J. Maxillofac. Surg. 5:267–297, 1977.

Fridën, J.M., Sjorström, M., and Eckblom, B. A morphological study of delayed muscle soreness. Experientia 37:506–507, 1981.

Frohlich, F.J. A longitudinal study of untreated Class II type malocclusions. Trans. Eur. Orthod. Soc. 137–151, 1961.

Fuchs, P. The muscular activity of the chewing apparatus during night sleep. An examination of healthy subjects and patients with functional disturbances. J. Oral Rehabil. 2:35–48, 1975.

Funakoshi, M., Fujita, N., and Takehana, S. Relations between occlusal interference and jaw muscle activities in response to changes in head position. J. Dent. Res. 55:684–690, 1976.

Funch, D.P., and Gale, E.N. Factors associated with nocturnal bruxism and its treatment. J. Behav. Mod. 31:385–397, 1980.

Furstman, L. The early development of the human temporomandibular joint. Am. J. Orthod. 49:672–682, 1963.

Gale, E.N. Behavioral approaches to temporomandibular disorders. Ann. Behav. Med. 8:11–16, 1986.

Gangorosa, L.P. Iontophoresis in Dental Practice. Chicago: Quintessence Publ. Co., 1983.

Gantt, D.G. Enamel thickness of primate teeth: its functional and phyletic implications. Ph.D. diss. abstr. 38/07 4244-A. Seattle: Washington University, 1977.

Gardner, E., Gray, D.J., and O'Rahilly, R. Anatomy. 2nd ed. Philadelphia: W.B. Saunders Co., 1963, pp. 845–847.

Gardiner, M.D. The Principles of Exercise Therapy. 3rd ed. London: G. Bell, 1973, pp. 41–61.

Garnick, J., and Ramfjord, S.P. Rest position. J. Prosthet. Dent. 12:895–911, 1962.

Gausch, K., and Kulmer, S. The role of retro-disclusion in the treatment of the TMJ patient. J. Oral Rehabil. 4:29–32, 1977.

Gerber, A. Kiefergelenk und Zahnokklusion. Dtsch. Zahnaerztl. Z. 26:119–141, 1971.

Gessel, A.H. Electromyographic biofeedback and tricyclic antidepressants in myofascial pain-dysfunction syndrome: psychological predictors of outcome. J. Am. Dent. Assoc. 91:1048–1052, 1975.

Gessel, A.H., and Alderman, M.M. Management of myofascial pain dysfunction syndrome of the temporomandibular joint by tension control training. Psychosomatics 12:302–309, 1971.

Ghia, J.N., Duncan, G.S., Scott, D.S., and Gregg, J.M. Therapeutic nerve blocks for chronic pain. Fam. Physician 20:74–78, 1979.

Ghia, J.N., Mao, W., Toomey, T.C., and Gregg, J.M. Acupuncture and chronic pain mechanisms. Pain 2:285–299, 1976.

Gibbs, C., and Lundeen, H. Jaw movements and forces during chewing and swallowing and their clinical significance. pp. 2–32 *In* H. Lundeen and C. Gibbs (eds.) Advances in Occlusion. Boston: John Wright, 1982.

Gibbs, C.H., Lundeen, H.C., Mahan, P.E., and Fujimoto, J. Chewing movements in relation to border movements at the first molar. J. Prosthet. Dent. 46:308–322, 1981a.

Gibbs, C.H., Mahan, P.E., Lundeen, H.C., Brehran, K., Walsh, E.K., and Holbrook, W.B. Occlusal forces during chewing and swallowing as measured by sound transmission. J. Prosthet. Dent. 46:443–449, 1981b.

Gibbs, C.H., Mahan, P.E., Lundeen, H.C., Brehran, K., Walsh, E.K., Sinkcwiz, S.L., and Ginsberg, S.B. Occlusal forces during chewing: influences of biting strength and food consistency. J. Prosthet. Dent. 46:561–567, 1981c.

Gibbs, C.H., Mahan, P.E., Mauderli, A., Lundeen, H.C., and Walsh, E.K. Limits of human bite strength. J. Prosthet. Dent. 56:226–229, 1986.

Gibbs, C.H., and Messerman, T. Jaw motion during speech. Am. Speech & Hearing Assoc. Report no. 7; 104–112, 1972.

Gibbs, C.H., and Suit, S.R. Movements of the jaw after unexpected contact with a hard object. J. Dent. Res. 52:810–814, 1973.

Gilboe, D.B. Centric relation as a treatment position. J. Prosthet. Dent. 50:685–689, 1983.

Glaros, A.G., and Rao, S.M. Effects of bruxism: a review of the literature. J. Prosthet. Dent. 38:149–157, 1977.

Glickman, I. Trauma from occlusion in the etiology of periodontal disease. *In* Clinical Periodontology. 4th ed. Philadelphia: W.B. Saunders Co., 1972.

Glickman, I., and Zander, H.A. Discussion of role of occlusion in the etiology and treatment of periodontal disease. J. Dent. Res. (Suppl.) 50:199, 1971.

Goharian, R.K., and Neff, P.A. Effect of occlusal retainers on temporomandibular joint and facial pain. J. Prosthet. Dent. 44:206–208, 1980.

Gold, N., Greene, C.S., and Laskin, D.M. TENS therapy for treatment of MPD syndrome. J. Dent. Res. 62 (Abstr. No. 676):244, 1983.

Goldberg, L.J. Masseter muscle excitation induced by stimulation of periodontal and gingival receptors in man. Brain Res. 32:369–381, 1971.

Goldberg, L.J. The effect of jaw position on the excitability of two reflexes involving the masseter muscle in man. Arch. Oral Biol. 17:565–576, 1972.

Goldberg, L.J., and Derfler, B. Relationship among recruitment order, spike amplitude, and twitch tension of single motor units in human masseter muscle. J. Neurophysiol. 40:879–890, 1977.

Goldman, H.M., and Cohen, D.W. Periodontal Therapy. 4th ed. St. Louis: C.V. Mosby Co., 1968.

Goldspink, G. The adaptation of muscle to a new functional length. *In* D.J. Anderson and B. Matthews (eds.) Mastication. Bristol: John Wright & Sons, 1976.

Goodall, J. Infant killing and canabalism in free living chimpanzees. Folia Primalologica 28:262–282, 1977.

Goodgold, J., and Eberstein, A. Electrodiagnosis of Neuromuscular Diseases. Baltimore: Williams & Wilkins, 1978.

Goodman, P., Greene, C.S., and Laskin, D.M. Response of patients with myofascial pain-dysfunction syndrome to work equilibration. J. Am. Dent. Assoc. 92:755–758, 1976.

Goodwin, G.M., and Luschei, E.S. Effects of destroying spindle afferents from jaw muscles on mastication in monkeys. J. Neurophysiol. 37:967–981, 1974.

Goodwin, G.M., and Luschei, E.S. Discharge of spindle afferents from jaw closing muscles during chewing in alert monkeys. J. Neurophysiol. 38:560–571, 1975.

Gossman, J.R., and Tarsitano, J.J. The styloid-stylohyoid syndrome. J. Oral. Surg. 35:555–560, 1977.

Gould, T.R.L., Melcher, A.H., and Brunette, D.M. Location of progenitor cells in peridontal ligament of mouse molar stimulated by wounding. Anat. Rec. 188:133–142, 1977.

Gould, T.R.L., Melcher, A.H., and Brunette, D.M. Migration and division of progenitor cell populations in periodontal ligament after wounding. J. Periodont. Res. 15:20–42, 1980.

Graf, H. Analysis of human jaw movement patterns by graphic computer display. pp. 323–329 *In* Y. Kawamura and R. Dubner (eds.) Oral-Facial Sensory and Motor Functions. Tokyo: Quintessence Publ. Co., 1981.

Graf, H., Grassl, H., and Aeberhard, H.J. A method for measurement of occlusal forces in three directions. Acta Helv. Odontol. 18:7–11, 1974.

Graf, H., and Zander, H. Tooth contact patterns in mastication. J. Prosthet. Dent. 13:1055–1066, 1963.

Greene, C.S. The relationship between research and clinical practice in treatment of myofascial pain dysfunction. Alpha Omegan 69:18–30, 1976.

Greene, C.S. Temporomandibular joint disorders. *In* J.W. Clark (ed.) Clinical Dentistry. Philadelphia: Harper & Row, 1984.

Greene, C.S., and Laskin, D.M. Meprobamate therapy for the myofascial pain dysfunction (MPD) syndrome: a double-blind evaluation. J. Am. Dent. Assoc. 82:587–590, 1971.

Greene, C.S., and Laskin, D.M. Splint therapy for the myofascial pain-dysfunction (MPD) syndrome: a comparative study. J. Am. Dent. Assoc. 84:624–628, 1972.

Greene, C.S., and Laskin, D.M. Long-term evaluation of conservative treatment for myofascial pain-dysfunction syndrome. J. Am. Dent. Assoc. 89:1365–1368, 1974.

Greene, C.S., Lerman, M.D., Sutcher, H.D., and Laskin, D.M. The TMJ pain-dysfunction syndrome: heterogeneity of the patient population. J. Am. Dent. Assoc. 79:1168–1172, 1969.

Greene, C.S., and Marbach, J.J. Epidemiologic studies of mandibular dysfunction: a critical review. J. Prosthet. Dent. 48:184–190, 1982.

Greene, C.S., and Turner, C. Mandibular dysfunction symptoms in a random population. J. Dent. Res. 62 (Spec. Issue A):304, 1983.

Greene, D.S., Turner, C., and Laskin, D.M. Long term outcome of TMJ clicking in 100 MPD patients. J. Dent. Res. 61:218, 1982.

Greenfield, B.E., and Wyke, B. Reflex innervation of the temporomandibular joint. Nature 211:940–941, 1966.

Greenwood, L.F., and Sessle, B.J. Pain, brain stem mechanisms, and motor function. pp. 108–119 *In* B.J. Sessle and A.G. Hannam (eds.) Mastication and Swallowing: Biological and Clinical Correlates. Toronto: University of Toronto Press, 1976.

Greenwood, P.H. Environmental effects on the pharyngeal mill of a cichlid fish, *Astatoreochronuis alluandi,* and their implications. Proc. Linn. Soc. (Lond.) 176:1–10, 1964.

Gregg, J.M. Central nervous system factors in the myofascial pain dysfunction syndrome. J. Ala. Dent. Assoc. 62:22–26, 1978.

Griffin, J.W., and McClure, M. Adverse responses to transcutaneous electrical nerve stimulation in a patient with rheumatoid arthritis. Phys. Ther. 61:354–355, 1981.

Griffiths, R.H. Report of the President's conference on the examination, diagnosis, and management of temporomandibular disorders. J. Am. Dent. Assoc. 106:75–79, 1983.

Grosfeld, O., and Czarnecka, B. Musculo-articular disorders of the stomatognathic system in school children examined according to clinical criteria. J. Oral Rehabil. 4:193–200, 1977.

Gross, A., and Gale, E.N. A prevalence study of the clinical signs associated with mandibular dysfunction. J. Am. Dent. Assoc. 197:932–936, 1983.

Gysi, A. The problem of articulation. Dent. Cosmos 52:1–19, 148–169, 403–418, 1910.

Haddad, A.W. The functioning dentition. pp. 146–183 *In* Y. Kawamura (ed.) Frontiers of Oral Physiology. Basel, Switzerland: S. Karger, 1974.

Hall, L.J. Physical therapy treatment results for 178 patients with temporomandibular joint syndrome. Am. J. Otol. 5:183–196, 1984.

Halpern, L.M. Psychotropic drugs and the management of chronic pain. Adv. Neurol. 4:539–545, 1974.

Halpern, L.M. Analgesic drugs in management of pain. Arch. Surg. 112:861–869, 1977.

Hamada, T., Kotani, H., Kawazoe, Y., and Yameda, S. Effect of occlusal splints on the EMG activity of masseter and temporal muscles in bruxism with clinical symptoms. J. Oral Rehabil. 9:119–123, 1982.

Hannam, A.G. Mastication in man. *In* P. Bryant, E. Gale, and J. Rugh (eds.) Oral Motor Behavior: Impact on Oral Conditions and Dental Treatment. Workshop Proceed-

ings, 16–17 May 1979. NIH Pub. no. 79-1845, Aug. 1979.
Hannam, A.G. Optimum occlusal relationships are essential for cranio-mandibular harmony. Position Paper. pp. 167–175 *In* I. Klineberg and B. Sessle (eds.) Oro-Facial Pain and Neuromuscular Dysfunction. Mechanisms and Clinical Correlates. Advances in the Biosciences. Oxford: Pergamon Press, 1984.
Hannam, A.G., De Cou, R.E., Scott, J.D., and Wood, W.W. The relationship between dental occlusion, muscle activity and associated jaw movement in man. Arch. Oral Biol. 22:25–32, 1977.
Hannam, A.G., and Matthews, B. Reflex jaw opening in response to stimulation of periodontal mechanoreceptors in the cat. Arch. Oral Biol. 14:415–419, 1969.
Hannam, A.G., Wood, W.W., De Cou, R.E., and Scott, J.D. The effects of working-side occlusal interferences on muscle activity and associated jaw movements in man. Arch. Oral Biol. 26:387–392, 1981.
Hansson, P., Ekblom, A., Thomsson, M., and Fjellner, B. Influence of naloxone on relief of acute oro-facial pain by transcutaneous electrical nerve stimulation (TENS) or vibration. Pain 24:323–329, 1986.
Hansson, P., and Ekblom, A. Transcutaneous electrical nerve stimulation (TENS) as compared to placebo TENS for the relief of acute oro-facial pain. Pain 15:157–165, 1983.
Hansson, T., and Milner, M. A study of the occurrence of symptoms of diseases of the temporomandibular joint, masticatory musculature, and related structures. J. Oral Rehabil. 2:313–324, 1975.
Hansson, T., and Öberg, T. Arthrosis and deviation in form in the temporomandibular joint: a macroscopic study on a human autopsy material. Acta Odontol. Scand. 35:167–174, 1977.
Hansson, T., Öberg, T., Carlsson, G.E., and Kopp, S. Thickness of the soft tissue layers and the articular disk in the temporomandibular joint. Acta Odontol. Scand. 35:77–83, 1977.
Haraldson, T., and Ingervall, B. Silent period and jaw jerk reflex in patients with osseointegrated oral implant bridges. J. Dent. Res. 87:365–372, 1979.
Haraldson, T., Karlsson, U., and Carlsson, G.E. Bite force and oral function in complete denture wearers. J. Oral Rehabil. 6:41–48, 1979.
Haraldson, T., and Mejersjö, C. Temporal arteritis: a report on two cases. Swed. Dent. J. 6:121–125, 1982.
Hargreaves, A.S., and Wardle, J.J.M. The use of physiotherapy in the treatment of temporomandibular disorders. Br. Dent. J. 155:121–124, 1983.
Harpman, J.A., and Woollard, H.H. The tendon of the lateral pterygoid muscle. J. Anat. 73:112–115, 1938.
Harrigan, W.F. Occlusion and surgery. Dent. Clin. North Am. 25:439–453, 1981.
Hartmann, E. Alcohol and bruxism. New Engl. J. Med. 301:333–334, 1979.
Hekneby, M. The load of the temporomandibular joint: physical calculations and analyses. J. Prosthet. Dent. 31:303–312, 1974.
Helkimo, M. Studies of function and dysfunction of the masticatory system. II. Index for anamnestic and clinical dysfunction and occlusal state. Swed. Dent. J. 67:101–121, 1974.
Helkimo, M. Various centric positions and methods of recording them. Chapt. 16 *In* G.A. Zarb, B. Bergman, J.A. Clayton, and H.F. MacKay (eds.) Prosthodontic Treatment for Partially Edentulous Patients. St. Louis: C.V. Mosby Co., 1978.
Helkimo, M.I., Bailey, J.O., Jr., and Ash, M.M., Jr. Correlations of electromyographic silent period duration and the Helkimo dysfunction index. Acta Odontal. Scand. 37:51–56, 1979.
Helm, S. Malocclusion in Danish children with adolescent dentition: an epidemiologic study. Am. J. Orthod. 54:352–366, 1968.
Helm, S. Prevalence of malocclusion in relation to development of the dentition. Acta Odontol. Scand. 28:(Suppl. 58):1–121, 1970.
Heløe, B., and Heiberg, A. A multiprofessional study of patients with myofascial pain-dysfunction syndrome. II. Acta Odontol. Scand. 38:119–128, 1980.
Henny, F.A. Intra-articular injection of hydrocortisone into the temporomandibular joint. J. Oral Surg. 12:314–320, 1954.
Hickey, J.C., Allison, M.L., Woelfel, J.B., Boucher, C.O., and Stacy, R.W. Mandibular movements in three dimensions. J. Prosthet. Dent. 13:72–92, 1963.
Hickey, J.C., Zarb, G.A., and Bolender, C.L. Boucher's Prosthodontic Treatment for Edentulous Patients. 9th ed. St. Louis: C.V. Mosby Co., 1985.
Hillsbery, K. Shark attack. Rolling Stone Aug 5:25–26, 28–29, 1982.
Hirschfeld, I. The individual missing tooth: a factor in dental and periodontal disease. J. Am. Dent. Assoc. 24:67–82, 1937.
Hoogmartems, M.J., Stuyck, J., Bockx, E., Cheng, N., Jacobs, G., Nijs, J., Vanderfacillie, J., Vanhoof, F., and Wonters, F. Stretch sensitivity of primary spindle endings in masseter and temporalis muscles: lateralization and association with unilateral preference pattern of mastication. Electromyogr. Clin. Neurophysiol. 20:369–381, 1980.
Houde, R. Clinical pharmacology (opiates and other compounds). pp. 191–203 *In* L.K.Y. Ng and J.J. Bonica (eds.) Pain, Discomfort and Humanitarian Care. New York: Elsevier, 1980.
Hussein, S.M., and McCall, W.D., Jr. Masseteric silent periods electrically evoked in normal subjects and patients with temporomandibular joint dysfunction. Exp. Neurol. 81:64–76, 1983.
Hylander, W.L. The human mandible: lever or link? Am. J. Phys. Anthropol. 43:227–242, 1975.
Hylander, W.L. Incisal bite force direction in humans and the functional significance of mammalian mandibular translation. Am. J. Phys. Anthropol. 48:1–8, 1978.
Hylander, W.L. An experimental analysis of temporomandibular joint reaction force in Macaques. Am. J. Phys. Anthropol. 51:433–456, 1979a.
Hylander, W.L. Functional anatomy. Chapt. 5 *In* B.G. Sarnat and D.M. Laskin (eds.) The Temporomandibular Joint. 3rd ed. Springfield: Charles C Thomas Publ., 1979b.
Ingersoll, W.B., and Kerens, E.G. A treatment for excessive occlusal trauma of bruxism. J. Am. Dent. Assoc. 44:22–27, 1952.
Ingervall, B. Studies of mandibular positions in children. Odont. Revy 19 (Suppl. 15):1–52, 1968.
Ingervall, B. Tooth contacts on the functional and nonfunctional side in children and young adults. Arch. Oral Biol. 17:191–200, 1972a.

Ingervall, B. Range of sagittal movement of the mandibular condyles and inclination of the condyle path in children and adults. Acta Odontol. Scand. 30:67–87, 1972b.

Ingervall, B. Prevalence of dental and occlusal anomalies in Swedish conscripts. Acta Odontol. Scand. 32:83–92, 1974.

Ingervall, B. Facial morphology and activity of temporal and lip muscles during swallowing and chewing. Angle Orthod. 46:372–380, 1976.

Ingervall, B., and Carlsson, G. Masticatory muscle activity before and after elimination of balancing side occlusal interferences. J. Oral Rehabil. 9:183–192, 1982.

Ingervall, B., and Helkimo, E. Masticatory muscle force and facial morphology in man. Arch. Oral Biol. 23:203–206, 1978.

Ingervall, B., Mohlin, B., and Thilander, B. Prevalence of symptoms of functional disturbances of the masticatory system in Swedish men. J. Oral Rehabil. 7:185–197, 1980.

Ingervall, B., Ridall, A., and Thilander, B. Changes in activity of the temporal muscles and lip muscles after surgical correction of mandibular prognathism. Int. J. Oral Surg. 8:290–300, 1979.

Ingervall, B., and Thilander, B. Relation between facial morphology and activity of the masticatory muscles. J. Oral Rehabil. 1:131–147, 1974.

Ingervall, B., and Thilander, B. Activity of temporal and masseter muscles in children with a lateral forced bite. Angle Orthod. 45:249–258, 1975.

Ingle, J.I. Alveolar osteoporosis and pulpal death associated with compulsive bruxism. Oral Surg. Oral Med. Oral Pathol. 13:1371–1381, 1960.

Ingle, J.I. Occupational bruxism and its relation to periodontal disease. J. Periodontol. 23:7–12, 1952.

Ireland, V.E. Disorders of the mandibular joint. Br. Dent. J. 115:287–291, 1963.

Isaacson, D. A clinical study of the condyle path. J. Prosthet. Dent. 9:927–935, 1959.

Isaacson, R.J. In response: oral health status in the United States: prevalence of malocclusion. J. Dent. Ed. 49:397, 1985.

Ito, T., Gibbs, C.H., Marquelles-Bonnet, R., Lupkiewicz, S.M., Young, H.M., Lundeen, H.C., and Mahan, P.E. Loading on the temporomandibular joints with five occlusal conditions. J. Prosthet. Dent. 56:478–483, 1986.

Jablonski, S. Illustrated Dictionary of Dentistry. Philadelphia: W.B. Saunders Co., 1982.

Jagger, R.G., and Carlsson, G.E. Temporomandibular pain-dysfunction and disorders of the parotid gland. Swed. Dent. J. 2:17–21, 1978.

Jameson, L.M., and Malone, W.F.P. Crown contours and gingival response. J. Prosthet. Dent. 47:620–624, 1982.

Jankelson, B. Neuromuscular aspects of occlusion. Dent. Clin. North Am. 23:157–168, 1979.

Janson, M. Long-term effects of orthodontic treatment. A functional, cephalometric and clinical study of Angle Class II, Division 1 malocclusion cases. Thesis. Norway: University of Bergen, 1981.

Jenkins, J. Preprosthodontic orthodontic treatment. Chapt. 13 *In* G.A. Zarb, B. Bergman, J.A. Clayton, and H.F. MacKay (eds.) Prosthodontic Treatment for Partially Edentulous Patients. St. Louis: C.V. Mosby Co., 1978.

Jenkins, G.N. The Physiology of the Mouth. 3rd ed. Philadelphia: Davis Co., 1966.

Jeter, T.S., Van Sickels, J.E., and Dolwick, M.F. Modified techniques for internal fixation of sagittal ramus osteotomies. J. Oral Maxillofac. Surg. 42:270–272, 1984.

Johanson, D.C., and Edey, M.A. Lucy: The Beginnings of Humankind. New York: Simon and Schuster, 1981.

Johanson, D.C., and White, T.D. A systematic assessment of early African hominids. Science 203:321–330, 1979.

Johanson, D.C., White, T., and Coppens, Y. A new species of the genus *Australopithecus* (Primates: Hominidae) from the Pilocene of eastern Africa. Kirtlandia no. 28: pp. 1–14, 1978.

Johnstone, D.R., and Templeton, M. The feasibility of palpating the lateral pterygoid muscle. J. Prosthet. Dent. 44:318–323, 1980.

Jolly, A. The evolution of primate behavior. Am. Sci. 73:230–239, 1985.

Jones, H.G. The primary dentition in *Homo sapiens* and the search for primitive features. Am. J. Phys. Anthropol. 5:251–282, 1947.

Kahn, J. Iontophoresis and ultrasound for postsurgical temporomandibular trismus and paresthesia. Phys. Ther. 60:307–308, 1980.

Kamen, S. Tardive dyskinesia: a significant syndrome for geriatric dentistry. Oral Surg. Oral Med. Oral Pathol. 39:52–57, 1975.

Kanter, F. The use of bite plates. pp. 300–306 *In* L. Schwartz (ed.) The Disorders of the Temporomandibular Joint. Philadelphia: W.B. Saunders Co., 1959.

Kao, F.F., and Kao, J.J. (eds.) Recent Advances in Acupuncture Research. New York: Institute for Advanced Research in Asian Science and Medicine, Inc., 1979.

Kaplan, R.L. Gnathology as a basis for a concept of occlusion. Dent. Clin. North Am., pp. 577–590, 1963.

Kardachi, B.J.R., Bailey, J.O., Jr., and Ash, M.M., Jr. A comparison of biofeedback and occlusal adjustment on bruxism. J. Periodontol. 49:367–372, 1978.

Kawamura, Y. Neurophysiologic background of occlusion. Periodontics 5:175–183, 1967.

Kawazoe, Y., Kotani, H., Hamada, T., and Yamada, S. Effect of occlusal splints on the electromyographic activities of masseter muscles during maximum clenching in patients with myofascial pain-dysfunction syndrome. J. Prosthet. Dent. 43:578–580, 1980.

Kaye, L.B., Moran, J.H., and Fritz, M.E. Statistical analysis of an urban population of 236 patients with head and neck pain. Part II. Patient symptomatology. J. Periodontol. 50:59–65, 1979.

Käyser, A.F. Shortened dental arches and oral function. J. Oral Rehabil. 8:457–462, 1981.

Keagy, R.D., and Keim, H.A. Intra-articular steroid therapy: repeated use in patients with chronic arthritis. Am. J. Med. Sci. 75:145–152, 1967.

Keefe, F.J., and Gil, K.M. Recent advances in the behavioral assessment and treatment of chronic pain. Ann. Behav. Med. 3:11–16, 1985.

Kempson, G.E., Tuke, M.A., Dingle, J.T., Barrett, A.J., and Horsfield, P.H. The effects of proteolytic enzymes on the mechanical properties of adult human articular cartilage. Biochem. Biophys. Acta 428:741–760, 1976.

Kimbel, W.H., White, I.D., and Johanson, D.C. Cranial morphology of *Australopithecus afarensis:* a comparative study based on a composite reconstruction of the adult skull. Am. J. Phys. Anthropol. 64:337–388, 1984.

Kindlova, M. Blood supply of the marginal periodontium in *Macacus Rhesus*. Arch. Oral Biol. 10:869–874, 1965.

Klineberg, I. Influence of temporomandibular articular mechanoreceptors on functional jaw movements. J. Oral Rehabil. 7:307–317, 1980.

Koerber, K.H. Elektronische Registrierung der Unterkieferbewegungen im normalen und okklusionsgestorten Gebiss. Dtsch. Zahnarztl. Z. 26:167–176, 1971.

Komori, E., Sugisaki, M., Tanabe, H., and Katoh, S. Discomalleolar ligament in the adult human. J. Craniomandib. Prac. 4:300–305, 1986.

Kopp, S. Topographical distribution of sulphated glycosaminoglysans in human temporomandibular joint disks. J. Oral Pathol. 5:265–276, 1976.

Kopp, S. Clinical findings in temporomandibular joint osteoarthrosis. Scand. J. Dent. Res. 85:434, 1977a.

Kopp, S. Constancy of clinical signs in patients with mandibular dysfunction. Community Dent. Oral Epidemiol. 5:94–98, 1977b.

Kopp, S. Temporomandibular joint osteoarthrosis. A histochemical and clinical study. Thesis. University of Göteborg, Sweden, 1977c.

Kopp, S. Topographical distribution of sulphated glycosaminoglysans in the surface layers of the human temporomandibular joint. J. Oral. Pathol. 7:283–294, 1978.

Kopp, S. Short term evaluation of counselling and occlusal adjustment in patients with mandibular dysfunction involving the temporomandibular joint. J. Oral Res. 6:101–109, 1979.

Kopp, S. Pain and functional disturbances of the masticatory system—a review of etiology and principles of treatment. Swed. Dent. J. 6:49–60, 1982.

Kopp, S., and Rockler, B. Variation in interpretation of radiographs of temporomandibular and hand joints. Dentomaxillofacial Radiogr. 7:95–102, 1978.

Kopp, S., and Wennenberg, B. Effects of occlusal treatment and intra-articular injections on TMJ pain and dysfunction. Acta Odontol. Scand. 39:87–96, 1981.

Kraus, B.S., Jordan, R.E., and Abrams, L. Dental Anatomy and Occlusion. Baltimore: Williams & Wilkins Co., 1969.

Kraus, H. The use of surface anesthesia in the treatment of painful motion. J. Am. Med. Assoc. 16:2582–2583, 1941.

Kraus, H. Muscle function and the temporomandibular joint. J. Prosthet. Dent. 13:950–955, 1963.

Kraus, H. Clinical Treatment of Back and Neck Pain. New York: McGraw-Hill, 1970.

Kraus, H. Trigger points. New York State J. Med. 73:1310–1314, 1973.

Krogh-Poulsen, W. Taendernes Morfologi. 3rd ed. Copenhagen: Munksgaard, 1958.

Krogh-Poulsen, W. Taendernes kontaktrelationer. *In* W. Krogh-Poulsen and O. Carlsen (eds.) Ortofunktion. Bidfunktion-Bettfysiologi. Copenhagen: Munksgaard, 1973.

Krogh-Poulsen, W. Klinisk undersøgelse. pp. 423–463 *In* W. Krogh-Poulsen and O. Carlsen (eds.) Bidfunktion/Bettfysiologi. Patofunktion. Copenhagen: Munksgaard, 1974.

Krogh-Poulsen, W.G., and Olsson, A. Management of the occlusion of the teeth. pp. 236–280 *In* L. Schwartz and C.M. Chayes (eds.) Facial Pain and Mandibular Dysfunction. Philadelphia: W.B. Saunders, Co., 1968.

Kubota, K. Motoneurone mechanisms: suprasegmental controls. pp. 60–75 *In* B.J. Sessle and A.G. Hannam (eds.) Mastication and Swallowing: Biological and Clinical Correlates. Toronto: University of Toronto Press, 1976.

Kundert, M., and Palla, S. Deutung und Fehldeutung in der okklusionsdiagnostischen Kiefergelenkradiologie. Schweiz. Mschr. Zahnheilk. 87:465–481, 1977.

Lamarre, Y., and Lund, J.P. Load compensation in human masseter muscles. J. Physiol. (Lond.) 253:21–35, 1975.

Lance, J.W. Mechanism and Management of Headache. 3rd ed. London: Butterworths, 1978.

Larson, C.R., Smith, A., and Luschei, E.S. Response characteristics of jaw muscle spindle and tooth mechanoreceptor afferents in monkeys during a controlled isometric biting task. pp. 175–185 *In* Y. Kawamura and R. Dubner (eds.) Oral-Facial Sensory and Motor Functions. Tokyo: Quintessence Publ. Co., 1981.

Larsson, E., and Ronnerman, A. Mandibular dysfunction symptoms in orthodontically treated patients ten years after the completion of treatment. Eur. J. Orthod. 3:1–6, 1981.

Lascelles, R.G. Atypical facial pain and depression. Br. J. Psychiat. 112:652–659, 1966.

Laskin, D.M. Etiology of the pain dysfunction syndrome. J. Am. Dent. Assoc. 79:147–153, 1969.

Laskin, D.M., and Greene, C. Influence of the doctor-patient relationship on placebo therapy for patients with myofascial pain-dysfunction (MPD) syndrome. J. Am. Dent. Assoc. 85:892–894, 1972.

Laskin, D.M., Ryan, W.A., and Greene, C.S. Incidence of temporomandibular symptoms in patients with major skeletal malocclusions: a survey of oral and maxillofacial surgery training programs. Oral Surg. Oral Med. Oral Pathol. 61:537–541, 1986.

Laskin, J.L., Wallace, W.R., and DeLeo, B. Use of bupivacaine hydrochloride in oral surgery—a clinical study. J. Oral Surg. 35:25–29, 1977.

Lawrence, T.N., Ellis, E., and McNamara, J.A. The frequency and distribution of skeletal and dental components in Class II orthognathic surgery patients. J. Oral Maxillofac. Surg. 43:29–34, 1985.

Lawson, R. Tooth replacement in the frog, *Rana temporaria*. J. Morph. 119:233–240, 1966.

Leavit, K. The needling effects in the relief of myofascial pain. Pain 6:83–90, 1979.

Le Gros Clark, W.E. History of the Primates. London: Trustees British Museum, 1965.

Leighton, B. Early recognition of normal occlusion. *In* J.A. McNamara, Jr. (ed.) The Biology of Occlusal Development. Ann Arbor: Center for Human Growth and Development, The University of Michigan. 1:147–167, 1977.

Levine, J.D., Gordon, N.C., and Fields, H.L. The mechanism of placebo analgesia. Lancet 2:654–657, 1978.

Lieb, M.M. Oral orthopedics. *In* H. Gelb (ed.) Clinical Management of Head, Neck and TMJ Pain and Dysfunction. Philadelphia: W.B. Saunders Co., 1977.

Liem, L.F. The pharyngeal jaw apparatus of the embiotocidae (Teleostei): a functional and evolutionary perspective. Copeia 2:311–323, 1986.

Lillegraven, J.A., Kielan-Jaworowska, Z., and Clemens, W.P. Mesozoic Mammals: The First Two Thirds of Mammalian History. Berkeley: Univ. of California Press, 1979.

Lindahl, L. Condylar fractures of the mandible. A longitudinal study. Thesis. Sweden: University of Göteborg, 1977.

Linden, R.W.A. Touch thresholds of vital and nonvital hu-

man teeth. Exp. Neurol. 48:387–390, 1975.
Linder-Aronson, S. Adenoids, their effect on mode of breathing and nasal airflow and their relationship to characteristics of the facial skeleton and the dentition. Acta Otolaryngol. Suppl. 265, pp. 1–132, 1970.
Lindhe, J., and Nyman, S. The role of occlusion in periodontal disease and the biological rationale for splinting in treatment of periodontitis. Oral Sci. Rev. 10:11–43, 1977.
Lindhe, J., and Svanberg, G. Influence of trauma from occlusion on progression of experimental periodontitis in the beagle dog. J. Clin. Periodontol. 1:3–14, 1974.
Lindqvist, B., and Heijbel, J. Bruxism in children with brain damage. Acta Odontol. Scand. 32:313–319, 1974.
Lindqvist, L.W., and Carlsson, G.E. Long-term effects on chewing with mandibular fixed prostheses on osseointegrated implants. Acta Odontol. Scand. 43:390–395, 1985.
Loeser, J.D., Black, R.G., and Christman, A. Relief of pain by transcutaneous stimulation. J. Neurosurg. 42:308–314, 1975.
Lous, I. The importance of referred pain in myogenic headache. Headache 16:119–122, 1976.
Lous, I., and Olesen, J. Evaluation of pericranial tenderness and oral function in patients with common migrane, muscle contraction headache and "combination headache." Pain 12:385–393, 1982.
Lovejoy, C.O. A reconstruction of the pelvis of AL-288 (Hadar formation Ethiopia). Am. J. Phys. Anthropol. 50:460, 1979.
Lovejoy, C.O. The origin of man. Science 211:341–350, 1981. (See also "Letters," Science 217:295–306, 1982.)
Lowe, A.A., and Johnston, W.D. Tongue and jaw muscle activity in response to mandibular rotations in a sample of normal and anterior open-bite subjects. Am. J. Orthod. 76:565–576, 1979.
Lund, J.P. Evidence for a central neural pattern generator regulating the chewing cycle. pp. 204–212 *In* D.J. Anderson and B. Matthews (eds.) Mastication. Bristol: John Wright & Sons, 1976.
Lund, J.P. Sensorimotor integration in the control of mastication. pp. 51–65 *In* I. Klineberg and B.J. Sessle (eds.) Oro-Facial Pain and Neuromuscular Dysfunction. Oxford: Pergamon Press Inc., 1985.
Lund, J.P., and Dellow, P.G. The influence of interactive stimuli on rhythmical masticatory movements in rabbits. Arch. Oral Biol. 16:215–223, 1971.
Lund, J.P., and Matthews, B. Responses of temporomandibular joint afferents recorded in the Gasserian ganglion of the rabbit to passive movements of the mandible. pp. 153–160 *In* Y. Kawamura and R. Dubner (eds.) Oral-Facial Sensory and Motor Functions. Tokyo: Quintessence Publ. Co., 1981.
Lund, J.P., and Olsson, K.A. The importance of reflexes and their control during jaw movement. Trends Neurosci. 6:458–463. 1983.
Lund, J.P., Richmond, F.J.R., Touloumis, C., Patry, Y., and Lamarre, Y. The distribution of Golgi tendon organs and muscle spindles in masseter and temporalis muscles of the cat. Neuroscience 3:259–270, 1978.
Lund, J.P., and Rossignol, S. Modulation of the amplitude of the digastric jaw opening reflex during the masticatory cycle. Neuroscience 6:95–98, 1981.
Lund, J.P., Smith, A.M., Sessle, B.J., and Murakami, T. Activity of trigeminal alpha and gamma motoneurons and muscle afferents during performance of a biting task. J. Neurophysiol. 42:710–725, 1979.
Lund, J.P., Touloumis, C., Patry, Y., Lamarre, Y., and Richmond, F. The distribution of Golgi tendon organs and muscle spindles in the masseter and temporalis muscles of the cat. Neuroscience 3:259–270, 1978.
Lund, P.C., Crivk, J.D., and Pagdanganen, R.T. Etidocaine—a new long-acting local anesthetic agent: a clinical evaluation. Anesth. Analg. 52:482–490, 1973.
Lundeen, H.C., Shryock, E.F., and Gibbs, C.H. An evaluation of mandibular border movements: their character and significance. J. Prosthet. Dent. 40:442–452, 1978.
Macalister, A.D. The development of the human temporomandibular joint. Aust. Dent. J. 59:21–27, 1955.
MacKenna, B.R., and Turker, K.S. Twitch tension in the jaw muscles of the cat at various degrees of mouth opening. Arch. Oral Biol. 23:917–920, 1978.
Magee, K.R. Bruxism related to levodopa therapy. J. Am. Med. Assoc. 214:147, 1970.
Magnusson, T. Mandibular dysfunction and recurrent headache. Thesis, Faculty of Odontology, University of Göteborg, Sweden, 1981.
Magnusson, T. Changes in recurrent headache and mandibular dysfunction after treatment with new complete dentures. J. Oral Rehabil. 9:95–105, 1982.
Magnusson, T., and Carlsson, G.E. Recurrent headaches in relation to temporomandibular joint pain-dysfunction. Acta Odontol. Scand. 36:333–338, 1978.
Magnusson, T., and Carlsson, G.E. Changes in recurrent headache and mandibular dysfunction after various types of dental treatment. Acta Odontol. Scand. 38:311–320, 1980a.
Magnusson, T., and Carlsson, G.E. Treatment of patients with functional disturbances in the masticatory system. A survey of 80 consecutive patients. Swed. Dent. J. 4:145–153, 1980b.
Magnusson, T., and Carlsson, G.E. A 2½-year follow-up of changes in headache and mandibular dysfunction after stomatognathic treatment. J. Prosthet. Dent. 49:398–402, 1983a.
Magnusson, T., and Carlsson, G.E. Occlusal adjustment in patients with persistent or recurrent signs of mandibular dysfunction after stomatognathic treatment. J. Prosthet. Dent. 49:706–710, 1983b.
Magnusson, T., and Enbom, L. Signs and symptoms of mandibular dysfunction after introduction of experimental balancing-side interferences. Acta Odontol. Scand. 42:129–135, 1984.
Mahan, P.E., Wilkinson, T.M., Gibbs, C.H., Mauderli, A., and Brannon, L.S. Superior and inferior bellies of the lateral pterygoid muscle EMG activity at basic jaw positions. J. Prosthet. Dent. 50:710–718, 1983.
Maitland, G.D. Peripheral Manipulation. 2nd ed. London: Butterworths, 1977, pp. 318–329.
Malmgren, O. Studies on the need and demand for orthodontic treatment. Swed. Dent. J. Suppl. 6, pp. 1–103, 1980.
Malow, R.M., Olson, R.E., and Greene, C.S. Myofascial pain dysfunction syndrome: a psychophysiological disorder. pp. 101–133 *In* C. Golden, S. Alcaparras, F. Strider, and B. Graber (eds.) Applied Techniques in Behavioral Medicine. New York: Grune and Stratton, 1981.
Mann, A.W., and Pankey, L.D. The P.M. philosophy of occlusal rehabilitation. Dent. Clin. North Am. Nov.:621–

636, 1963.
Manns, A., Miralles, R., and Guerrero, F. The changes in electrical activity of the postural muscles of the mandible upon varying the vertical dimension. J. Prosthet. Dent. 45:438–445, 1981.
Manns, A., Miralles, R., and Palazzi, C. EMG, bite force, and elongation of the masseter muscle under isometric voluntary contractions and variations of vertical dimension. J. Prosthet. Dent. 42:674–682, 1979.
Manns, A., and Spreng, M. EMG amplitude and frequency at different muscular elongations under constant masticatory force or EMG activity. Acta Physiol. Lat. Am. 27:259–271, 1977.
Marbach, J. Phantom bite syndrome. Am. J. Psychiatry 134:476–479, 1978.
Marshall, W.G. The relationship between the meniscus of the TMJ and the anterior ligament of the malleus. J. Dent. Res. 54:649 (Abstr. no. 26), 1975.
Martin, R. Review of "The Comparative Biology and Evolutionary Relationships of Tree Shrews." W.P. Lackett (ed.) Science 211:813, 1981.
Matthews, B.F. Collagen/chondroitin sulphate ratio of human articular cartilage related to function. Br. Med. J. 2:1295, 1952.
McCall, W.D., Jr., Bailey, J.O., and Ash, M.M. A quantitative measure of mandibular joint dysfunction: phase plane modelling of jaw movement in man. Arch. Oral Biol. 21:685–689, 1976.
McCall, W.D., Jr., Gale, E.N., and Uthman, A.A. The variability of EMG silent periods in TMJ patients. J. Oral Rehabil. 8:103–105, 1981.
McCall, W.D., Jr., Uthman, A.A., and Mohl, N.D. Symptom severity and EMG silent periods. J. Dent. Res. 57:709–714, 1978.
McCarty, W. Diagnosis and treatment of internal derangements of the articular disc and mandibular condyle. pp. 145–168 *In* W.K. Solberg and G.T. Clark (eds.) Temporomandibular Joint Problems: Biologic Diagnosis and Treatment. Chicago: Quintessence Publ. Co., 1980.
McCollum, B.B. Considering the mouth as a functioning unit as the basis of a dental diagnosis. J. South. Calif. Dent. Assoc. 5:268–276, 1938.
McCollum, B.B. Fundamentals involved in prescribing restorative dental remedies. Dent. Items Interest 61:522–533, 641–648, 724–736, 852–863, 942–950, 1939.
McCollum, B.B., and Stuart, C.E. A Research Report. South Pasadena, Calif.: Scientific Press, 1955.
McHenry, H.M. Relative cheek-tooth size in Australopithecines. Am. J. Phys. Anthropol. 64:297–306, 1984.
McLain, J.B., and Proffitt, W.R. Oral health status in the United States: prevalence of malocclusion. J. Dent. Ed. 49:386–396, 1985.
McLean, J.W. The science and art of dental ceramics. pp. 99–124 *In* J.F. Bates, D.J. Neill, and H.W. Preiskel (eds.) Restoration of the Partially Dentate Mouth. Chicago: Quintessence Publ. Co., 1984.
McNamara, D.C. Inhibitory effects in the masticatory neuromusculature of human subjects in a median occlusal position. Arch. Oral Biol. 21:329–331, 1976.
McNamara, J.A., Jr. The independent functions of the two heads of the lateral pterygoid muscles. Am. J. Anat. 138:197–206, 1973.
McNamara, J.A., Jr. Components of Class II malocclusion in children 8–10 years of age. Angle Orthod. 51:177–202, 1981.
McNamara, J.A., Jr. A method of cephalometric evaluation. Am. J. Orthod. 86:449–469, 1984a.
McNamara, J.A., Jr. Dentofacial adaptations in adult patients following functional regulator therapy. Am. J. Orthod. 85:57–71, 1984b.
McNamara, J.A., Jr., Bookstein, F.L., and Shaughnessy, T.G. Skeletal and dental changes following functional regulator therapy on Class II patients. Am. J. Orthod. 88:91–110, 1985.
McNamara, J.A., Jr., and Carlson, D.S. Quantitative analysis of temporomandibular joint adaptations to protrusive function. Am. J. Orthod. 76:593–611, 1979.
Mehringer, E.J. The use of speech patterns as an aid in prosthodontic reconstruction. J. Prosthet. Dent. 13:825–836, 1963.
Mejersjö, C., and Carlsson, G.E. Long-term results of treatment for temporomandibular joint pain-dysfunction. J. Prosthet. Dent. 49:809–815, 1983.
Mejersjö, C., and Carlsson, G.E. Analysis of factors influencing the long-term effect of treatment of TMJ-pain dysfunction. J. Oral Rehabil. 11:289–297, 1984.
Melcher, A.H. Periodontal ligament. pp. 204–239 *In* S.N. Bhaskar (ed.) Orban's Oral Histology and Embryology. 9th ed. St. Louis: C.V. Mosby Co., 1980.
Melcher, A.H., and Eastoe, J.E. The connective tissues of the periodontium. pp. 167–343 *In* A.H. Melcher and W.H. Bowen (eds.) Biology of the Periodontium. New York: Academic Press, 1969.
Meyenberg, M., Kubik, S., and Palla, S. Relationships of the muscles of mastication to the articular disc of the temporomandibular joint. Helv. Odont. Acta 30:1–20, 1986.
Mikami, D.B. A review of psychogenic aspects and treatment of bruxism. J. Prosthet. Dent. 37:411–419, 1977.
Miller, W.A. Pulp calcifications in a Taurodont tooth. Br. Dent. J. 126:456–459, 1968.
Miller, W.A. The tooth enamel of *Latimeria Chalumnae*. Nature (Lond.) 221:1242, 1969.
Miller, W.A., and Radnor, C.J.P. Tooth replacement patterns in young *Caiman sclerops*. J. Morphol. 130:501–510, 1970.
Miller, W.A., and Radnor, C.J.P. Tooth replacement in the Bowfin (*Amia calva:* Holostei). J. Morphol. 140:381–396, 1973.
Miller, W.A., and Rowe, D.J. Variations in tooth replacement patterns in adult *Necturus maculosus*. J. Morphol. 140:63–76, 1973.
Moffett, B. The morphogenesis of the temporomandibular joint. Am. J. Orthod. 52:401–415, 1966.
Moffett, B. Classification and diagnosis of temporomandibular joint disturbances. *In* W.K. Solberg and G.T. Clark (eds.) Temporomandibular Joint Problems: Biologic Diagnosis and Treatment. Chicago: Quintessence Publ. Co., 1980.
Moffett, B.C. The prenatal development of the human temporomandibular joint. no. 243 *In* Contributions to Embryology. Washington: Carnegie Institute, 1957.
Moffett, B.C. The temporomandibular joint. Chapt. 6 *In* J.J. Sherry (ed.) Complete Denture Prosthodontics. New York: McGraw-Hill, 1962.
Moffett, B.C., Johnson, L.C., McCabe, J.B., and Askew, H.C. Articular remodeling in the adult human temporomandibular joint. Am. J. Anat. 115:119–142, 1964.
Moffett, B.C., Lent, C.J., McCabe, J.B., and Askew, H.C.

Articular remodelling in the human adult temporomandibular joint. Am. J. Anat. 115:119–147, 1964.
Mohl, N.D. The role of head posture in mandibular function. pp. 97–111 *In* W.K. Solberg and G.T. Clark (eds.) Abnormal Jaw Mechanics: Diagnosis and Treatment. Chicago: Quintessence Publ. Co., 1984.
Mohlin, B. Prevalence of mandibular dysfunction and relation between malocclusion and mandibular dysfunction in a group of women in Sweden. Eur. J. Orthod. 5:115–123, 1983.
Mohlin, B., and Kopp, S. A clinical study of the relationship between malocclusions, occlusal interferences and mandibular pain and dysfunction. Swed. Dent. J. 2:105–112, 1978.
Moldofsky, H., Scarisbrick, P., Englan, R., and Smyth, H. Musculoskeletal symptoms and non-REM sleep disturbances in patients with "Fibrositis Syndrome" and healthy subjects. Psychosom. Med. 37:341–351, 1975.
Molin, C., Edman, G., and Schalling, D. Psychological studies of patients with mandibular pain dysfunction syndrome (MDS). II. Tolerance for experimentally induced pain. Sven. Tandlak. Tidskr. 66:15–23, 1973.
Møller, E. The chewing apparatus. Acta Physiol. Scand. 69 (Suppl. 280):1–229, 1966.
Møller, E. Evidence that the rest position is subject to servocontrol. pp. 72–80 *In* D.J. Anderson and B. Matthews (eds.) Mastication. Bristol: John Wright & Sons, 1976.
Molnar, S. Human tooth wear, tooth function and cultural variability. Am. J. Phys. Anthropol. 34:175–189, 1971.
Molnar, S., and Gantt, D.G. Functional implications of primate enamel thickness. Am. J. Phys. Anthropol. 86:447–454, 1977.
Moloney, F., and Howard, J.A. Internal derangements of the temporomandibular joint: anterior repositioning splint therapy. Aust. Dent. J. 31:30–39, 1986.
Mongini, F. Remodelling of the mandibular condyle in the adult and its relationship to the condition of the dental arches. Acta Anat. 82:437–453, 1972.
Mongini, F. Dental abrasion as a factor in remodeling of the mandibular condyle. Acta Anat. 92:292–300, 1975.
Mongini, F. Condylar remodeling after occlusal therapy. J. Prosthet. Dent. 43:568–577, 1980.
Mongini, F. Combined method to determine the therapeutic position for occlusal rehabilitation. J. Prosthet. Dent. 47:434–439, 1982.
Mongini, F. Abnormalities in condylar and occlusal positions. pp. 23–43 *In* W.K. Solberg and G.T. Clark (eds.) Abnormal Jaw Mechanics: Diagnosis and Treatment. Chicago: Quintessence Publ. Co., 1983.
Mongini, F., and Capurso, U. Factors influencing the pantographic tracings of mandibular border movements. J. Prosthet. Dent. 48:585–598, 1982.
Monson, G.S. Occlusion as applied to crown and bridgework. J. Natl. Dent. Assoc. 7:399–413, 1920.
Monson, G.S. Some important factors which influence occlusion. J. Am. Dent. Assoc. 9:498–503, 1922.
Monson, G.S. Applied mechanics to the theory of mandibular movements. Dent. Cosmos 74:1039–1053, 1932.
Moorrees, C.F.A., and Kean, M.R. Natural head position: a basic consideration for analysis of cephalometric radiographs. Am. J. Phys. Anthropol. 16:213–234, 1958.
Moorrees, C.F.A., and Reed, R.B. Changes in dental arch dimensions expressed on the basis of tooth eruption as a measure of biologic age. J. Dent. Res. 44:129–141, 1965.
Moss, M.L. Cartilage. Chapt. 6 *In* R.O. Greep (ed.) Histology. 2nd ed. New York: McGraw-Hill, 1966.
Moss, R.A., Hammer, D., Adams, H.E., Jenkins, J.O., Thompson, K., and Haber, J. A more efficient biofeedback procedure for treatment of nocturnal bruxism. J. Oral Rehabil. 9:125–131. 1982.
Moss, R.A., Wedding, D., and Sanders, S.H. The comparative efficacy of relaxation training and masseter EMG feedback in the treatment of TMJ dysfunction. J. Oral Rehabil. 10:9–17, 1983.
Murphy, T.R. The relationship between attritional facets and the occlusal plane in aboriginal Australians. Arch. Oral Biol. 9:269–280, 1964.
Murphy, W.A. Arthrography of the temporomandibular joint. Radiol. Clin. North Am. 19:365–377, 1981.
Myers, D.E., and McCall, W.D., Jr. Head pain as a result of experimental ischemic exercise of the temporalis muscle. Headache 23:113–116, 1983.
Nadler, S.C. Detection and recognition of bruxism. J. Am. Dent. Assoc. 61:472–479, 1960.
Nanda, R., and Sugawara, J. Mandibular adaptations following total maxillary osteotomy in adolescent monkeys. Am. J. Orthod. 83:485–494, 1983.
Nanda, R., Sugawara, J., and Topazian, R.G. Effect of maxillary osteotomy on subsequent craniofacial growth in adolescent monkeys. Am. J. Orthod. 83:391–407, 1983.
Nicol, B.R., Somes, G.W., Ellinger, C.W., Unger, J.W., and Fuhrman, J. Patient response to variations in denture technique. II. Five-year cephalometric evaluation. J. Prosthet. Dent. 41:368–372, 1979.
Noble, H.W. Comparative functional anatomy of the temporo-mandibular joint. *In* G.A. Zarb and G.E. Carlsson (eds.) Temporomandibular Joint Function and Dysfunction. Copenhagen: Munksgaard, 1979.
Nyman, S., and Lindhe, J. A longitudinal study of combined periodontal and prosthetic treatment of patients with advanced periodontal disease. J. Periodontol. 50:163–169, 1979.
Öberg, T. Radiology of the temporomandibular joint. pp. 49–68 *In* W.K. Solberg and G.T. Clark (eds.) Temporomandibular Joint Problems: Biologic Diagnosis and Treatment. Chicago: Quintessence Publ. Co., 1980.
Öberg, T., and Carlsson, G.E. Macroscopic and microscopic anatomy of the temporomandibular joint. Chapt. 3 *In* G.A. Zarb and G.E. Carlsson (eds.) Temporomandibular Joint Function and Dysfunction. St. Louis: C.V. Mosby Co., 1979.
Öberg, T., Carlsson, G.E., and Fajers, C.M. The temporomandibular joint: a morphological study on a human autopsy material. Acta Odontol. Scand. 29:349–384, 1971.
Olkinuora, M. Bruxism: a review of the literature on, and a discussion of studies of bruxism and its psychogenesis and some new psychological hypotheses. Suomen Hammaslaakarisseuran Toimituksia 65:312–324, 1969.
Olkinuora, M. A psychosomatic study of bruxism with emphasis on mental strain and familiar predisposition factors. Proc. Finn. Dent. Soc. 68:110–123, 1972.
Omnell, K.H. Radiology of the TMJ. Chapt. 8 *In* W.B. Kirby (ed.) Current Advances in Oral Surgery. Vol. 3. St. Louis: C.V. Mosby Co., 1980.
O'Neil, R. Relief of chronic facial pain by transcutaneous electrical nerve stimulation. Br. J. Oral Surg. 19:112–115, 1981.

Oppenheim, H., and Wing, M. Benign hypertrophy of masseter muscle. Arch. Otolaryngol. 70:207–210, 1959.
Orban, B., and Weinman, J. Signs of traumatic occlusion in average human jaws. J. Dent. Res. 13:216, 1933.
O'Ryan, F., and Epker, B.N. Deliberate surgical control of mandibular growth: a biomechanical theory. Oral Surg. Oral Med. Oral Pathol. 53:2–18, 1982.
Österberg, T., and Carlsson, G.E. Symptoms and signs of mandibular dysfunction in 70-year-old men and women in Göteborg, Sweden. Community Dent. Oral Epidemiol. 7:315–321, 1979.
Österberg, T., and Steen, B. Relationship between dental state and dietary intake in 70-year-old males and females in Göteborg, Sweden: a population study. J. Oral Rehabil. 9:509–521, 1982.
Öwall, B., and Møller, E. Oral tactile sensibility during biting and chewing. Odont. Rev. 25:327–346, 1974.
Palla, S. Eine Studie über die Kondylenposition in Roentgenbild. Schweiz. Mschr. Zahnheilk. 87:304–315, 1977.
Parsons, M.T., and Boucher, L.J. The bilaminar zone of the meniscus. J. Dent. Res. 45:59–61, 1966.
Paulsen, H.U. Changes in sagittal molar occlusion during growth. Danish Dent. J. 75:1258–1267, 1971.
Perry, H.T., Lammie, G.A., Main, J., and Teuscher, G.W. Occlusion in a stress situation. J. Am. Dent. Assoc. 60:626–633, 1960.
Persson, M., and Sundell, S. Facial morphology and open bite deformity in amelogenesis imperfecta. A roentgencephalometric study. Acta Odontol. Scand. 40:135–144, 1982.
Peyer, B. Comparative Odontology. R. Zangerl (ed.) Chicago: The University of Chicago Press, 1968.
Picton, D.C. Experimental evidence on the role of abnormal contacts in the etiology of periodontal disease. *In* D.J. Anderson and B. Matthews (eds.) Mastication. Bristol: John Wright & Sons, 1976.
Picton, D.C.A., and Wills, D.J. Viscoelastic properties of the periodontal ligament and mucous membrane. J. Prosthet. Dent. 40:263–272, 1978.
Pinto, O.F. A new structure related to the temporomandibular joint and middle ear. J. Prosthet. Dent. 12:95–103, 1962.
Pinto, O.F. Temporomandibular joint problems in underwater activities. J. Prosthet. Dent. 16:772–781, 1966.
Polson, A.M., and Heijl, L.C. Occlusion and periodontal disease. Dent. Clin. North Am. 24:783–795, 1980.
Polson, A.M., Meitner, S.W., and Zander, M.A. Trauma and progression of marginal periodontitis in squirrel monkeys. J. Periodont. Res. 11:279–289, 1976.
Popovich, F., and Grainger, R.M. Burlington orthodontic research centre progress report. Series 2:5–42, 1957–1959.
Popovich, F., and Thompson, G.W. Thumb- and finger-sucking: its relation to malocclusion. Am. J. Orthod. 63:148–155, 1973.
Posselt, U. Studies on the mobility of the human mandible. Acta Odontol. Scand. 10:1–150, 1952.
Posselt, U. Treatment of bruxism by bite guards and bite plates. J. Can. Dent. Assoc. 29:773–778, 1963.
Posselt, U. Physiology of Occlusion and Rehabilitation. 2nd ed. Philadelphia: F.A. Davis Co., 1968.
Poswillo, D.E. The late effects of mandibular condylectomy. Oral Surg. 33:500–511, 1972.
Poswillo, D.E. Congenital malformations: prenatal experimental studies. pp. 127–179 *In* B.G. Sarnat and D.M. Laskin (eds.) The Temporomandibular Joint. A Biological Basis for Clinical Practice. Springfield: Charles C Thomas Publ., 1979.
Proffit, W.R., Epker, B.N., and Ackerman, J.L. Systematic description of dentofacial deformities: the data base. pp. 105–154 *In* W.H. Bell, W.R. Proffit, and R.P. White (eds.) Surgical Correction of Dentofacial Deformities. Vol. I. Philadelphia: W.B. Saunders Co., 1980.
Proffit, W.R., Fields, H.W., and Nixon, W.L. Occlusal forces in normal- and long-face adults. J. Dent. Res. 62:566–571, 1983.
Pullinger, A.G., Solberg, W.K., Hollender, L., and Guichet, D. Tomographic analysis of mandibular condyle position in diagnostic subgroups of temporomandibular disorders. J. Prosthet. Dent. 55:723–729, 1986.
Pullinger, A.G., Hollender, L., Solberg, W.K., and Peterson, A. A tomographic study of mandibular condyle position in an asymptomatic population. J. Prosthet. Dent. 53:706–713, 1985.
Raft, D., Toomey, T., and Gregg, J.M. Behavior modification and haloperodol in chronic facial pain. South. Med. J. 72:155–159, 1979.
Rak, Y. Australopithecine taxonomy and phylogeny in light of facial morphology. Am. J. Phys. Anthropol. 66:281–287, 1985.
Ramfjord, S.P. Dysfunctional temporomandibular joint and muscle pain. J. Prosthet. Dent. 11:353–374, 1961a.
Ramfjord, S.P. Bruxism, a clinical and electromyographic study. J. Am. Dent. Assoc. 62:36–58, 1961b.
Ramfjord, S.P., and Ash, M.M. Periodontology and Periodontics. Philadelphia: W.B. Saunders Co., 1979.
Ramfjord, S., and Ash, M.M. Significance of occlusion in the etiology and treatment of early, moderate, and advanced periodontitis. J. Periodontol. 52:511–517, 1981.
Ramfjord, S.P., and Ash, M.M. Occlusion. 3rd ed. Philadelphia: W.B. Saunders Co., 1983.
Ramfjord, S.P., and Blankenship, J.R. Increased occlusal vertical dimension in adult monkeys. J. Prosthet. Dent. 45:74–83, 1981.
Randow, K., Carlsson, K., Edlund, J., and Öberg, T. The effect of occlusal interference on the masticatory system. Odontol. Rev. 27:245–255, 1976.
Ransjö, K., and Thilander, B. Perception of mandibular position in cases of temporomandibular joint disorders. Scand. Dent. J. 71:134–144, 1963.
Rao, S.M., and Glaros, A.G. Electromyographic correlates of experimentally induced stress in diurnal bruxists and normals. J. Dent. Res. 58:1872–1878, 1979.
Raustia, A.M., Pohjola, R.T., and Virtanen, K.K. Acupuncture compared with stomatognathic treatment for TMJ dysfunction. Part I. A randomized study. J. Prosthet. Dent. 54:581–585, 1985.
Ready, L.B., and Hare, B. Drug problems in chronic pain patients. Anesthesiology Rev. 6:28–31, 1979.
Ready, L.B., Kozody, R., Barsa, J.E., and Murphy, T.M. Trigger point injections vs. jet injection in the treatment of myofascial pain. Pain 15:201–206, 1983.
Reding, G.R., Rubright, W.C., and Zimmerman, S.O. Incidence of bruxism. J. Dent. Res. 45:1198–1204, 1966.
Reding, G.R., Zepelin, H., Robinson, J.E., Jr., Zimmerman, S.O., and Smith, V.H. Nocturnal teeth-grinding: all-night psychophysiologic studies. J. Dent. Res. 47:786–797, 1968.

Reemer, K.R., Mamandas, A.H., Hunter, W.S., and Way, D.C. Cephalometric changes associated with treatment using the activator, the Frankle appliance and fixed appliance. Am. J. Orthod. 88:363–372, 1985.

Rees, L.A. The structure and function of the mandibular joint. Br. Dent. J. 96:125–133, 1954.

Rensberger B. Facing the past. Science 81, 2(8):40–51, 1981.

Richmond, G., Rugh, J.D., Dolfi, R., and Wasilewsky, J.W. Survey of bruxism in an institutionalized mentally retarded population. Am. J. Ment. Defic. 88:418–421, 1984.

Ricketts, R.M. Variations of the temporomandibular joint as revealed by cephalometric laminography. Am. J. Orthod. 36:877–898, 1950.

Ricketts, R.M. Clinical implications of the temporomandibular joint. Am. J. Orthod. 52:416–439, 1966.

Ricketts, R.M. Occlusion—the medium of dentistry. J. Prosthet. Dent. 21:39–60, 1969.

Rieder, C.E. Possible premature degenerative temporomandibular joint disease in violinists. J. Prosthet. Dent. 35:662–664, 1976.

Riise, C., and Ericsson, S.G. A clinical study of the distribution of occlusal tooth contacts in the intercuspal position at light and hard pressures in adults. J. Oral Rehabil. 10:473–480, 1983.

Riise, C., and Sheikholeslam, A. The influence of experimental interfering occlusal contacts on the postural activity of the anterior temporal and masseter muscles in young adults. J. Oral Rehabil. 9:419–425, 1982.

Ringqvist, M. Isometric bite force and its relation to dimensions of the facial skeleton. Acta Odontol. Scand. 31:35–42, 1973.

Robinson, J.E., Reding, G.R., Zepelin, H., Smith, V.H., and Zimmerman, S.O. Nocturnal teeth-grinding: a reassessment for dentistry. J. Am. Dent. Assoc. 78:1308–1311, 1969.

Robinson, M. The temporomandibular joint: theory of reflex controlled nonlever action of the mandible. J. Am. Dent. Assoc. 33:1260–1271, 1946.

Rocabado, M. Diagnosis and treatment of abnormal craiocervical and craniomandibular mechanics. pp. 141–159 *In* W.K. Solberg and G.T. Clark (eds.) Abnormal Jaw Mechanics: Diagnosis and Treatment. Chicago: Quintessence Publ. Co., 1984.

Romer, A.S. Vertebrate Paleontology. Chicago: University of Chicago Press, 1966.

Rosen, J.S. Self-monitoring in the treatment of diurnal bruxism. J. Behav. Ther. Exp. Psychiatry 12:347–350, 1981.

Rosenbaum, C.H., McDonald, R.E., and Levitt, E.E. Occlusion of cerebral-palsied children. J. Dent. Res. 45:1696–1700, 1966.

Ross, R.B. Developmental anamolies and dysfunctions of the temporomandibular joint. pp. 119–154 *In* G.A. Zarb and G.E. Carlsson (eds.) Temporomandibular Joint Function and Dysfunction. Copenhagen: Munksgaard, 1979.

Ross, R.B., and Johnston, M.C. Cleft Lip and Palate. Baltimore: The Williams & Wilkins Co., 1972.

Roydhouse, R.H. The temporomandibular joint: upward force of the condyles on the cranium. J. Am. Dent. Assoc. 50:166–172, 1955.

Rugh, J.D. Variation in human masticatory behavior under temporal constraints. J. Comp. Physiol. Psych. 80:169–174, 1972.

Rugh, J.D. Muscle activity studies in MPD in the natural environment. J. Dent. Res. 61:175 (Abstract no. S-24), 1982.

Rugh, J.D. Psychological factors in the etiology of masticatory pain and dysfunction. pp. 85–94 *In* D. Laskin, W. Greenfield, E. Gale, J. Rugh, P. Neff, C. Alling, and W. Ayer (eds.) The President's Conference on the Examination, Diagnosis and Management of Temporomandibular Disorders. Chicago: American Dental Association, 1983.

Rugh, J.D., and Drago, C.J. Vertical dimension: a study of clinical rest position and jaw muscle activity. J. Prosthet. Dent. 45:670–675, 1981.

Rugh, J.D., Jacobs, D.T., Taverna, R.D., and Johnson, R.W. Psychophysiological changes and oral conditions. pp. 19–83 *In* L.K. Cohen and P.S. Bryant (eds.) Social Sciences and Dentistry. Vol. II. Chicago: Quintessence Publ. Co., 1984.

Rugh, J.D., and Johnson, R.W. Temporal analysis of nocturnal bruxism during EMG feedback. J. Periodontol. 52:263–265, 1981.

Rugh, J.D., and Johnson, R.W. Vertical dimension discrepancies and masticatory pain/dysfunction. pp. 117–133 *In* W.K. Solberg and G.T. Clark (eds.) Abnormal Jaw Mechanics: Diagnosis and Treatment. Chicago: Quintessence Publ. Co., 1984.

Rugh, J.D., and Lemke, R.R. Significance of oral habits. pp. 947–966 *In* J.D. Matarazzo, S.M. Weiss, J.A. Herd, N.E. Miller, and S.M. Weiss (eds.) Behavioral Health: A Handbook of Health Enhancement and Disease Prevention. New York: John Wiley & Sons, 1984.

Rugh, J.D., and Robbins, J.W. Oral habit disorders. pp. 179–202 *In* B.D. Ingersoll (ed.) Behavioral Aspects in Dentistry. New York: Appleton-Century-Crofts, 1982.

Rugh, J.D., and Solberg, W.K. Measurement of human oral forces. Behav. Res. Meth. Instru. 4:125–128, 1972.

Rugh, J.D., and Solberg, W.K. Electromyographic studies of bruxist behavior before and during treatment. J. Calif. State Dent. Assoc. 3:56–59, 1975.

Rugh, J.D., and Solberg, W.K. Psychological implications in temporomandibular pain and dysfunction. Oral Sci. Rev. 7:3–30, 1976.

Rugh, J.D., and Solberg, W.K. Psychological implications in temporomandibular pain and dysfunction. pp. 239–268 *In* G.A. Zarb and G.E. Carlsson (eds.) Temporomandibular Joint: Function and Dysfunction. Copenhagen: Munksgaard, 1979.

Rugh, J.D., and Solberg, W.K. Oral health status in the United States: temporomandibular disorders. J. Dent. Educ. 49:398–405, 1985.

Sadowsky, G., and BeGole, E.A. Long-term status of temporomandibular joint function and functional occlusion after orthodontic treatment. Am. J. Orthod. 78:201–212, 1980.

Sanson, G.D. The evolution and significance of mastication in the Macropodidae. Austral. Mamm. 2:23–28, 1978.

Sanson, G.D. Evolution of feeding adaptions in fossil and recent macropodids. Melbourne: Monash University Press, 1982.

Sarnat, B.G., and Laskin, D.M. (eds.) The Temporomandibular Joint: A Biological Basis for Clinical Practice. 3rd ed. Springfield: Charles C Thomas Publ., 1980.

Satoh, T., and Harada, Y. Electrophysiological study on tooth-grinding during sleep. Electroencephalogr. Clin.

Neurophysiol. 35:267–275, 1973.
Savalle, W.P.M. Some aspects about the morphology of the capsule of the temporomandibular joint in man. J. Oral Rehabil. 12:545–546, 1984.
Schärer, P. Bruxism. *In* Y. Kawamura (ed.) Frontiers of Oral Biology. Basel, Switzerland: S. Karger, 1974.
Schärer, P., Legault, J.V., and Zander, H.A. Mastication under anesthesia. Helv. Odontol. Acta 10:130–134, 1966.
Schärer, P., and Stallard, R.E. The effect of an occlusal interference on the tooth contact occurrence during mastication. Helv. Odontol. Acta 10:49–56, 1966.
Schärer, P., Stallard, R.E., and Zander, H.A. Occlusal interferences and mastication: an electromyographic study. J. Prosthet. Dent. 17:438–439, 1967.
Schluger, S., Yuodelis, R.A., and Page, R.C. Periodontal Disease. Philadelphia: Lee & Febiger, 1977.
Schoeninger, M.J. Diet and the evolution of modern human form. Am. J. Phys. Anthropol. 58:37–52, 1982.
Schuyler, C.H. Principles employed in full denture prosthesis which may be applied in other fields of dentistry. J. Am. Dent. Assoc. 16:2045–2054, 1929.
Schuyler, C.H. Fundamental principles in the correction of occlusal disharmony, natural and artificial. J. Am. Dent. Assoc. 22:1193–1202, 1935.
Schuyler, C.H. Correction of occlusal disharmony of natural dentition. N.Y. Dent. J. 13:445–462, 1947.
Schuyler, C.H. Factors of occlusion applicable to restorative dentistry. J. Prosthet. Dent. 3:772–782, 1953.
Schuyler, C.H. Factors of occlusion to be observed in everyday practice. J. Am. Dent. Assoc. 57:221–231, 1958.
Schuyler, C.H. An evaluation of incisal guidance and its influence in restorative dentistry. J. Prosthet. Dent. 9:374–378, 1959.
Schuyler, C.H. Factors contributing to traumatic occlusion. J. Prosthet. Dent. 11:708–715, 1961.
Schuyler, C.H. The function and importance of incisal guidance in oral rehabilitation. J. Prosthet. Dent. 13:1011–1029, 1963.
Schwartz, L. Pain associated with the temporomandibular joint. J. Am. Dent. Assoc. 51:394–397, 1955.
Schwartz, L. Disorders of the Temporomandibular Joint. Philadelphia: W.B. Saunders Co., 1959.
Schwartz, L., and Chayes, C.M. Facial Pain and Mandibular Dysfunction. Philadelphia: W.B. Saunders Co., 1969.
Schweitzer, J.M. Concepts of occlusion: a discussion. Dent. Clin. North Am. 649–671, 1963.
Scott, D.S., and Gregg, J.M. Myofascial pain of the temporomandibular joint: a review of the behavioral-relaxation therapies. Pain 9:231–241, 1980.
Scott, J.H., and Symons, N.B.B. Introduction to Dental Anatomy. 8th ed. Edinburgh: Churchill Livingstone, 1977.
Selby, A. Physiotherapy in the management of temporomandibular disorders. Aust. Dent. J. 30:273–280, 1985.
Seltzer, S. Pain Control in Dentistry. Philadelphia: J.B. Lippincott Co., 1978.
Sessle, B.J. Identification of alpha and gamma trigeminal motoneurons and effects of stimulation of amygdala, cerebellum, and cerebral cortex. Exp. Neurol. 54:303–322, 1977.
Sessle, B.J., and Greenwood, L.F. Peripheral influences on alpha and gamma motoneurons. pp. 174–183 *In* D.J. Anderson and B. Matthews (eds.) Mastication. Bristol: John Wright & Sons, 1976.
Sessle, B.J., and Gurza, S.C. Jaw movement-related activity and reflexly induced changes in the lateral pterygoid muscle of the monkey *Macaca Fascicularis*. Arch. Oral Biol. 27:167–173, 1982.
Sessle, B.J., and Schmitt, A. Effects of controlled tooth stimulation on jaw muscle activity in man. Arch. Oral Biol. 17:1597–1607, 1972.
Sheppard, I.M., and Sheppard, S.M. Range of condylar movement during mandibular opening. J. Prosthet. Dent. 15:263–271, 1965.
Sherrington, C.S. The integrative action of the nervous system. London: Archibald Constable, 1906.
Sherrington, C.S. Reflexes elicitable in the cat from pinna vibrissae and jaws. J. Physiol. 51:404–431, 1917.
Shore, N.A. TMJ Dysfunction and Occlusal Rehabilitation. 2nd ed. Philadelphia: J.B. Lippincott Co., 1976.
Sicher, H. Temporomandibular articulation in mandibular overclosure. J. Am. Dent. Assoc. 30:131–139, 1948.
Sicher, H., and DuBrul, E.L. Oral Anatomy. 6th ed. St. Louis: C.V. Mosby Co., 1975, p. 138.
Silness, J. Fixed prosthodontics and periodontal health. Dent. Clin. North Am. 24:317–329, 1980.
Simons, E.L. A source for comparison of *Ramapithecus* with *Australopithecus* and *Homo*. S. Afr. J. Sci. 64:92–112, 1968.
Simons, E.L. Man's immediate forerunners. Philos. Trans. R. Soc. Lond. B 292:21–41, 1981.
Skiba, T.J., and Laskin, D.M. Masticatory muscle silent periods in patients with MPD syndrome before and after treatment. J. Dent. Res. 60:699–706, 1981.
Slots, J. Subgingival microflora and periodontal disease. J. Clin. Periodontol. 6:351–382, 1979.
Smith, D.M., McLachlan, K.R., and McCall, W.D., Jr. A numerical model of temporomandibular joint loading. J. Dent. Res. 65:1046–1052, 1986.
Smith, M.M. Enamel in the oral teeth of *Latimeria chalumnae* (*Pisces:* Actinistia): a scanning electron microscope study. J. Zool. (Lond.) 185:355–369, 1978.
Smith, R.J. Mandibular biomechanics and temporomandibular joint function in primates. Am. J. Phys. Anthropol. 49:341–350, 1978.
Sokoloff, L. The Biology of Degenerative Joint Disease. Chicago: The University of Chicago Press, 1969, pp. 24–30.
Solberg, W.K. Epidemiology, incidence and prevalence of temporomandibular disorders: a review. pp. 30–39 *In* D. Laskin, W. Greenfield, E. Gale, J. Rugh, P. Neff, C. Alling, and W. Ayer (eds.) The President's Conference on the Examination, Diagnosis and Management of Temporomandibular Disorders. Chicago: American Dental Association, 1983.
Solberg, W.K. Temporomandibular disorders: masticatory myalgia and its management. Br. Dent. J. 160:351–356, 1986.
Solberg, W.K., Clark, G.T., and Rugh, J.D. Nocturnal electromyographic evaluation of bruxism patients undergoing short term splint treatment. J. Oral Rehabil. 2:215–233, 1975.
Solberg, W.K., and Rugh, J.D. The use of biofeedback devices in the treatment of bruxism. S. Calif. Dent. Assoc. J. 40:852–853, 1972.
Solberg, W.K., Woo, M.W., and Houston, J.B. Prevalence of mandibular dysfunction in young adults. J. Am. Dent. Assoc. 98:25–34, 1979.

Spee, F.G. The condylar path of the mandible along the skull. Arch. Anat. Physiol. 16:285–294, 1890 (in German); J. Am. Dent. Assoc. 100:670–675, 1980 (English translation).

Spiessl, B. Rigid internal fixation after sagittal split osteotomy of the ascending ramus. *In* B. Spiessl (ed.) New Concepts in Maxillofacial Bone Surgery. 1st ed. New York: Springer-Verlag, 1976.

Stallard, H., and Stuart, C.E. What kind of occlusion should recusped teeth be given? Dent. Clin. North Am. Nov.:591–606, 1963.

Standlee, J.P., Caputo, A.A., and Ralph, J.P. Stress trajectories within the mandible under occlusal loads. J. Dent. Res. 56:1297–1302, 1977.

Standlee, J.P., Caputo, A.A., and Ralph, J.P. The condyle as a stress-distributing component of the temporomandibular joint. J. Oral Rehabil. 8:391–400, 1981.

Steger, E., Deponte, V., and Windhorst, C.H. Anatomische Untersuchung zur Frage des sogenannten Costensyndroms. Dtsch. Zahnarztl. Z. 29:531–535, 1974.

Stern, J.T., and Susman, R.L. The Locomotor Anatomy of *Australopithecus afarensis*. Am. J. Phys. Anthropol. 60:279–317, 1983.

Sternbach, R.A. Pain Patients: Traits and Treatments. New York: Academic Press, 1974.

Stewart, H.F., and Stratmeyer, M.E. An Overview of Ultrasound Theory, Measurement, Medical Applications and Biological Effects. Rockville, Md.: U.S. Dept. of Health and Human Services, 1982.

Storey, A.T. Physiology of a changing vertical dimension. J. Prosthet. Dent. 12:912–921, 1962.

Storey, A.T. Physiology of occlusion. pp. 38–56 *In* N.H. Rowe (ed.) Proc. Symposium on Occlusion: Research in Form and Function. Ann Arbor: University of Michigan, 1975.

Storey, A.T. Interactions of alimentary and upper respiratory tract reflexes. pp. 23–31 *In* B.J. Sessle and A.G. Hannam (eds.) Mastication and Swallowing. Toronto: University of Toronto Press, 1976.

Storey, A.T. Controversies related to temporomandibular joint function and dysfunction. pp. 433–457 *In* G.A. Zarb and G.E. Carlsson (eds.) Temporomandibular Joint: Function and Dysfunction. Copenhagen: Munksgaard, 1979.

Stuart, C.E., and Stallard, H. Oral Rehabilitation and Occlusion. San Francisco: University of California, 1959.

Stuart, C.E., and Stallard, H. Principles involved in restoring occlusion to natural teeth. J. Prosthet. Dent. 10:304–313, 1960.

Svanberg, G. Influence of trauma from occlusion on the periodontium of dogs with normal or inflammed gingivae. Odontol. Rev. 25:165–178, 1974.

Svanberg, G., and Lindhe, J. Vascular reactions in the periodontal ligament incident to trauma from occlusion. J. Periodontol. 1:58–69, 1974.

Symons, N.B.B. The development of the human mandibular joint. J. Anat. 86:326–332, 1952.

Tallgren, A. Changes in adult face height due to aging, wear and loss of teeth and prosthetic treatment. Acta Odontol. Scand. 15:1–122 (Suppl. 24), 1957.

Taylor, C.B., Zlutnick, S.I., Corley, M.J., and Flora, J. The effects of detoxification, relaxation and brief supportive therapy in chronic pain. Pain 8:319–329, 1980.

Teaford, M.K., and Walker, A. Quantitative differences in dental micro wear and comment on the presumed diet of *Sivapithecus*. Am. J. Phys. Anthropol. 64:191–200, 1984.

Ten Cate, A.R. Oral Histology: Development, Structure and Function. St. Louis: C.V. Mosby Co., 1980.

Thaller, J.L. The use of the Cornell Index to determine the correlation between bruxism and the anxiety state: a preliminary report. J. Periodontol. 31:138–140, 1960.

Thilander, B. Innervation of the temporomandibular joint capsule in man. Trans. Royal Sch. Dent. Stockholm and Umea, 7:9–67, 1961.

Thilander, B. Innervation of the temporomandibular disc in man. Acta Odontol. Scand. 22:151–156, 1964.

Thomas, L. The Lives of a Cell. New York: Bantam Books, 1974.

Thomson, H. Mandibular dysfunction syndrome. Br. Dent. J. 107:243–250, 1971.

Timmis, D.P., Aragon, S.B., and Van Sickels, J.E. Masticatory dysfunction with rigid and nonrigid osteosynthesis of sagittal split osteotomies. Oral Surg. Oral Med. Oral Pathol. 62:119–123, 1986.

Toller, P. Non-surgical treatment of dysfunctions of the temporomandibular joint. Oral Sci. Rev. 7:70–85, 1976.

Travell, J. Temporomandibular joint pain referred from muscles of the head and neck. J. Prosthet. Dent. 10:745–763, 1960.

Travell, J.G., and Simons, D.G. Myofascial Pain and Dysfunction: The Trigger Point Manual. Baltimore: Williams & Wilkins, 1983.

Trenouth, M.J. The relationship between bruxism and temporomandibular joint dysfunction as shown by computer analysis of nocturnal tooth contact patterns. J. Oral Rehabil. 6:81–87, 1979.

Trinkaus, E., and Howells, W.W. The Neanderthals. Sci. Am. 241(6):118–133, 1979.

Troelstrup, B., and Møller, E. Electromyography of the temporalis and masseter muscles in children with unilateral cross-bite. Scand. J. Dent. Res. 78:425–430, 1970.

Tseng, T.C., and Wang, S.C. Locus of action of centrally acting muscle relaxants, diazepam, and tybamate. J. Pharmacol. Exp. Therap. 178:350–360, 1971.

Van Steenberghe, D., and deVries, J.H. The development of a maximal clenching force between two antagonistic teeth. J. Periodont. Res. 13:91–97, 1978a.

Van Steenberghe, D., and deVries, J.H. The influence of local anesthesia and occlusal surface area on the forces developed during repetitive maximal clenching efforts. J. Periodont. Res. 13:270–274, 1978b.

Vargervig, K., and Harvold, E. Response to activator treatment in Class II malocclusions. Am. J. Orthod. 88:242–251, 1985.

Vernallis, F.F. Teeth-grinding: some relationships to anxiety, hostility and hyperactivity. J. Clin. Psychol. 11:389–391, 1955.

Villarosa, G.A., and Moss, R.A. Oral behavioral patterns as factors contributing to the development of head and facial pain. J. Prosthet. Dent. 54:427–430, 1985.

Waerhaug, J. The infrabony pocket and its relationship to trauma from occlusion and subgingival plaque. J. Periodontol. 50:355, 1979a.

Waerhaug, J. The angular bony defect and its relationship to trauma from occlusion and downgrowth of subgingival plaque. J. Clin. Periodontol. 6:61, 1979b.

Walker, A. Functional anatomy of oral tissues: mastication and deglutition. Chapt. 8 *In* J.H. Shaw, E.A. Sweeney, C.C. Cappuccino, and S.M. Meller (eds.) Textbook of

Oral Biology. Philadelphia: C.V. Mosby Co., 1978.
Walker, A., Leakey, J.M., and Brown, F.H. 2.5 Myr *Australopithecus boisei* from West of Lake Turkana, Kenya. Nature (Lond.) 322:517–522, 1986.
Walker, W.E. Prosthetic dentistry: the glenoid fossa; the movements of the mandible; the cusps of the teeth. Dent. Cosmos 38:34–43, 1896.
Wänman, A., and Agerberg, G. Headache and dysfunction of the masticatory system in adolescents. Cephalalgia 6:247–255, 1986.
Washburn, H.B. History and evolution of the study of occlusion. Dent. Cosmos 67:223–237, 1925.
Watt, D.M., and Wakabayashi, Y. Study of a classification of occlusion. J. Oral Rehabil. 5:101–110, 1978.
Weinberg, L.A. What we really see in a TMJ radiograph. J. Prosthet. Dent. 30:898–913, 1973.
Weinberg, L.A. Anterior condylar displacement: its diagnosis and treatment. J. Prosthet. Dent. 34:195–207, 1975.
Weinberg, L. Temporomandibular joint function and its effect on concepts of occlusion. J. Prosthet. Dent. 35:553–566, 1976.
Weinberg, L.A. Posterior unilateral condylar displacement: its diagnosis and treatment. J. Prosthet. Dent. 37:559–569, 1977.
Weinberg, L.A. Role of condylar position in TMJ dysfunction-pain syndrome. J. Prosthet. Dent. 41:636–643, 1979.
Weinberg, L.A. The etiology, diagnosis, and treatment of TMJ dysfunction-pain syndrome. Part II: Differential diagnosis. J. Prosthet. Dent. 43:58–70, 1980a.
Weinberg, L.A. The etiology, diagnosis, and treatment of TMJ dysfunction-pain syndrome. Part III: Treatment. J. Prosthet. Dent. 43:186–196, 1980b.
Weinberger, B.W. Orthodontics: An Historical Review of Its Origin and Evolution. Vol. II. St. Louis: C.V. Mosby Co., 1926, p. 674.
Wessberg, G.A., Carroll, W.L., Dinham, R., and Wolford, L.M. Transcutaneous electrical stimulation as an adjunct in the management of myofascial pain-dysfunction syndrome. J. Prosthet. Dent. 45:307–314, 1981.
Westerman, R.A. Muscles and motoneurons. pp. 21–49 *In* I. Klineberg and B. Sessle (eds.) Oro-Facial Pain and Neuromuscular Dysfunction. Oxford: Pergamon, 1985.
Westesson, P.-L. Double-contrast arthrography and internal derangement of the temporomandibular joint. Swed. Dent. J., Suppl. 13, 1982.
Whillis, J. The development of synovial joints. J. Anat. 74:277–283, 1940.
White, T.D., Johansen, D.C., and Kimbel, W.H. *Australopithecus africanus:* its phyletic position reconsidered. S. Afr. J. Sci. 77:445–470, 1981.
Wickwire, N.A., Gibbs, C.H., Jacobson, A.P., and Lundeen, H.C. Chewing patterns in normal children. Angle Orthod. 51:48–60, 1981.
Widdowson, T.W. Special or Dental Anatomy and Physiology and Dental Histology, Human and Comparative. Vol. 2. 7th ed. London: Staples Press Ltd., 1946.
Widmalm, S.-E. The silent period in the masseter muscle of patients with TMJ dysfunction. Acta Odontol. Scand. 34:43–52, 1976.
Widmer, C.G. Jaw-opening reflex activity in the inferior head of the lateral pterygoid muscle in man. Arch. Oral Biol. 32:135–142, 1987.
Winstanley, R.B. The hinge-axis: a review of the literature. J. Oral Rehabil. 12:135–159, 1985.
Woda, A., Vigneron, P., and Kay, D. Nonfunctional and functional occlusal contacts: a review of the literature. J. Prosthet. Dent. 42:335–341, 1979.
Wolf, S. The pharmacology of placebos. Pharmacol. Rev. 132:91–92, 1959.
Wolff, H.G. Headache and Other Head Pain. New York: Oxford University Press, 1963.
Wolford, G., Walker, G., Schendel, S.A., et al. Mandibular deficiency syndrome: clinical delineation and therapeutic significance. Oral Surg. Oral Med. Oral Pathol. 45:329–348, 1978.
Wood, W.W., Gelfant, H., and Hannam, A.G. Effect of occlusal reconstruction on the reproducibility of chewing movements. J. Prosthet. Dent. 46:181–184, 1981.
Wood, W.W., Takada, K., and Hannam, A.G. The electromyographic activity of the inferior part of the human lateral pterygoid muscle during clenching and chewing. Arch. Oral Biol. 31:245–253, 1986.
Wooten, J.W. Physiology of the temporomandibular joint. Oral Surg. Oral Med. Oral Pathol. 21:543–553, 1966.
Worth, H.M. Radiology of the temporomandibular joint. *In* G.A. Zarb and G.E. Carlsson (eds.) Temporomandibular Joint: Function and Dysfunction. Copenhagen: Munksgaard, 1979.
Wright, D.M., and Moffett, B.C. The postnatal development of the human temporomandibular joint. Am. J. Anat. 141:235–250, 1974.
Xhonga, F.A. Bruxism and its effect on the teeth. J. Oral Rehabil. 4:65–76, 1977.
Yale, S.H., Allison, B.D., and Hauptfuehrer, J.D. An epidemiological assessment of mandibular condyle morphology. Oral Surg. Oral Med. Oral Pathol. 21:169–177, 1966.
Yavelow, I., Forster, I., and Wininger, M. Mandibular relearning. Oral Surg. Oral Med. Oral Pathol. 36:632–641, 1973.
Yemm, R. A comparison of the electrical activity of masseter and temporal muscles of human subjects during experimental stress. Arch. Oral Biol. 16:269–273, 1971a.
Yemm, R. Comparison of the activity of left and right masseter muscles of normal individuals and patients with mandibular dysfunction during experimental stress. J. Dent. Res. 50:1320–1323, 1971b.
Yemm, R. Reflex jaw opening following electrical stimulation of oral mucous membrane in man. Arch. Oral Biol. 17:513–523, 1972a.
Yemm, R. Stress-induced muscle activity: a possible etiologic factor in denture soreness. J. Prosthet. Dent. 28:133–140, 1972b.
Yemm, R. Neurophysiologic studies of temporomandibular joint dysfunction. Oral Sci. Rev. 7:31–53, 1976a.
Yemm, R. The role of tissue elasticity in the control of mandibular resting posture. pp. 81–89 *In* D.J. Anderson and B. Matthews (eds.) Mastication. Bristol: John Wright & Sons, 1976b.
Yemm, R. Neurophysiologic studies of temporomandibular joint dysfunction. pp. 215–237 *In* G.A. Zarb and G.E. Carlsson (eds.) Temporomandibular Joint: Function and Dysfunction. Copenhagen: Munksgaard, 1979.
Yemm, R. A neurophysiological approach to the pathology and etiology of temporomandibular dysfunction. J. Oral Rehabil. 12:343–353, 1985.
Yemm, R., and Berry, D.C. Passive control in mandibular

rest position. J. Prosthet. Dent. 22:30–36, 1969.
Yuodelis, R.A. The morphogenesis of the human temporomandibular joint and its associated structures. J. Dent. Res. 45:182–191, 1966.
Zander, H.A., and Polson, A.M. Present status of occlusion and occlusal therapy in periodontics. J. Periodontol. 48:540–544, 1977.
Zarb, G.A. Oral motor patterns and their relation to oral prostheses. J. Prosthet. Dent. 47:472–478, 1982.
Zarb, G.A. Nonsurgical treatment of rheumatoid and degenerative arthritis of the TMJ. pp. 33–136 *In* D. Laskin, W. Greenfield, E. Gale, J. Rugh, P. Neff, C. Alling, and W. Ayer (eds.) The President's Conference on the Examination, Diagnosis and Management of Temporomandibular Disorders. Chicago: American Dental Association, 1983.
Zarb, G.A., Bergman, B., Clayton, J.A., and MacKay, H.F. Prosthodontic Treatment for Partially Edentulous Patients. St. Louis: C.V. Mosby Co., 1978.
Zarb, G.A., and Carlsson, G.E. The Temporomandibular Joint: Function and Dysfunction. Copenhagen: Munksgaard, 1979.
Zarb, G.A., and Speck, J.E. The treatment of mandibular dysfunction. pp. 373–396 *In* G.A. Zarb and G.E. Carlsson (eds.) Temporomandibular Joint: Function and Dysfunction. Copenhagen: Munksgaard, 1979.
Zarb, G.A., and Thompson, G.W. Assessment of clinical treatment of patients with temporomandibular joint dysfunction. J. Prosthet. Dent. 24:542–553, 1970.
Zarb, G.A., and Thompson, G.W. The treatment of patients with temporomandibular joint pain dysfunction syndrome. J. Can. Dent. Assoc. 41:410–417, 1975.
Zimmerman, A.A. An evaluation of Costen's syndrome from an anatomic point of view. pp. 82–110 *In* B.G. Sarnat (ed.) The Temporomandibular Joint. Springfield, Ill.: Charles C Thomas Publ., 1951.

Index

A

Aborigines, Australian, dentition 145, 170–171
Acromegaly 224
Acupuncture 349
Alveolar process 73
American Academy of Denture Prosthetics 19
American Association of Dental Schools 16
American Dental Association 16, 335
Analgesics 346–348, 353
Anesthetics,
  adjuvants 344–346
  local 352–353
Anorexia nervosa 211
Anticonvulsants 355
Antidepressants 354–355
Anti-inflammatories 353–354
Antimigraines 355
Antipsychotics 355
Anxiolytics 354, 356
Articular capsule 87, 88
Articular disk 84, 88, 92, 94
Articular eminence 86, 91
Articulators, 137–140, 140–141
  history of 163
  types 138

B

Beckwith-Wiedemann syndrome 363
Behavior modification, 331–335
  behavioral extinction 332
  behavioral substitutes 332
  biofeedback 333–335, 335
  general relaxation theory 336–337
  massed practice 333
  patient selection 337–338
  reinforcement theory 331–332
  self-monitoring 332–333
Behavioral therapy, 329–338
  principles 329–331
Bennett movement 90, 133, 136, 137, 144
Biofeedback,
  devices 333–334, 335
  in electromyography 113
Bite. *See* Crossbite, Deep bite, Dual bite, Open bite, Overbite, Overjet, Scissors bite.
Bite force 147
Brain stem 116, 117
Bruxism,
  electromyography 112
  nocturnal, 249–256
    described 252, 253
    diagnosis 255–256
    etiology 254
    in children 253
    prevalence 252–253
    sequelae 249–252
  therapy effectiveness 278
  tooth wear 210, 212, 213, 280

C

Canine guidance 63
Cementocytes 72
Cementum,
  cellular 72
  described 73
Cheek, protection 68
Chewing,
  electromyography 110–111, 113
  mandibular movements 144, 146
Chimpanzee 37
Cleft lip 309
Cleft palate 309
Condyle,
  described 83, 84, 85, 88, 91, 92
  fracture, dentition effects 225
  movements 145–147
  traumatic, surgery 362
Coronoid process disorders 205

Coronoplasty. *See* Occlusal adjustment, therapy.
Cranial arteritis. *See* Temporal arteritis.
Crossbite 49, 50, 51
Curricular Guidelines in Occlusion 16
Curve of Spee 60, 61
Curve of Wilson 60, 61, 170
Cusps,
  centric-holding 63
  guiding 66
  intercuspal position 62, 63, 64, 287–288, 296
  supporting 63, 65, 66

D

Deep bite 49, 50, 51, 54
Deglutition, 153–155
  See also Swallowing.
Dental arch 58, 59, 60, 61
Dental disease, differential diagnosis 204
Dental treatment, occlusal effects 225–226
Dentition, 57–69
  adult natural 57–69
  dental treatment effects 225–226
  development relations 55
  esthetics 69
  form and function relations 55
  ideal 57
  mixed 43
  natural, characteristics 57–69
  normal 57
  occlusal problems 209–225
  occlusal variations 209–225
  permanent,
    eruption chronology 46
    jaw relations 60
    variations 48
  primary,
    attrition 45
    described 43, 44
    eruption chronology 44
    leeway space 46, 47
    posterior 45
    primate space 45, 47
  self-protective features 67, 68
Denture, partial, fixed 306, 307
Denture, partial, removable 306, 307, 308
Diagnosis, differential,
  masticatory system dysfunction 203–207
  occlusal problems 185–207
  pain 203–207
Diagnosis, oral 179–184
Disclusion, organized 174
Diurnal parafunction, 256–260
  described 256
  etiology 258–259
  evaluation 259–260
  sequelae 257–258
Dog 33
Dogfish 27, 28
Drug abuse 356
Drug detoxification 356
Dual bite 198

E

Ear disorders 204
Electromyography, 108–113
  and biofeedback 113
  bruxism 112
  chewing 110–111, 113
  equipment 108–109
  jaw reflexes 112, 113
  malocclusion 112
  occlusion and 109–113
  pitfalls and problems 109
  postural rest position 112
  swallowing 110–111, 113
  techniques 108
  temporomandibular disorders 112
Esthetics,
  dentition 69
  facial 359–361
Examination,
  clinical signs and symptoms 185–189
  masticatory system 198–207
  occlusal problems 185–207
  radiographic signs 189
Exercise therapy, 340–344
  anesthetic adjuvants 344–346
  for neck 343–344
  muscle strengthening 343
  relearning rotation exercise 340–341
  stretching 342

F

Face,
  developmental relations 55
  esthetics 359–361
  form and function relations 55
  growth 52
  reflexes 120
Face-bows 139
Fibers,
  alveolar crest 74
  alveolingual 71
  apical 74
  circular 71
  dentogingival 71
  dentoperiosteal 71
  horizontal 74
  interradicular 74
  oblique 74
  oxytalan 74
  Sharpey's 71, 72, 73, 75
  transseptal 71
Finger-sucking 56
Fruit, tooth wear from 212
Functional outer aspect 65
Functionalism,
  controversies 174–175
  history of 168, 169

G

Gagging 124
Giant cell arteritis. *See* Temporal arteritis.
Gingiva,
  described 71
  fiber groups 71, 72
  free 71
  lamina propria 71
  marginal 71
  tissue protection 67
  tooth form relations 67
Glossary. *See* Terminology.
Gnathology,
  controversies 174–175
  history of 163, 166–168, 169
Guiding inclines 65

H

Hanau's quint 67
Headache,
  differential diagnosis 206–207
  etiology 251
Heat 349
Hemifacial microsomia 362
Hypercementosis 191, 193

I

Indians, California, dentition 171
Injection, trigger point 345–346
Intermediate plexus 77
Interocclusal appliance therapy, 271–284
  clinical effectiveness 275–277
  cognitive awareness theory 273
  maxillomandibular theory 272, 274
  occlusal disengagement theory 271
  symptom-specific effectiveness 277–280
  temporomandibular joint repositioning theory 273
  theory 271–274
  vertical dimension theory 271
Iontophoresis 347–348

J

Jaw,
  growth 52, 53, 54
  reflexes, 118–120
    cyclic 126, 127
    electromyography 112, 113
Jaw relation,
  development 47
  mixed dentition, molars 46
  permanent dentition 60
  primary, posterior teeth 45
  record, prosthodontics 322
  sagittal 46

L

Lamina dura 73, 74, 191

Larynx, reflexes 121
Leopard 33
Lip,
  and neutral zone 62
  protection 68
The Lives of a Cell 377
Lizard,
  blue tongue 28, 29
  monitor 28, 29

M

Malocclusion,
  Angle system, defined 164
  electromyography 112
  functional, 218–223
    morphologic aspects 223–224
  morphologic, 217–218
    functional predisposing 223–224
Mammal,
  masticatory system, 31–35, 35–41
    bipedal hominids 37
    carnivore 32, 33
    features of 31
    herbivore 33, 34
    human 35
    omnivore 35
    primate 35–41
  skull 33, 34
Mandible,
  growth 52, 53, 54
  intercuspal position 62, 63, 64
  postural rest position 112, 128
Mandibular fossa 86, 91, 94
Mandibular movement, 89, 90, 91, 92, 129–141
  Bennett 90, 133, 136, 137, 144
  border, 129, 135, 145
    frontal plane 132
    horizontal plane 133, 134, 136
    sagittal plane 129, 130, 131, 144
  examination 201
  functional 134, 135
  in chewing cycle 144, 146
  in mastication 143–145, 146
  joint morphology 135, 136
  limits of 130
  range of 201
  tooth morphology 135
Mastication, 143–152
  clinical implications 152
  development of 149
  efficiency 148
  forces 147–148
  learning of 149
  mandibular movements 143–145
  muscle activity 151
  neurological control 150–151
  rhythmic 125–127
Masticatory system,
  adaptation 18
  anatomy 18, 25–175
  clinical examination 198–207
  defined 17
  dysfunction, 177–261
    behavioral therapy 329–338
    differential diagnosis 203
    exercise therapy 340–344
    interocclusal appliance therapy 271–284
    occlusal adjustment therapy 285–303
    operative therapy 321–324
    orthodontic therapy 324–327
    pharmacological therapy 351–357
    physical therapy 339–350
    prosthodontic therapy 305–321
    skeletal 373
    surgical therapy 359–375
    therapy 263–375
  function 18
  human 35
  mammal 31–35, 35–41
  morphology 18
  occlusal problems 177–261
    See also Occlusion, problems.
  pain 203
  pain-dysfunction 199, 202
  patient history and 198–199
  physiology 23–175
  primate 35–41
  temporomandibular joint examination 200
  theoretically ideal 180–181
  tooth loss effects 216
  traumatic injuries 204
  variability 18

vertebrate,
comparative anatomy 27–41
evolution 27–41
lower 27–31
Maxilla,
alveolar process growth 52, 53
growth 52, 53
tuberosities 52, 53
Meckel's cartilage 82, 83
Mudpuppy 28, 29
Muscle,
cervical group 106
digastric 105
facial group 106
infrahyoid group 106
lateral pterygoid 104
masseter 103
masticatory, manipulation 349
medial pterygoid 104
suprahyoid group 105
temporalis 103
tensor palatini 102
tensor tympani 83, 102
Muscles, 97–114
action potential 102
activity, 108–113
of mastication 151
described 97–102
electrical properties 102
electromechanical coupling 102
examination 200–201
facial, organization 116, 117
fatigue 101
force-velocity 98, 99
free nerve endings 108
hypertrophy, from bruxism 251
innervation 102
jaw-closing 103–104
jaw-opening 104–105
length-tension 98, 99
molecular structure 100, 101
motor units 101
muscle spindles 106–108
neuromuscular junction 100, 101
neurosensory receptors 106–108
of mandibular function 103–106
oral, organization 116, 117
physiological properties 98–101
relaxants 355–356
tendon organs 108
tetanus 99, 100
twitch 99, 100
Myalgia, therapy effectiveness 278, 279

N

Necturus maculosis. *See* Mudpuppy.
Nerves,
cranial, organization 117, 118
spinal, organization 117, 118
Neuralgia 206
Neuromuscular system, 115–128
study problems 115–116
tooth loss effects 217
Neutral space 61, 62
Neutral zone 61, 62
Nomenclature. *See* Terminology.

O

Occlusal adjustment,
appliance-determined 296
armamentarium 293
diagnostic cast procedure 294
excursive 299
indications, natural teeth 292
intercuspal position 296
mandibular manipulation 297–299
objectives, natural teeth 292
patient management 293–294
principles 294–296
procedures, 293–301
sequence 300–302
recontouring 295, 296, 299
retruded contact position 297
therapy, 285–303
abnormal mandibular occlusal position 286–287
avoidance of tooth contact 286
behavioral effects of 287
theories 285–287
traumatic occlusal contact 285
Occlusal contacts, 62, 64
diagnosis 192–193

examination sequence 194–196
intercuspal position 287–288
lateral guidance 289, 290
protrusive guidance 289, 291
recognition of 287–292
retruded position 219–221, 225
retrusive guidance 291–292
Occlusal force,
periodontal response 79, 227–233
periodontal sensory receptors and 79
Occlusal interferences, 194
between RCP and ICP 194, 195, 196, 197
during excursive movements 194, 197
nonworking side 221
retruded contact position 219–221
working side 221, 222, 223
Occlusal morphology 65, 217–218, 322
Occlusal parafunction, 249–261
described 249
Occlusal relationships 62, 63, 64, 65
Occlusal surfaces 62, 66
Occlusal table 65, 66
Occlusal therapy,
objectives 305
operative 321–324
orthodontic 324–327
principles 379
prosthodontic 305–321
traditional 305–328
Occlusion,
anomalies 48, 49, 50, 51, 52, 217–218
balanced,
defined 162
described 66
determinants of 67
history of 163–166, 168–169
canine-protected 172–173
centric 62, 173, 312–314
Class I 43
Class II 47
concepts of, 161–175
current 171–175
history of 163–171
course organization 16
curriculum guidelines 16
defined 15
development of 43–53
diagnosis 179–184
disorders 18
distal 47, 51
electromyography and 109–113
group function 172–173
incisal guidance 63
introduction to 15–23
mesial 51
mutual protection,
criteria 327
defined 163
described 172–173, 174
history of 169
natural dentition 166–168
neutral 43
nonphysiologic,
clinical signs 265, 266
controversy in 265
overview 182–184
pathologic conditions in 183
periodontal conditions in 183
temporomandibular
disorders in 183–184
therapy, 263–283, 265, 266
sequence 270
waiting period 266
tooth loss sequelae 212–217
normal 48
periodontal sensory receptors and 79
physiologic,
adaptation 265, 266
criteria 181–182, 377–378
overview 181–182
progression to nonphysiologic 212–217
posterior guidance 63
postnormal 47
problems,
differential diagnosis 185–207
examination 185–207
See also Masticatory systems,
occlusal problems.
structural problems 266–267
teaching objectives 15, 16
temporomandibular
disorders and 268–270, 377–383
temporomandibular joint
relations 137–141, 235–248
terminology 19–23
theoretically ideal,

centric stop location 64
criteria 180–181
defined 48
overview 180–181
therapeutic,
described 378
objectives 305, 310
overview 184
traumatic,
and periodontitis 230
clinical diagnosis 229–230
primary 227
radiography 229–230, 231, 232
response range 228
secondary 227
therapy 230–233
Occlusocranial relationships 58, 59
Open bite,
described 49, 50
development of 54
examination 198
occurrence 51
Operative therapy 321–324
Orthodontic force, root resorption from 72
Orthodontic therapy 324–327
biologic price 326
objectives 324
preprosthetic 325, 326
sequelae 327
Orthodontics, and orthognathic surgery 363–372
Orthognathic surgery,
and orthodontics 363–372
defined 359
for temporomandibular joint problems 373–375
procedures 367
timing of 361–367
Osteoarthritis 203
Osteoarthrosis 96
Overbite 48, 63
Overjet 48, 49, 51, 63

P

Pain-dysfunction,
masticatory system 199, 202
Palate, reflexes 121
Parotid gland diseases 204–205
Pathology, oral, nonphysiologic occlusion 183
Patient history 198–199
Patient management 293–294
Periodontal diseases, nonphysiologic occlusion 183
Periodontal ligament, 72
adaptive response 73, 78
blood supply 76
collagen fibers 74
function 77, 80
ground substance 75, 78
histology 74, 76, 77
principal fibers 74
remodeling 77
sensory innervation 78
Periodontal sensory receptors 78, 79
Periodontal space changes 191
Periodontitis, traumatic occlusion and 230
Periodontium, 71–80
fiber groups 74
histology 72, 75, 76
occlusal force response 79, 227–233
structure 71–77
tissue protection 68
Pharmacological therapy, 351–357
agents for 352–356
principles 351–352
Pharynx, reflexes 121
Physical therapy, 339–350
agents for 339
in temporomandibular disorders 339–340
methods 339
Placebo 269, 356–357
Plane,
facial 58
mandibular 58
of occlusion 58
Profile, cephalometric measurement 53
Prognathism, cephalometric measurement 53
Prosthodontic therapy, 305–321
axial force 314–317, 318
clefts 309
freedom of contact 317–319, 319–321
interocclusal distance 309–312, 314, 315, 316

jaw relations 312–314, 314–317
retruded closure 312–314, 316
tooth loss 306, 307, 308

R

Reflexes,
facial 120
horizontal jaw 119
jaw 118–120
jaw-closing 118, 119
jaw-opening 118
jaw-unloading 119
regulation of activity, 121–125, 126
central 121, 122, 123, 126
peripheral 123, 124, 126, 127
simple 116
synergies 124, 125, 126
tongue 120
vagal 121
Respiration, 155–156
dental aspects 155
Retrodiscal pad 91, 94
Rheumatoid arthritis 203

S

Scissors bite 51
Sheep 34
Shrew, tree 31
Sinus disorders 204
Skull,
human 38, 39, 40
mammal, carnivore 33
primate 37, 39, 40
vertebrate, lower 28, 29, 30, 31
Soft tissue,
changes 189
protection 68
Speech, 156–160
mechanism of 157
natural 156
sound production, 157
consonants 157, 158, 159, 160
diphthongs 160
sibilants 160
vowels 157
Spinal cord 116
Splints, stabilization,
adjustment 282
design 274–275, 280, 281
insertion 280, 281
postinsertion instructions 283
Study casts, 137–140
articulated 193
mounting 140, 193
Styloid-stylohyoid syndrome 205
Surgical therapy, 359–375
Swallowing,
electromyography 110–111, 113
force 155
tooth effects 155
types 154
See also Deglutition.
Synovial membrane 94

T

TENS. *See* Transcutaneous electrical nerve stimulation.
Temporal arteritis 205
Temporomandibular joint, 81–96
adaptation 95
and occlusal function 235–248
anomalies,
congenital 247
overdevelopment 247
postnatal 247–248
underdevelopment 247
unilateral hyperplasia 247
articular tissue 84, 86, 87, 88, 90, 91
biomechanics 90
blood supply 95
components 81–83
composition 90, 91
development 81–83
examination 200
function 83–90
histology 90–94
masticatory force effects 88, 91, 92
nerve supply 95
osteoarthrosis 96
otological relations 83

pain 203
radiography 84, 85
relation to occlusion 66, 268
structure 82, 83–90
tooth relations 137–141

Temporomandibular disorders,
bruxism and 251
degenerative. *See* Temporomandibular disorders, osteoarthrosis.
disk dislocation 244–247
diurnal parafunction and 258
electromyography 112
etiology 380–382
in nonphysiologic occlusion 183–184
internal derangement 244–247
mechanical displacement theory 380–381
muscle theory 381–382
neuromuscular theory 381
occlusion and 377–383
osteoarthrosis 235–239
physical therapy 339–340
psychophysiological theory 382
rheumatoid arthritis 239–242
signs and symptoms 268
skeletal disharmony and 373
surgery for 373–375
tooth loss effects 216–217
traumatic arthritis 242–244
treatment objectives 268

Temporomandibular joint ligament 88, 89, 90

Terminology, of occlusion 19–23

Therapeutic concepts 265–270

Thielmann's formula 67

Thomas, Lewis 377

Tongue,
and neutral zone 62
protection of 68
reflexes 120

Tooth,
abrasion 210
attrition, 209, 210, 214, 215
bruxism 280
erosion 211
eruption, developmental patterns 47
fremitus 186
interproximal contacts 187–188
interproximal space 186, 187, 188–189
loss,
adverse effects 212–217
treatment needs 266
loss of substance 209–212
migration 213
mobility 186
percussive sounds 189
premature loss 187–188, 189
primary, premature loss 51
root,
fracture 191
resorption, orthodontic force 72, 192
temporomandibular joint relations 137–141
wear,
bruxism and 251
diagnosis 211–212, 213, 214
occlusal 144, 189, 190, 210–211, 212, 213, 214, 215

Transcutaneous electrical nerve stimulation 346

Trismus,
postinjection 206
therapy effectiveness 279

Tupia glis. *See* Shrew, tree.

U

Ultrasound 347

V

Vapocoolant spray 344, 345

Varanus. *See* Lizard, monitor.

Vertebrate,
lower,
masticatory system 27–31
skull 28, 29, 30, 31
masticatory system,
comparative anatomy 27–41
evolution 27–41

S. DELUCA